THE DENTAL PULP

BIOLOGIC CONSIDERATIONS IN DENTAL PROCEDURES
Third Edition

Samuel Seltzer, D.D.S.
Director, Maxillofacial Pain Control Center,
School of Dentistry, Temple University;
Henry Isiah Door Professor of Research
and Teaching in Dental Science;
Professor Emeritus of Endodontology, School of Dentistry,
Temple University, Philadelphia, Pennsylvania

I.B. Bender, D.D.S.
Professor Emeritus of Endodontics,
School of Dental Medicine, University of Pennsylvania;
Chairman Emeritus, Department of Dentistry,
Albert Einstein Medical Center, Philadelphia, Pennsylvania

Ishiyaku EuroAmerica, Inc., Publishers

NOTICE

Dentistry is an ever-changing science. As new research and clinical experience broaden our knowledge, changes in treatment are required. The editors and the publisher of this work have made every effort to ensure that the procedures herein are accurate and in accord with the standards accepted at the time of publication.

THE DENTAL PULP

BIOLOGIC CONSIDERATIONS IN DENTAL PROCEDURES

Third Edition

Book Editor: Gregory Hacke, D.C.

Copyright © 1990 by Ishiyaku EuroAmerica, Inc.
Copyright © 1984 by J.B. Lippincott Company
Copyright © 1975, 1965 by J.B. Lippincott Company

All rights reserved. No part of this publication may be reproduced or transmitted by any means, electronic, mechanical, or otherwise, including photocopying and recording, or by any information storage or retrieval system, without permission–in writing–from the publishers.

Ishiyaku EuroAmerica, Inc.
716 Hanley Industrial Court, St. Louis, Missouri 63144

Library of Congress Catalogue Number 90-055420

Seltzer, Samuel, D.D.S.
Bender, I.B., D.D.S.
The Dental Pulp
Biologic Considerations In Dental Procedures
Third Edition

ISBN 0-912791-86-1

Ishiyaku EuroAmerica, Inc.
St. Louis • Tokyo

Composition by: Jackie Buchanan at Characters, Collinsville, IL, 618/344-2958

THIS BOOK IS AFFECTIONATELY DEDICATED
TO OUR WIVES AND CHILDREN,
RUTH, STEVEN, AND ROCHELLE SELTZER AND
LILLIAN AND ANDREW BENDER AND SUSAN BLUMSTEIN

PREFACE

Rapid advances in the basic sciences and the development of sophisticated instrumentation have had a profound effect on our knowledge of every organ in the body. The dental pulp is no exception. There are technical difficulties in deriving information from the pulp, an organ or tissue that is difficult to see because it is encased by the hardest materials in the body. Some of these difficulties have been overcome by ingenious research since the publication of our last two editions. The objective of the third edition of *The Dental Pulp* remains the same as that of the first two: to advocate the use of clinical procedures that are based on scientific facts. As always, the purpose of this text is to correlate clinical practice with basic science. Ultimately, an underpinning of basic science leads to the most effective clinical treatment. The rapid development of scientific information is of little value if it cannot be applied clinically.

Every chapter in the third edition has been updated. Some chapters have been completely rewritten and others have been combined for brevity and clarity. Many of the illustrations are new, having been gathered both from our own investigations and from investigators from various scientific disciplines. In view of the overwhelming number of new investigations in the fields of circulatory and nerve physiology in the pulp, we sought and received the cooperation and assistance of Syngcuk Kim, D.D.S., Ph.D., Columbia University, New York, to assist us in rewriting Chapters 5 and 6.

As in the two previous editions, the keynote of the present text is prevention of pulpal injury. Preventive measures are discussed extensively in the chapters on pulpal irritants. The scientific literature is replete with controversial and sometimes contradictory findings. An attempt has been made to describe and discuss controversial treatment methods with the goal of delineating their effects on the pulp. Wherever the evidence has appeared to be equivocal, the disparities have been presented. Under those circumstances, the choice of treatment is left to the reader's discretion. However, we take a definite stand where the evidence, in our opinion and clinical experience, is valid.

Throughout the text we have endeavored to present reasons for clinical procedures based on available scientific data. We hope this text will help those who are interested not only in how, but also in why a procedure is done. The present edition also clarifies some muddled and cloudy areas that existed in the previous editions. To summarize, we are modifying the quote from the first edition, "This is a big issue about a little tissue," to "This little tissue has created a big issue."

We express our thanks and appreciation to Mitchell Weinberg for his tireless and devoted assistance in the preparation of this text. We also thank the multitude of investigators who have contributed to our bibliography on the dental pulp. Without their investigations, this new edition would not have been needed.

SAMUEL SELTZER
I.B. BENDER

PREFACE TO THE FIRST EDITION

For many years, dentists have regarded dentin merely as a hard tissue that is cut for restorative procedures, not as part of a vital tissue that reacts to injury. Actually, cutting of the dentin and the odontoblastic processes which traverse the tubules involves exposure of living pulp cells to irritation.

Moreover, it has been believed by many that, once the root of the tooth is formed, the pulp has served its function and, following the completion of root end formation, no longer serves a useful purpose. In fact, the pulp has been considered to be a nuisance, giving rise to pain, on manipulative procedures, and complications of periapical inflammation when severely injured.

In order to understand the kind of tissue of which the dental pulp is composed, we have begun with the embryogenesis of the pulp. Inasmuch as the dentin is the hard tissue which is manufactured by the pulp, we felt it important to delve into the biology of the dentin. Since the dental pulp is a connective tissue, we thought it necessary to review connective tissues generally, as a background to our discourse on the pulp as a connective tissue. Also, the blood and the nerve supplies of the pulp are discussed.

In recent years, a large number of studies have shown that manipulative dental procedures, such as cutting of the dentin at various rotatory speeds, taking of impressions, application of drugs and insertion of restorations, affect the pulp. In addition, the processes of caries, erosion and attrition also affect the pulp. Formerly, it was believed that, once a pulp was injured, it could not recover. The contents of the chapters in this book, with numerous references to the works of other investigators, show that, on the contrary, the pulp has great recuperative powers. Thus, if the traumatic insults to the dentin and the pulp can be kept to a minimum or if restorative procedures can be modified to reduce injury, the likelihood of pulp recovery is enhanced.

In the chapters on microbial, mechanical, chemical, thermal and radiant irritants, we have presented documentary evidence of how the pulp reacts to injury. The pulp reacts to the irritant with an inflammatory response similar to that of any other connective tissue. A separate chapter was written to describe inflammation, so that a clearer understanding of pulp inflammation may be obtained.

In describing connective tissue and inflammation, we have incorporated various scientific data from allied fields, including histochemistry and biochemistry. By making use of information furnished by modern research tools such as electron microscopy, electrophoresis and radioautography, we feel that we have made our presentation more meaningful to both the student and the practitioner.

Frequently, carious and mechanical pulp exposures are treated by pulp capping and pulpotomy procedures. The indications and the contraindications, together with the tissue reactions to these procedures, are discussed.

All bodily tissues age; the dental pulp is no exception. The retrogressive changes which result from physiologic and pathologic processes are discussed in detail.

The classification of pulp diseases from a histologic standpoint, which is presented, varies somewhat from previous classifications. An understanding of this classification is needed for the reader to comprehend the clinical correlations which follow.

Finally, the relationship of clinical findings to histologic diagnosis and significant aids for differential diagnosis of pulp conditions are discussed. We are hopeful that our text will help to clarify some previously fuzzy areas and, also, will stimulate further interest in the biology of the dental pulp, on the part of dental students, clinicians and research workers.

This text differs from others that are presently available, in that it attempts to bridge the gap between the basic sciences and clinical practice. In most of the chapters, significant clinical correlations have been presented whenever data were available. For the undergraduate student, histology becomes more meaningful when it is clinically correlated. For the general practitioner, the clinical aspects of dentistry assume greater significance when the histologic background is understood.

We are also aware that, if a text on the dental pulp is to be complete, studies of the effects of orthodontic tooth movement and periodontal disease on the pulp should be included. We feel that, in these disciplines of dentistry, sparse information on interrelationships is available. Therefore, two separate chapters dealing with conclusions drawn from human material have been included, in order to make the text more complete.

A course entitled The Biology of the Dental Pulp has been, and is now being, presented to students of the School of Dental Medicine, University of Pennsylvania, our home base. When asked for criticism of the course at its completion, one of our students wrote, "This is a big issue about a little tissue." We believe that this aptly sums up what we have done.

We wish to thank Miss Rita Cherry and Mrs. Frances Parker, our secretaries, for their wonderful cooperation in typing the manuscript so many times. We are especially indebted to our endodontic resident Dr. Harold Nazimov and to Dr. Jerry Smith, endodontic graduate student, for their unflagging assistance. We apologize to their wives for the countless evenings devoted to this labor rather than to their families.

Mrs. Elizabeth Odenheimer, our chief technician, we thank especially, for her tireless devotion to the duties that seem to multiply so rapidly in a project such as this.

Our thanks also go to Drs. Richard Moodnik and Walter Soltanoff, who took the trouble to record and transcribe many of our lectures. Those notes served as a framework on which our book was built.

Finally, of Ruth Seltzer and Steve, and of Lillian Bender, Andrew and Susan, who bore with us during the long months of deprivation, we humbly beg forgiveness. Were it not for their encouragement, perhaps we might never have completed the text. It is to them that we fondly dedicate this book.

SAMUEL SELTZER
I.B. BENDER

CONTENTS

1   THE DEVELOPMENT OF THE DENTIN AND THE DENTAL PULP   1

    Enzymes, 3
    Odontoblasts and Dentin Formation, 4
    Clinical Correlations, 11

2   DENTIN   41

    Initiation of Dentinogenesis, 41
    Mechanism of Dentinogenesis, 42
    Chemical Structure, 53
    Secondary Dentin, 54
    Radioautography, 55
    Width of Dentinal Tubules, 58
    Metabolic Interchanges, 59

3   CONNECTIVE TISSUE   64

    The Fibers of Connective Tissue, 64
    Ground Substance, 68
    Cells, 69
    Systemic Factors That Affect Connective Tissue, 71

4   THE PULP AS CONNECTIVE TISSUE   78

    The Cells of the Pulp, 78
    Fibers, 96
    Ground Substance, 97
    Systemic Factors That Affect the Pulp, 99
    Tumor Transplantation, 101

5 THE CIRCULATION OF THE PULP — 105

Systemic Circulation, 105
Microcirculation, 105
Control of Blood Flow, 111
Lymphatics, 121
Clinical Correlations, 124
Changes Due to Inflammation, 127

6 THE NERVE SUPPLY OF THE PULP AND PAIN PERCEPTION — 131

Physiology of Neural Conduction, 131
Innervation of the Teeth, 134
Theories of Tooth Pain Perception, 140

7 INFLAMMATION AND INFECTION — 152

Acute Inflammation, 152
Chronic Inflammation, 159
Antibodies, 162
Repair, 165
Enzymes in Inflammation, 167
Action of Hormones, 168
Role of Vitamins, 169
Role of Proteins, 170
Infection, 170

8 PULP IRRITANTS: MICROBIAL — 173

Dental Caries, 173
Carious Dentin, 173
Microorganisms in Carious Dentin, 176
Defense Against Caries, 177
Inflammation Under Caries, 178
The Dynamics of the Development of Pulpitis from Dental Caries, 181
Indirect Pulp Capping, 188
Anachoresis, 189
Bacterial Invasion as a Result of Pressure, 190
Bacteremia Associated With Operative Manipulation, 191
Periodontal Involvement, 191
Systemic Infections, 192

9 MECHANICAL AND THERMAL IRRITANTS — 195

"Dentistogenic" (Iatrogenic) Pulpitis, 195
Depth of Cavity Preparations, 197
Relationship of Depth of Preparation to Reparative Dentin Formation, 199
Speed of Rotation, 199
Heat and Pressure, 200
Dry Cavity Preparation, 201
Nature of Cutting Instrument, 201
Size of Wheels and Burs, 202
Coolants, 203
Extensiveness of Preparation, 205
Other Physical Traumata, 207
The Effect of Tooth Movement on the Dental Pulp, 210

10 CHEMICAL IRRITANTS — 215

Dentin Sterilizing Agents, 215
Cleansing and Drying Medicaments, 218
Desensitizing and Remineralizing Agents, 219
Cavity Liners and Temporary and Permanent Filling Materials (and Related Procedures), 225

11 PERMANENT RESTORATIONS — 238

Permanent Restorative Materials, 238
Crown and Bridge Procedures, 246
Marginal Leakage, 247
Marginal Percolation, 248
Evaluation of All Filling Materials, 249

12 PULPITIS FROM OPERATIVE PROCEDURES 252

Odontoblasts, 252
Acute Pulpitis, 254
Chronic Pulpitis, 260
Repair, 263
The Dynamics of Pulp Inflammation
   Following Operative Procedures, 266
Cumulative Effects of Irritants, 267

13 RADIANT IRRITANTS 274

X-Irradiation, 274
Laser Beam, 277
Radium, 277
Strontium, 278
Cobalt, 278

14 PULP CAPPING AND PULPOTOMY 281

Indications for Pulp Capping, 281
Indications for Pulpotomy, 281
Physical Phenomena Associated With
   Mechanical Pulp Exposures, 282
Factors That Affect Outcome of Pulp Capping
   or Pulpotomy, 283
Histopathology, 286
Drugs in Pulp Capping and Pulpotomy, 289
Apexification Procedures, 297

15 THE INTERRELATIONSHIP OF PULP AND PERIODONTAL DISEASE 303

Lateral and Accessory Canals:
   Anatomic Considerations, 303
The Effect of Periodontal Disease on the
   Dental Pulp, 306
Atrophic Changes (Pulposis), 309
Inflammatory Changes, 311
Resorptions, 312
Toxic Products, 312
Effects of Periodontal Treatment and
   Local Medication, 314
The Effect of Pulp Lesions on
   Periodontal Lesions, 317
Correlation of Periodontal Involvement
   With Pain, 317
Correlation of Periodontal Involvement
   With Age, 319
Correlation of Periodontal Lesions and
   Thermal Responses, 319
The Pulpal-Periodontal Syndrome, 319

16 RETROGRESSIVE AND AGE CHANGES OF THE DENTAL PULP 324

Decrease in Cellular Components, 325
Dentinal Sclerosis, 325
Dead Tracts in the Primary Dentin, 327
Decrease in Number and Quality of
   Blood Vessels and Nerves, 327
Formation of Secondary Dentin, 328
Formation of Reparative Dentin, 329
Interference With Matrix Formation and
   Mineralization, 334
Atrophy (Pulposis), 338
Dystrophic Mineralization, 339
Denticles, 343
Increase in Number and Thickness of
   Collagen Fibers (Fibrosis), 344
Clinical Correlations of Induced Pulp
   Aging, 345
Artifacts, 346

17 HISTOLOGIC CLASSIFICATION OF PULP DISEASES 349

Classification, 349
Difficulties in Classification, 359

18 DIFFERENTIAL DIAGNOSIS 361

Subjective Findings, 361
Objective Findings, 362

Other Diagnostic Aids, 363

19 CLINICAL DIAGNOSIS 373

Subjective Symptoms (Patient's Complaints): Relationship of Pain to Histologic Findings, 374
Objective Findings: Relationship of Clinical Tests to Histopathologic Findings, 377

Classification for Clinical Diagnosis, 383
Classification for Therapeutic Purposes, 383

INDEX 387

1
THE DEVELOPMENT OF THE DENTIN AND THE DENTAL PULP

For convenience, the development of the teeth will be described in stages, although there is no sharp demarcation between one stage and the next.

Tooth development begins about the sixth week of fetal life. At that time, the oral epithelium is composed of two layers: a basal layer of epithelial cells that are rather columnar, and a surface layer of flattened epithelial cells. These are separated from the underlying connective tissue by a basement membrane.

Bud Stage. After the sixth week, a thickening of the epithelial layer occurs, owing to rapid proliferation of some cells of the basal layer. This is known as the dental lamina and is the primordium or the precursor of the enamel organ. Shortly, there appear within the dental lamina ten small, rounded thickenings in each jaw. These are the future tooth buds which are known as the bud stage of develoment (Fig. 1–1).

Cap Stage. Following the bud stage, rhythmic (circadian) cell division results in an unequal proliferation of some of the epithelium (Gasser et al, 1972), forming the cap stage (Fig. 1–2, *left*). The deep surface of the bud begins to invaginate and several layers become apparent. These are the inner dental epithelium, which is a layer of tall epithelial cells at the concavity, and the outer dental epithelium, which is a single layer of short epithelial cells on the outside. In the center, the cells become separated by an increased amount of intercellular, mucoid fluid rich in glycogen, as demonstrated by the periodic acid-Schiff (PAS) reaction. These cells are called the stellate reticulum or enamel pulp. The proliferated epithelium is attached to the dental lamina by a strand of epithelium, and this epithelium continues to grow and proliferate in the connective tissue.

About the eighth week of fetal life, the first beginning of the dental papilla is seen (Fig. 1–2, *right*). This is a condensation of connective tissue under the inner dental epithelium, which will become the future dental pulp. The cells in the dental papilla at first are large and rounded or polyhedral, with pale cytoplasm and large nuclei. As the pulp matures, the cells take on a spindle shape. Metachromatic ground substance (acid mucopolysaccharides) is present in great abundance (Fullmer, 1972). In addition, glycogen deposits of considerable size accumulate in the cytoplasm of undifferentiated mesenchyme cells but not in the fibroblasts or odon-

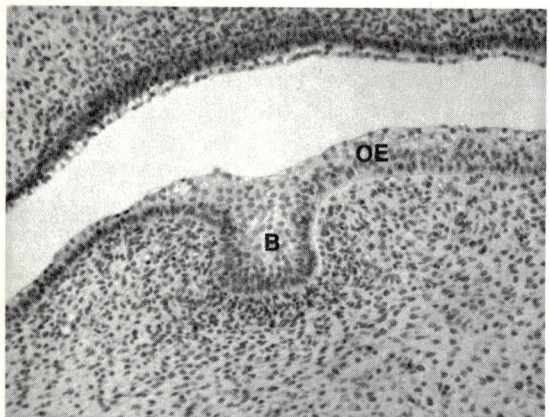

FIG. 1-1 Bud stage. B, tooth bud, about 7th week in utero. OE, oral epithelium. ×50.

toblasts (Russell, 1967), suggesting that the glycogen is depleted during differentiation (Garant, 1968). The glycogen may provide the energy for subsequent protein synthesis of the fibroblasts of the dental pulp. Concurrently, the mesenchyme surrounding the outside of the developing tooth condenses and becomes more fibrous. This tissue is known as the dental sac. The dental sac cells will form the tissues of the periodontium, which consist of the periodontal ligament, cementum, and alveolar bone (Ten Cate, 1975).

Bell Stage. The next stage, in which changes occur in the enamel organ, is known as the bell stage (Fig. 1-3).

The invagination deepens, and a series of interactions between the epithelial and mesenchymal cells occurs, resulting in differentiation of the cells of the inner dental epithelium into tall columnar cells called ameloblasts (Slavkin, 1974). The exchange of inductive information between epithelium and mesenchyme takes place across a basement membrane. This membrane is also known as the membrana preformativa or basal lamina. The ameloblasts will be instrumental in forming enamel. The cells of the dental papilla underlying the ameloblasts differentiate into odontoblasts, which will elaborate dentin. Next to the inner dental epithelium, several layers of low squamous cells begin to appear. This layer is known as the stratum intermedium (Fig. 1-4). Hunt and Paynter (1963) found by radioautography that the cells of the stratum intermedium in the guinea pig molar give rise to the cells of the stellate reticulum.

As develoment continues, the cells of the stratum intermedium become star shaped, with long, anastomosing processes. The cells of the outer dental epithelium flatten and the surface becomes folded.

The dental lamina proliferates at its deep end to give rise to the permanent tooth successor. It then disintegrates between the enamel organ and the oral epithelium (Fig. 1-4).

FIG. 1-2 Cap stage. *(A)* The enamel organ (EO) of an 11-week-old fetus. DL, dental lamina. DP, dental papilla. *(B)* A higher magnification of the dental papilla (DP), which will become the dental pulp.

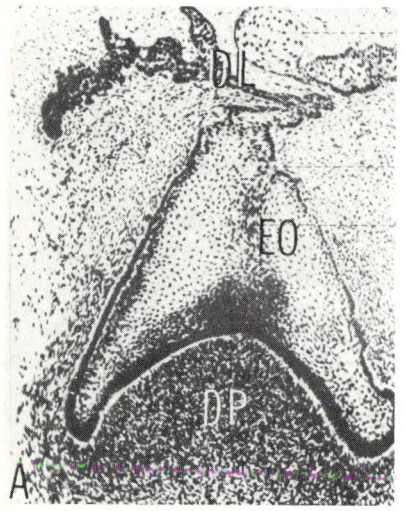
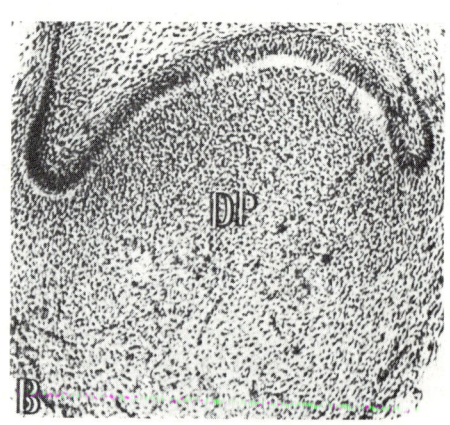

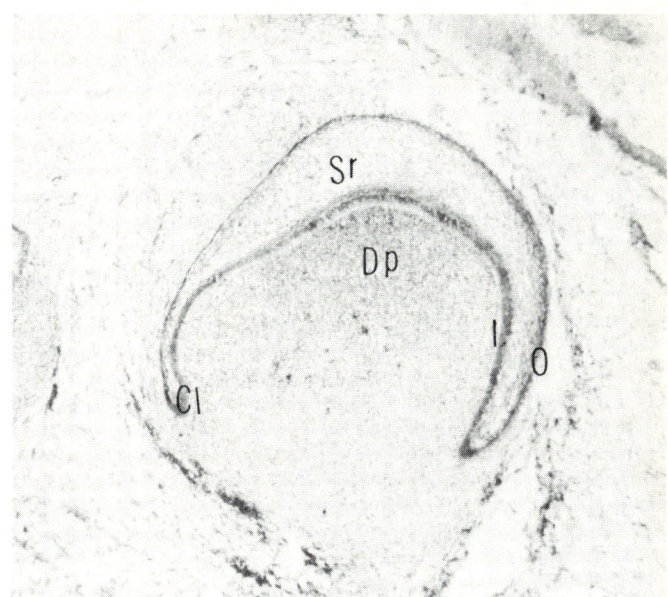

FIG. 1-3 Bell stage of tooth development, about 14th week in utero. Connective tissue condensation under inner dental epithelium (I) is the dental papilla (Dp). Between the inner dental epithelium and the outer dental epithelium (O) is the stellate reticulum (Sr). Cl, cervical loop. ×54.

ENZYMES

Hydrolytic Enzymes

Hydrolytic enzyme activities of human tooth germs at various stages of development and young erupted permanent teeth have been studied by Matthiessen (1966) and Ten Cate (1967).

Alkaline phosphatase activity was found in the bud stage. In the cap stage, the activity was most pronounced in the stellate reticulum and stratum intermedium and absent in the ameloblastic layer. According to Yoshiki and Kurahashi (1971) and Lunt and Noble (1972), the alkaline phosphatase is localized mainly to the surface of the plasma membrane (Fig. 1-5). In the bell stage, a distinct reaction was found in the dental papilla. In the odontoblastic layer, the alkaline phosphatase activity began after differentiation of the odontoblasts.

Acid phosphatase activity was found in all of the cells of the enamel organ during the bud stage. In the cap stage, strong activity was seen in the outer and inner dental epithelia; weaker reactions were present in the stellate reticulum. At the bell stage, all layers except the reticulum showed distinct reactions. The cells of the dental papilla showed moderate acid phosphatase activity which increased, especially in the odontoblasts, with the onset of dentinogenesis.

Unspecific esterase activity corresponded to that of acid phosphatase in the bud and cap stages. In the bell stage, the unspecific esterase increased in the outer, and decreased in the inner, dental epithelium. Mild reactions were present in the stratum intermedium. Reaction was minimal in the reticular layer. The cells of the dental papilla showed slight unspecific esterase activity. After differentiation, the odontoblasts showed intense activity.

Adenosine triphosphatases (ATPase) were found to be prominent in the ameloblasts and stratum intermedium of the incisors of young mice. The odontoblasts and pulp cells exhibited moderate activity (Severson, 1968). Later, in the odontoblastic and subodontoblastic layers, ATPase activity was found to be highest when mineralization begins (Guo and Messer, 1976).

Oxidative Enzymes

Differentiating odontoblasts exhibited marked activity with respect to succinic dehydrogenase, lactic dehydrogenase, glucose-6-phosphate dehydrogenase, diphosphopyridine nucleotide diaphorase (DPNH) and triphosphopyridine nucleotide diaphorase (TPNH; Fullmer, 1963).

Lactate dehydrogenase isoenzymes have also been detected in the odontoblastic layer of the developing teeth of the mouse (Roberts and

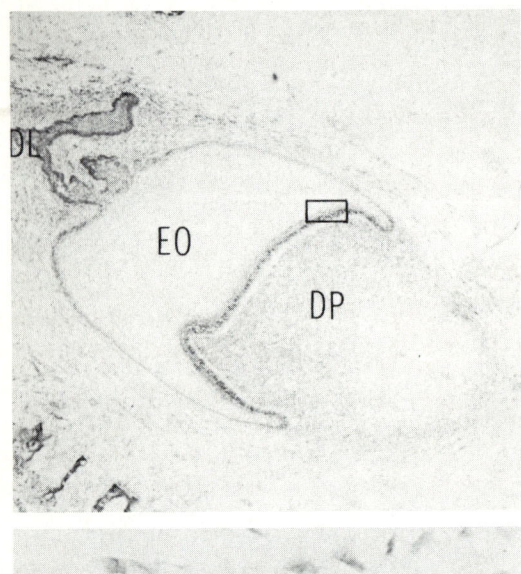

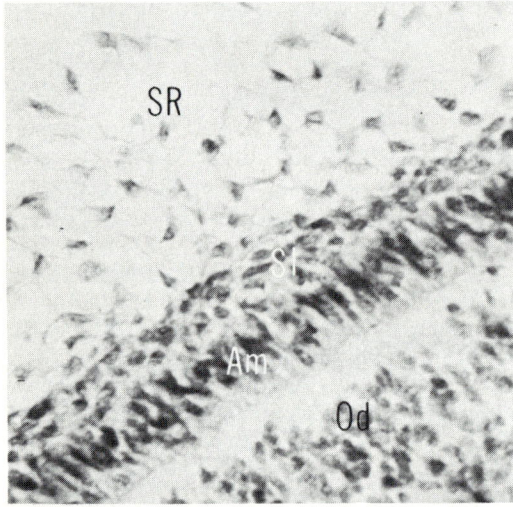

FIG. 1-4 Advanced bell stage of tooth development. *(Top)* Tooth germ, consisting of dental pulp (DP) and enamel organ (EO), still connected to the dental lamina (DL). ×54. *(Bottom)* Higher magnification of region outlined by rectangle in top picture. The ameloblasts (Am) have differentiated into tall, columnar cells. Above the ameloblastic layer is the stratum intermedium (SI) and the stellate reticulum (SR). The odontoblasts (Od) are separated from the ameloblasts by a basement membrane. ×540.

Strachan, 1967) and the rat (Linde and Ljunggren, 1970).

The presence of these enzymes indicates that the energy for odontoblastic metabolism is produced by a strictly anaerobic metabolic pathway. However, partially deficient aerobic metabolism may also occur, since measurements of pulpal respiration over successive 10-minute intervals revealed noticeable variation of rates as well as brief periods of suspension of oxygen consumption. A higher uptake of oxygen occurred in odontoblasts that were actively manufacturing dentin (Fisher, 1967).

Biologic Role

The exact biologic significance of the role of alkaline phosphatase is still conjectural. It has been implicated in the mineralization process (Robison, 1923), the transport of metabolites through cell membranes (Verzár and McDougall, 1936), the synthesis of fibrous proteins (Bradfield, 1950), the formation of acid mucopolysaccharides (Ten Cate, 1959), the process of cell differentiation (Lunt and Noble, 1972), and the mediation of the transport of glucose (Anagnostopoulos and Matsudaira, 1958).

The biologic role of acid phosphatase and unspecific esterase is also controversial. Acid phosphatases have been shown to be related to protein synthesis (Burstone, 1960) or reversed pinocytosis (Fearnhead, 1961). Most investigators believe these enzymes are characteristically present in cellular lysosomes that are involved in intracellular digestion (De Duve, 1959).

Adenosine-5'-triphosphate (ATP) is involved in energy-requiring reactions and processes (Le Bell, 1981). Measurements of ATP are used to study the metabolism of cells and to detect cell death (Stewart and Arie, 1973).

Dehydrogenases are generally regarded as a measure of metabolic activity. The energy needed for cellular differentiation and mineralization is based on the activity of the dehydrogenases (Larmas and Larmas, 1976). However, their role in various biologic processes has not been specifically defined.

Since ATPase activity increases when mineralization begins (Severson, 1971), the enzyme is probably involved in calcium transport in the pulp (Messer and Guo, 1979).

ODONTOBLASTS AND DENTIN FORMATION

The formation of a layer of high columnar cells becomes evident in the dental papilla. The nuclei of these cells lie close to the cells of the inner dental epithelium; the cytoplasm has become basophilic and PAS positive. These cells are the odontoblasts, which have differentiated

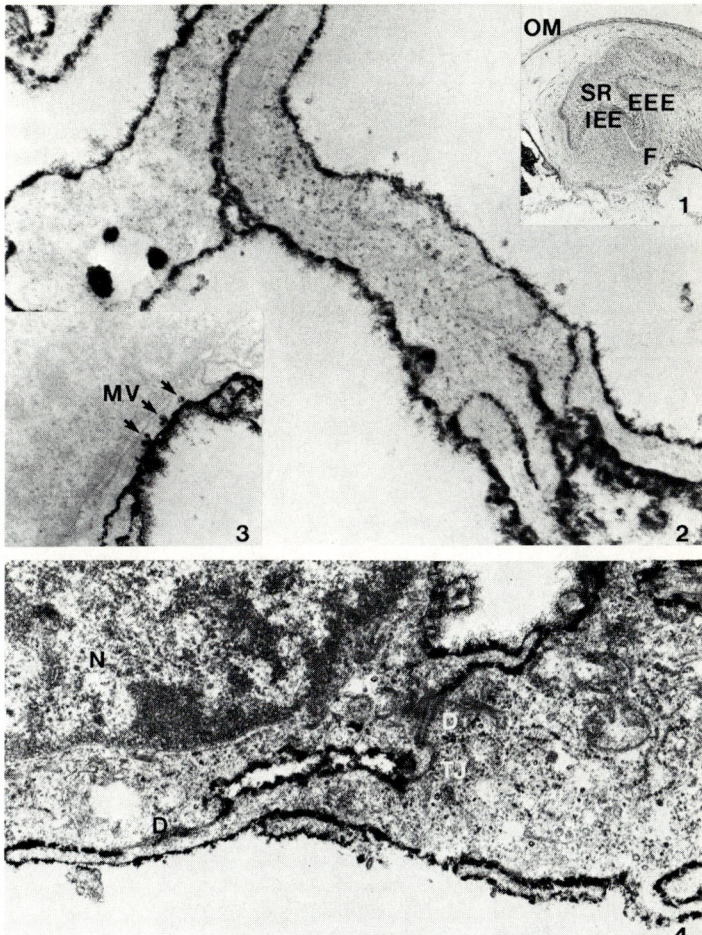

FIG. 1-5 *(Top, right)* Cryostat section of enamel organ, cap stage. Stellate reticulum cells (SR) are beginning to show separation. IEE, internal enamel epithelium; EEE, external enamel epithelium; F, follicle; OM, oral mucosa. ×40. *(Top left, center right)* Alkaline phosphatase reaction in stellate reticulum cells, localized on plasma membranes of both free and contacting sufaces over almost the entire cell periphery. ×30,000. *(Left, center)* Positive reaction in microvesicles (MV) immediately below the cell surface. ×30,000. *(Bottom)* The enzyme reaction product is absent where desmosomes (D) or tight junctions (TJ) exist between stellate reticulum cells. N, nucleus. Stained uranyl acetate/lead citrate. ×30,000. (Lunt DA, Noble HW: Localization of alkaline phosphatases in human cap-stage enamel organs by electron histochemistry. Arch Oral Biol 17:761, 1972)

from the cells in the pulp. According to Hurmerinta et al (1980), this differentiation is based on the interaction of cell surface macromolecules, such as sulfated glycosaminoglycans, with extracellular matrix. The odontoblasts are rich in alkaline phosphatase, which appears to be associated with the deposition of dentin matrix (Larmas and Thesleff, 1980). The odontoblasts shortly begin to secrete a matrix that is collagenous. This matrix is known as predentin or uncalcified dentin or dentinoid, and represents the beginning of hard tissue formation in the tooth (Fig. 1-6).

This first extracellular matrix formed by the odontoblasts contains fibronectin, a tissue glycoprotein involved in adhesion of cells (Linde et al, 1982). Eventually, the initial matrix will form the organic constituent of the first dentin, called mantle dentin.

As dentin is deposited at the distal end of the cell, the odontoblast becomes displaced in a pulpal direction. During this pulpward movement, the odontoblast forms a continually elongating cytoplasmic process. Thus, the odontoblast develops into a cell with two distinct parts, the cell body and the odontoblastic process. The cell body is concerned with synthesis of predentin, and the cell process is engaged in the deposition of the product (Reith, 1968; Fig. 1-7). Both prosecretory and secretory granules are found in the Golgi region and in both the apical portion of the odontoblast and its process (Fig. 1-8). The contents of the granules are subsequently released into the predentin by exocytosis.

The endoplasmic reticulum consists of vesicles of various types. Ribonucleoprotein granules accumulate on the surface of the endoplasmic reticulum, indicating that it is involved in protein (collagen) elaboration. These dense granules are believed to originate from the Golgi apparatus (Garant et al, 1968; Reith, 1968).

FIG. 1-7 Odontoblastic process of young odontoblast (yOP) showing dense bodies (DB) and vesicles (V). Arrows mark filaments that connect to apical junctional complexes of odontoblasts. Filaments occupy a plane that corresponds to location of the odontoblastic-predentinal membrane; filaments also demarcate synthetic portion of odontoblast *(above)* containing rough-surfaced endoplasmic reticulum (rER) and mitochondria (M) from discharge portion of cell below, namely, the process. Predentin contains thin collagen fibrils adjacent to odontoblast (rectangle 1) and thick collagen fibrils (rectangle 2) at mineralization front (MF). ×18,000. (Reith EJ: Collagen formation in developing molar teeth of rats. J Ultrastruct Res 21:383, 1968)

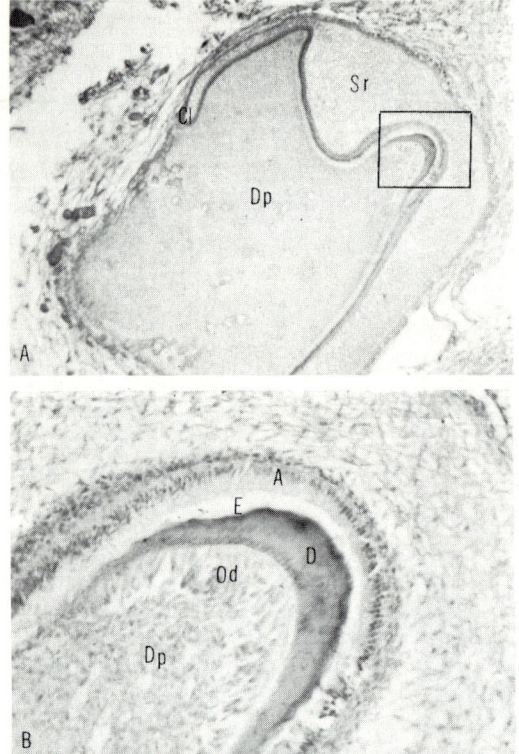

FIG. 1-6 Early stage of dentin formation in the bell stage of tooth development of a 5-month-old fetus. *(A)* Tooth germ, consisting of dental pulp (Dp) and enamel organ. Cl, cervical loop; Sr, stellate reticulum. ×54. *(B)* Higher magnification of area outlined by square in *(A)*. Odontoblasts (Od) of the dental pulp (Dp) have elaborated dentin (D). Ameloblasts (A) have produced thin layer of enamel (E). ×240.

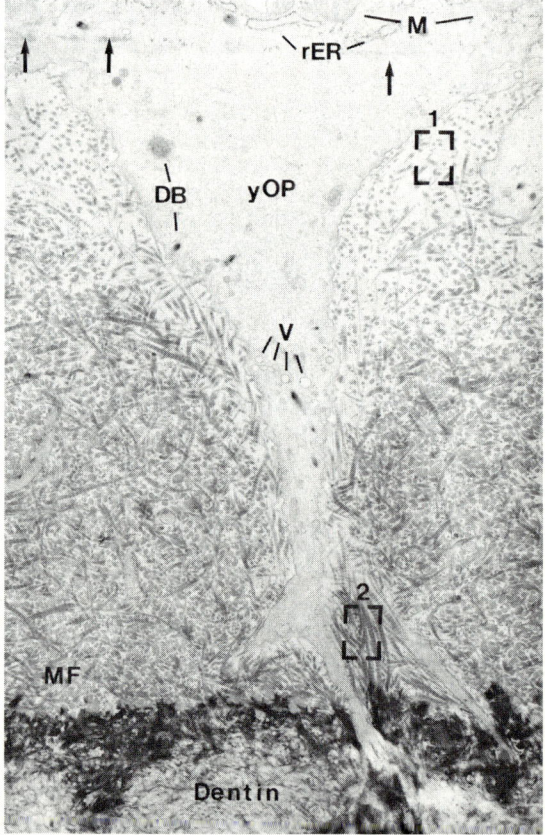

In electron microscopic examinations of tooth buds from fetuses 3 to 5 months old, Frank and Nalbandian (1963) noted that the odontoblasts assume elongated forms prior to matrix elaboration. Within the cell body, there is an extensive increase in cytoplasmic organelles, such as ergastoplasm (endoplasmic reticulum), Golgi complex and mitochondria (Fig. 1-9). In addition to these organelles, the cell bodies and processes of rat molar odontoblasts have been shown to contain centrioles with rudimentary cilia, lysosomes, multivesicular bodies, and well-developed networks of microfilaments and microtubules. Cross bridges or side arms are present between the microtubules and microfibrils (Garant, 1972; Fig. 1-10).

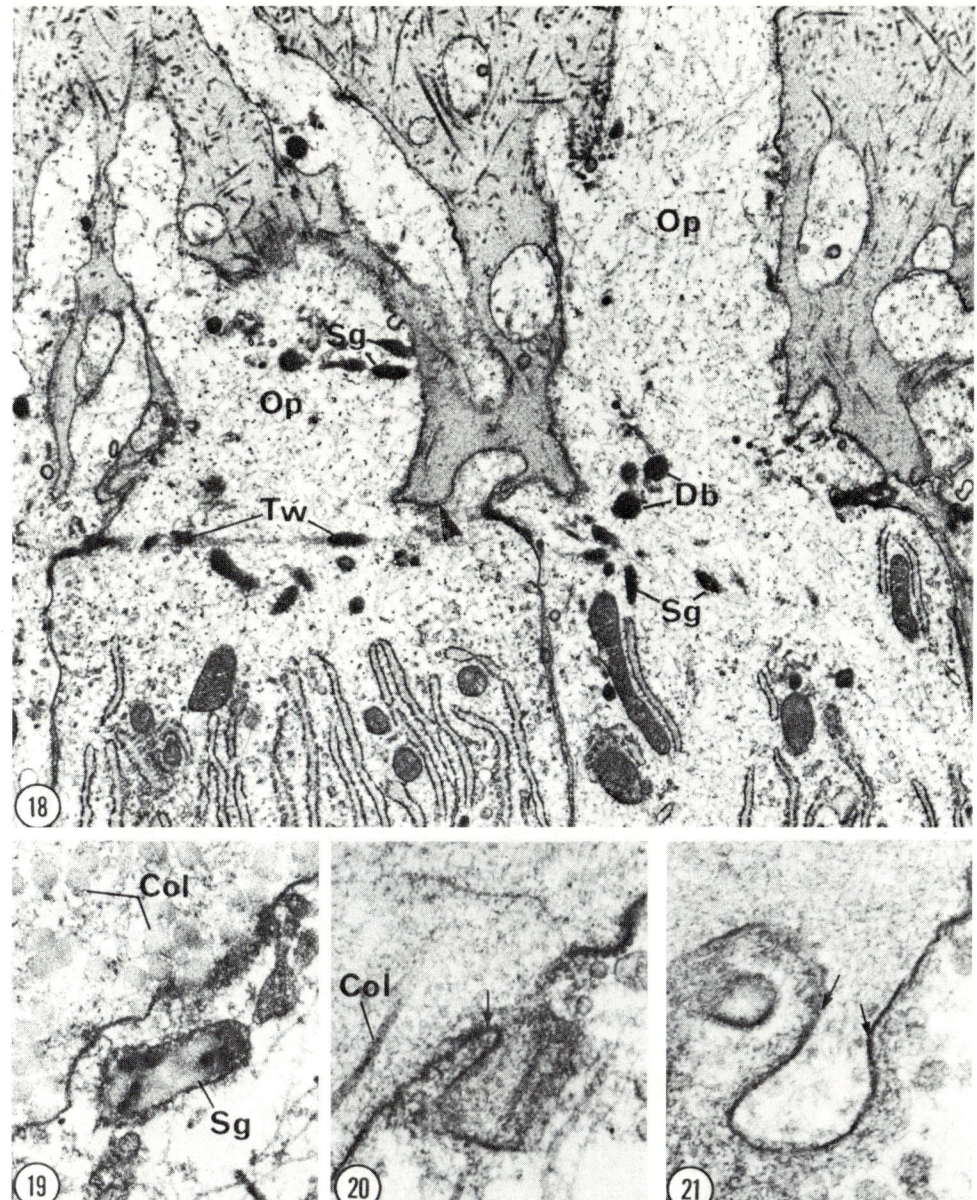

FIG. 1-8 Portions of odontoblast processes *(Top)* and presumed steps in the release of content of secretory granules *(Bottom)*. *(Top)* Apical regions of odontoblasts showing profiles of odontoblast processes (Op) and their minor branches in various planes of section. In the cell at left, the terminal web (Tw) is taken as the boundary between cytoplasm and odontoblast process. Secretory granules (Sg) and dense bodies (Db) are regular components of the process; however, the rough endoplasmic reticulum is excluded. The proximal predentin is finely granular and shows randomly arranged collagen fibrils. These become abundant in distal predentin *(top of frame)*. On the external surface of the plasmalemma, particularly in the proximal portions of the odontoblast process, where secretory granules are frequently encountered, electron-dense accumulations may be distinguished (arrowhead). Other elements occasionally detected in predentin are not believed to be typical collagen fibrils but rather aggregates of tropocollagen or procollagen molecules. ×14,400. *(Bottom, left)* Secretory granule (Sg) in a portion of odontoblast process (lower right) with nearby predentin (upper left) routinely stained with uranyl acetate and lead citrate. The secretory granule shows a

(Continued)

7

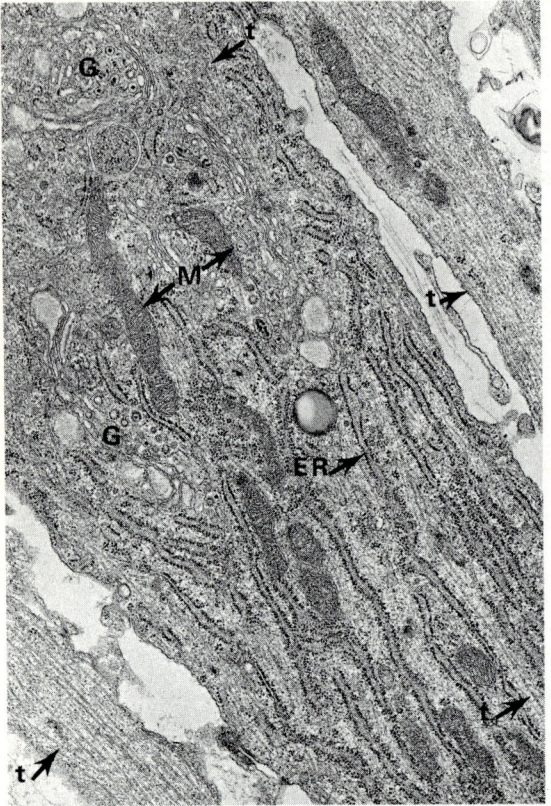

FIG. 1-9 Cytoplasm of several odontoblasts, showing well developed network of microtubules (t). ER, endoplasmic reticulum; G, Golgi apparatus; M, mitochondria. ×17,000. (Garant PR: The organization of microtubules within rat odontoblast processes revealed by perfusion fixation with glutaraldehyde. Arch Oral Biol 17:1047, 1972)

The Golgi complex is intimately associated with the endoplasmic reticulum and is related to secretory function (Palade, 1975). According to Weinstock and Leblond (1974), the Golgi apparatus consists of interconnected stacks of flattened fenestrated saccules, usually four per stack.

In their studies, Weinstock and Leblond (1974) injected tritium-labeled proline intravenously into rats. Within 2 minutes, the label was found in the rough endoplasmic reticulum, indicating that this was the site of synthesis of the polypeptide precursors of collagen, the proalpha chains. These chains give rise to procollagen molecules, assembled in the Golgi apparatus. Such procollagen molecules have been detected by Weinstock (1977) as centrosymmetrical cross-bonded structures within the predentin and dentin matrix of rat incisors.

The mitochondria, which are situated in close relationship to the endoplasmic reticulum, are made up of double membranes, of which the folded inner membrane gives rise to cristae mitochondriales, containing an assembly of cytochromes, which are the energy reservoir of the cell.

Centrioles appear in the electron microscope as cylindrical bodies whose walls consist of parallel tubular structures. They are usually found in pairs, lying near each other at each pole of the cell. They self-replicate prior to cell division (DeHarven and Dustin, 1960).

Lysosomes are structures that contain a number of digestive enzymes such as acid phosphatases, as well as others that break down proteins and nucleic acids (Gianetto and De Duve, 1955).

(Continued)
moderately electron-dense homogeneous content that resembles in staining properties the collagen fibrils (Col) distinguishable in the adjacent predentin matrix. Electron-dense particles are also present in the granule. The granule lies adjacent to the plasmalemma. Cytoplasmic filaments are at lower right. ×60,000. *(Bottom, middle).* Secretory granule in the proximal portion of the odontoblast process. The limiting membrane of the granule may be seen confluent with the plasma membrane of the process (arrow). There is evidence of the presence of filament bundles (arrowhead) of the same length as those observed in cylindrical Golgi saccules. Presumably, extrusion of the granule content into the predentin matrix (upper left) will ensue. A collagen fibril (Col) and threads of various sizes may be seen in the predentin. ×60,000. *(Bottom, right)* Secretory granule discharge in a region of the odontoblast process similar to that seen in top figure (arrowhead). The granule membrane is continuous with, and part of, the plasmalemma in the region between the arrows. The regular pattern of electron-dense accumulations on the external surface of the plasmalemma are seen. A clear area within which delicate threads are visible in various planes of section may be identified in the central region. ×60,000. (Weinstock M, Leblond CP: Synthesis, migration, and release of precursor collagen by odontoblasts as visualized by radioautography after (3H) proline administration. J Cell Biol 60:93, 1974)

THE DEVELOPMENT OF THE DENTIN AND THE DENTAL PULP

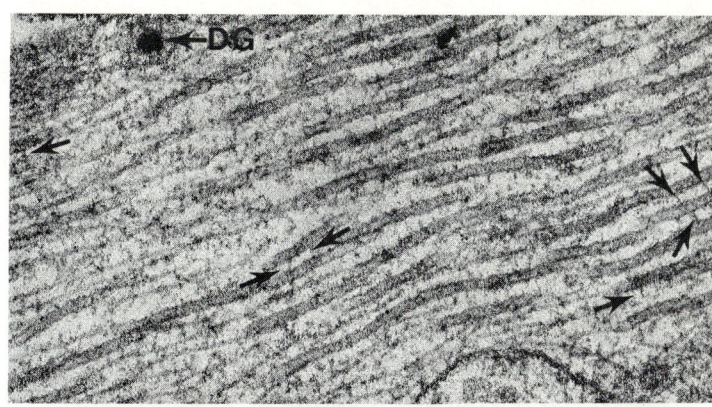
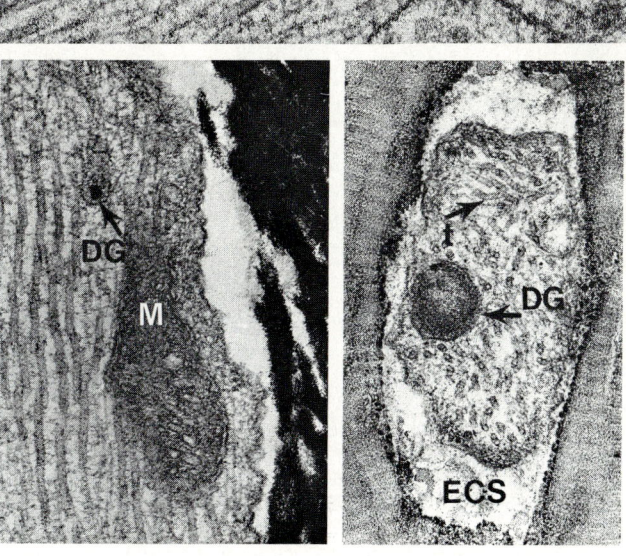

FIG. 1-10 *(Top)* High magnification of part of an odontoblast process, showing side arms (arrows) projecting from microtubules. Similar structures contact the cytoplasmic filaments. DG, dense granule. ×120,000. *(Bottom, left)* Enlarged area of odontoblast process, depicting mitochondria (M) and dense granule (DG) in zone of mineralized dentin. ×90,000. *(Bottom, right)* Cross section of odontoblast process in demineralized dentin. A dense granule (DG) and numerous microtubules are contained within the process. ECS, extracellular space. ×60,000. (Garant PR: The organization of microtubules within rat odontoblast processes revealed by perfusion fixation with glutaraldehyde. Arch Oral Biol 17:1047, 1972)

The microtubules are believed to serve a cytoskeletal function designed to maintain cell shape or participate in effecting changes in cell shape, such as extension and retraction of pseudopods (MacGregor and Stebbins, 1970). Garant has postulated that, as more and more dentin is deposited, the microtubules may be required for the elongation of the odontoblastic process. The microtubules may also play a role in the intracellular transport of water and small ions (Slautterbach, 1963) and in the saltatory (abrupt) movements of larger particles (Bikle et al, 1966). Thus, the cytoplasmic granules may be transported from the Golgi apparatus to deeper areas in the odontoblastic process by the microtubule network.

Although the odontoblasts are for the most part close to each other, in some places, microvilli project into narrow intercellular spaces. Bundles of collagen fibers can be seen between some of the cells during the formation of mantle dentin. These fibers are known as von Korff fibers, and they extend from the subodontoblastic layer to the predentin (Reith, 1968; see Figs. 2–4 and 2–5). As dentinogenesis proceeds, von Korff fibers become less numerous. Closely related to the cell membrane of the odontoblastic process is a second group of collagenous fibers. These fibers quickly become the predominant fiber type (Fig. 1–7).

Transition from Dental Papilla to Dental Pulp

The dentin continues to be elaborated in a rhythmic fashion. From this stage forward, the dental papilla becomes the dental pulp. The boundary between the inner dental epithelium and the odontoblasts forms the outline of the future dentinoenamel junction (Fig. 1–11).

The junction of the inner and the outer dental

10 | THE DENTAL PULP

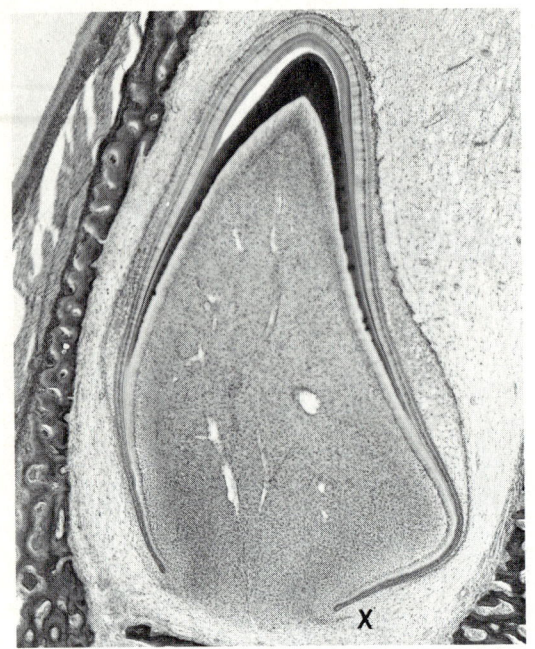

FIG. 1-11 In appositional stage of development of premolar teeth, dentinoenamel and cementoenamel junctions are demarcated and crown form is apparent. X, Hertwig's sheath. ×12. PAS and hematoxylin stain. (Grant D, Bernick S: Morphodifferentiation and structure of Hertwig's root sheath in the cat. J Dent Res 50:1580, 1971. Copyright by the American Dental Association. Reproduced by permission)

epithelia at the basal margin of the enamel organ represents the future cementoenamel junction. This joined epithelium proliferates and gives rise to Hertwig's epithelial root sheath, which is concerned with root development. Hertwig's sheath has been studied morphologically, radioautographically and histochemically in various animals and in humans. Such studies have shown that following the bud stage, the sheath becomes progressively narrower and longer to form a pseudopodlike extension into the connective tissue. The cells of the inner dental epithelium are separated from the developing pulpal tissue by an intact PAS-positive basement membrane (Grant and Bernick, 1971) (Fig. 1-12).

In both the early and the late stages of root development of dog teeth, the ends of the odontoblastic processes grow outwards. The processes eventually become embedded in new matrix. According to Owens (1978b), these pro-jections unite with islands of cementum, thus appearing to play an active role in the fusion of dentin and cementum. Hertwig's root sheath persists throughout root formation. With the onset of cementogenesis, the continuity of the root sheath is disrupted by proliferation of fibroblasts. Many epithelial cells fail to move away from the root surface and appear to be involved in some collagen production, which unites cementum and dentin matrixes (Owens, 1978a). Remnants of Hertwig's root sheath persist as epithelial rests–cell rests of Malassez. Continued dentin deposition results in narrowing of the apical foramen (Fig. 1-13). Following the formation of dentin, the enamel begins to be elaborated.

Blood Supply

According to Saunders (1966) and to Cutright (1970), the blood supply of the developing tooth bud originates from an oval or circular reticulated plexus in the alveolar bone. This plexus gradually enlarges and assumes the shape of the developing tooth. A series of blood vessels, arising from the plexus, grow into the dental papilla,

FIG. 1-12 Hertwig's sheath (point X, from Fig. 1-11) is made up of inner, intermediate, and outer epithelial layers. An intact PAS-positive membrane over the dental papilla surface rounds the loop end and then appears to fade and disappear on the dental sac (DS) surface. DP, dental papilla. PAS and hematoxylin. ×500. (Grant D, Bernick S: Morphodifferentiation and structure of Hertwig's root sheath in the cat. J Dent Res 50:1580, 1971. Copyright by the American Dental Association. Reproduced by permission)

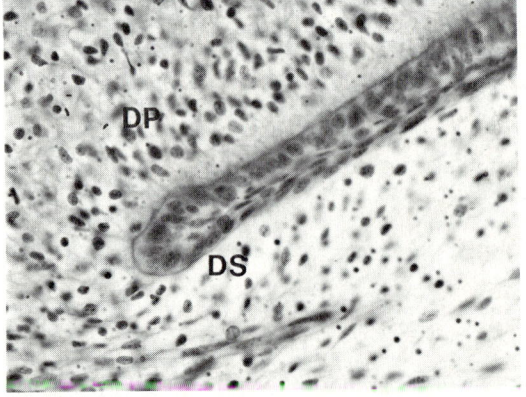

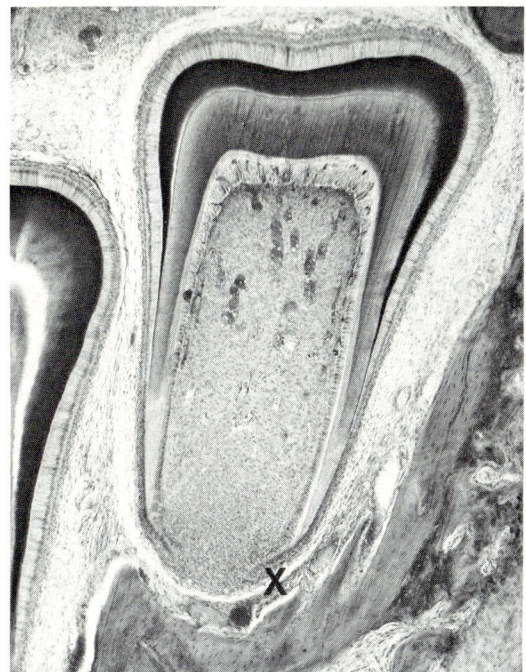

FIG. 1-13 Progressive narrowing of apical foramen is apparent in a permanent incisor at beginning root formation. Note the bulbous appearance of Hertwig's sheath (X) at the apical foramen. PAS and hematoxylin stain. ×10. (Grant D, Bernick S: Morphodifferentiation and structure of Hertwig's root sheath in the cat. J Dent Res 50:1580, 1971. Copyright by the American Dental Association. Reproduced by permission)

where they remain as the future pulpal vessels. Tobin (1972) injected the vascular systems of maxillae and mandibles of 50 human fetuses with an India ink–formalin suspension. Under a dissecting microscope, the blood supplies of the developing teeth were then studied and correlated with the extent of mineralization of the teeth. Branches of vessels in the basal wall of the dental sac were observed to course through the dental papilla to the developing dentin and to the lateral areas of the dental papilla (Fig. 1-14). The pulpal artery terminated at the pulpodentinal junction in a plexus of small vessels. With continued tooth development, the encircling plexus is transformed into the vascular plexus of the periodontal ligament. The blood vessels of the periodontal plexus of the deciduous teeth connect with those of the developing permanent teeth.

Nerve Supply

During crown formation in the early developmental period, a few axons enter the dental papilla. Peripheral nerve plexuses do not develop. During the eruptive stage, there is a rapid development of sensory innervation to form the plexus of Raschkow and terminals in the odontoblastic layer. Gradually, as the teeth mature, root formation is completed and the root foramina narrow. Axon numbers and densities increase and dentin becomes innervated (Byers, 1980).

CLINICAL CORRELATIONS

Certain disorders, such as nutritional disturbances, congenital defects, and infections, have an influence on the developing teeth. The disturbances affect certain portions of the teeth, depending on the stage of tooth development at the time of their occurrence. Thus, the tooth tissues may be affected at any of the following stages, which summarize the development of the tooth:

1. Thickening of the epithelium (initiation)
2. Proliferation of the epithelial tissue into the connective tissue
3. Histodifferentiation of the cells
4. Morphodifferentiation of the cells
5. Apposition of hard structures

One single stage does not occur at any particular time, and several stages are present simultaneously. A disturbance in any one of the stages of development will produce a characteristic lesion discernible either in a histologic section or by clinical observation.

ENAMEL FORMATION

In the deciduous dentition, a substantial amount of enamel has already been formed at the time of birth. Enamel formation is completed between 1½ months after birth for the maxillary central incisor and 11 months after birth for the maxillary second molar. The times for the completion of enamel formation vary in the other deciduous teeth (Table 1-1; Lunt and Law, 1974).

For the permanent teeth, enamel formation has already begun in utero for the mandibular central and lateral incisors and for the maxillary

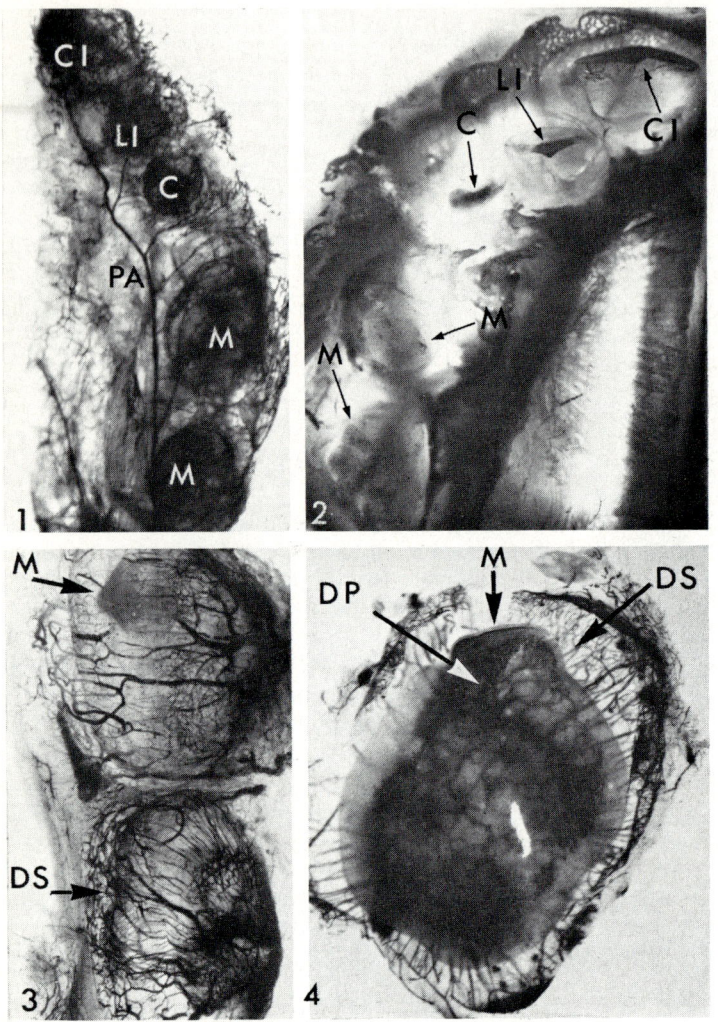

FIG. 1-14 *(Top, left)* Fetus, 19 weeks: Oral view, right side of palate, showing the palatine artery (PA) and its branches to the developing tooth germs. ×5. *(Top, right)* Fetus, 18½ weeks: Oral view, left side of palate (gingiva and superficial part of dental sacs removed), showing the mineralization of the cusps (black arrow) in the various tooth germs. ×10. *(Bottom, left)* Fetus, 18 weeks: Two intact molar dental sacs (buccal view), showing mineralization (M) on a developing cusp and the blood vessels in the wall of the dental sacs (DS). ×8. *(Bottom, right)* Fetus, 17 weeks: Isolated dental sac from which the oral part was removed, showing the mineralization of a cusp (M), and the vessels in the wall of the dental sac (DS) and in the dental papilla (DP). No vessels from the wall of the dental sac traversed the stellate reticulum (made transparent by clearing oil) to the mineralized or nonmineralized area of the dental cusps. Compare with Fig. 2-1 for vessels and mineralization in other tooth germs. ×12. (Tobin CE: Correlation of vascularity with mineralization in human fetal teeth. Anat Rec 174:371, 1972)

and mandibular first molars. Enamel formation is completed between about 3 years for the maxillary and mandibular first molars and about 7½ years for the maxillary and mandibular second molars (Oliver et al, 1963). Times of completion of enamel formation vary for the other teeth (Fig. 1-15).

TOOTH SIZE

The sizes and shapes of the teeth are genetically controlled, and the teeth of males differ from those of females in many developmental aspects. In males, the teeth are usually larger; also, they calcify later and erupt later than they do in females. In addition, closure of the apices of teeth occurs at a later age in males than in females (Garn et al, 1965).

NEOPLASMS

If a disturbance in proliferation develops, an ameloblastoma or other tumor may form.

Ameloblastomas are considered to be odontogenic tumors of ectodermal origin, the cells of which have the property of differentiation into enamel epithelium without actually forming enamel. The tumor develops from the dental lamina or from the enamel organ itself.

Other tumors such as odontogenic myxomas and fibromas may form from the embryonic or the adult mesenchymal cells of the tooth germ.

TABLE 1-1
Lunt and Law's Suggested Chronology for the Calcification of the Deciduous Dentition

DECIDUOUS TOOTH	HARD TISSUE FORMATION BEGINS (FERTILIZATION AGE IN UTERO, WEEKS)		AMOUNT OF ENAMEL FORMED AT BIRTH	ENAMEL COMPLETED (MONTHS AFTER BIRTH)	ROOT COMPLETED (YEAR)
MAXILLARY					
Central incisor	14	(13–16)	Five sixths	1½	1½
Lateral incisor	16	(14⅔–16½)	Two thirds	2½	2
Canine	17	(15–18)	One third	9	3¼
First molar	15½	(14½–17)	Cusps united; occlusal completely calcified plus one half to three fourths crown height	6	2½
Second molar	19	(16–23½)	Cusps united; occlusal incompletely calcified; calcified tissue covers one fifth to one fourth crown height	11	3
MANDIBULAR					
Central incisor	14	(13–16)	Three fifths	2½	1½
Lateral incisor	16	(14⅔–)	Three fifths	3	1½
Canine	17	(16–)	One third	9	3¼
First molar	15½	(14½–17)	Cusps united; occlusal completely calcified	5½	2¼
Second molar	18	(17–19½)	Cusps united; occlusal incompletely calcified	10	3

(Lunt RC, Law DB: A review of the chronology of calcification of deciduous teeth. JADA 89:599, 1974. Copyright by the American Dental Association. Reprinted by permission)

FIG. 1-15 Chronology of enamel formation. Each bar represents the development of a single tooth, plotted against age. The left margin of the bar represents the beginning of enamel formation, the right margin represents its completion. (Oliver WJ, Owings CL, Brown WE, Shapiro AB: Hypoplastic enamel associated with the nephrotic syndrome. Pediatrics 32:399, 1963)

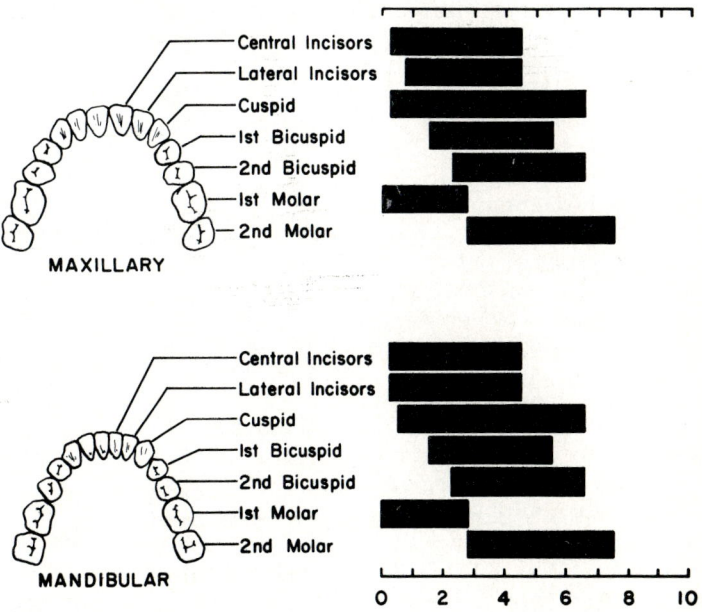

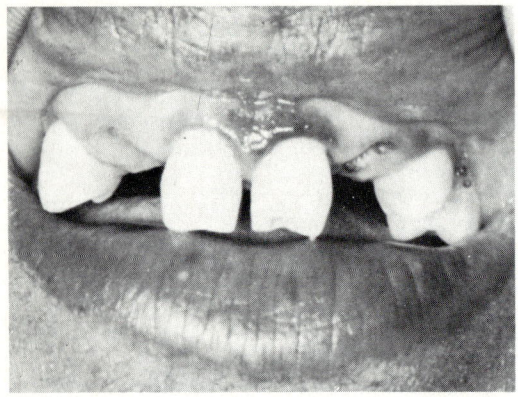

FIG. 1-16 Notched incisors, characteristic of a congenital syphilitic.

When the stellate reticulum undergoes degeneration, a space is formed that becomes lined with stratified squamous epithelium. Subsequently, this lesion is designated as a primordial cyst. Microscopically, such a cyst contains keratin (Gorlin, 1970).

INFECTIONS

Infections may affect the stages of histodifferentiation, morphodifferentiation, and maturation.

Systemic Infections. The systemic infection syphilis causes the formation of hutchinsonian teeth, which are characteristically shovel-shaped or notched anterior teeth (Fig. 1-16) or mulberry molars. Saunders (1957) has shown that the spirochetes of syphilis enter the blood vessels in the areas where the tooth is being formed, interfering with the stages of differentiation and maturation, resulting in the malformations.

Exanthematous fevers such as rubella, chickenpox, measles and scarlet fever also affect the development of the teeth. These infections are associated with high fevers affecting the stages of histodifferentiation and morphodifferentiation. Since they affect tissues of ectodermic origin, the enamel is altered. The ameloblasts are sensitive to, and are injured by, high temperatures, resulting in pitting of the enamel (Kreshover, 1960). In infants with congenital rubella, the most prominent resultant dental anomalies are hypoplastic, or partial or total aplastic enamel of the deciduous teeth. Also, tooth eruption is delayed (Guggenheimer et al, 1971).

Since the enamel is continuously elaborated in a rhythmic fashion, it is possible to estimate the age at which the fever occurred by the location of the pitted region on the enamel surface of the tooth (Fig. 1-15). For example, the presence of a pitted or eroded line in anteriors enables the observer to estimate the specific age at which the patient had measles, chickenpox, or scarlet fever. Thus, the enamel—and, frequently, the dentin—presents a clue as to when a systemic disturbance took place. Similar effects occur in bone, but become erased because there is continuous deposition and resorption. In enamel, only deposition occurs.

Skeletal and dental deformities result from viral infections in experimental animals. The pulps of developing teeth of young hamsters infected with a small DNA virus were found by Garant et al (1980) to contain a round cell infiltration near the cervical loops. Focal degeneration of the odontoblastic layer and adjacent pulp, caused by the virus particles, was also found.

In other experiments, mice were infected with tumor-inducing SE polyoma virus at birth (Cohen and Shklar, 1965) and within 12 hours of birth (Fleming, 1963). Tumor cells invaded the dentinal tubules and interfered with amelogenesis. Cohen and Shklar found that the viruses had a striking affinity for the teeth and bones, causing gross malformations and necrotic pulps.

Local infections of deciduous teeth for short periods (up to 6 weeks) were not found to influence odontogenesis of the permanent central incisor successors in studies by Andreasen and Riis (1978). However, long-standing infections that cause periapical abscesses may affect the succeeding tooth bud. The spread of such infections may be enhanced by the direct connection of the pulpal and periodontal vasculature of the deciduous teeth with the vascular plexus surrounding the developing permanent teeth (Cutright, 1970). In these circumstances, the formation of the enamel of the permanent teeth is impeded, resulting in hypoplasia and hypomineralization (Binns and Escobar, 1967; Kaplan et al, 1967; Matsumiya, 1968). In addition, the teeth become discolored. These teeth are called Turner teeth (Fig. 1-17). Other effects on the permanent successors may be impaction, rotation, ectopic eruption, or interference with normal eruption sequence. In extreme cases, exfoliation of the permanent tooth bud may result.

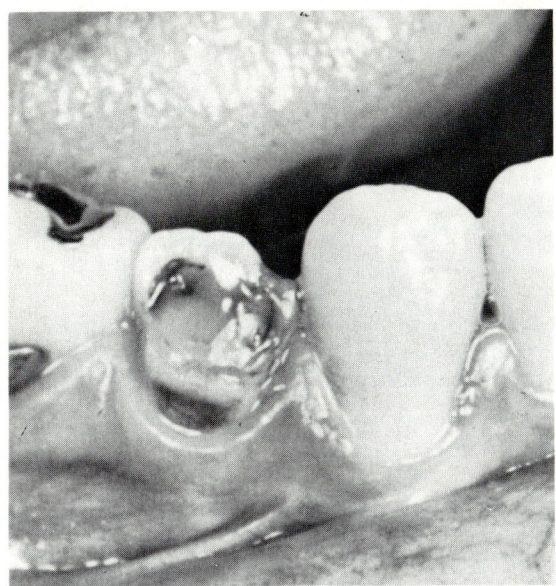

FIG. 1-17 A Turner tooth. Enamel formation of the lower first bicuspid has been impeded because of inflammation of its predecessor, the deciduous first molar.

TRAUMA FROM MECHANICAL OR PHYSICAL INJURIES

Because of the close relationship of the root apices of the primary teeth with the tooth buds of the permanent successors, trauma to the primary teeth is easily transmitted to the developing permanent teeth (Fig. 1-18). The trauma may cause no damage, or it may interfere with further tooth development, resulting in various malformations (Fig. 1-19). Such aberrations have been produced experimentally in the teeth of animals. They range from slight disturbances in enamel mineralization, through changes in morphology of crown or root, to sequestration of the entire tooth bud (Levy, 1968; Cutright, 1971; Suckling, 1980). Andreasen et al (1971), Andreasen and Ravn (1971), and vanGool (1973) studied the effects of traumatic injuries to the primary teeth on the permanent successors by clinical, radiographic, histologic, microradiographic and electron microscopic techniques. They found the following range of disturbances to occur:

- White or yellow-brown discoloration of enamel
- Discoloration of enamel and horizontal enamel hypoplasia
- Crown dilaceration
- Odontomalike malformation
- Root duplication
- Vestibular root angulation
- Lateral root angulation or dilaceration
- Partial or complete arrest of root formation
- Sequestration of entire tooth germ
- Ectopic, premature, or delayed eruption or impaction

The type of malformations that resulted from the injury depended on the severity of the injury and the stage of tooth formation at the time of the injury (Figs. 1-20, 1-21, and 1-22). Disturbances in morphology were usually accom-

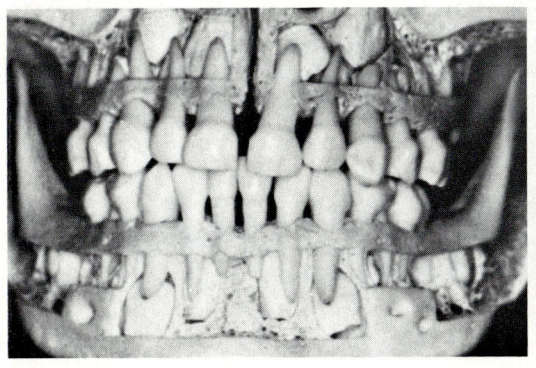
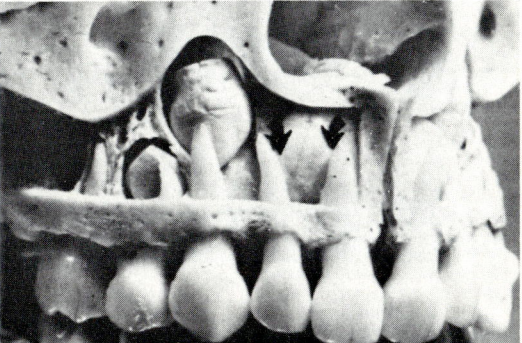

FIG. 1-18 Skull of a 5-year-old child, revealing the relationship between primary and permanent teeth. Note that both the central and the lateral primary incisor are close to the permanent central incisor (arrows). (Andreasen JO, Sundström B, Ravn JJ: The effect of traumatic injuries to primary teeth on their permanent successors. I. A study of 117 injured permanent teeth. Scand J Dent Res 79:219, 1971)

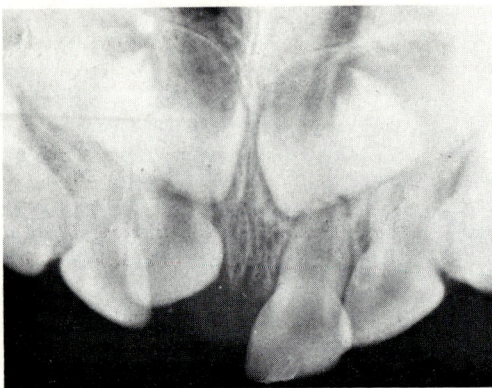 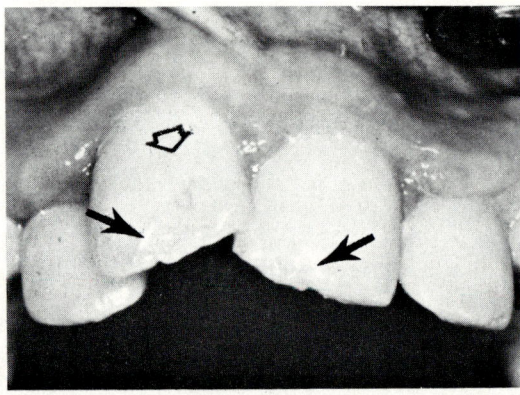

FIG. 1-19 Enamel hypoplasia affecting involved and noninvolved permanent incisors. *(Left)* Intrusion of a primary right central incisor at the age of 3 years. *(Right)* At follow-up 10 years later both central incisors demonstrated incisal defects in the enamel (solid arrows); furthermore, the right central incisor shows a yellow discoloration of the vestibular enamel (arrow). (Andreasen JO, Ravn JJ: The effect of traumatic injuries to primary teeth on their permanent successors. II. Scand J Dent Res 79:284, 1971)

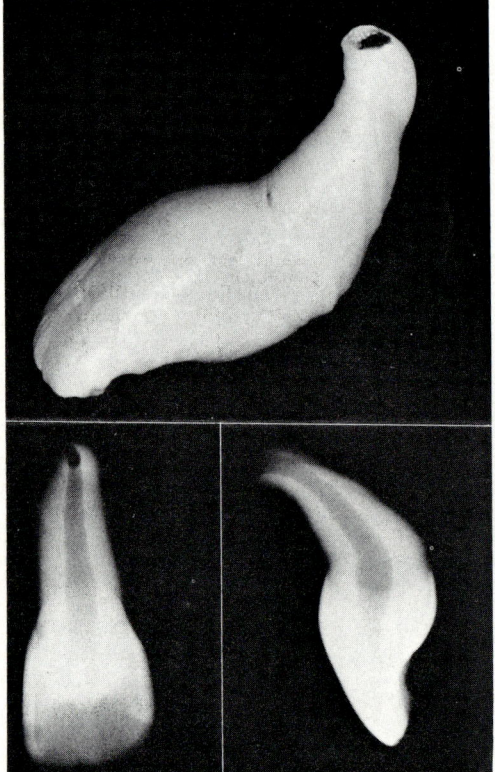 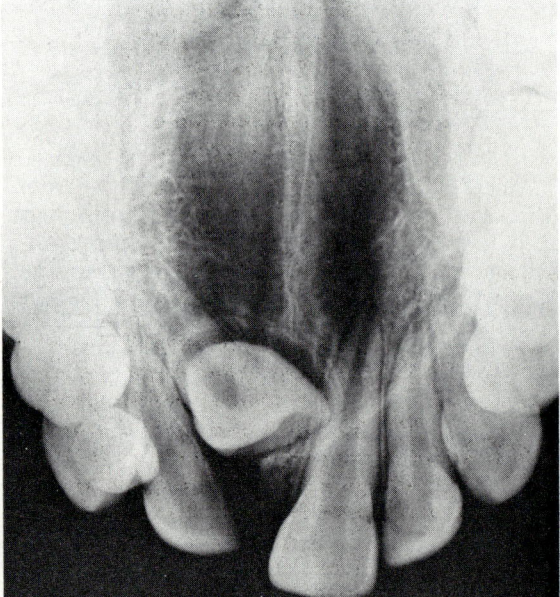

FIG. 1-20 *(Top, left)* Dilacerated incisor. *(Right)* Occlusal roentgenogram. *(Bottom, left and center)* Anteroposterior and lateral views; note that the dilaceration is not visible in the anteroposterior view. (van Gool AV: Injury to the permanent tooth germ after trauma to the deciduous predecessor. Oral Surg 35:2, 1973)

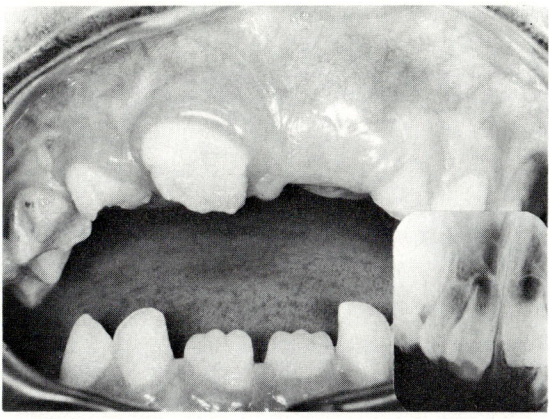

FIG. 1-21 Hypoplasia of the central and lateral maxillary right incisors. *(Inset)* Routine dental film. (van Gool AV: Injury to the permanent tooth germ after trauma to the deciduous predecessor. Oral Surg 35:2, 1973)

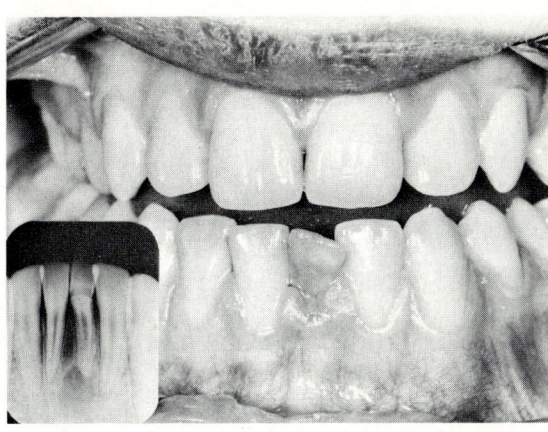

FIG. 1-22 Dilaceration of the lower left central incisor. *(Inset)* Roentgenogram shows apical granuloma. (van Gool AV: Injury to the permanent tooth germ after trauma to the deciduous predecessor. Oral Surg 35:2, 1973)

panied by disturbances in mineralization (Fig. 1-23).

White discolorations of enamel exhibited a decrease in mineral content and were not attributable to a specific type of injury. Yellow-brown discolorations resulted from the incorporation of hemoglobin breakdown products into the mineralizing enamel matrix.

Practically all of the other malformations resulted from intrusive luxation, with or without impaction, or exarticulation of the primary teeth. These injuries occurred from less than 1 year to 7 years of age.

NUTRITIONAL DISORDERS

Among other systemic disturbances affecting tooth development are nutritional disorders such as protein malnutrition, deficiency of essential fatty acids, and various vitamin and mineral deficiencies.

The developing tooth germs of both experimental animals and humans are vulnerable to severe nutritional deprivations, resulting in cellular and morphologic alterations. The eruption and gross appearance of the teeth may be affected (Enwonwu, 1973).

All nutritional deficiencies may potentially cause disturbances in amelogenesis because the ameloblasts are a sensitive group of cells.

Protein malnutrition of young rats resulted in alteration of the shape and anatomic relationships of the jaws, development of smaller teeth, delay in eruption, and overcrowding and malocclusion, as compared to controls (Tonge and McCance, 1965; DiOrio, 1969; Shaw, 1970). Calcium uptake and the rate of dentin apposition and mineralization is reduced (Nakamoto et al, 1979; Glick and Rowe, 1981).

Fat-free diets caused degenerative changes in the odontoblasts of rats; as a result, the dentin formed was poorly mineralized (Prout and Tring, 1973). In addition, the lipid composition of the enamel and dentin was found to be altered (Prout and Atkin, 1973).

Vitamin A deficiency, an infrequent clinical entity in the United States, interferes with the stage of histodifferentiation. Deficiency of vitamin A affects the metabolism of the cells of the inner dental epithelium (the ameloblasts) and interferes with their enzyme systems. Normally, the ameloblasts are columnar in shape and secrete substances necessary for the formation of the enamel. When vitamin A is missing, the ameloblasts do not differentiate into columnar cells and their secretory function is impaired. A morphogenetic relationship exists between cells, with one cell or a group of cells affecting other cells and stimulating their development. Dentin deposition is necessary for ameloblastic differentiation, and the presence

phorus, lack of vitamin D resulted in a reduction of tooth mass and absolute weight of the mineral deposited (Ferguson and Hartles, 1966). The pulp chambers usually remained large, presumably from disturbances in mineralization (Marks et al, 1965). By contrast, in exanthematous fevers, only the enamel becomes affected. Another difference between the effects of vitamin D deficiency and those of the exanthematous fevers is that vitamin D deficiencies are usually present over a longer period of time, and hence wider areas are affected (Fig. 1-24). In exanthematous fevers, high temperatures usually last for only 2 to 5 days. Interference with enamel formation would thus be short lived and cause only a small region of disturbance.

Vitamin E (tocopherol) deficiency has been shown to cause enamel hypoplasia, defects in tooth form and retardation of eruption rate of rats' teeth (Nelson and Chaudhry, 1966). In addition, the teeth were depigmented. Thus far, there have been no reported instances of human dental defects due to deficiency of vitamin E.

Trace Elements

Subcutaneous administration of a large number of anions and cations has been shown, by microradiography, to induce alterations in the mineralization of rat incisor dentin and enamel (Eisenmann and Yaeger, 1969). The effects of most of the ions were temporary. Some ions affected enamel predominantly; some exerted their effects primarily on dentin. A large number of ions affected both enamel and dentin. The effects either were nonspecific or were due to interferences with specific cells, matrixes, or enzymes.

Magnesium is needed for the synthesis of ground substance and collagen fibers and as a source of energy for the mineralization process. Magnesium is an essential mineral for enamel formation in rats, and its lack represents another factor to be considered in disturbances of enamel formation (Becks and Furuta, 1941; Trowbridge and Seltzer, 1967). So far, the effects of magnesium deficiency in human teeth have not been reported.

CHANGES DUE TO BIRTH

The rhythmic maturation and mineralization of the hard tissues of the teeth before birth depend on intrauterine metabolism. The materials

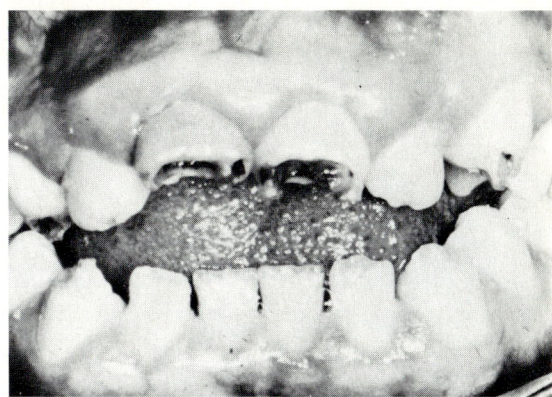

FIG. 1-24 The teeth of a child with rickets. Note severe hypoplasia of anterior teeth.

needed for mineralization of the developing teeth in utero are derived from the mother. Part of the calcium transferred to the fetus has been stored in the maternal skeletal system. During fetal tooth development, the calcium traverses the placental barrier and is deposited in the dentin (Goren and Gerstner, 1965).

At the time of birth, there is a sudden and complete change in the metabolic process, and tooth formation is affected. The rhythmic deposition of the dentin and the enamel is disturbed, and this disturbance is registered by an increased incremental spacing, the so-called neonatal line (Fig. 1-25). The neonatal line represents disturbances in physiologic activity at birth and during the succeeding 3 to 4 day period. Changes take place in the direction of the enamel prisms, and there is a wider zone of reduced crystal density at the postnatal side of the neonatal line (Whittaker and Richards, 1978). Schour (1941) demonstrated this incremental pattern by injecting alizarin red S into rats. Dentin that mineralized before or after the dye was administered was not stained. Similar interference in mineralization is demonstrable by parenteral administration of tetracycline into rats, dogs, and humans. The antibiotic is incorporated into the developing dentin and results in less mineralization and the appearance of striations. The pattern of tetracycline lines in dentin follows the growth increments of the tooth and provides an excellent indicator of the rate of growth.

Neonatal lines are found in the deciduous and permanent teeth that are being formed at the time of birth. Teeth undergoing mineralization

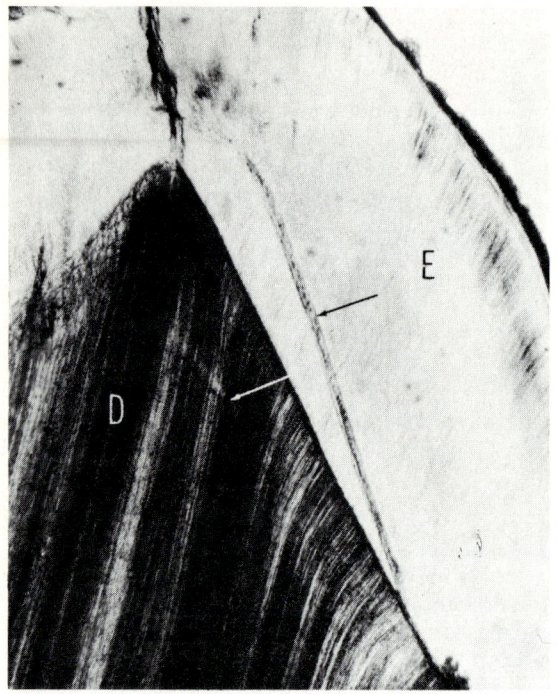

FIG. 1-25 Ground section of a deciduous molar; neonatal lines, indicated by arrows, in the enamel (E) and the dentin (D). (Courtesy of Dr. Maury Massler, Chicago)

and maturation at that time are affected. Inasmuch as every permanent first molar has already begun mineralization before birth (Christiansen and Kraus, 1965), the neonatal line is present in the first permanent molar and is not present in the deciduous teeth, which have already been formed in utero.

CONGENITAL DEFECTS

Human cell nuclei contain 23 pairs of chromosomes. The chromosomes contain linearly arranged desoxyribonucleic acid (DNA) molecules plus ribonucleic acid (RNA) and basic proteins. The primary hereditary material is generally believed to be DNA (Glass, 1962).

The DNA-coded information governs the synthesis of messenger RNA, which transmits the coded message to cytoplasmic ribosomes. Recent advances have made it possible to find and purify the stretch of DNA that encodes the RNA (Brown, 1973). The ribosomes translate the message into amino acid sequences. Each amino acid has one or more specific "code words" determined by a sequence of three nucleotides. Mutations that change the type of nucleotide or alter the nucleotide sequence result in alterations of protein structure (Crick, 1962).

The genetic code governs embryologic differentiation and development and the synthesis of structural proteins and enzymes. The enzymes regulate biochemical pathways.

Inherited defects of the teeth and oral structures may result from defects of single genes or variations affecting multiple genes arranged along the chromosomes, or numeric or morphologic alteration of the chromosomes themselves.

The end results of genetic variation may include effects on specific teeth or on the entire dentition. For a complete review and description of the manifestations of genetic diseases in the human dental pulp, the interested reader is referred to Witkop, 1973.

Down's Syndrome

Down's syndrome is a genetic disorder caused by an extra copy of chromosome 21, a small acrocentric chromosome, or a specific segment of it. A number of physical and mental characteristics are associated with this disorder. Included are moderate growth retardation and some signs of premature aging (Van Keuren et al, 1982).

Tooth size is affected by Down's syndrome. Townsend (1983) found that deciduous teeth in affected patients tend to be larger in certain dimensions. Permanent teeth, however, were found to be significantly smaller. The incidence of taurodontism is increased (Jaspers, 1981).

Anodontia and Supernumerary Teeth

If there is a disturbance in initiation, the clinical condition of anodontia, or absence of teeth, occurs (Fig. 1-26). This condition may be total or partial. Total anodontia is relatively uncommon (Brothwell et al, 1963). The most common form of partial anodontia is congenital absence of the mandibular and maxillary second premolars, laterals, and third molars (Grahnen, 1956; Hunstadbraten, 1973). Garn et al (1963) have pointed out that polymorphism in the number of human teeth is not an isolated phenomenon but, instead, is fundamentally related to the size, the development, and the timing of mineralization of the dentition as a whole. In patients with Down's syndrome (mongolism) the incidence of congenital anodontia is increased.

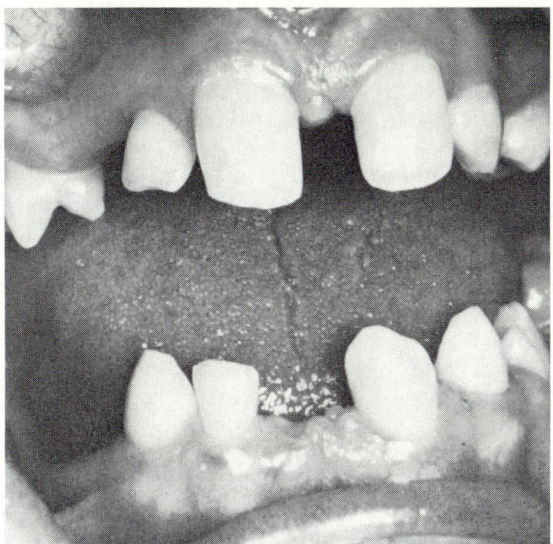

FIG. 1-26 Partial anodontia.

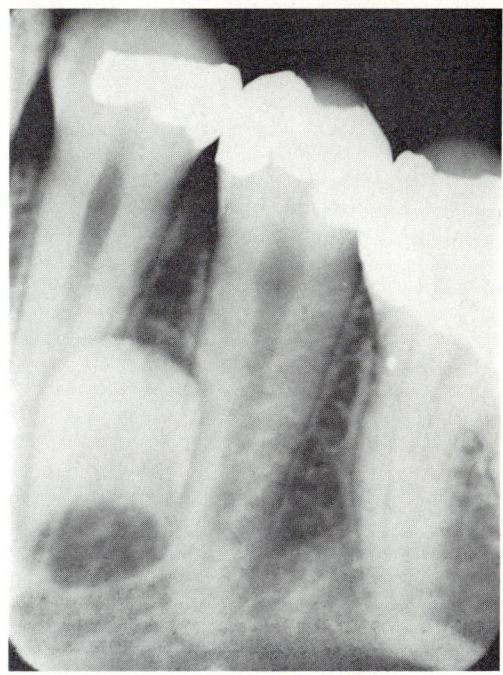

FIG. 1-27 The development of a supernumerary lower bicuspid.

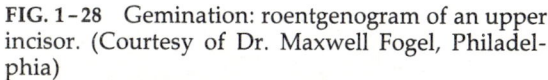

FIG. 1-28 Gemination: roentgenogram of an upper incisor. (Courtesy of Dr. Maxwell Fogel, Philadelphia)

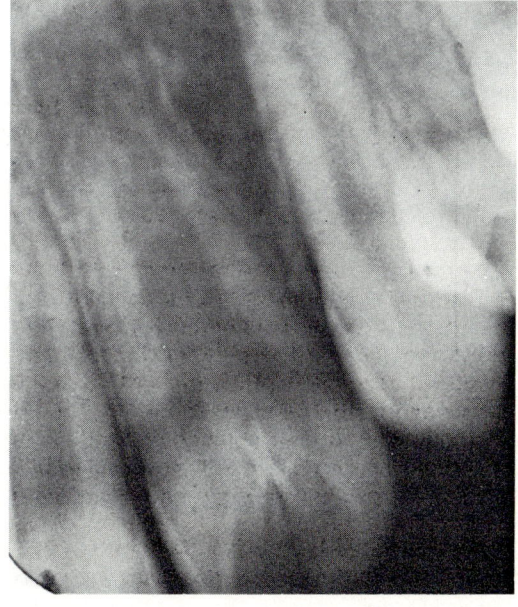

According to Graber (1978), congenital absence of teeth is inherited. It is passed on to each generation by an autosomal dominant pattern with incomplete penetrance and variable expressivity. Graber has postulated that, in many cases, this anomaly may be a microform of systemic ectodermal dysplasia.

If an excessive amount of stimulation occurs during initiation and proliferation, supernumerary teeth are formed (Fig. 1-27). A supernumerary tooth may develop from the dental lamina as a completely separate entity, or it may result from a dichotomy of an existing tooth germ (Berkovitz and Thompson, 1973).

The presence of supernumerary teeth is associated in high incidence (50%) with incomplete cleft lip, with or without accompanying anomalies such as alveolar and palatal clefts. Patients with complete cleft lips show an extremely low incidence of supernumerary teeth (Nagai et al, 1965).

Occasionally, a tooth germ divides during the period of the development of the teeth, resulting in the formation of a double crown with a single root. This condition is called gemination (Fig. 1-28).

Should the crowns of two separate tooth buds fuse during development, the result is a bifid crown with two root canals in one root. Such an anomaly is called fusion.

The roots of two separate teeth may fuse after

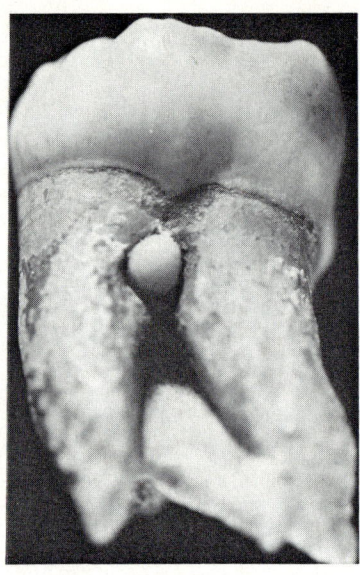

FIG. 1-29 Enamel pearl. (Cavanha AO: Enamel pearls. Oral Surg 19:373, 1965)

the development of the crowns has been completed. Such a condition, a rarely encountered anomaly, is called concrescence.

Hertwig's root sheath normally does not produce enamel. Occasionally, however, small enamel droplets, called enamel pearls, are formed on the surfaces of or between the roots (Cavanha, 1965; Fig. 1–29).

Matrix formation and maturation of teeth may be affected by various congenital defects.

Hereditary Enamel Hypoplasia and Hypocalcification

According to Weinmann et al (1945), hereditary enamel hypoplasia is an enamel defect characterized by a deficiency in quantity of enamel; hereditary enamel hyocalcification is characterized by a deficiency in mineralization of a normal quantity of enamel.

Amelogenesis Imperfecta. It has been found that different mutations are responsible for producing similar-appearing traits. Thus, classifications of amelogenesis imperfecta have been made that are based on the mode of inheritance as well as morphologic, radiologic and histologic features (Rushton, 1965; Winter et al, 1969; Witkop, 1972).

In the hypoplastic type, the disease is inherited as a sex-linked dominant trait. In men, the enamel is one eighth to one fourth the normal thickness. In women, the defect may be different and less severe. Vertical bands of hypoplastic enamel may alternate with vertical bands of enamel approaching normal thickness (Witkop, 1964).

The affected tooth looks discolored because of the lack of enamel. The color of a tooth depends on the presence of (1) the enamel, which is blue or white; (2) the dentin, which is yellow; and (3) the pulp, which is pink. Changing the characteristics or the volume of any one of these tooth components causes changes in tooth color.

In amelogenesis imperfecta, the tooth looks darker as well as dirty and stained, not only because the enamel is missing but also because the uncovered dentin is stained more readily by foodstuffs.

Scanning electron micrographs of the hypoplastic areas reveal numerous pits and craters intermixed with smoother, less affected surfaces (Sauk et al, 1972b). The defects primarily involve mineralization of the enamel prism sheaths (Sauk et al, 1972a; Kerebel and Daclusi, 1976). On occasion, the hypoplastic enamel of some teeth that undergo rapid attrition may be found in conjunction with pulp mineralizations, characteristics similar to those of enamel and dentin dysplasia (Gertzman et al, 1979).

Another type of amelogenesis imperfecta, termed hypomaturation, has been described by Witkop and Rao (1971) and by McLarty et al (1973). This condition occurs both as an autosomal recessively inherited trait and as an X-linked disorder. In this type, enamel is formed of normal thickness, but it is harder than normal enamel. It has a mottled opaque white to yellow-brown or red-brown color and it tends to chip away from the underlying dentin (Fig. 1–30). The enamel defects are found in the rod structure and in the enamel rod sheaths. Scanning electron micrographs show a fibrous pattern of structureless enamel rods and interprismatic voids (Witkop et al, 1973).

A rarer type of amelogenesis imperfecta, hypomaturation type, has been described by Witkop (1965) as *snow-capped teeth*. Clinically, there is hypomaturation confined to the incisal and occlusal thirds of the crowns. Several such cases have been described by Escobar et al (1981). Their examinations of the teeth by scanning electron microscopy revealed that, after acid etching, the enamel prisms were identical to those of normal teeth, suggesting that the

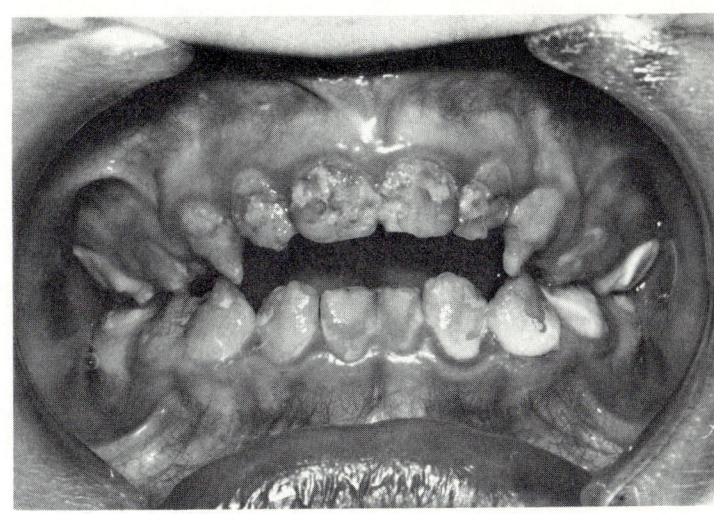

FIG. 1-30 Deciduous dentition has mottled yellow-brown enamel, similar to that seen in the permanent teeth of this patient's sister. Deciduous teeth also show evidence of resorption prior to eruption: note especially cuspids. White material, most noticeable on the patient's left, is heavy calculus. Note the anterior open-bite; this is frequently seen in various types of amelogenesis imperfecta. No carious lesions are present. (Witkop CJ, Jr, Kuhlmann W, Sauk J: Autosomal recessive pigmented hypomaturation amelogenesis imperfecta. Oral Surg 36:367, 1973)

structural defect was confined to the dissolved outer prismless enamel layer.

Hypoplasia of the enamel and other morphologic tooth irregularities can be produced by sickle-cell anemia (Soni, 1966); it may be related to a variety of congenital brain defects such as cerebral palsy, as well as to epilepsy, ocular fibroplasia, nephrosis, and Down's syndrome (trisomy G, mongolism; Cohen et al, 1970).

Dentinogenesis Imperfecta (Hereditary Opalescent Dentin)

A common congenital defect is dentinogenesis imperfecta (hereditary opalescent dentin), a defect in dentin formation.

Opalescent dentin may occur in conjunction with or without osteogenesis imperfecta. It has been suggested that, in order to distinguish between the two, the term dentinogenesis imperfecta be used for the variety accompanying osteogenesis imperfecta, and opalescent dentin be used only when the bones are not involved (Witkop, 1973; Shields et al, 1973; Giasanti and Budnick, 1975). According to Witkop (1957) and Bixler et al (1969), opalescent dentin is transmitted as an autosomal dominant trait. It occurs in both sexes, but it is found more frequently in the female. Eruption is delayed, and, when the affected teeth erupt, they are slightly bluish, changing gradually to purplish-opalescent or amber. Only a small amount of dentin is formed initially, and most of the tooth is made up of pulp tissue (Fig. 1-31). In the absence of dentin, the underlying yellow is missing. The

FIG. 1-31 Dentinogenesis imperfecta. (A) and (B) Roentgenograms reveal a small quantity of dentin formed and delayed eruption of teeth ((A) 11½ years; (B) 8 years). (C) Later stage, showing filling-in of pulp canals with dentin. (Courtesy of Dr. Morris Kelner, Philadelphia)

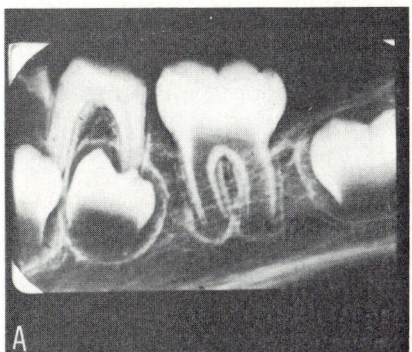
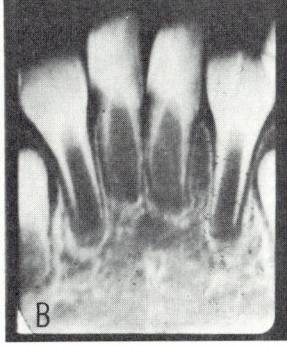
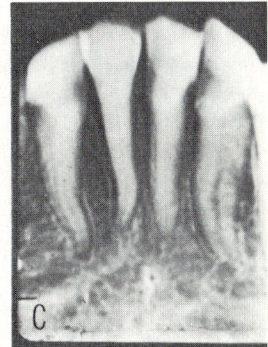

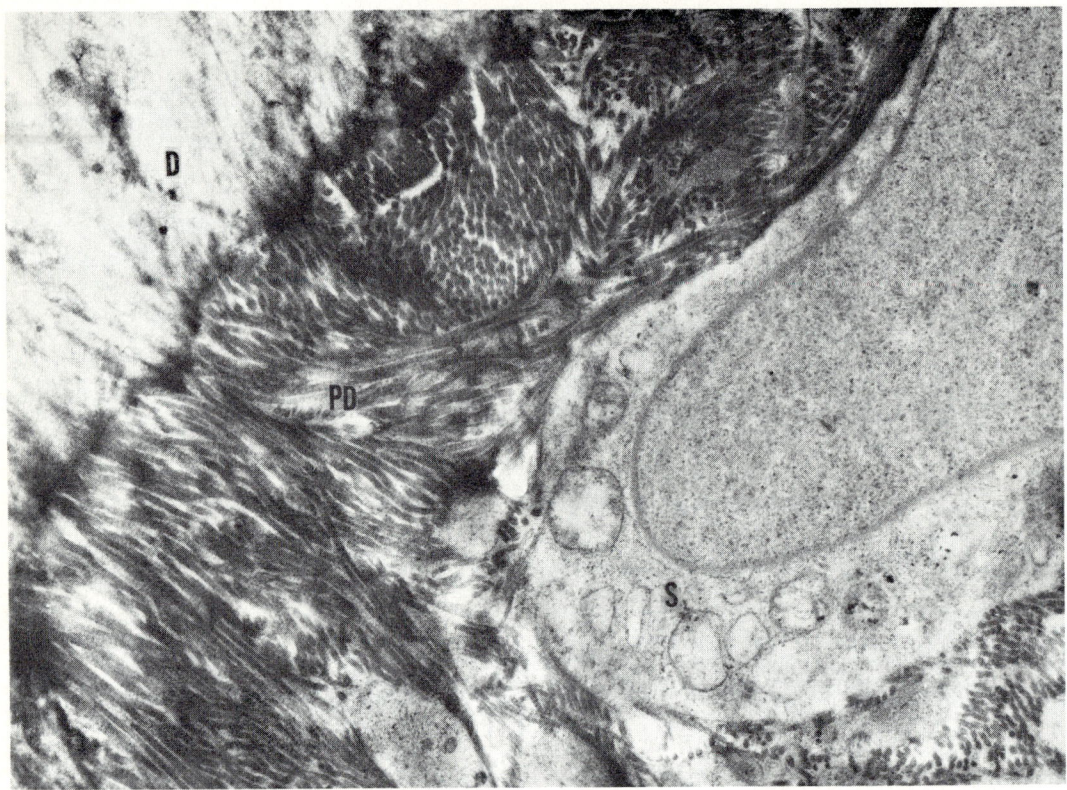

FIG. 1-32 Junction between scleroblasts and irregular dentin in a tooth from human dentinogenesis imperfecta, showing bundles of coarse collagen fibrils forming a predentinlike layer (PD) and irregular dentin (D). Note oval scleroblasts (S) with sparse cytoplasm and few organelles. Odontoblast processes are not present. Phosphotungstic acid and lead citrate. ×12,000. (Herold RC: Fine structure of tooth dentine in human dentinogenesis imperfecta. Arch Oral Biol 17:1009, 1972)

color is also affected because there is more pulp tissue that contains many blood vessels. Frequently, the vessels rupture and there are slight hemorrhages. The roots appear inordinately short. The odontoblasts do not differentiate properly and, hence, are smaller and reduced in number when seen in histologic sections. Function of the odontoblasts is affected, and, in time, they degenerate and other pulp cells take over their function. They rapidly elaborate an amorphous, nontubular type of dentin, which tends to occlude the entire pulp chamber and root canal (Fig. 1-32). In some regions, irregular, wide tubules are found that are ready pathways for the passage of microorganisms.

In dentinogenesis imperfecta, less mineralization occurs; hence, the teeth are much softer. According to Kerebel et al (1981), the mineral phase of the dentin consists of a carbonated apatite with crystallites of normal size, but they are less numerous than in normal dentin. There are losses of calcium, phosphorus, and magnesium and a higher calcium/phosphate ratio and water content.

There is a tendency for the enamel, which is normal, to chip off such teeth, because the dentinoenamel junction, normally a scalloped region physically holding the enamel and the dentin together, is a straight line. Crowns of the teeth are more subject to fracture. Generally, however, caries susceptibility is low.

Dentin changes, strikingly similar to those seen in dentinogenesis imperfecta, have been reported to occur in the teeth of patients afflicted with Cooley's anemia (Soni et al, 1966). Such changes involved the formation of atypical, poorly mineralized, dentin resembling osteodentin and the presence of unusual inclusion bodies in the dentinal tubules. Cementum hyperplasia also occurred.

A rare case of dentinogenesis imperfecta with dens invaginatus has been reported by Kerebel et al (1983).

Dentinal Dysplasia

Dentin dysplasia is a rare autosomal dominant disorder. Two types of dentin dysplasia, I and II, have been reported by Witkop (1975), who prefers the term radicular dentin dysplasia for Type I and coronal dentin dysplasia for Type II.

The defects of dentinal dysplasia (Type I) are present in all the teeth of both the deciduous and the permanent dentitions. The crowns of the teeth are normally shaped, but the roots are usually short, blunted, or absent. The color of the teeth may be normal, or, in some patients, may have a brown or blue tinge with an opalescent sheen. The teeth are usually crowded in the arch. In the deciduous dentition, total pulpal obliteration by amorphous (dysplastic) dentin or pulp stones usually results (Melnick et al, 1980). In the permanent teeth, a pulpal remnant, demilune in appearance, may remain. Root canals become obliterated by dentin of peculiar cascade pattern (Sauk et al, 1972). Concomitantly, periapical radiolucencies develop, despite the absence of dental caries (Wesley et al, 1976; Tidwell and Cunningham, 1979; Petrone and Noble, 1981).

A rare, anomalous type of dentinal dysplasia (Type II) has been reported by Shields et al (1973) and by Melnick et al (1977). The pulp chambers of the deciduous teeth became obliterated, but in the permanent teeth dentinal hypertrophy produced a thistle-tube pulp configuration together with pulp stones. The anterior maxillary teeth were the most severely affected. The permanent teeth may or may not be discolored (Fig. 1-33).

Giasanti and Allen (1974) reported on the findings in another family with dentinal dysplasia in which the deciduous teeth resembled those found in hereditary opalescent dentin or dentinogenesis imperfecta. The teeth of the permanent dentition resembled those described for pulpal dysplasia.

A new syndrome, dentin dysplasia with sclerotic bone and skeletal anomalies, has been reported by Morris and Augsburger (1977). They found that abnormalities of Hertwig's root teeth were associated with this syndrome.

Dens Invaginatus (Dens in Dente). Invagination of the mineralized portion of the tooth can occur within both the crown and the root of the tooth, although crown invaginations are much more common (Fig. 1-34). In the latter, there is a deep invagination of the lingual pit of the tooth, resulting in an enamel-lined cavity inside the tooth. The invagination may remain confined within the root as a blind sac, or it may communicate with the pulp or penetrate laterally or apically to the periodontal ligament. The orifice of the cavity is on the lingual surface. Most commonly, the upper lateral incisor is afflicted, although on rare occasions other teeth may be involved. The affected tooth may appear normal on the labial surface, but usually it is wide, bulky, and deformed (barrel shaped). There is strong evidence that the condition is genetically determined.

The pulps of such teeth frequently undergo inflammatory and degenerative changes with eventual pulp necrosis.

Other Hypoplasias and Morphologic Tooth Irregularities

Taurodontism is the term used to describe a variation in the form of multirooted teeth in which the body of the tooth is enlarged and the roots are reduced in size. Such teeth have large pulp chambers with the furcation areas displaced apically; there is no constriction at the level of the cementoenamel junction. Both deciduous and permanent molars are affected (Fig. 1-35). The condition may be inherited but the genetics are confusing; the condition may be associated with other systemic or structural abnormalities (Goldstein and Gottlieb, 1973; Sauk and Delaney, 1973), such as amelogenesis imperfecta (Congleton and Burkes, 1979).

Ectodermal dysplasia includes an extensive number of conditions in which there are disturbances in both formation and function of ectodermally derived structures. Various groups of ectodermal dysplasias have been described by Freire-Maia (1971). These groups include those with hair defects, nail defects, abnormal dentitions, and altered sweating. At least two of these dysplasias are included in most types of ectodermal dysplasia. According to Witkop et al (1975), there is a heterogeneous group in which the presenting sign is usually hypodontia. Another type of hypodontia, which includes congenital nail dysplasia, has been reported by Hudson and Witkop (1975).

The tricho-dento-osseous syndrome is an autosomal dominant disorder in which the hair and teeth are abnormal. The dental anomalies consist of amelogenesis imperfecta, taurodontism,

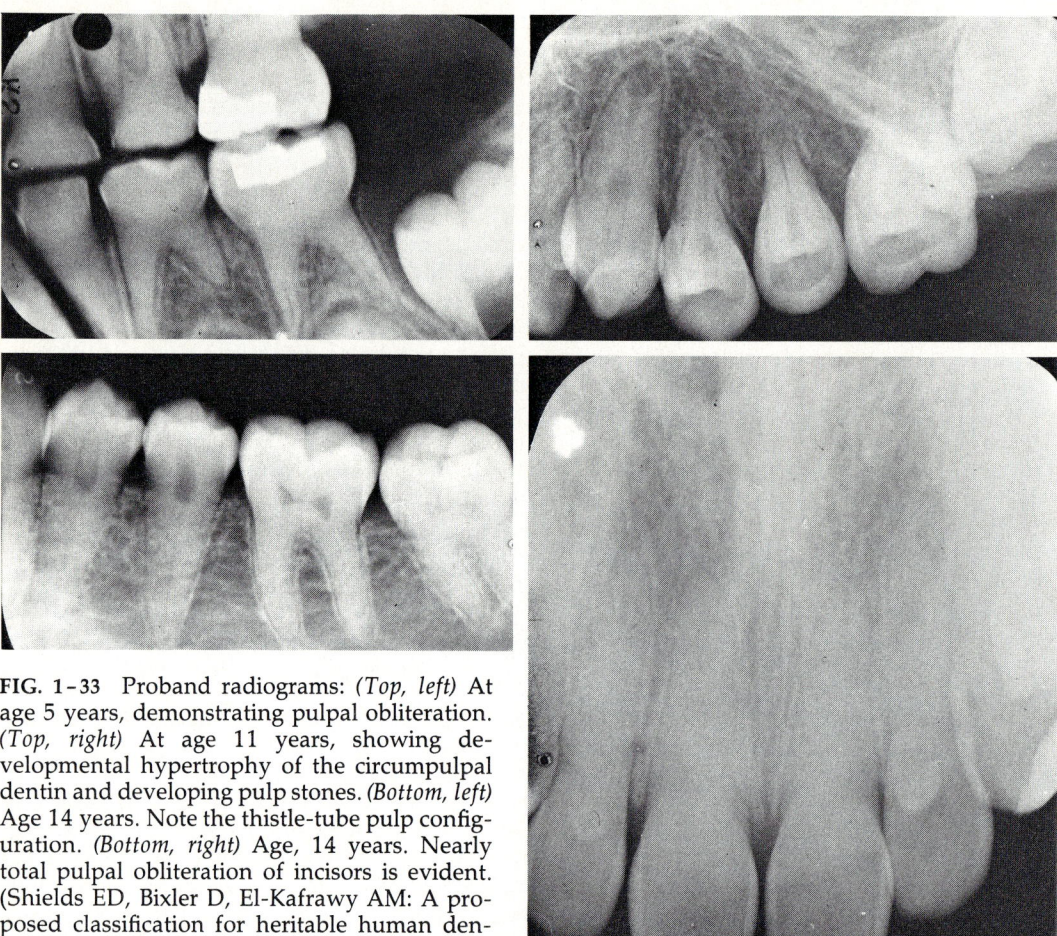

FIG. 1-33 Proband radiograms: *(Top, left)* At age 5 years, demonstrating pulpal obliteration. *(Top, right)* At age 11 years, showing developmental hypertrophy of the circumpulpal dentin and developing pulp stones. *(Bottom, left)* Age 14 years. Note the thistle-tube pulp configuration. *(Bottom, right)* Age, 14 years. Nearly total pulpal obliteration of incisors is evident. (Shields ED, Bixler D, El-Kafrawy AM: A proposed classification for heritable human dentine defects with a description of a new entity. Arch Oral Biol 18:543, 1973)

periapical inflammations, delayed eruption, and impacted teeth (Gulmen et al, 1976). Jorgenson and Warson (1973) have postulated that this syndrome may be caused by the product of a mutant gene acting on the dental epithelia.

Pulpal dysplasia is a dominantly inherited trait that bridges the gap between those conditions exhibiting abnormally enlarged pulp chambers and those with mineralization in the pulp space. The color of the teeth is normal. The pulp chambers are gradually reduced and eventually obliterated by pulp stones (Witkop, 1973).

Regional odontodysplasia is a bizarre developmental anomaly in tooth formation. Although not hereditary, it may represent a somatic mutation affecting adjacent teeth in a segment of the dental arches. Local vascular defects, such as facial nevi, may be involved in the etiology (Walton et al, 1978). The follicles of the developing teeth are hyperplastic and their connective tissues contain mineralized cementum (Sapp and Gardner, 1973). Both deciduous and permanent teeth can be affected, most frequently the maxillary anteriors (Sadeghi and Ashrafi, 1981). The afflicted teeth appear smaller than normal, with short roots. Pulp chambers and root canals are often markedly enlarged. The pulps become mineralized and may eventually become necrotic; periapical pathosis may develop. Histologically, the enamel is thinner than normal (Lustmann and

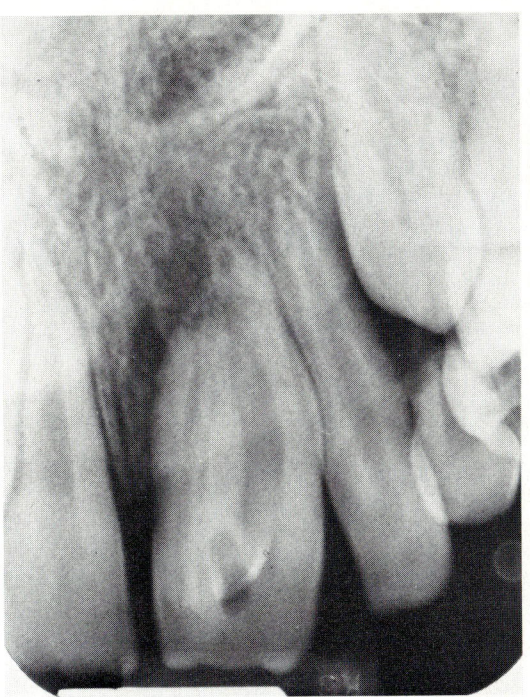
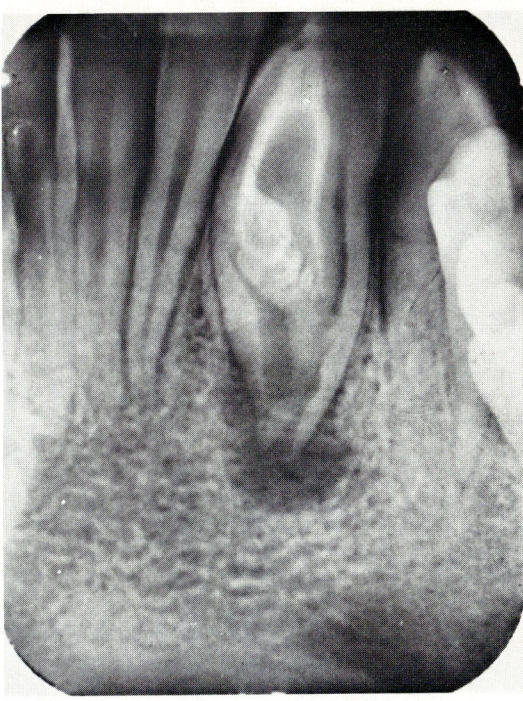

FIG. 1-34 Two examples of dens invaginatus. (*Left,* courtesy of Dr. Jack Ginsberg, Cinnaminson, N.J.; *Right,* courtesy of Dr. George Biron, Norristown, Pa.)

Ulmansky, 1976) and hypoplastic, owing to a decrease in the number of ameloblasts (Kerebel and Kerebel, 1981, 1982). The dentin is amorphous (Gardner and Sapp, 1977).

Radiographs of such teeth have a ghostlike quality (Fig. 1-36) because of the marked decrease in radiodensity (Hintz and Peters, 1972; Gardner and Sapp, 1973; Pinkham and Burkes, 1973).

Hypophosphatasia is a rare familial disorder characterized by a deficiency of the enzyme alkaline phosphatase. According to Bruckner et al (1962), the disease usually appears during the first few years of life and is usually fatal. Generally, those patients who survive the first year have a good prognosis but exhibit residual skeletal deformities. Dentally, there is premature loss of deciduous incisors, owing to aplasia of the cementum. Houpt et al (1970) and Beumer et al (1973) studied histologically the exfoliated or extracted deciduous teeth from children afflicted with hypophosphatasia. In addition to the sparsity of cementum, there was extensive, unrepaired external root resorption, increased size of pulp chambers, reduction in the number of odontoblasts, abnormally wide predentin zones, and abundance of interglobular dentin (Figs. 1-37 and 1-38). All of these observations suggested impaired mineralization.

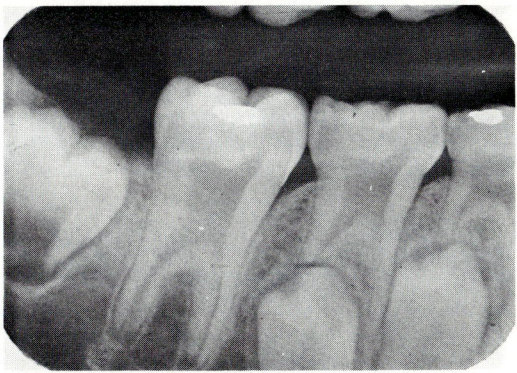

FIG. 1-35 Root form classification: Mesotaurodont. (Goldstein E, Gottlieb MA: Taurodontism: Familial tendencies demonstrated in eleven of fourteen case reports. Oral Surg 36:131, 1973)

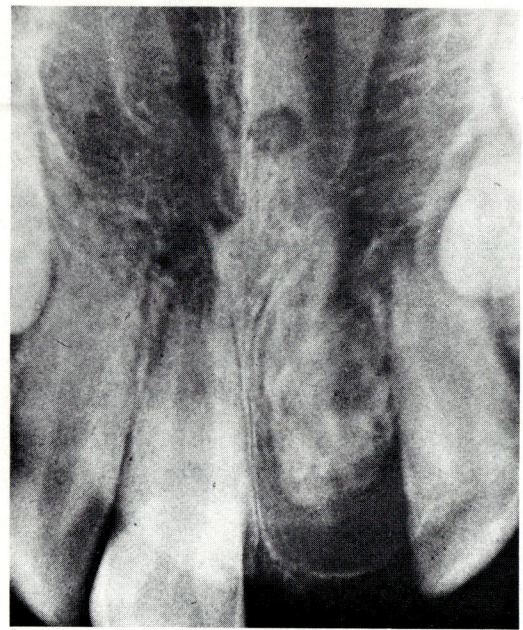

FIG. 1-36 Regional odontodysplasia. Roentgenogram of the affected central incisor area. (Pinkham JR, Burkes EJ: Odontodysplasia. Oral Surg 36:841, 1973)

Hereditary (familial) hypophosphatemia (vitamin D–resistant rickets) is a systemic disease of inborn error of metabolism, secondary to defective renal-tubular reabsorption of phosphate. The disease is sex-linked with hypophosphatemia as the essential trait, affecting both males and females. Both sexes transmit the abnormal trait to their offspring. Females, affected with the X-linked dominant trait, transmit the disease to one half of their sons and to one half of their daughters. On the other hand, the affected male transmits the disease to all the daughters but not to the sons. Characteristically, the rickets is refractory to the usual therapeutic doses of vitamin D. In addition to a poorly mineralized skeleton, dental defects such as hypoplastic enamel and numerous areas of interglobular dentin are manifest (Tracy et al, 1971; Nikiforuk and Fraser, 1979; Fig. 1-39). These defects may be the first manifestations of the disease. In young patients, the pulp chambers tend to be large, with prominent pulp horns extending to the dentinoenamel junction (Fig. 1-39). With vitamin D therapy, the pulp chambers and root canals become obliterated by deposition of dentin. The pulps of the affected teeth tend to become necrotic following the loss of enamel over the pulp horns. Periapical abscesses may then develop (Archard and Witkop, 1966; Rakocz et al, 1982; Fig. 1-39).

Congenital (erythropoietic) porphyria is a rare entity in which porphyrins are deposited in both the enamel and the dentin of deciduous and permanent teeth. Periodic exacerbations of the disease result in the localization of uroporphyrin in discrete bands, especially in the dentin, as determined by fluorescent microscopy (Trodahl et al, 1972). The amount varies with the severity and the duration of the disease.

EFFECTS OF DRUGS

Antibiotics

The teeth of animals and humans have been shown to incorporate tetracyclines that were administered to the young animal or the growing child during development. Such antibiotic administration has been used to treat a variety of childhood illnesses, including cystic fibrosis (Primosch, 1980).

The tetracycline molecule has an affinity for heavy metal ions; it chelates with calcium. Thus, tetracycline is incorporated into any tissue that

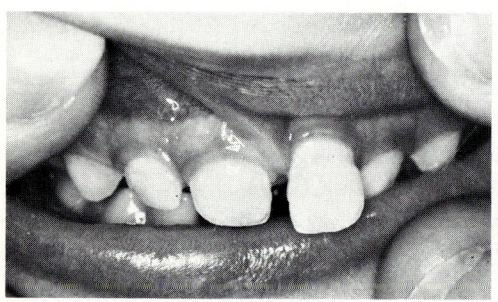
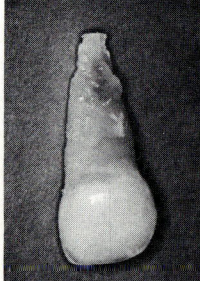

FIG. 1-37 *(Left)* Hypophosphatasia in a child 3½ years old. The left central incisor appears to be extruding, and it exfoliated spontaneously 1 month later. Note the absence of inflammatory periodontal disease. *(Right)* Note the absence of periapical root resorption in the exfoliated left central incisor. (Beumer J, Trowbridge HO, Silverman S, Eisenberg E: Childhood hypophosphatasia and the premature loss of teeth. Oral Surg 35:631, 1973)

is mineralizing when the drug is given. Such incorporation occurs regardless of whether the drug is administered in diverse amounts, in a single dose, or in divided doses over several days (Bevelander and Nakahara, 1966). Furthermore, tooth disorders may be induced by a variety of tetracycline analogues (Fig. 1–40; McIntosh and Storey, 1970; Moffitt et al, 1974).

Tetracycline administration to young pigs and goats from birth to 3 to 10 weeks has not been found to disturb the structure or mineralization of dentin (Kawasaki and Fearnhead, 1975).

Oral doses of demethylchlortetracycline, administered to monkeys for 7 days, had no effect on dentin apposition, although bone growth was inhibited (Yen and Shaw, 1975). However, ultrastructural changes of the odontoblasts and ameloblasts in experimental animals are dose dependent (Kruger, 1975).

The teeth of the human fetus are susceptible

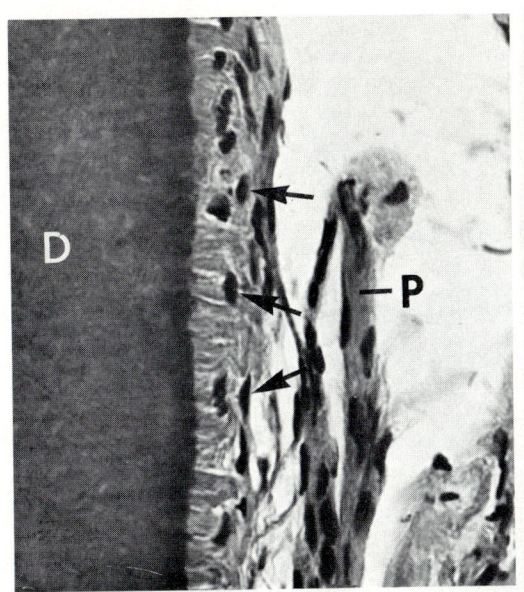
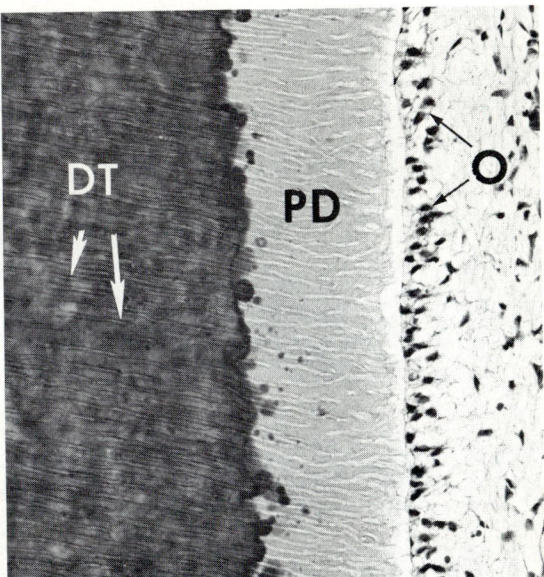
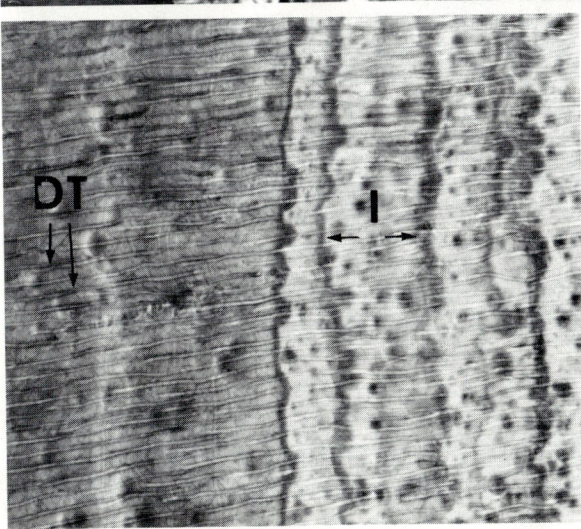

FIG. 1–38 *(Top, left)* Deciduous incisor, showing an attempt at cementogenesis. Remnants of the periodontal ligament (P) can be seen along the root surface. Cells resembling cementoblasts (arrows) are embedded in a mesh of collagen fibers. D, Dentin. Masson's trichrome stain. ×625. *(Top, right)* Deciduous incisor, demonstrating impaired calcification of dentin. Note the increased width of the predentin (PD). The dentinal tubules (DT) are prominent, and the odontoblasts (O) are reduced in number and appear atrophic. Hematoxylin and eosin. ×250. *(Bottom)* Deciduous incisor, demonstrating incomplete calcification of dentin. Note the prominent dentinal tubules (DT) and pronounced incremental lines (I). Hematoxylin and eosin. ×250. (Beumer J, Trowbridge HO, Silverman S, Eisenberg E: Childhood hypophosphatasia and the premature loss of teeth. Oral Surg 35:631, 1973)

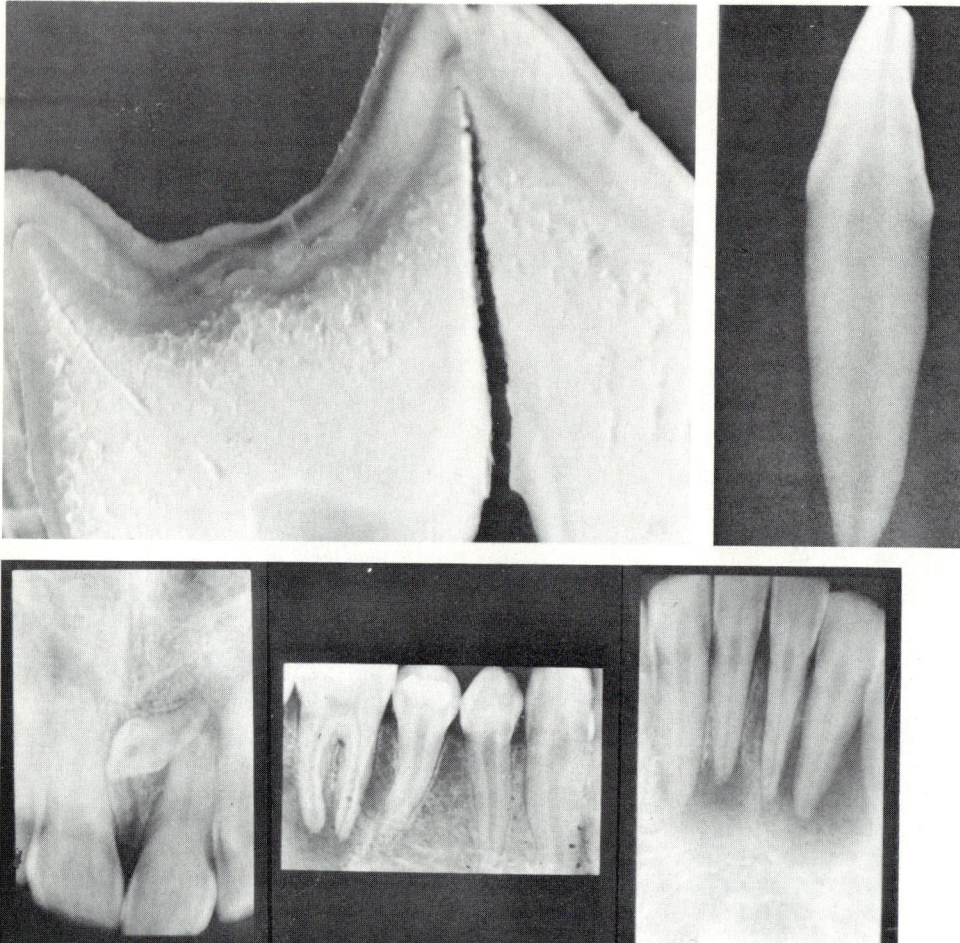

FIG. 1-39 *(Top, left)* Ground section of unerupted premolar shows large pulp horn extending to the dentinoenamel junction. Enamel overlying this tract is hypoplastic. Dentin is composed of calcospherites of interglobular mineralization (Witkop CJ: Manifestations of genetic diseases in the human pulp. In Siskin M (ed): The Biology of the Human Dental Pulp. St. Louis, CV Mosby, 1973). *(Top, right)* Radiograph of central incisor, taken from proximal side. Pulp is exposed. *(Bottom)* Three of five cases of hypophosphatemic vitamin D–resistant rickets from a single family with teeth manifesting periapical lesions in molars. Radiographs disclose pulp spaces extending to the dentinoenamel region in all teeth, including supernumerary *(left)*. This extension is a characteristic of hereditary hypophosphatemia. Periapical lesions in lower anteriors *(right)* are the first to be observed, most likely owing to the rapidly attrited incisal surfaces. (Courtesy of Dr. Shelly Lamm, Ithaca, N.Y.)

to the injurious effects of the antibiotic as early as the 28th week of gestation. The permanent teeth can become pigmented and hypoplastic if the tetracycline is administered to children between the ages of 2 months and 2 years. Both enamel matrix formation and mineralization may be affected (Fig. 1–41; Baker, 1972).

Both macroscopic and microscopic changes occur, mainly in the dentin of deciduous and, rarely, that of permanent teeth. Macroscopically, there is intense yellow staining of the dentin caused by incorporation and retention of the antibiotic. Microscopically, the dentin exhibits a yellow coloration and a golden-yellow fluorescence in bands corresponding to the dose and the administration pattern. The enamel does not appear to be stained by the tetracyclines, although small amounts are incorporated, but mineralization is inhibited and hypoplasia may result (Bennett and Law, 1965; Baker, 1972; Fig. 1–42).

The electron microscopic studies of tetracycline-induced enamel and dentin defects in rat incisors by Nylen et al (1972) and Kruger (1975) indicate that the tetracyclines achieve their principal effects on enamel formation by injuring the presecretory ameloblasts and odontoblasts. The injured cells cause hypoplastic lesions, which lead in turn to disturbances in mineralization.

Other antibiotics, such as lincomycin, have been reported to have no adverse effects on the developing dentition of the rat (Turner, 1970).

Colchicine, Vinblastine, and Vincristine

Microtubules are involved in the secretion of collagen by hard tissue forming and other cells. They are found in ameloblasts and odontoblasts as well as other eukaryotic cells and are thus involved in enamel and dentin matrix formation (Akita et al, 1983). Colchicine, vinblastine, and vincristine disrupt microtubule assembly by binding to tubulin, resulting in odontoblastic and fibroblastic damage and inhibition of dentinogenesis (Kudo, 1975; Stene and Koppang, 1980; Senzaki, 1980; Mataki, 1981). Interferences with the eruption rates of rat mandibular incisors have also been reported to be a consequence of injections of colchicine and vinblastine (Chiba et al, 1980).

Diphenylhydantoin

Epileptics receiving long-term diphenylhydantoin (DPH) may develop osteomalacia or rickets due to an accelerated vitamin D metabolism (Reynolds, 1975). Robinson et al (1978) found that long-term administration of DPH to rats reduced the size of the incisors and most of the molars. They suggested that in addition to the anticonvulsant-induced osteomalacia, DPH may induce a state of "pseudohypoparathyroidism" by inhibiting the action of parathyroid hormone on bones and teeth.

ENDOCRINE HORMONES

Endocrine hormones play an important role in the development of the teeth, particularly prior to eruption. The roots of the teeth, especially,

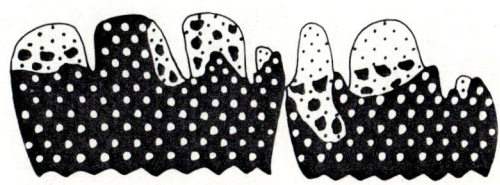
Tetracycline

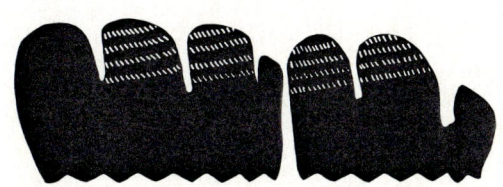
Chlortetracycline

FIG. 1-40 Effect on molar development of tetracycline hydrochloride and chlortetracycline at a daily dosage of 100 mg/kg administered intraperitoneally from day 4 to day 23 after birth. (McIntosh HA, Storey E: Tetracycline-induced tooth changes. 4. Discoloration and hypoplasia induced by tetracycline analogues. Med J Aust 1:114, 1970)

are affected. Once a tooth is completely formed, endocrines do not affect it.

Thyroid Hormones. The hormones elaborated by the thyroid gland affect the eruption of the teeth and their structure. Eruption time, dentin, and root development are retarded in hypothyroidism in rats following thyroidectomy (Ziskin et al, 1940).

Administration of low dosages of the goitrogen propylthiouracil had no effect on dentinogenesis of the molar teeth of immature male albino rats (Johannessen, 1966).

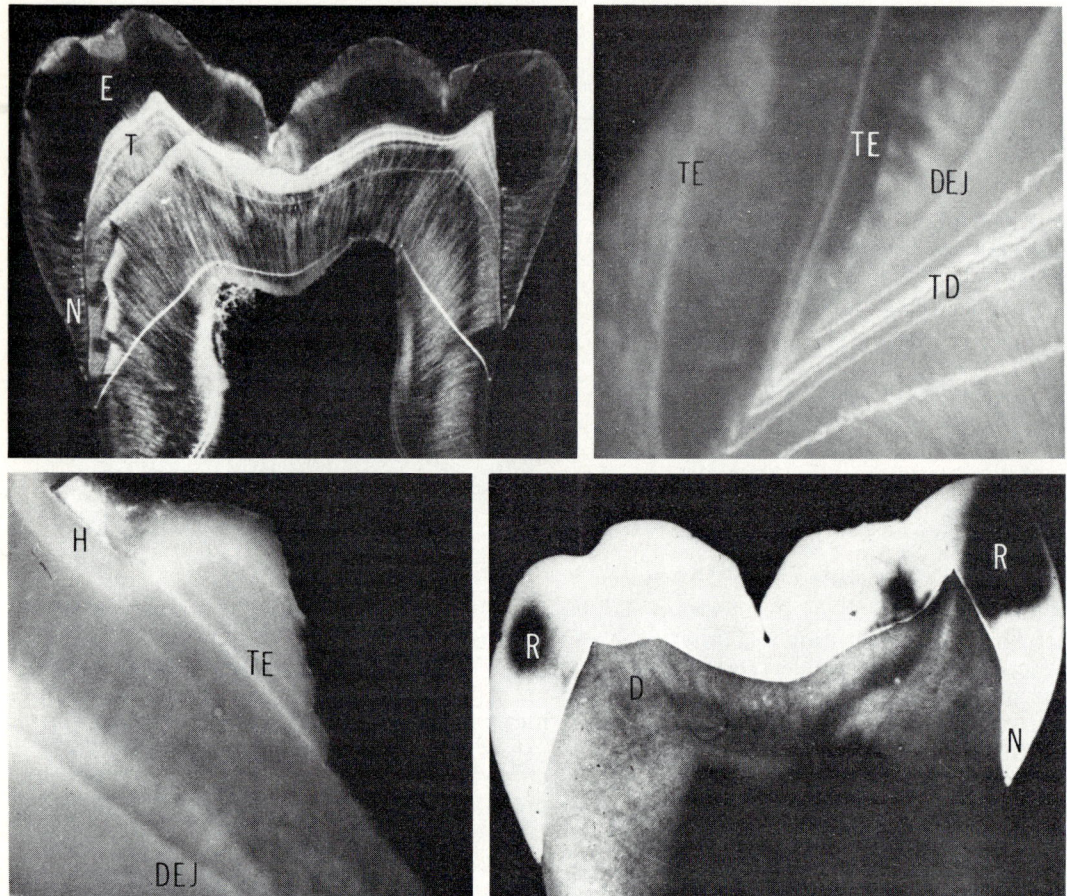

FIG. 1-41 Severely tetracycline-discolored first permanent molars. *(Top, left)* The affected enamel (E) is located in areas corresponding with the fluorescent lines (T) in the crown dentin. The affected enamel differs in appearance from the normal enamel (N) situated in the cervical part of the crown. Ultraviolet light. ×10. *(Top, right)* Fluorescent lines in the crown dentin (TD) are paired with prominent but less noticeable fluorescent lines (TE) in the adjoining enamel. DEJ, dentin-enamel junction. Ultraviolet light. ×40. *(Bottom, left)* This molar is hypoplastic as well as severely tetracycline-discolored. Fluorescent lines in the enamel (TE) are in close association with the diffusely fluorescent hypoplastic defect (H). DEJ, dentin-enamel junction. Ultraviolet light. ×40. *(Bottom, right)* Microradiograph of a severely tetracycline-discolored first permanent molar crown. The radiolucent areas (R) correspond to the areas of diffusely discolored opaque enamel and are sharply contrasted with the remaining mineralized areas of normal enamel (N) and dentin (D). ×10. (Baker KL: The fluorescent, microradiographic, microhardness and specific gravity properties of tetracycline-affected human enamel and dentine. Arch Oral Biol 17:525, 1972)

An examination by Hinrichs (1966) of the teeth of 36 human patients with cretinism and juvenile hypothyroidism revealed few striking morphologic changes. Four cases exhibited hypocalcification; enamel hypoplasia was found in five patients. The most significant finding, in eight cases, was retardation of eruption. With the administration of thyroid therapy, the eruption of the teeth was accelerated.

Experimental hyperthyroidism in newborn rats caused precocious tooth eruption. In normal adult rats, injections of thyroxine produced an increased eruption rate of the incisors (Hoskins, 1927).

Parathyroid Hormone. The parathyroid gland controls calcium and phosphorus metabolism of the body. The parathyroid hormone lowers the serum phosphorus by decreasing tubular reabsorption of phosphate. The hormone also elevates the serum calcium by inducing bone resorption and promoting reabsorption of calcium from the renal tubules (Bartter, 1964). Occasionally, when the thyroid gland is removed, the parathyroids, which lie deep in the thyroid tissue, are accidentally ablated and hypoparathyroidism may result. This condition can cause an interference in mineralization of the roots of teeth that have not yet fully formed.

Radiographic examination of patients suffering from hypoparathyroidism discloses early closure of the root ends. The affected roots are shorter than those of adjacent teeth that matured before the disease developed.

Disturbances in enamel mineralization may occur but are seldom observed in hypoparathyroidism, since the disease rarely occurs before age 12. However, disturbances in dentin mineralization of the roots in the region of the apex can occur, producing blunt, short roots. The poor mineralization of the dentin results from alteration of the protein-mucopolysaccharide complex of the dentinal matrix (Bernick, 1969).

Pituitary Hormones. The pituitary growth hormone controls the basic process of the growth of teeth, whereas the thyroid hormone controls differentiation and maturation of ameloblasts and odontoblasts.

Following hypophysectomy, Schour and Van Dyke (1932) and Becks et al (1946) found that a thickening of the dentinal walls at the expense of the pulp chamber was a constant pathognomonic symptom of hypophysectomy. However, mineralization of the dentin was found to be disturbed, as disclosed by histochemical stains (Bernick, 1967).

Radiologic studies of the jaws and teeth of 48 cases of pituitary dwarfism by Kosowicz and Rzymski (1977) revealed that there was delayed shedding of the deciduous teeth, delayed eruption of the permanent teeth, complete absence of the third molar tooth buds, and underdevelopment of the jaw bones.

Replacement therapy with growth hormone and thyroxine in hypophysectomized rats produced corrective effects of eruption rate and restoration of the completely atrophied enamel organ.

Overproduction of the growth hormone in the

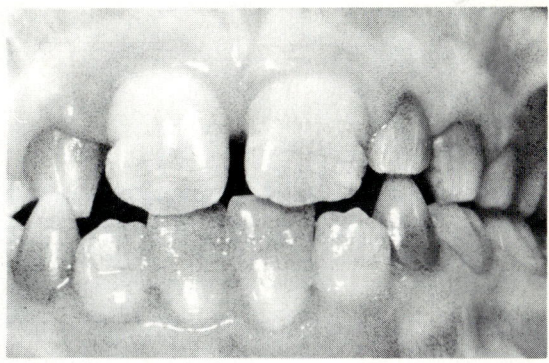

FIG. 1-42 Example of dentition demonstrating enamel hypoplasia in direct association with tetracycline discoloration. (Primosch RE: Tetracycline discoloration, enamel defects, and dental caries in patients with cystic fibrosis. Oral Surg 50:301, 1980)

adult (hyperpituitarism) may lead to the clinical state of acromegaly. In acromegaly the teeth are large, and the roots are long, in proportion to the enlarged bones. The teeth are yellow, with an increased density in the dentin and enamel.

Underproduction of growth hormone in the child is exemplified by Simmond's syndrome or progeria. This disease is often spoken of as pituitary senility. Among its many interesting clinical characteristics are the features of senility, such as baldness, loose thin skin, angina pectoris, and arteriosclerosis. The teeth erupt early and are soon lost. The patient generally dies of senile disease before 18 years of age (Album and Hope, 1958).

Pituitary deficiency in the adult is characterized by the Fröhlich syndrome, in which there is marked adiposity. The teeth and their pulps are not affected, since the disease develops after the teeth are formed.

Estrogenic Hormones. Administration of estrogenic hormones to rats results in inhibition of linear bone growth and an osteosclerosislike appearance of the shafts of the long bones. Mineralization of the dentin is also affected, resulting in an increased number of poorly calcified, interglobular areas (Bernick and Ershoff, 1964).

Gonadal Hormones. Since the gonads begin to function after complete development of the teeth, the hormones of these glands have no effect on histodifferentiation, maturation, or eruption of teeth. However, the dentin of

34 | THE DENTAL PULP

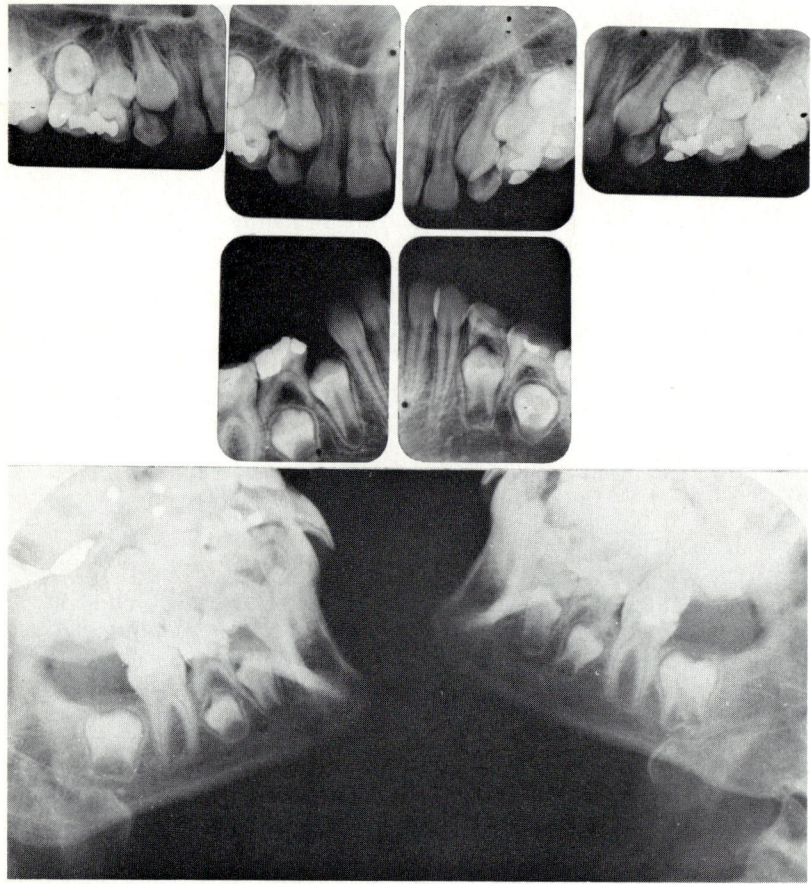

FIG. 1-43 *(Top and bottom)* Roentgenograms taken at age 9½ years of child's jaw that had been irradiated at age 5 months with 400 R. *(Top)* Note slightly advanced development of lower left second premolar and second molar. *(Bottom)* Extraoral roentgenograms of mandible. (Weyman J: The effect of irradiation on developing teeth. Oral Surg 25:623, 1968)

gonadectomized rats was found to be poorly mineralized, as characterized by an increased number of interglobular spaces (Bernick, 1968).

Corticosteroids (Cortisone). Growth was retarded in newborn rats given immunosuppressive levels of cortisone. The ameloblasts and odontoblasts were small. The net result was a retardation of amelogenesis and dentinogenesis (Nakamoto and Wilson, 1968). However, in other studies (Anneroth and Bloom, 1966), glucocorticoid-treated rats exhibited the formation of excessive quantities of hard tissue in the incisors, and Ball (1977) found that there was no reduction in the rate of dentin deposition in hypercorticoid rats.

X-IRRADIATION

Undifferentiated cells are more responsive to irradiation than differentiated cells; thus, the young, differentiating, but not yet dentin-producing odontoblasts and the ameloblasts of rats are the most radiosensitive of the cells of the developing tooth germ. Single and fractional radiation doses ranging from 300 R to 1500 R were administered. Above the 600 R dose level, disturbances in dentinogenesis in the form of niche formation and osteodentin production oc-

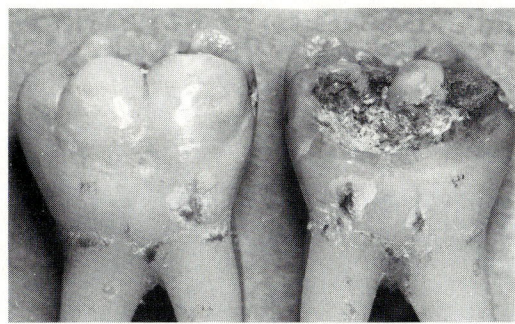
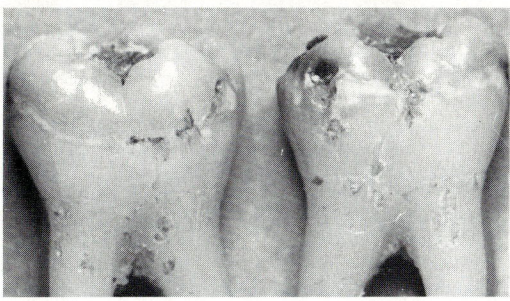
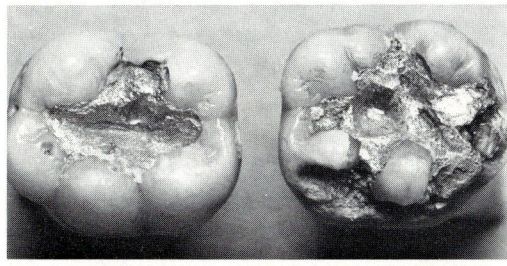

FIG. 1-44 Lower first permanent molars after extraction. *(Top)* Buccal view; *(middle)* lingual view; *(bottom)* occlusal view. (Weyman J: The effect of irradiation on developing teeth. Oral Surg 25:623, 1968)

curred in the newly differentiating odontoblasts (Collett and Thonard, 1965; Adkins, 1967). Interference in amelogenesis was evidenced by the development of enamel hypoplasia (Lindvall et al, 1972).

In developing human teeth, the damage depends on the amount, source, and type of radiation, exposure factors, and the stage of development at the time of radiation (Kimeldorf et al, 1963). At the earliest stage of tooth development, amelogenesis may be affected, resulting in hypoplastic enamel lesions (Figs. 1-43 and 1-44). Heavy doses at the earliest stages of tooth development may cause agenesis. Between the two extremes, various malformations may occur, ranging from dwarfing of the teeth to cessation of amelogenesis and dilaceration of the roots.

The eruption of human teeth with short roots has occurred as a result of x-irradiation. Complete inhibition of further root formation results.

BIBLIOGRAPHY

Adkins KF: The effect of 1200 r of x-radiation on dentinogenesis in the mandibular teeth of rats. Arch Oral Biol 12:1569, 1967

Akita H, Kagayama M, Sato R: Light and electron microscopy of the effects of colchicine and vinblastine on maturing rat ameloblasts in vivo. Arch Oral Biol 28:263, 1983

Album MM, and Hope JW: Progeria. Oral Surg 9:985, 1958

Anagnostopoulos C, Matsudaira H: In Ichihara K (ed): Proceedings of the International Symposium on Enzyme Chemistry, Tokyo-Kyoto, p 166. New York, Academic Press, 1958

Andreasen JO, Ravn JJ: The effect of traumatic injuries to primary teeth on their permanent successors. II. A clinical and radiographic follow-up study of 213 teeth. Scand J Dent Res 79:284, 1971

Andreasen JO, Riis I: Influence of pulp necrosis and periapical inflammation of primary teeth on their permanent successor. Int J Oral Surg 7:178, 1978

Andreasen JO, Sunström B, Ravn JJ: The effect of traumatic injuries to primary teeth on their permanent successors. I. A clinical and histologic study of 117 injured permanent teeth. Scand J Dent Res 79:219, 1971

Anneroth G, Bloom G: Structural changes in the incisors of cortisone-treated rats. J Dent Res 45:229, 1966

Archard HO, Witkop CJ, Jr: Hereditary hypophosphatemia (vitamin D-resistant rickets) presenting primary dental manifestations. Oral Surg 22:184, 1966

Baker KL: The fluorescent, microradiographic, microhardness and specific gravity properties of tetracycline-affected human enamel and dentine. Arch Oral Biol 17:525, 1972

Ball PC: Lack of effect of excess glucocorticoid hormone on the rate of dentin deposition in rats. J Dent Res 56:685, 1977

Bartter FC: Parathyroid hormones and phosphate metabolism. J Dent Res 43:1098, 1964

Baume LJ, Becks H, Ray JC, Evans HM: Hormonal control of tooth eruption. II. The effects of hypophysectomy on the upper rat incisor following progressively longer intervals. J Dent Res 33:91, 1954b

Becks H, Collins DA, Simpson ME, Evans HM: Changes in the central incisors of the hypophysectomized female rats after different postoperative periods. Arch Path 41:457, 1946

Becks H, Furuta W: Effect of magnesium deficient diets on oral and dental tissues. II. Changes in the enamel structure. JADA 28:1083, 1941

Bennett IC, Law DB: Incorporation of tetracycline in

developing dog enamel and dentin. J Dent Res 44:788, 1965

Berkovitz BKB, Thomson P: Observations on the etiology of supernumerary upper incisors in the albino ferret (*Mustela Putorius*). Arch Oral Biol 18:457, 1973

Bernick S: Histochemical study of dentin in parathyroidectomized rats. J Dent Res 48:1251, 1969

Bernick S: Histochemical study of dentin in gonadectomized rats. J Dent Res 47:1176, 1968

Bernick S: Histochemical study of dentine in rats following hypophysectomy. Oral Surg 23:680, 1967

Bernick S, Ershoff BH: Histochemical study of dentine in estrogen-treated rats. Oral Surg 18:249, 1964

Beumer J, Trowbridge HO, Silverman S, Jr, Eisenberg E: Childhood hypophosphatasia and the premature loss of teeth. Oral Surg 35:631, 1973

Bevelander G, Nakahara H: The effect of diverse amounts of tetracycline on fluorescence and coloration of teeth. J Dent Res 68:114, 1966

Bikle D, Tilney LG, Porter HR: Microtubules and pigment migration in the melanophores of *Fundulus heteroclitus*. Protoplasma 61:322, 1966

Binns WH, Escobar A: Defects in permanent teeth following pulp exposure of primary teeth. J Dent Child 34:4, 1967

Bixler D, Conneally PM, Christen AG: Dentinogenesis imperfecta: Genetic variations in a six-generation family. J Dent Res 48:1196, 1969

Bradfield JGR: The localization of enzymes in cells. Biol Rev 25:113, 1950

Brothwell DR, Carbonell VM, Goose DH: Dental Anthropology. London, Pergamon Press, 1963

Brown DD: The isolation of genes. Sci Am 229:21, 1973

Bruckner, RJ, Rickles NH, Porter DR: Hypophosphatasia with premature shedding of teeth and aplasia of cementum. Oral Surg 15:1351, 1962

Burstone MS: Hydrolytic enzymes in dentinogenesis and osteogenesis. In Sognnaes RF (ed): Calcification in Biological Systems. Publ 64, Am Ass Adv Sci, Washington, DC, 1960

Byers MR: The development of sensory innervation in dentin. J Comp Neurol 191:413, 1980

Cavanha AD: Enamel pearls. Oral Surg 19:373, 1965

Chiba M, Takizawa K, Ohshima S: Dose-response effects of colchicine and vinblastine on unimpeded eruption rates of the rat mandibular incisor. Arch Oral Biol 25:115, 1980

Christensen GJ, Kraus BS: Initial calcification of the human permanent first molar. J Dent Res 44:1338, 1965

Cohen MM, Blitzer FJ, Arvystas MG, Bonneau RH: Abnormalities of the permanent dentition in trisomy G. J Dent Res 49:1386, 1970

Cohen MM, Shklar G: Deformities of the craniofacial and dental complex in the H-1 virus modified hamster. Oral Surg 17:533, 1964

Cohen MM, Shklar G: Pulpal pathosis in mice infected with polyoma virus. Oral Surg 20:245, 1965

Collett WK, Thonard JC: The effect of fractional radiation on dentinogenesis in the rat. J Dent Res 44:84, 1965

Congleton J, Burkes EJ, Jr: Amelogenesis imperfecta with taurodontism. Oral Surg 48:540, 1979

Crick FHC: The genetic code. Sci Am 207:66, 1962

Cutright DE: The morphogenesis of the vascular supply to the permanent teeth of macaca rhesus. Oral Surg 30:284, 1970

Cutright DE: The reaction of permanent tooth buds to injury. Oral Surg 32:832, 1971

deBeer GR: The differentiation of neural crest cells into visceral cartilages and odontoblasts in amblystoma, and a re-examination of the germ-layer theory. Proc Roy Soc [Ser B] 134:377, 1947

De Duve C: Lysosomes, a new group of cytoplasmic particles. In Hayashi T (ed): Subcellular Particles. New York, Ronald Press, 1959

DeHarven E, Dustin P, Jr: Centre Nationale de la Recherche Scientifique (Paris). Colloque No. 189, 1960

DiOrio LP: Influence of protein malnutrition on growth and development of dental structures of infant rats. Master's thesis, Massachusetts Institute of Technology, June, 1969

Eisenmann DR, Yaeger JA: Alterations in the formation of rat dentine and enamel induced by various ions. Arch Oral Biol 14:1045, 1969

Eklund G, Stalhane I, Hedegard B: A study of traumatized teeth in children aged 7–15 years. Swed Dent J 69:179, 1976

Enwonwu CO: Influence of socio-economic conditions on dental development in Nigerian children. Arch Oral Biol 18:95, 1973

Escobar VH, Goldblatt LI, Bixler D: A clinical, genetic, and ultrastructural study of snow-capped teeth: amelogenesis imperfecta, hypomaturation type. Oral Surg 52:607, 1981

Fearnhead RW: Secretory products of ameloblasts. In Boyd JD, Johnson FR, Lever JD (eds): Electron Microscopy in Anatomy. London, Arnold, 1961

Ferguson HW, Hartles RL: The effect of diets deficient in calcium or phosphorus in the presence and absence of supplements of vitamin D on the incisor teeth and bone of adult rats. Arch Oral Biol 11:1345, 1966

Fisher AK: Respiratory variations within the normal dental pulp. J Dent Res 46:424, 1967

Fleming HS: SE polyoma-virus tumor and the teeth. J Dent Res 42:1405, 1963

Frank RM, Nalbandian J: Comparative aspects of development of dental hard structures. J Dent Res 42:422, 1963

Freire-Maia N: Ectodermal dysplasias. Hum Hered 21:309, 1971

Fullmer HM: Dehydrogenases in developing teeth of rats. J Histochem Cytochem 11:641, 1963

Fullmer HM: Histochemical studies of the acid mucopolysaccharides. Oral Surg 3:976, 1972

Garant PR: The organization of microtubules within rat odontoblast process revealed by perfusion fixation with glutaraldehyde. Arch Oral Biol 17:1047, 1972

Garant PR, Baer PN, Kilham L: Electron microscopic localization of virions in developing teeth of young hamsters infected with minute virus of mice. J Dent Res 59:80, 1980

Garant PR, Szabo G, Nalbandian J: The fine structure of the mouse odontoblast. Arch Oral Biol 13:857, 1968

Gardner DG, Sapp JP: Regional odontodysplasia. Oral Surg 35:351, 1973

Gardner DG, Sapp JP: Ultrastructural, electron-probe, and microhardness studies of the controversial amorphous areas in the dentin of regional odontodysplasia. Oral Surg 44:549, 1977

Garn SM, Lewis AB, Kerewsky RS, Jegart K: Sex differences in intraindividual tooth-size communalities. J Dent Res 44:476, 1965

Garn SM, Lewis AB, Vicinus JH: Third molar polymorphism and its significance to dental genetics. J Dent Res 42:1344, 1963

Gasser RF, Scheving LE, Pauly JE: Circadian rhythms in the cell division rate of the inner enamel epithelium and in the uptake of ^{3}H-thymidine by the root tip of rat incisors. J Dent Res 51:740, 1972

Gertzman GBR, Gaston G, Quinn I: Amelogenesis imperfecta; local hypoplastic type with pulpal calcification. JADA 99:637, 1979

Gianetto R, De Duve C: Comparative study of the binding of acid phosphatase, β-glucuronidase and cathepsin by rat-liver particles. Biochem J 59:433, 1955

Giasanti JS, Allen JD: Dentin dysplasia, Type II, or dentin dysplasia, coronal type. Oral Surg 38:911, 1974

Giasanti JS, Budnick SD: Six generations of hereditary opalescent dentin: report of case. JADA 90:439, 1975

Glass HB: The biochemical basis of human heredity. In Witkop CJ, Jr (ed): Genetics and Dental Health. pp 1–16. New York, McGraw-Hill, 1962

Glick PL, Rowe DJ: Effects of chronic protein deficiency on the formation of the rat incisor teeth. Arch Oral Biol 26: 459, 1981

Goldstein E, Gottlieb MA: Taurodontism: familial tendencies demonstrated in eleven of fourteen case reports. Oral Surg 36:131, 1973

Goren A, Gerstner R: Autoradiographic localization in fetal oral tissues of maternally stored calcium 45. J Dent Res 44:1272, 1965

Gorlin RJ: Thoma's Oral Pathology, 6th ed, p 456. St. Louis, Mosby, 1970

Graber LW: Congenital absence of teeth: a review with emphasis on inheritance patterns. JADA 96:266, 1978

Grahnen H: Hypodontia in the permanent dentition. A clinical and genetic investigation. Odont Revy 7, Suppl 3, 1956

Grant D, Bernick S: Morphodifferentiation and structure of Hertwig's root sheath in the cat. J Dent Res 50:1580, 1971

Guggenheimer J, Nowak AJ, Michaels RM: Dental manifestations of the rubella syndrome. Oral Surg 32:30, 1971

Gulmen S, Pullon P, O'Brien LW: Tricho-dento-osseous syndrome. J Endodont 2:117, 1976

Guo MK, Messer HH: Properties of Ca^{2+}-, Mg^{2+}-activated adenosine triphosphatase from rat incisor pulp. Arch Oral Biol 21:637, 1976

Hedegard B, Stalhane I: A study of traumatized permanent teeth in children aged 7–15 years. Swed Dent J 66:43, 1973

Herold RC: Fine structure of tooth dentine in human dentinogenesis imperfecta. Arch Oral Biol 17:1009, 1972

Hinrichs EH: Dental changes in juvenile hypothyroidism. J Dent Child 33:167, 1966

Hintz CS, Peters RA: Odontodysplasia. Report of an unusual case and a review of the literature. Oral Surg 34:744, 1972

Hoskins MM: The effects of acetyl thyroxin on the teeth of newborn rats. Proc Soc Exp Biol Med 25:55, 1927–1928

Houpt MI, Kenny FM, Listgarten M: Hypophosphatasia: Case reports. J Dent Child 37:38, 1970

Hudson CD, Witkop CJ, Jr: Autosomal dominant hypodontia with nail dysgenesis. Report of twenty-nine cases in six families. Oral Surg 39:409, 1975

Hunstadbraten K: Hypodontia in the permanent dentition. J Dent Child 40:115, 1973

Hunt AM, Paynter KJ: The role of cells of the stratum intermedium in the development of the guinea pig molar. A study of cell differentiation and migration using tritiated thymidine. Arch Oral Biol 8:65, 1963

Hurmerinta K, Thesleff I, Saxén L: In vitro inhibition of mouse odontoblast differentiation by vitamin A. Arch Oral Biol 25:385, 1980

Jaspers MT: Taurodontism in the Down syndrome. Oral Surg 51:632, 1981

Johannessen LB: Effects on food intake, somatic growth and dentinogenesis in immature male albino rats of a low dose of propylthiouracil without, and together with, desiccated thyroid. Arch Oral Biol 11:983, 1966

Jorgenson RJ, Warson RW: Dental abnormalities in the tricho-dento-osseous syndrome. Oral Surg 36:693, 1973

Kaplan NL, Zach L, Goldsmith ED: Effects of pulpal exposure in the primary dentition on the succedaneous teeth. J Dent Child 34:237, 1967

Kawasaki K, Fearnhead RW: On the relationship between tetracycline and the incremental lines in dentine. J Anat 119:49, 1975

Kerebel B, Daculsi G: Amelogenesis imperfecta-etude structurale, ultrastructurale et radiocristallographique. J Biol Buccale 4:43, 1976

Kerebel B, Daculsi G, Menanteau J, Kerebel LM: The inorganic phase in dentinogenesis imperfecta. J Dent Res 60:1655, 1981

Kerebel B, Kerebel LM: Enamel in odontodysplasia. Oral Surg 52:404, 1981

Kerebel B, Kerebel LM, Daculsi G, Doury J: Dentinogenesis imperfecta with dens in dente. Oral Surg 55:286, 1983

Kerebel B, Kerebel LM.: Structural, ultrastructural, microradiographic, and electron-probe studies of an unusual case of regional odontodysplasia. J Dent Res 61:1056, 1982

Kimeldorf DJ, Jones DC, Castanera TJ: The radiobiology of teeth (a review). Radiat Res 20:518, 1963

Kosowicz J, Rzymski K: Abnormalities of tooth development in pituitary dwarfism. Oral Surg 44:853, 1977

Kreshover SJ: Metabolic disturbances in tooth formation. In Metabolism of oral tissues. Ann NY Acad Sci 85:161, 1960

Kruger BJ: Dose-dependent ultrastructural changes induced by tetracycline in developing dental tissues of the rat. J Dent Res 54:822, 1975

Kudo N: Effects of colchicine on the secretion of matrices of dentine and enamel in the rat incisor. Autoradiographic study using 3H-proline. Calc Tiss Res 18:37, 1975

Larmas L, Larmas M: A histochemical study of various dehydrogenases in human tooth ontogeny. Arch Oral Biol 21:371, 1976

Larmas M, Thesleff I: Biochemical study of changes in

non-specific alkaline phosphomonoesterase activity during mouse tooth ontogeny. Arch Oral Biol 25:791, 1980

Le Bell Y: Ca^{2+}- and Mg^{2+}-activated ATP hydrolysis in human tooth pulp. J Dent Res 60:128, 1981

Levy BA: Effects of experimental trauma on developing first molar teeth in rats. J Dent Res 47:323, 1968

Linde LA, Ljunggren AE: Lactate dehydrogenase isoenzymes in odontoblasts from rat incisors. Arch Oral Biol 15:549, 1970

Linde A, Johansson S, Jonsson R, Jontell M: Localization of fibronectin during dentinogenesis in rat incisor. Arch Oral Biol 27:1069, 1982

Lindvall A-M, Omnell K-Å, Schildt BE: The effect of roentgen irradiation on the formation of enamel and dentin in maxillary rat incisors. Scand J Dent Res 80:253, 1972

Lunt DA, Noble HW: Localization of alkaline phosphatases in human cap stage enamel organs by electron histochemistry. Arch Oral Biol 17:761, 1972

Lunt RC, Law DB: A review of the chronology of calcification of deciduous teeth. JADA 89:599, 1974

Lustmann J, Ulmansky M: Structural changes in odontodysplasia. Oral Surg 41:193, 1976

Macgregor HG, Stebbins H: A massive system of microtubules associated with cytoplasmic movement in telotrophic ovarioles. J Cell Sci 6:431, 1970

McIntosh HA, Storey E: Tetracycline-induced tooth changes. 4. Discoloration and hypoplasia induced by tetracycline analogues. Med J Aust 1:114, 1970

McLarty EL, Giansanti JS, Hibbard ED: X-linked hypomaturation type of amelogenesis imperfecta exhibiting lyonization in affected females. Oral Surg 36:678, 1973

Marks SC, Lindahl RL, Bawden JW: Dental and cephalometric findings in vitamin D resistant rickets. J Dent Child 32:259, 1965

Mataki S: Comparison of the effect of colchicine and vinblastine on the inhibition of dentinogenesis in rat incisors. Arch Oral Biol 26:955, 1981

Matsumiya S: Experimental pathological study on the effect of treatment of infected root canals in the deciduous tooth on growth of the permanent tooth germ. Int Dent J 18:546, 1968

Matthiessen ME: Enzyme histochemistry of the prenatal development of human deciduous teeth. 1. Alkaline phosphatase, acid phosphatase and unspecific AS-esterase. Acta Anat 63:523, 1966

Melnick M, Eastman JR, Goldblatt LI, Michaud M, Bixler D: Dentin dysplasia, Type II: A rare autosomal dominant disorder. Oral Surg 44:592, 1977

Melnick M, Levin LS, Brady J: Dentin dysplasia type I: A scanning electron microscope analysis of the primary dentition. Oral Surg 50:335, 1980

Messer HH, Guo MK: Lack of relation of pulp Ca^{2+}-, Mg^{2+}- ATPase to mineralization rate in rat incisor dentine in response to vitamin D and calcium intake. Arch Oral Biol 24:271, 1979

Moffitt JM, Cooley RO, Olsen NH, Hefferren JJ: Prediction of tetracycline-induced tooth discoloration. JADA 88:547, 1974

Morris ME, Augsburger RH: Dentine dysplasia and skeletal anomalies inherited as an autosomal dominant trait. Oral Surg 43:267, 1977

Nagai I, Fujiki Y, Fuchihata H, Yoshimoto T: Supernumerary tooth associated with cleft lip and palate. JADA 70:642, 1965

Nakamoto T, Mallak HM, Miller SA: The effect of protein-energy malnutrition on the growth of tooth germs in newborn rats. J Dent Res 58:1115, 1979

Nakamoto T, Wilson RH: The growth rate of tooth germ in newly-born rats injected with cortisone acetate. Arch Oral Biol 13:1107, 1968

Nelson MA, Chaudhry AP: Effects of tocopherol (vitamin E)-deficient diet on some oral, para-oral, and hematopoietic tissues of the rat. J Dent Res 45:1072, 1966

Nikiforuk G, Fraser D: Etiology of enamel hypoplasia and interglobular dentin: The roles of hypocalcemia and hypophosphatemia. Metab Bone Dis Rel Res 2:17, 1979

Nylen MU, Omnell A, Löfgren C-G: An electron microscopic study of tetracycline-induced enamel defects in rat incisor enamel. Scand J Dent Res 80:384, 1972

Oliver WJ, Owings CL, Brown WE, Shapiro BA: Hypoplastic enamel associated with the nephrotic syndrome. Pediatrics 32:399, 1963

Osman M, Ruch J-V: Behavior of odontoblasts and basal lamina of trypsin or EDTA-isolated mouse dental papillae in short-term culture. J Dent Res 60:1015, 1981

Owens PDA: Odontoblast processes during late root development of premolar teeth in dogs. Arch Oral Biol 23:237, 1978b

Owens PDA: Ultrastructure of Hertwig's epithelial root sheath during early root development in premolar teeth in dogs. Arch Oral Biol 23:91, 1978a

Palade G: Intracellular aspects of the process of protein synthesis. Science 189:347, 1975

Petrone JA, Noble ER: Dentin dysplasia type I: a clinical report. JADA 103:891, 1981

Pinkham JR, Burkes EJ, Jr: Odontodysplasia. Oral Surg 36:841, 1973

Primosch RE: Tetracycline discoloration, enamel defects, and dental caries in patients with cystic fibrosis. Oral Surg 50:301, 1980

Prout RES, Atkin ER: Effect of diet deficient in essential fatty acid on fatty acid composition of enamel and dentine of the rat. Arch Oral Biol 18:583, 1973

Prout RES, Tring FC: Dentinogenesis in incisors of rats deficient in essential fatty acids. J Dent Res 52:462, 1973

Rakocz M, Keating J, Johnson R: Management of the primary dentition in vitamin D-resistant rickets. Oral Surg 54:166, 1982

Reith EJ: Collagen formation in developing molar teeth of rats. J Ultrastruct Res 21:383, 1968

Reynolds EH: Chronic anti-epileptic toxicity: A review. Epilepsia (Boston) 16:319, 1975

Roberts RW, Strachân DS: Quantitation of lactate dehydrogenase of developing molar teeth of the mouse. J Dent Res 46:522, 1967

Robison R: The possible significance of hexosephosphoric esters in ossification. Biochem J 17:286, 1923

Robinson PB, Rowe DJF, Harris M: The effects of diphenylhydantoin and vitamin D deficiency on developing teeth in the rat. Arch Oral Biol 23:137, 1978

Ruch J-V, Karcher-Djuricic V, Gerber R: Quelques aspects du rôle de la prédentine dans la différentiation des adamantoblastes. Arch Anat Microsc Morphol Exp 61:127, 1972

(eds): Alzheimer's Disease, Down's Syndrome, and Aging. Ann NY Acad Sci 396:55, 1982

Verzár F, McDougall EJ: Absorption from the Intestine. London, Longmans Green, 1936

Walton JL, Witkop CJ, Jr, Walker PO: Report of three cases with vascular nevi overlying the adjacent skin of the face. Oral Surg 92:676, 1978

Weinmann JP, Svoboda JF, Woods RW: Hereditary disturbances of enamel formation and calcification. JADA 32:397, 1945

Weinstock M: Centrosymmetrical cross-banded structures in the matrix of rat incisor predentin and dentin. J Ultrastruct Res 61:218, 1977

Weinstock M, Leblond CP: Synthesis, migration, and release of precursor collagen by odontoblasts as visualized by radioautography after (3H) proline administration. J Cell Biol 60:92, 1974

Wesley RK, Wysocki GP, Mintz SM, Jackson J: Dentin dysplasia type I. Clinical, morphologic, and genetic studies of a case. Oral Surg 41:516, 1976

Weyman J: The effect of irradiation on developing teeth. Oral Surg 25:623, 1968

Whittaker DK, Richards D: Scanning electron microscopy of the neonatal line in human enamel. Arch Oral Biol 23:45, 1978

Winter GB, Lee KW, Johnson NW: Hereditary amelogenesis imperfecta; a rare autosomal dominant type. Brit Dent J 127:157, 1969

Witkop CJ, Jr: Genes, chromosomes and dentistry. JADA 68:846, 1964

Witkop CJ, Jr: Manifestations of genetic diseases in the human pulp. In Siskin M (ed): The Biology of the Human Dental Pulp, pp 25–63. St. Louis, CV Mosby, 1973

Witkop CJ, Jr, Wolf RO: Hypoplasia and intrinsic staining of enamel following tetracycline therapy. JAMA 185:1008, 1963

Witkop CJ, Jr: Genetic diseases of the oral cavity. In Tiecke RW (ed): Oral Pathology, pp 786–843. New York, McGraw-Hill, 1965

Witkop CJ, Jr: Genetics. Schweiz Mschr Zahnheilk 82:917, 1972

Witkop CJ, Jr: Hereditary defects of dentin. Dent Clin North Amer 19:29, 1975

Witkop CJ, Jr, Brearly LJ, Gentry WC: Hypoplastic enamel, onycholysis, and hypohidrosis inherited as an autosomal dominant trait; a review of ectodermal dysplasia syndromes. Oral Surg 39:71, 1975

Witkop CJ, Jr, Kuhlmann W, Sauk J: Autosomal recessive pigmented hypomaturation amelogenesis imperfecta. Report of a kindred. Oral Surg 36:367, 1973

Witkop CJ, Jr, Rao S: Inherited defects in tooth structure. In Bergsma D (ed): Birth Defects. Vol 7, pp 153–184. Original Article Series, Part XI, Orofacial Structures. National Foundation-March of Dimes. Baltimore, Williams and Wilkins, 1971

Yen PK-J, Shaw JH: Effects of repeated oral doses of dimethylchlortetracycline on bones and dentin of young rhesus monkeys. J Dent Res 54:358, 1975

Yoshiki S, Kurahashi Y: A light and electron microscopic study of alkaline phosphatase activity in the early stage of dentinogenesis in the young rat. Arch Oral Biol 16:1143, 1971

Ziskin D, Applebaum E, Salmon TN: The effect of thyroparathyroidectomy at birth and at 7 days on dental and skeletal development of rats. J Dent Res 19:93, 1940

Ziskin D, Applebaum E: The effect of thyroidectomy upon growing and thyroid stimulation on permanent dentition of rhesus monkeys. J Dent Res 20:21, 1941

Ruch J-V, Karcher-Djuricic V, Gerber R: Les déterminismes de la morphogenèse et des cytodifferentiations des ébauches dentaires de souris. J Biol Buccale 1:45, 1973

Rushton MA: Hereditary enamel defects. Proc R Soc Med 57:53, 1965

Russell DL: The distribution of glycogen in bovine dental pulp. J Dent Res 46:1182, 1967

Sadeghi EM, Ashrafi MH: Regional odontodysplasia: Clinical, pathologic, and therapeutic considerations. JADA 102:336, 1981

Samuels LD: Uptake of radium-226 from drinking water into human deciduous teeth. Arch Oral Biol 11:581, 1966

Sapp JP, Gardner DG: Regional odontodysplasia: An ultrastructural and histochemical study of the soft-tissue calcifications. Oral Surg 36:383, 1973

Sauk JJ, Jr, Cotton WR, Lyon HW, Witkop, CJ: Electron-optic analysis of hypomineralized amelogenesis imperfecta in man. Arch Oral Biol 17:771, 1972a

Sauk JJ, Jr, Lyon HW, Trowbridge HO, Witkop CJ, Jr: An electron optic analysis and explanation for the etiology of dentinal dysplasia. Oral Surg 33:763, 1972

Sauk JJ, Delaney JR: Taurodontism, diminished root formation, and microcephalic dwarfism. Oral Surg 36:231, 1973

Sauk JJ, Vickers RA, Copeland JS, Lyon HW: The surface of genetically determined hypoplastic enamel in human teeth. Oral Surg 34:60, 1972b

Saunders RL de C: Microradiographic studies of human adult and fetal dental pulp studies. In X-ray Microscopy and Microradiography, p 561. New York, Academic Press, 1957

Saunders RL de C: X-ray microscopy of the periodontal and dental pulp vessels in the monkey and in man. Oral Surg 22:503, 1966

Schour I: Neonatal line in the enamel and dentin of the human deciduous teeth and first permanent molar. JADA 23:1946, 1936

Schour I: Vital staining of growing bones and teeth with alizarine red S. J Dent Res 20:411, 1941

Schour I, Van Dyke HB: Changes in teeth following hypophysectomy. I. Changes in the incisor of the white rat. Am J Anat 50:397, 1932

Senzaki H: A histological study of reparative dentinogenesis in the rat incisor after colchicine administration. Arch Oral Biol 25:737, 1980

Severson AR: Histochemical demonstration of adenosine triphosphatase in dental tissue. J Dent Res 47:1201, 1968

Severson AR: Histochemical demonstration of nucleoside triphosphate hydrolysis in the mouse dentition. Acta Histochem 40:86, 1971

Shaw JH: Marginal protein deficiency during the reproductive cycle in rats: influence on body weight and development of skulls and teeth of offspring. J Dent Res 49:350, 1970

Shields ED, Bixler D, El-Kafrawy AM: A proposed classification for heritable human dentine defects with a description of a new entity. Arch Oral Biol 18:543, 1973

Slavkin HC: Embryonic tooth formation. Oral Sci Rev 4:1, 1974

Slavkin HC, Bringas P: Epithelial-mesenchymal interactions during odontogenesis. IV. Morphogenical evidence for direct heterotypic cell-cell contacts. Dev Biol 50:428, 1976

Slautterbach DB: Cytoplasmic microtubules. I. Hydra. J Cell Biol 18:367, 1963

Soni NN: Microradiographic study of dental tissues in sickle-cell anemia. Arch Oral Biol 11:561, 1966

Soni NN, Barbee FE, Ferguson AD, Parrish BA: Microradiographic study of odontologic tissues in Cooley's anemia. J Dent Res 45:281, 1966

Soni NN, Henry JL, Silberkweit M, Coombs BP: Polarized light and microradiographic study of dental tissue in dentinogenesis imperfecta. J Dent Res 46:434, 1967

Soni NN, Marks SS: Microradiographic and polarized-light study of dental tissues in vitamin D-resistant rickets. Oral Surg 23:755, 1967

Stewart JE, Arie J: Depletion of glycogen and adenosine triphosphate as major factors in the death of lobsters (Homarus americanus) infected with Gaffkya homari. Can J Microbiol 19:1103, 1973

Stene T, Koppang HS: Autoradiographic investigation of dentin production in rat incisors after vincristine administration. Scand J Dent Res 88:104, 1980

Suckling G: Defects of enamel in sheep resulting from trauma during tooth development. J Dent Res 59:1541, 1980

Ten Cate AR: Development of the periodontal membrane and collagen turnover. In Poole DFG, Stack MV (eds). Eruption and Occlusion, pp 281–289, London, Butterworth, 1975

Ten Cate AR: The histochemistry of human tooth development. Proc Nutr Soc 18:65, 1959

Ten Cate AR: A histochemical study of the human odontoblast. Arch Oral Biol 12:963, 1967

Thesleff I, Lehtonen E, Saxén L: Basement membrane formation in transfilter tooth culture and its relation to odontoblast differentiation. Differentiation 10:71, 1978

Tidwell E, Cunningham CJ: Dentinal dysplasia: Endodontic treatment, with case report. J Endodont 5:372, 1979

Tobin CE: Correlation of vascularity with remineralization in human fetal teeth. Anat Rec 174:371, 1972

Tonge CH, McCance RA: Severe undernutrition in growing and adult animals. 15. The mouth, jaws and teeth of pigs. Br J Nutr 19:361, 1965

Townsend GC: Tooth size in children and young adults with Trisomy 21 (Down) syndrome. Arch Oral Biol 28:159, 1983

Tracy WE, Steen JC, Steiner JE, Buist NRM: Analysis of dentine pathogenesis in vitamin D-resistant rickets. Oral Surg 32:38, 1971

Trodahl JN, Schwartz S, Gorlin RJ: The pigmentation of dental tissues in erythropoietic (congenital) porphyria. J Oral Pathol (Copenhagen) 1:159, 1972

Trowbridge H, Seltzer JL: Formation of dentin and bone matrix in magnesium-deficient rats. J Periodont Res 2:147, 1967

Turner HJ: Effects of lincomycin on developing rat dentition. JADA 81:77, 1970

vanGool AV: Injury to the permanent tooth germ after trauma to the deciduous predecessor. Oral Surg 35:2, 1973

Van Keuren ML, Goldman D, Merril CR: Protein variations associated with Down's Syndrome, chromosome 21, and Alzheimer's disease. In Sinex FM, Merril CR

sections. Intense staining occurs in highly calcified tissues. It has also been used to localize sialic acid.

Colloidal iron (Hale's method) has been used to identify acid mucopolysaccharides, but this method is not specific, since neutral polysaccharides may also be stained by it.

For a detailed description of the histochemical characteristics of some of the tooth tissues, refer to Zerlotti and Yaeger (1967).

MECHANISM OF DENTINOGENESIS

The materials needed for mineralization of the dentin are derived from blood vessels in the dental papilla. Tobin (1972) correlated the blood supplies of the developing teeth with the extent of their mineralization (Fig. 2–1).

The blood vessels increased in size and complexity as the degree of mineralization increased. With the progression of mineralization, other pulpal vessels enlarged and apparently became the primary nutritional channels for further growth and mineralization of the dentin and enamel. However, Path and Meyer (1977) have determined, by the isotope fractionization method, that pulpal blood flow in the developing teeth of dogs did not depend on the stage of oral development. In addition, autoradiographic studies by Wennberg and Bawden (1978) apparently indicated that the pulpal route did not supply significant amounts of calcium to the rapidly mineralizing enamel. Apparently, minerals diffuse into the hard structures from the surrounding tissues. In Tobin's studies, no vessels were found in the stellate reticulum, on the outer surface of the ameloblasts, or in proximity to the formed enamel.

Dentinogenesis begins when preodontoblasts polarize to form secreting odontoblasts. The basement membrane (basal lamina, membrana preformativa), derived from the inner dental epithelium, controls the polarization of the odontoblasts. Ruch et al (1976) have shown that when the basement membrane was removed by trypsin digestion, the odontoblasts were unable to polarize. The components of the basement membrane that are involved in polarization are collagen (Types I and IV), fibronectin, and laminin (Lesot et al, 1981).

When the odontoblasts are ready to elaborate dentin, many metachromatic granules accumulate within their cytoplasm. These granules are collagen precursors that contain both protein and ground substance as well as enzymes of various types. Presently, the contents of the granules are extruded extracellularly (Fig. 2–2; Weinstock and Leblond, 1974), and they become collagen fibrils (Fig. 2–3). Predentin collagen fibrils vary in diameter from 200 Å at the base of the odontoblastic process to about 700 Å at the mineralization front, and they vary in thickness. They are welded together by carbohydrate-protein combinations called glycosaminoglycans. The glycosaminoglycans are sulfated, including heparin sulfate (Branford White, 1978), and chondroitin-4-sulfate (Embery and Smalley, 1980). They can be detected by electron microscopy after the dentin is treated with cationic dyes (Goldberg and Septier, 1983). Other noncollagenous components of the dentin matrix include phosphoproteins (phosphophoryns; Curley-Joseph and Veis, 1979; Butler et al, 1979), plasma proteins (Thomas and Leaver, 1975), and various glycoproteins (Thomas and Leaver, 1977; Smith and Leaver, 1979, 1981).

It has generally been believed that the matrix of the first-formed, or mantle, dentin also contains coarse fiber bundles, known as von Korff fibers (Fig. 2–4). When viewed in the light microscope, these silver-stained fiber bundles appear to originate in the pulp and course between the odontoblasts to become incorporated into the dentinal matrix (Fig. 2–5). On the other hand, electrophoretic studies of bovine molar dentin by Lechner and Kalnitsky (1981) have indicated that von Korff fibers consist solely of Type I collagen, which is synthesized by odontoblasts. Type III collagen, a pulpal component, is absent in dentin, strongly suggesting that pulp collagen fibers do not become embedded in dentin. According to Ten Cate et al (1970) and Ten Cate (1978), von Korff fibers are actually silver-impregnated ground substance between the separated odontoblasts (Fig. 2–5).

Chemical changes in the predentin occur just prior to mineralization. The fibers lose their argyrophilic properties, alkaline phosphatase decreases, and the staining characteristics of the mucopolysaccharides change (Kiguel, 1965). There is loss of affinity for colloidal iron and a positive PAS reaction, indicating the presence of glycoprotein. The exact mechanism of dentin mineralization is still not clear. According to one theory, through the mediation of alkaline phos-

trix formed some days later had a diffuse reaction of low intensity (Fig. 2-17).

The newly synthesized proteins of the dentinal matrix are initially incorporated into the developing dentin as discrete bands. During subsequent stages of dentin formation, the labeled dentin proteins remain fixed in position.

Interglobular Dentin

Normally, the dentin is mineralized by fusion of small globules of hydroxyapatite, known as calcospherites. During the formation of calcospherites, both radial and collagen-oriented crystals are formed simultaneously. The mineralization of dentin is brought about by the initiation and growth of calcospherites (Shellis, 1983). They can be seen readily in predentin as round, basophilic spheres (Fig. 2-18, left). When dentin is treated with papain, an internal concentric banding of the calcospherites becomes visible (Quigley et al, 1965; Fig. 2-18, right). Should globular fusion fail to occur, unmineralized or hypomineralized areas persist between the globules. Such areas are termed interglobular dentin. Dentinal tubules pass through these less mineralized areas without interruption. Interglobular dentin is found mainly in the coronal portion of the tooth near the dentinoenamel junction. As a result of congenital disease or nutritional or hormonal deficiencies, dentin mineralization is affected, resulting in increased areas of interglobular dentin (see Chap. 1).

Tomes' Granular Layer

A thin layer of dentin adjacent to the cementum appears granular in ground sections of the teeth. This is called Tomes' granular layer. Microradiographic, polarized light, phase-contrast, and scanning electron microscope studies of this layer have been made by Shackleford (1971; Fig. 2-19). He found that it consisted of a narrow zone of hypomineralized, hyperorganic dentinal matrix. One component of Tomes' layer appears to be fibrillar in nature. The dentinal tubules pass through Tomes' layer and terminate in the cementum. According to Owens (1973), administration of tetracycline causes labeling of the dentin. The tetracycline bands pass from the dentin through the granular layer and then turn coronally.

Although the exact function of Tomes' granular layer has not been elucidated, Shackleford believed that, in dogs, it protected the tooth from sudden insults or large occlusal forces transferred to the dentin by way of the periodontal ligament.

FIG. 2-18 *(Left)* Scanning electron micrograph: calcospherites of predentin. *(Right)* Decalcified section of human dentin, after papain digestion. Note the lightly stained circular areas, identified as calcospherites. Harris H & E stain. (Quigley MB, Starrs JW, Zwarych PD: Demonstration of calcospherites in mature human dentin. J Dent Res 44:794, 1965. Copyright by the American Dental Association. Reproduced by permission)

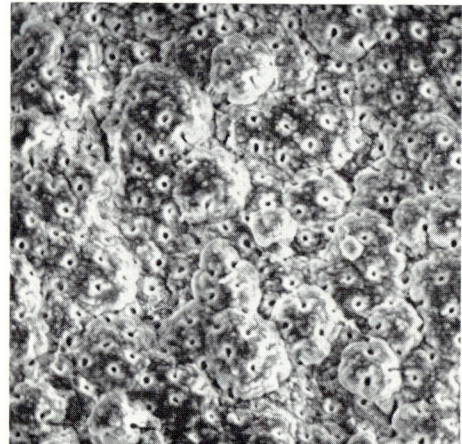
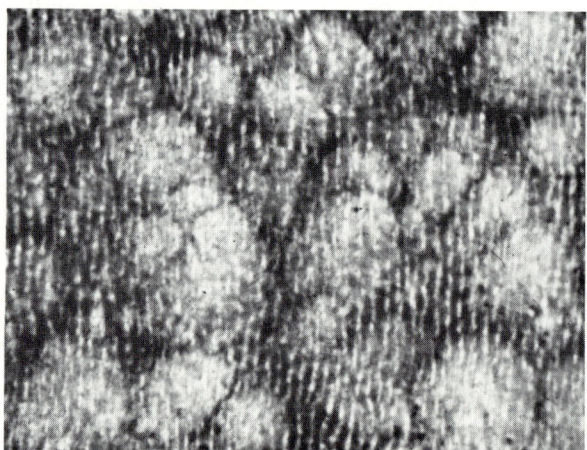

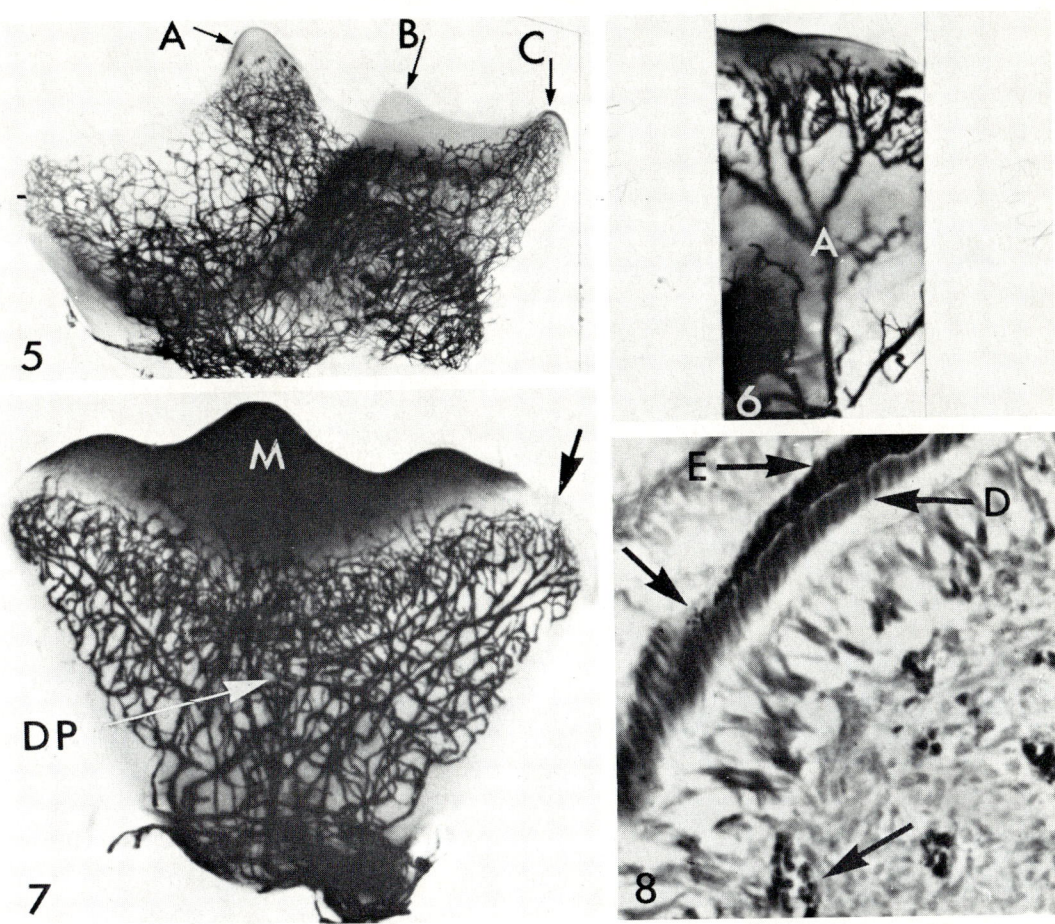

FIG. 2-1 *(Top, left)* Fetus, 18 weeks: Lingual view, isolated molar tooth germ, showing the papillary vessels and the extent of mineralization in 3 developing cusps. In *A*, there is little mineralization of the cusp, although the papillary vessels to this cusp are well formed. In cusp *B*, there is no evidence of mineralization or growth of papillary vessels, whereas in *C* definite mineralization at the tip of the cusp has occurred, and papillary vessels extend to the area of the dentin. ×10. *(Top, right)* Fetus, 18 weeks: The helical form of a central pulpal artery (A) extended through the papilla and divided into "segmental" branches which form a plexus of vessels subjacent to the dentin. (Compare *bottom, left*.) ×8. *(Bottom, left)* Fetus, 17 weeks: Central incisor tooth germ, showing complete injection of the papillary vessels (DP), mineralization of the cusp, (M) and nonmineralized area (arrow) superficial to the plexus of papillary vessels. ×8. *(Bottom, right)* Fetus, 17 weeks: Injected vessels at the dentino-pulpal border (lower arrow) and at the edge of the developing enamel (upper arrow). The latter vessels coursed through the pulp to the outer surface of the developing dentin (D) and enamel (E). ×15. (Tobin CE: Correlation of vascularity with mineralization in human fetal teeth. Anat Rec 174:371, 1972)

phatase, the ground substance or matrix becomes a calcium phosphate acceptor and mineralization begins. The alkaline phosphatase in dentin is located primarily in the plasma membranes of the odontoblastic processes (Yoshiki and Kurahashi, 1971; Granström and Linde, 1972, 1977). However, other odontoblastic cellular organelles, such as lysosomes, mitochondria, Golgi saccules, and vesicles, probably also contain alkaline phosphatase (Weinstock and Leblond, 1974; Läikkö and Larmas, 1980). Initially, calcium is bound, and then the phosphate.

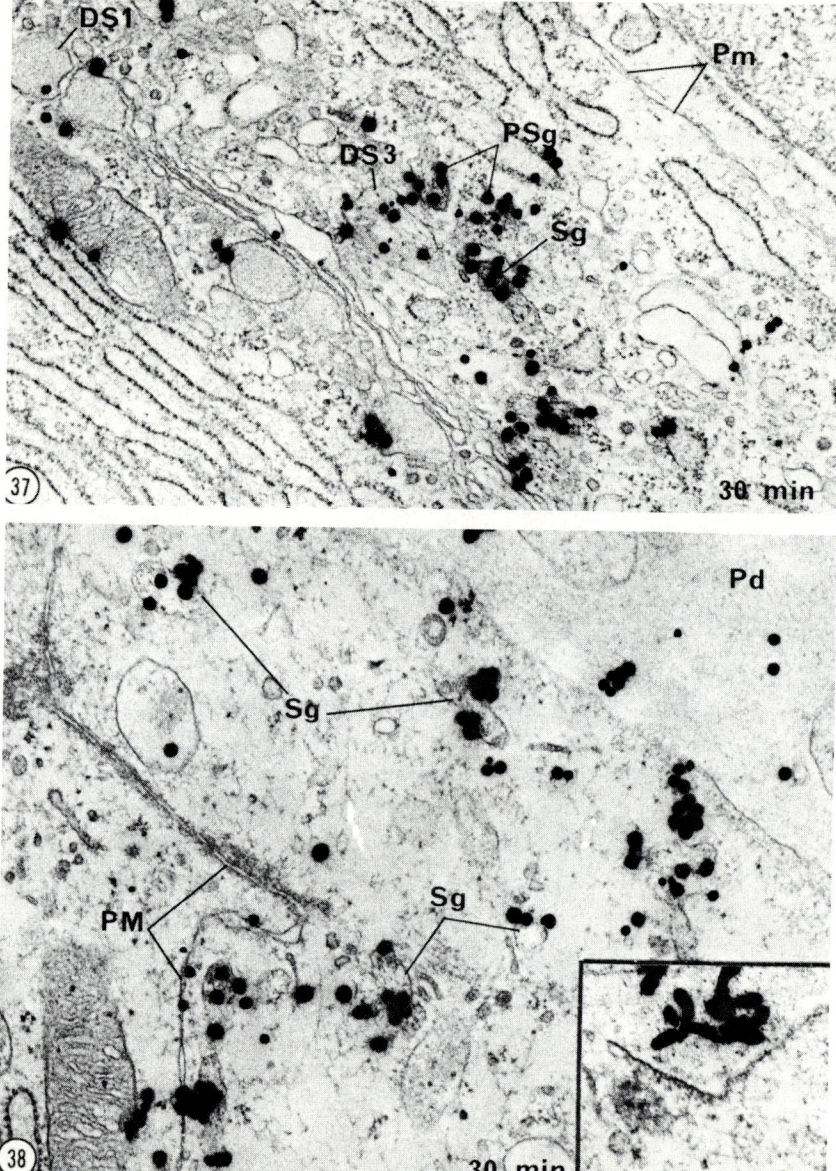

FIG. 2-2 Radioautographs of portions of odontoblasts after (^{3}H) proline injection. *(Top)* Golgi region of an odontoblast from an animal sacrificed 30 minutes after injection (4-month exposure). Silver grains predominate over profiles identified as prosecretory (PSg) and secretory (Sg) granules on one side of the Golgi apparatus. Some silver grains are still present over the rER and the distended portions of saccules (DS1 and DS4). The abundance of grains over the granules suggests that radioactivity is concentrated within them. Pm, plasma membrane. ×40,000. *(Bottom)* Apical region of odontoblast from an animal sacrificed 30 minutes after injection. The distribution of radioactivity is depicted over that area of the cell and the base of the odontoblast process (4 month exposure). Clusters of silver grains may be seen over the secretory granules (Sg) routinely found in this region. A few silver grains are also present over predentin

(Continued)

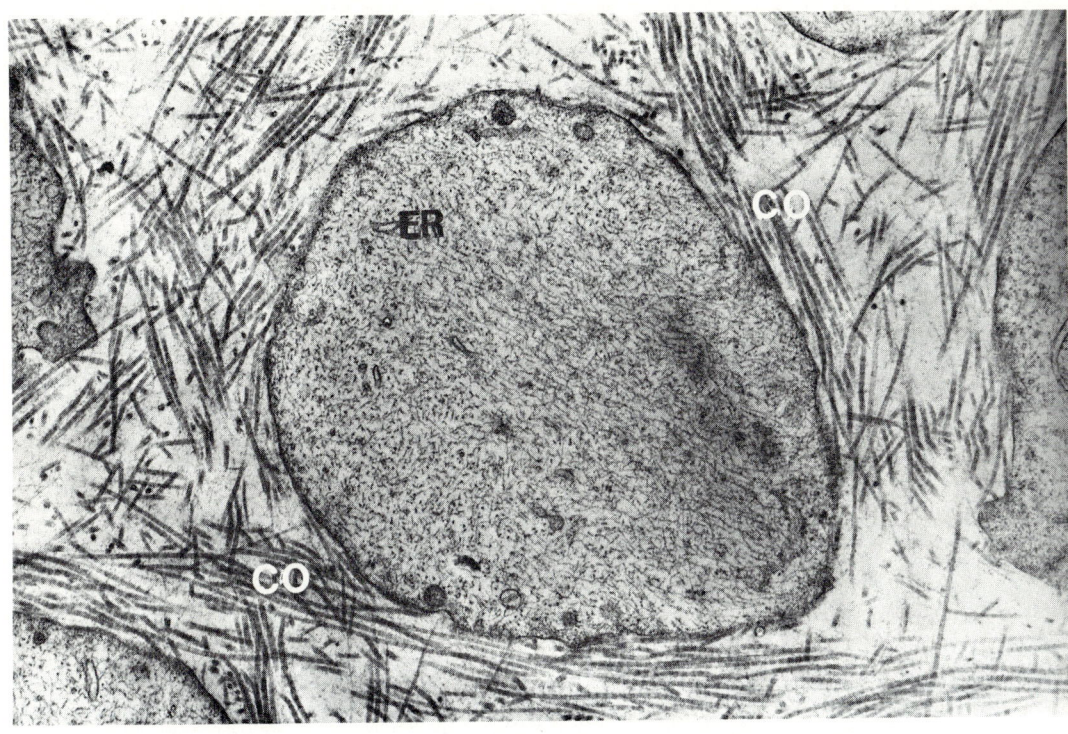

FIG. 2-3 Transverse section through the predentin layer. Odontoblastic processes, limited by a cell membrane, contain a cytoplasmic mass rich in small filaments, ribosomelike structures and some scarce endoplasmic reticulum vesicles (ER). Numerous collagen fibrils (CO) embedded in a transparent ground substance separate adjacent odontoblastic processes. ×28,000. (Frank RM: Ultrastructure of human dentine. Third Europ Symp Calc Tiss 17:259, 1966)

It is generally believed that dicalcium phosphate is formed first. In the theory of epitaxy, an oriented growth of inorganic apatite crystals occurs in the fibrous protein matrix. The nuclei produced are lodged firmly in the matrix both on and inside the fibers of the intertubular and the peritubular matrices, and they continue to grow. They are transformed to tricalcium phosphate, calcium carbonate, and apatites.

Light and electron microscope studies and electron microscope analyses (Reith, 1976; Boyde and Reith, 1977; and Boyde et al, 1978) indicate that some calcium passes through and between the odontoblasts. Such findings suggest a cellular role for dentin mineralization. Amorphous and crystalline material (probably hydroxyapatite; Takuma et al, 1977) accumulates in small membrane-bound bodies (matrix vesi-

---

(Continued)
(Pd), indicating that labeled collagen precursors have already been deposited there. Pm, plasma membrane. *Inset* depicts invagination of the plasmalemma at the base of the odontoblast process. Thirty minutes after (^{3}H) proline injection label is present over the content of that invagination. Moderately electron-dense accumulations are present on the cell surface. ×40,000. *Inset,* Elon ascorbic acid development. ×60,000. (Weinstock M, Leblond CP: Synthesis, migration, and release of precursor collagen by odontoblasts as visualized by radioautography after (^{3}H) proline administration. Cell Biol 60:92, 1974)

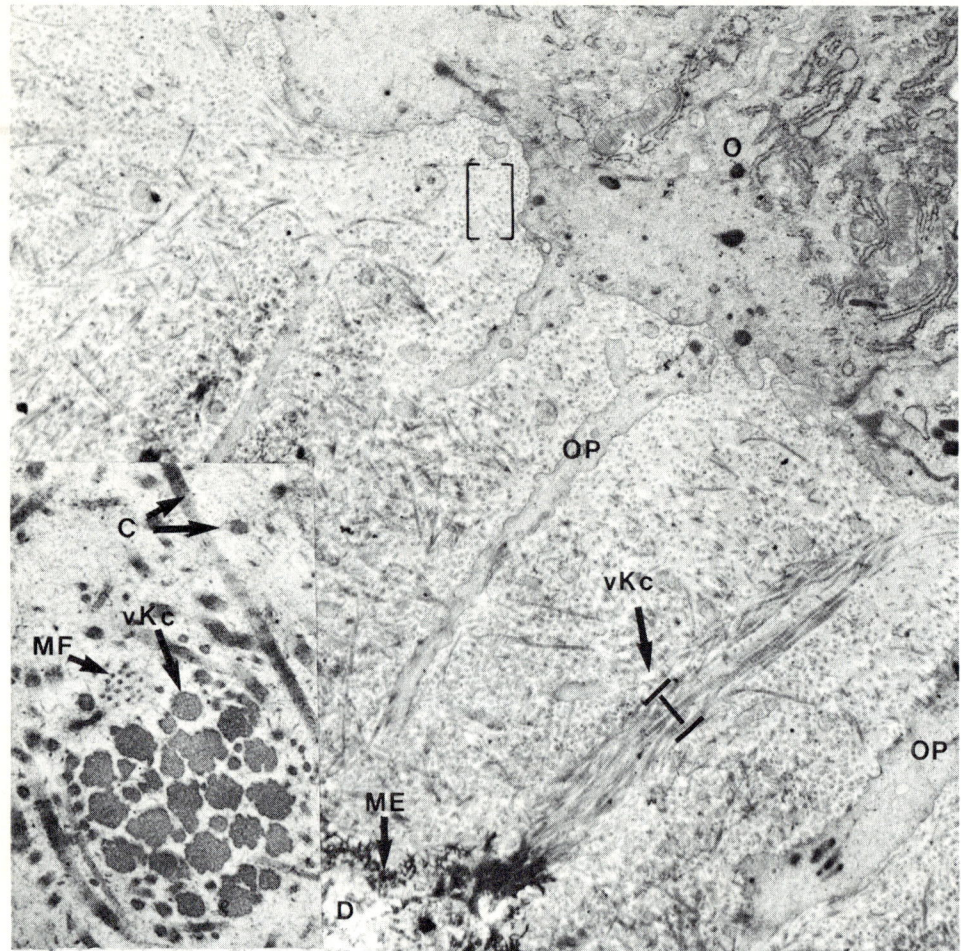

FIG. 2-4 Von Korff's fibers (vKc) traversing the predentin. Collagen fibrils of the von Korff's fiber are thick throughout the length of the fiber. In contrast, other collagen fibrils of predentin (bracketed rectangle) are thin near odontoblasts (O) and thick near mineralization front (MF). OP, odontoblastic process. ×18,400. *(Inset)* Cross section of von Korff's fiber showing thick collagen fibril (vKc, arrow) and thin microfibrils (MF). Contrast collagen fibril of von Korff's fiber to other collagen fibril (C) in predentin. ×40,500. (Courtesy of Dr. E. J. Reith, Temple University, Philadelphia).

cles) within and between the odontoblasts. The crystals eventually extend beyond the borders of the cell membrane and join with other such crystal fronts to form small lakes or globules of mineralized dentin (Eisenmann and Glick, 1972).

The presence of calcium in abacus bodies (Golgi elements) and secretory granules of the odontoblasts has been demonstrated by histochemical and x-ray analyses (Reith, 1976; Appleton and Morris, 1979). The calcium is bound to a dentin precursor, possibly precursor collagen, within the Golgi saccules (Fig. 2-6). The abacus bodies are ultrastructural manifestations of this binding. Probably these intracellular seeded sites facilitate the extracellular mineralization that follows. On electron microscopic examination, the ratio of collagen to ground substance increases closer to the mineralization front (see Fig. 1-7). The collagen appears to become associated with glycoprotein, concomitant with mineralization (Weinstock, 1972).

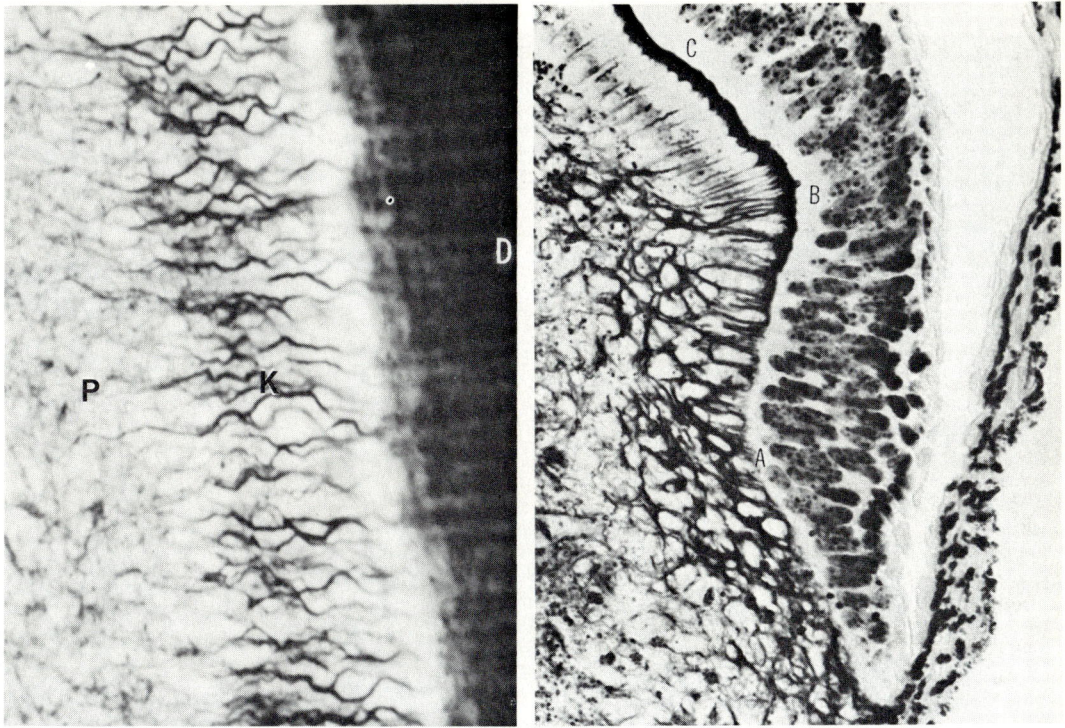

FIG. 2-5 *(Left)* Precollagenous fibers, or von Korff fibers (K), coursing from pulp (P) to mature dentin (D). Silver stain. ×960. *(Right)* Cervical loop region of the first molar tooth germ of a day-old mouse, showing the presence and distribution of von Korff fibers. In the area marked A, the von Korff fibers terminate against the internal dental epithelium without any change in width. In the area marked B, the terminal fanning of von Korff fibers is illustrated. In the area marked C, the reduction in number of von Korff fibers is apparent. Bulk impregnated with silver and Epon embedded. ×1050. (Ten Cate AR, Melcher AH, Pudy G, Wagner D: The nonfibrous nature of the von Korff fibres in developing dentine: A light and electron microscope study. Anat Rec 168:491, 1970)

FIG. 2-6 Golgi region of odontoblast showing abacus bodies. Numbers from 1 to 5 show presumed progression of young (1) to increasingly mature (5) abacus body. Bottom part of number touches abacus body. GS, Golgi saccule. ×15,000. (Courtesy of Dr. E. J. Reith, Temple University, Philadelphia).

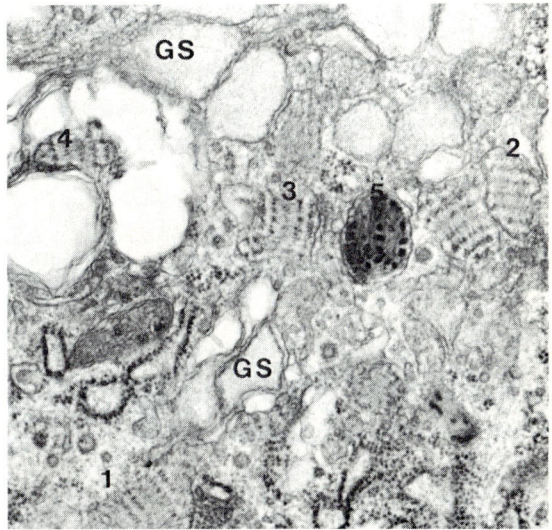

Subsequently, in the mature dentin a peritubular matrix differentiates around the cell membrane of the odontoblastic process (Fig. 2-7), and the pH becomes alkaline. This matrix is a fibrillar network with a higher electron density than that of the intertubular substance (Frank, 1966).

The peritubular matrix, which can be seen at a distance of about 60 μ to 100 μ from the predentin-dentin junction, rapidly attains a high level of mineralization (Figs. 2-8 and 2-9). Such rapid mineralization results in a gradual narrow-

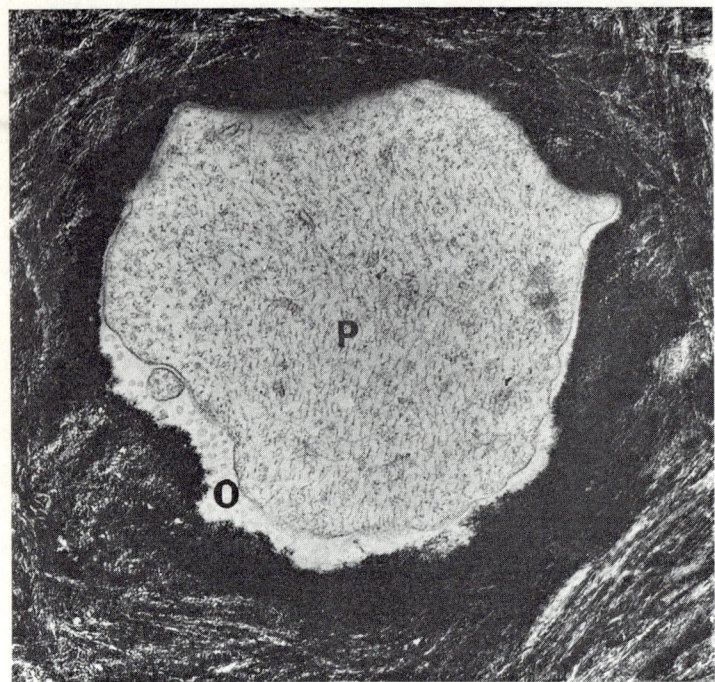

FIG. 2-7 Transverse section through a dentinal tubule. Between the cytoplasmic odontoblastic process (P), limited by a cell membrane, and the calcified wall of the tubule (in black), an organic periodontoblastic space (O) can be seen. It contains cross-sectioned collagen fibers embedded in ground substance as well as a cross-sectioned lateral extension of the process. ×52,000. (Frank RM: Ultrastructure of human dentine. Third Europ Symp Calc Tiss 17:259, 1966)

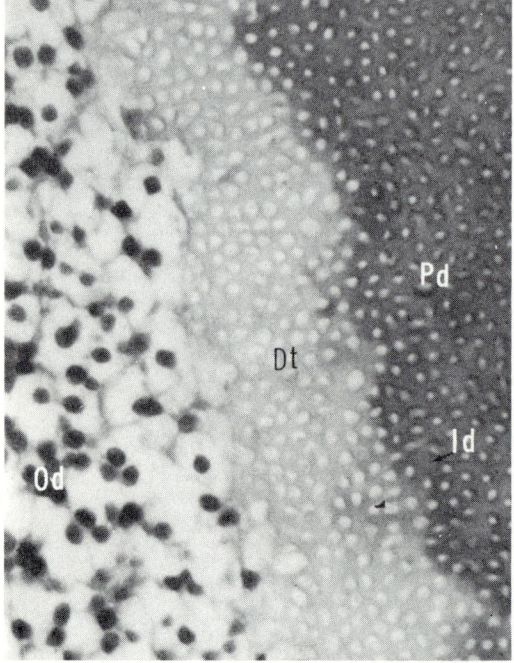

FIG. 2-8 Cross section of dentinal tubules (Dt) at pulpo-dentinal junction. The peritubular dentin (darker regions around the tubules—Pd) is more highly mineralized than the intertubular dentin (Id). Odontoblasts (Od) form a syncytium. ×960.

ing of the dentinal tubules. In adult teeth, mineralization of the intertubular matrix begins at a distance of 20 μ to 25 μ from the predentin-dentin junction.

The microradiographic* studies of Mjör (1966a) indicate that the zone of dentin close to the dentin-predentin border is highly mineral-

* Microradiography is used for the study of mineralized tissues. It is based on the absorption of x-rays. When x-rays pass through a section of tissue, they are absorbed to varying degrees, depending on the atomic number of the material in the section, the amount of substance and the energy (wavelength) of the x-rays. The technique consists of exposing ground sections of teeth to x-rays and recording the exposure on a film with a fine-grained emulsion. After the film is developed, the micrograph can be examined in the light microscope. Differences in degree of mineralization, as depicted by variations in degree of grayness, can be measured by a densitometer (Mjör and Pindborg, 1973).

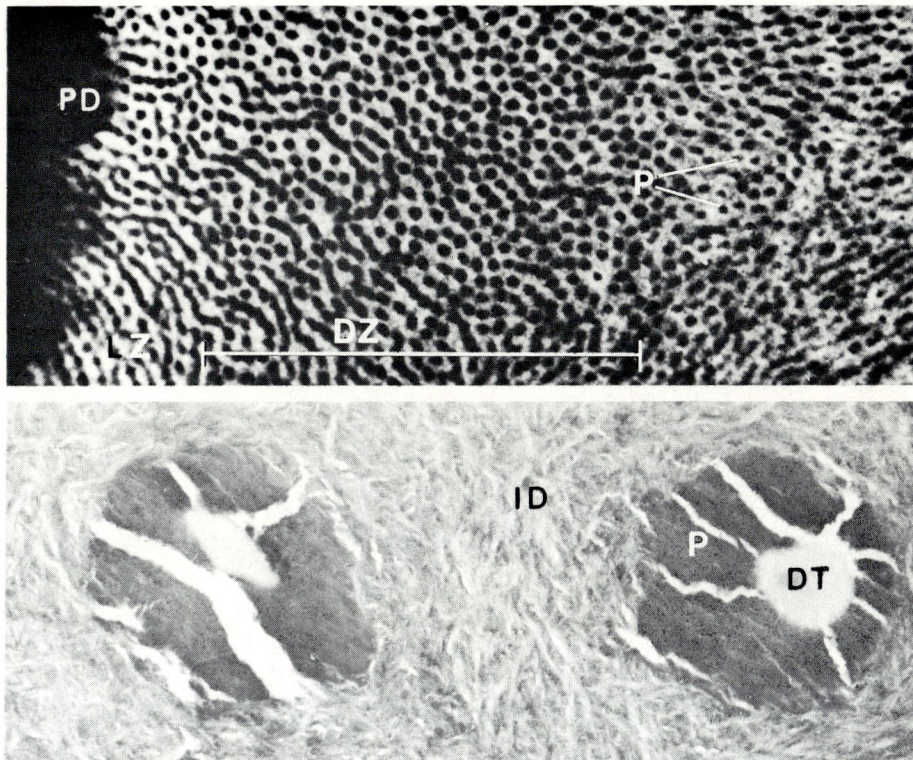

FIG. 2-9 *(Top)* Microradiograph of undemineralized section, showing cross-sectioned dentinal tubules. Note that the intertubular dentin is darker (less mineralized) in the dark zone (DZ) than in the light zone (LZ). Tubules with highly mineralized peritubular dentin, P, are absent in the dark and the light zones but they regularly are found more peripherally. PD, predentin. ×450. *(Bottom)* Electron micrograph showing dentinal tubule (DT). peritubular dentin (P) and intertubular dentin (ID). Peritubular dentin is highly mineralized, and it therefore cracks easily during the preparation of ultrathin sections, as shown here. ×12,000. (Mjör IA, Pindborg JJ: Histology of the Human Tooth. Copenhagen, Munksgaard, 1973)

ized (Figs. 2-10 and 2-11). The width of this zone depends on the age and the stage of development of the tooth. Adjacent to this highly mineralized zone, a broad zone with low mineral content was found. Variations in the mineralization of these two zones was considered to be due mainly to variations in the mineralization of the intertubular matrix. A third and a fourth zone, representing the major portion of the dentin, contained highly mineralized peritubular matrices. Acid mucopolysaccharides were present at the mineralization sites.

Rapid mineralization of the peritubular matrix at further distances results in a gradual narrowing of the dentinal tubules (Fig. 2-12).

Electron microprobe analyses indicate considerable variation in the mineralization of dentin (Fig. 2-13). In young teeth, the peritubular matrix is less mineralized than the intertubular matrix. With age, the peritubular dentin becomes more mineralized (Miller et al, 1971). Thus, it appears that dentin is initially mineralized, in the developmental stage, at the predentin-dentin junction. Here the intertubular dentin mineralizes. Farther peripherally, a second mineralization front occurs in the peritubular matrix. Thus, further physiologic mineralization (sclerosis) of the dentinal tubules continues throughout life.

The hydroxyapatite crystals of dentin have

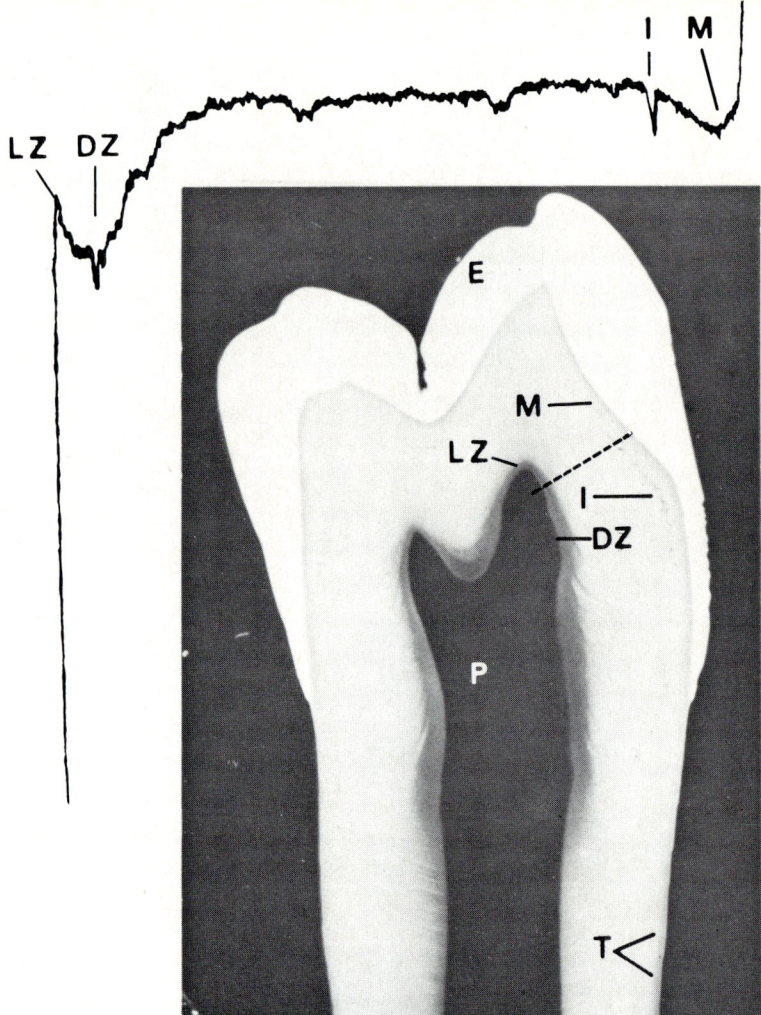

FIG. 2-10 Microradiograph of undemineralized section of tooth. Dotted line indicates position of densitometric reading, i.e., curve showing degree of grayness on the microradiograph. M, mantle dentin; I, interglobular dentin; DZ, dark (less mineralized) zone near pulp (note that it branches into the dentin); LZ, light (more mineralized) zone near pulp; P, pulp and predentin (which is unmineralized); T, Tomes' granular layer; E, enamel. ×6. (Mjör IA, Pindborg JJ: Histology of the Human Tooth, Copenhagen, Munksgaard, 1973)

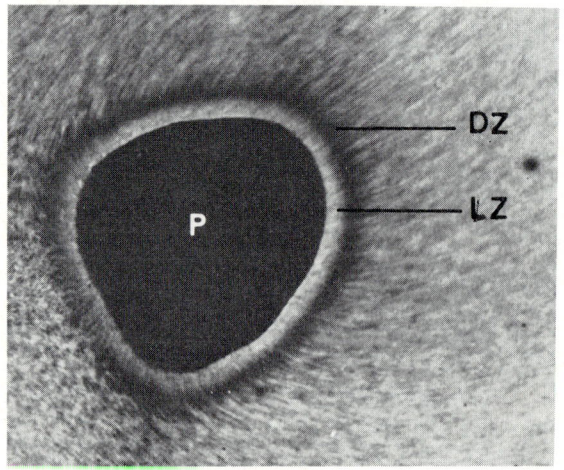

FIG. 2-11 Microradiograph of undemineralized section prepared through a pulp horn. P, pulp and predentin (which is unmineralized); DZ, dark (less mineralized) zone near pulp; LZ, light (more mineralized) zone near pulp. ×60. (Mjör IA, Pindborg JJ: Histology of the Human Tooth, Copenhagen, Munksgaard, 1973)

been estimated to be up to 2000 Å in length and 20 Å to 180 Å in thickness.

Studies with the scanning and transmission electron microscopes indicate that the crystal structure of the peritubular dentin is different from that of the intertubular dentin. The peritubular crystals are small, equal-sided, and approximately 250 Å in size (Lester and Boyde, 1968). The crystals of intertubular dentin are larger, hexagonal plates of hydroxyapatite, 1000 Å in length and 20 Å to 35 Å in thickness, which appear needle shaped when viewed edge-on (Johansen, 1964; Fig. 2–14).

Once the matrix becomes mineralized, mature dentin is formed. Under normal circumstances, there is always a lag in the mineralization of the dentin matrix. Thus, a thin layer of unmineralized dentin, or predentin, is present in sections of normally functioning teeth (see Figs. 2–10 and 2–11). Alterations in the width and quality of this layer indicate irregularities in pulp metabolism due to disease processes or drugs. Dentin thus consists of a matrix composed of protein and sulfated acid mucopolysaccharides into which calcium and phosphorus salts are deposited.

Dentin is elaborated as a tubular structure in a rhythmic fashion (Kawasaki et al, 1980). Larsson and Linde (1971) have suggested that such rhythmic dentin deposition is controlled by the

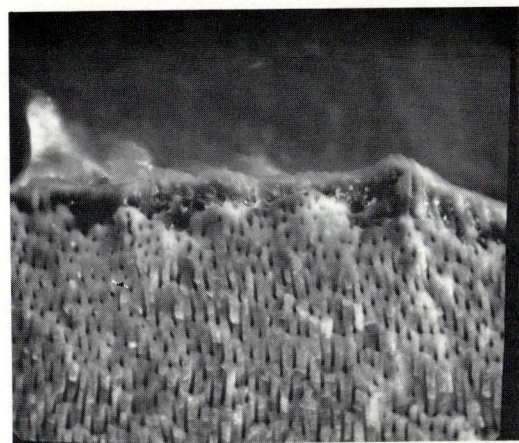

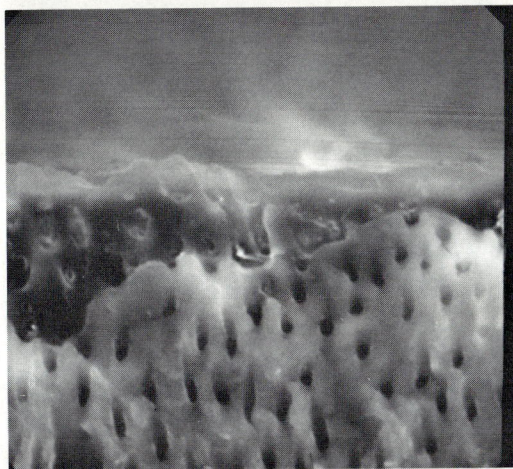

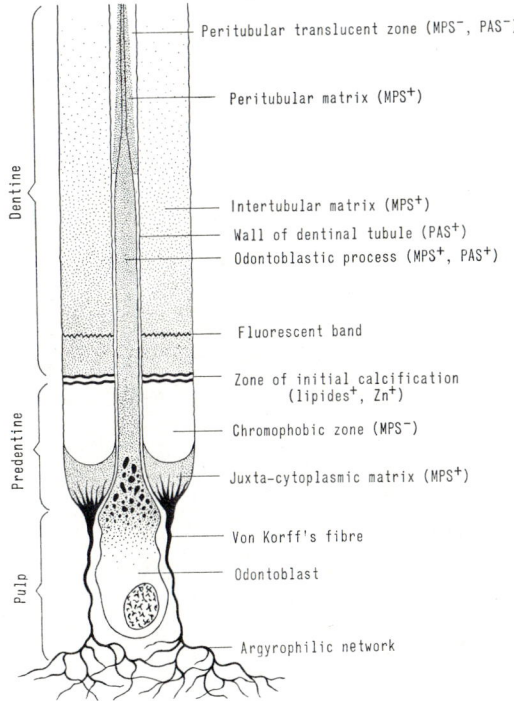

FIG. 2-12 Histochemical assessment of dentinogenesis (Fiore-Donno G, Baume LJ: Etude histochimique de la dentinogenése humaine. Helv odont acta 10 (Suppl IV):141, 1966)

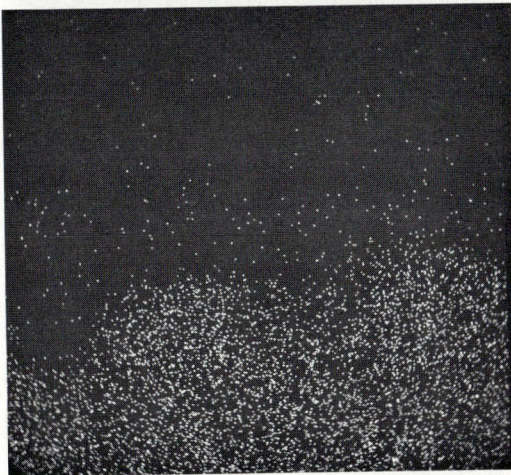

FIG. 2-13 Scanning electron microscope study of dentin. *(Top)* Coronal dentin of mature tooth. ×600. *(Middle)* Higher magnification. ×1800. *(Bottom)* Electron microprobe analysis of calcium distribution in middle figure. White dots represent calcium.

2
DENTIN

Dentin is one of the mineralized tissues in the body. The teeth and their supporting structures contain four of these tissues, namely, enamel, dentin, cementum, and bone. The fifth tissue that may mineralize is cartilage. Pathologic mineralizations also occur within the dental pulp.

The dentin is involved in disease processes of the dental pulp, as well as in endodontic therapy.

INITIATION OF DENTINOGENESIS

Dentin formation is initiated by a specialized group of cells, the odontoblasts, which differentiate from cells of the dental papilla at about the eighth or the ninth week of fetal life. Odontoblasts are cells that are believed to be derived from the mesoderm, the germ layer from which the connective tissues of the body are derived. However, there is a mounting body of evidence that the origin of the odontoblasts may be the neural crest (deBeer, 1947; Symons, 1955). When these cells are about to elaborate dentin, they assume a tall, columnar appearance and metachromatic granules appear in their cytoplasm (See Fig. 1–7).

The Use of Tissue Stains. The terms basophilia, acidophilia, and metachromasia are in widespread use in the dental literature and perhaps should be defined. All proteins are made up of combinations of amino acids, and they have both acidic and basic or hydroxyl groups present. A substance that is stained by the basic radical of the dye is basophilic. A substance that is stained by the acid radical of the dye is acidophilic. Most cells are basophilic, that is, they are stained bluish by hematoxylin. The term metachromasia refers to staining that is different from the color of the dye. For instance, a stain such as toluidine blue is bluish, but it stains certain tissues pinkish or violet rather than bluish. This color change indicates metachromasia, a property of polysaccharides of high molecular weight.

Various other stains are employed to study the chemical characteristics of tissue components. A brief description of these stains, which are mentioned throughout this text, follows:

Periodic Acid-Schiff (PAS) is used to identify glycogen and carbohydrate-protein complexes containing galactose, fucose, and hexosamine. The color developed in tissue sections varies, depending on the quantity and availability of the carbohydrates present.

Alcian Blue is used to locate acid mucopolysaccharides and to identify calcium in tissue

circadian rhythmic activity of peripheral adrenergic neurons that produce variations in the blood flow to the odontoblasts. The tubules proceed from the dentinoenamel junction pulpward in a curving, recurving S-shaped course. As a result of this, cutting of the tubules at one end near the enamel causes reactions in the pulp subjacent to the cut tubules.

The dentin is not as hard as the enamel, since it has a much higher organic content. Hence, it can be cut more easily. When dentin is demineralized, the remaining organic matrix stains pinkish with eosin. The dentin has a consistency similar to that of cartilage, and, when demineralized, it can be bent or compressed and will spring back into shape. Dentin has a high degree of elasticity, and this property is utilized in a number of operative procedures, such as plugging gold foil, in which it yields slightly under the force of the mallet blow and traps the foil.

Whenever the dentin is damaged (by abrasion, erosion, attrition, dental caries or operative procedures), some reaction takes place within the pulp, because the dentinal tubules contain odontoblastic processes that are extensions of pulp cells and, in the crown, extend the length of the tubules up to the dentinoenamel junction and, sometimes, even slightly into the enamel. Thus, it is impossible to cut the dentin without affecting the pulp in some way.

The dentin contains both precollagenous and collagenous fibers and, possibly, some atypical collagen fibrils (Warshawsky, 1972; Fig. 2–15). The precollagenous fibers (von Korff fibers) are young, immature collagenous fibers and ground substance that stain black with silver salts (see Fig. 2–5). They are therefore known as argyrophilic fibers, that is, they "like" silver and attract it. They may reach 2000 Å in thickness.

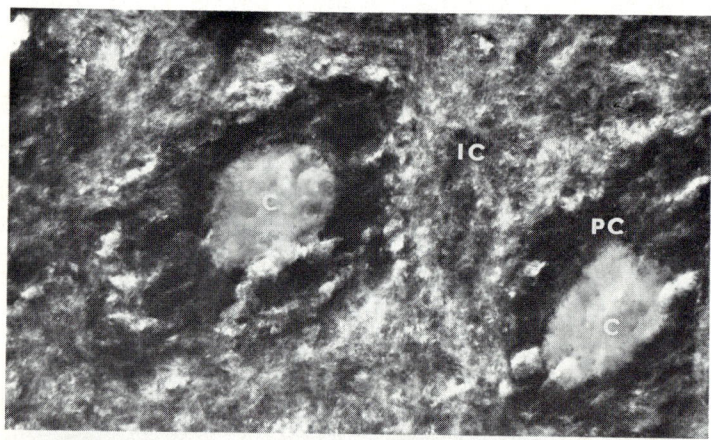

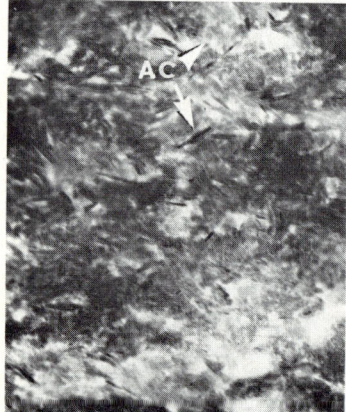

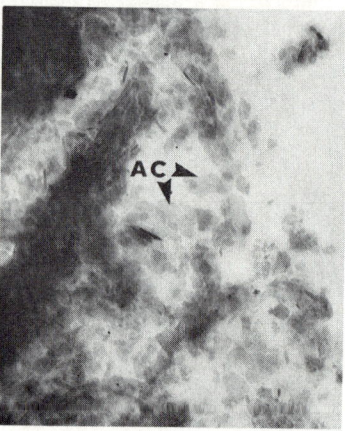

FIG. 2-14 Permanent human dentin from erupted teeth, inorganic phase. (Top) Cross section of dentinal canals (C) surrounded by a hypermineralized pericanalicular zone (PC); intercanalicular areas (IC) are less densely mineralized. ×16,000 approx. (Bottom, left) Section of intercanalicular matrix; individual apatite crystallites (AC) are seen in edge and broad surface views. ×75,900 approx. (Bottom, right) Broad surface view of apatite crystallites (AC) from edge of section. ×99,000 approx. (Johansen E: Microstructure of enamel and dentin. J Dent Res 43:1007, 1964. Copyright by the American Dental Association. Reproduced by permission)

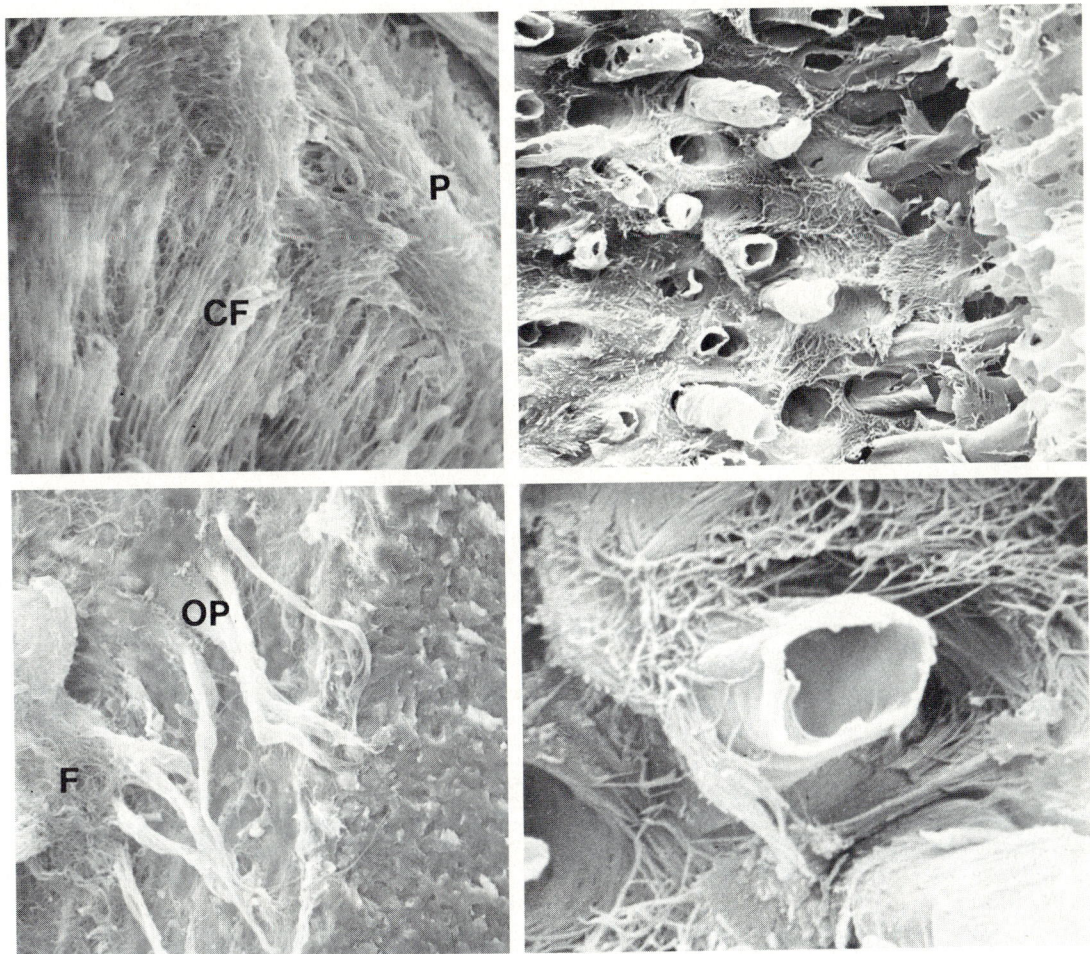

FIG. 2-15 *(Top, left)* Collagenous fibers (CF) of dentin. P, pulp. ×600. *(Bottom, left)* Network of fibrils (F) in dentin. OP, odontoblastic processes. ×600. *(Top, right)* Exposed predentin. Pulp tissue to the right with interrupted processes. The tubule apertures contain the other end of the fractured, tubelike processes. Underneath, the processes are continuous. A network of fibrils is seen between the tubules. The fibrils close to the process are coated with an amorphous material contributing to a membranous structure surrounding the cytoplasmic process. ×2200. *(Bottom, right)* Detail from picture at *top, right*. The process is surrounded by a network of fibrils closely attached to the process. ×11,000. (Pictures at right, top and bottom, from Brännström M, Garberoglio R: The dentinal tubules and the odontoblast processes. Acta odont scand 30:291, 1972)

CHEMICAL STRUCTURE

Dentin is composed of approximately 70% inorganic matter, 18% organic matter, and 12% water (Mjör, 1972). The inorganic portion is mainly hydroxyapatite. The bulk of the organic portion (approximately 90%) is composed of collagen. This collagen has a low metabolic turnover (Borggreven et al, 1979).

The amino acid content of dentin collagen has been analyzed by a variety of analytic methods that include microbiologic assay, quantitative paper chromatography, and ion-exchange methods. From these analyses, it appears that the main protein constituent of dentin has a composition similar to that of collagen from other mammalian tissues, especially bone and tendon. Four amino acids account for two thirds of the

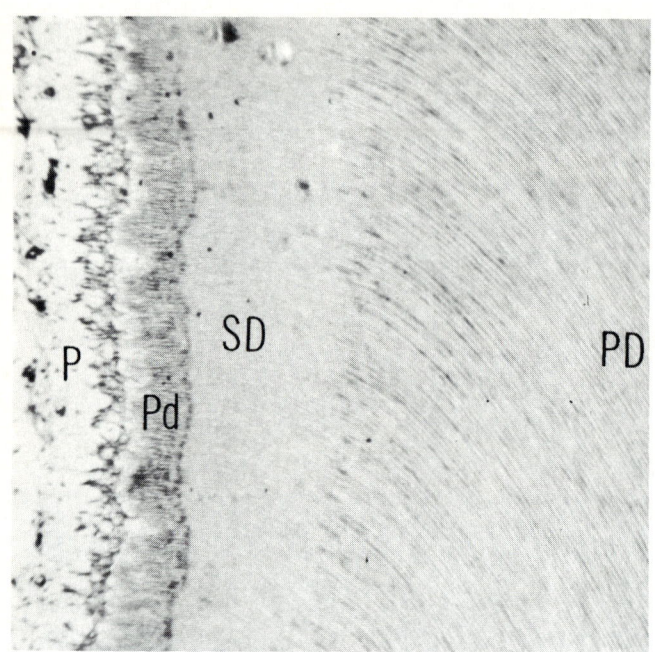

FIG. 2-16 Between primary dentin (PD) and secondary dentin (SD), a slight change in the direction of the tubules may be observed. Predentin (Pd) is elaborated continuously by the odontoblasts of the pulp (P). ×54.

total number of residues. These are glycine (approximately 1 in 3), alanine (1 in 9), proline (1 in 8.5) and hydroxyproline (1 in 10; Eastoe, 1963). Because of the amino acid content of dentin, radioactive amino acids such as tritiated glycine and proline have been used for the study of the synthesis of dentinal matrix (Carneiro and Leblond, 1959; Young, 1962; Slavkin et al, 1967). Even the minute quantities of some amino acids that are present in dentinal collagen, such as histidine (0.47%; Piez, 1961) are detected radioautographically in the odontoblasts and the immediate dentinal matrix 1 hour after isotope injection (Hwang et al, 1963).

Dentin also contains a small quantity (less than 1%) of citrate, an organic anion that is widely distributed in mineralized tissues. In addition, dentin contains a small fraction of albumin (Okamura, 1983), and of lipid components that have been demonstrated by histochemical reactions (Sognnaes and Wislocki, 1950), paper chromatography (Dirksen, 1962), and various extraction methods (Allred, 1968). Cholesterol, cholesterol esters, various glycerides, fatty acids, and various phospholipids have been identified (Dirksen and Marinetti, 1970; Odutuga and Prout, 1973). The lipids, which are located in the peritubular matrix, become unmasked by dental caries (Allred, 1966a,b).

SECONDARY DENTIN

Secondary dentin is elaborated after tooth eruption; it is similar to primary dentin but differs in that there is a change in the direction of the tubules. This change is visible in histologic sections (Fig. 2-16). Dentin is deposited continuously by the pulp tissue.

Various investigators have reported differences in the quantity of daily dentin deposition in animals. Schour (1960) estimated that dentin forms at a rate of 16 μm/day in rats, and about 4 μm/day in macaque monkeys. Others (Rölling and Melson, 1979; Wennberg et al, 1982) have reported a 0.8 μm daily deposit of secondary dentin in monkey teeth.

In man, Schour has claimed that 4 μm of secondary dentin is deposited daily. As a result of such continuous deposition, the volume of the pulp becomes progressively smaller with age. Investigations using labeled compounds that participate in dentin matrix formation, such as ^{35}S-sulfate (Bélanger, 1958), ^{14}C-glucose (Kumamoto and Leblond, 1958; Leblond, Bélanger, and Greulich, 1955), ^{3}H-methionine (Karpishka, Leblond, and Carneiro, 1959), and ^{3}H-leucine (Carneiro and Leblond, 1959) demonstrate the incremental or layered character of dentin deposition by radioautography (Fig. 2-17).

RADIOAUTOGRAPHY

A radioautograph is made by placing a histologic section or a slab of tooth structure that contains radioactive materials in close contact with a photographic emulsion. The alpha and beta particles emitted from the tagged material strike the silver bromide crystals contained in the photographic emulsion, thereby producing a latent image. This is the same process as that which occurs when an ordinary photograph is made, except that, in the latter, the radiation is in the range of the visible spectrum. The film is then developed and fixed. Darkened areas on the emulsion correspond to the distribution of the isotope in the section of the tooth.

In the labeled carbon experiments, the tagged carbon in glucose, which was incorporated into the matrix, was no longer demonstrable in the matrix as time went by, because the matrix containing the isotope was subsequently mineralized. The new matrix that was elaborated after the glucose administration did not contain the isotope. This experiment demonstrated the continuous deposition of dentin throughout life. A similar demonstration of continuous dentin deposition was made by Young and Greulich (1963), using tritiated glycine in rats and by Tiber (1971), using ^{3}H-leucine, in rhesus monkeys. The portion of the dentin matrix formed at the time of the ^{3}H-glycine or ^{3}H-leucine administration was intensely labeled. By contrast, ma-

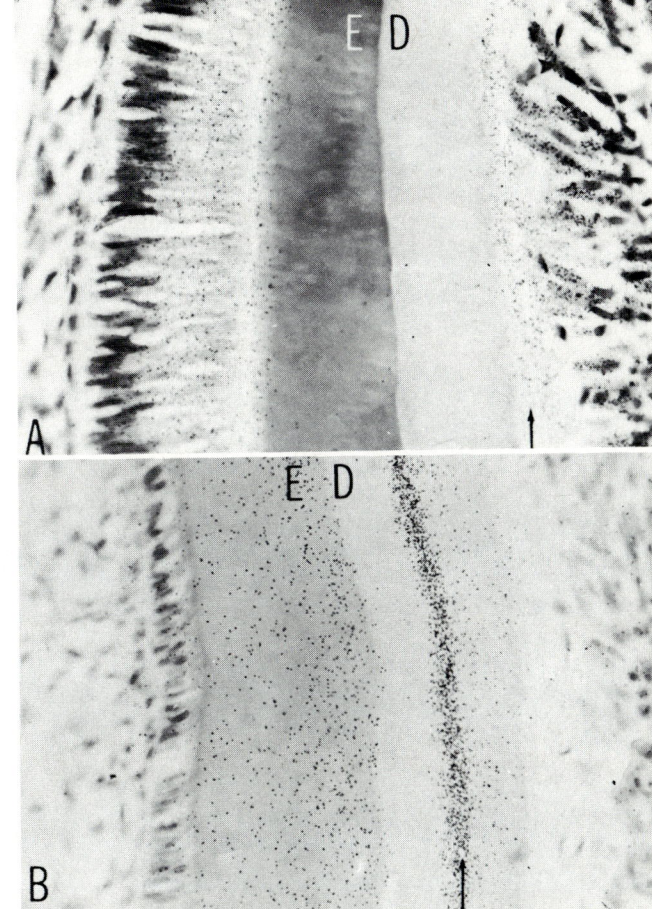

FIG. 2-17 (A) Dentin and enamel matrices, from rat sacrificed 1 hour after administration of glycine-^{3}H. The reaction of odontoblasts seen at 30 minutes has been partially transferred to the newly formed predentin (arrow). Similarly, a reactive layer of newly formed enamel matrix is apparent at the apices of the ameloblasts. ×275. (B) Dentin and enamel matrices, from rat sacrificed 96 hours after administration of glycine-^{3}H. The major reaction band in dentin matrix (arrow) and the diffusely labeled dentin matrix formed subsequent to the early postinjection period are clearly illustrated. Preinjection dentin matrix is unlabeled. Enamel matrix is diffusely labeled, but the reaction is more intense in the region of the dentinoenamel junction. ×260. (Young RW, Greulich CK: Distinctive autoradiographic patterns of glycine incorporation in rat enamel and dentine matrices. Arch Oral Biol 8:509, 1963)

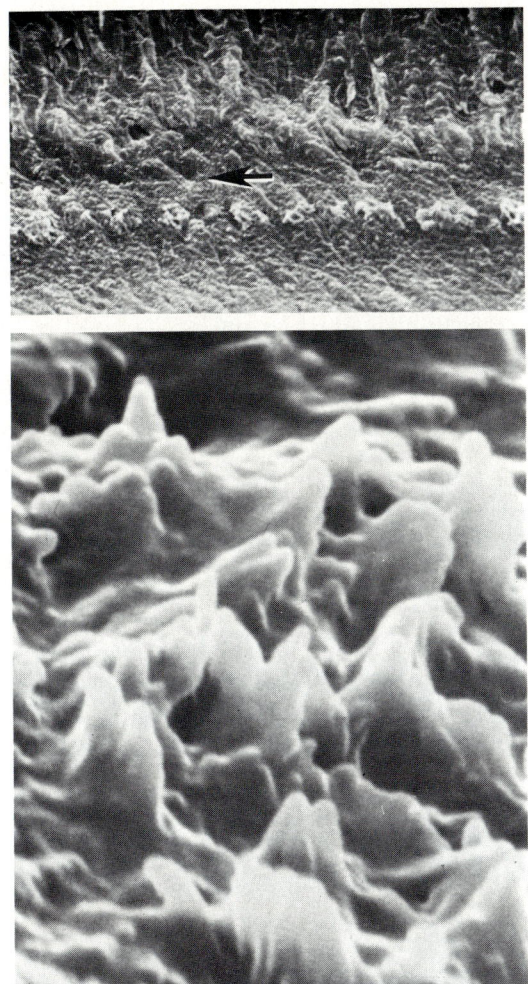

FIG. 2-19 *(Top)* Scanning electron micrograph of demineralized tooth in cross section. Tomes' granular layer appears as elevated focal areas below cementodentinal junction (arrow). ×1000. *(Bottom)* Scanning electron micrograph of demineralized tooth in cross section. One of the Tomes' "granules" shows exposed fibrils oriented longitudinally in the tooth. ×22,000. (Shackleford JM: The structure of Tomes' granular layer in dog premolar teeth. Anat Rec 170:357, 1971)

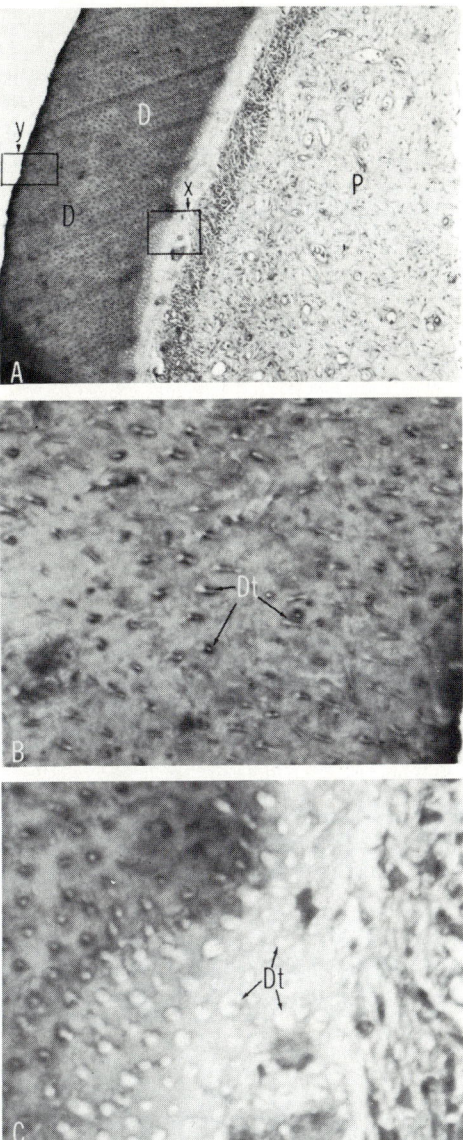

FIG. 2-20 Width of dentinal tubules. *(A)* Cross section of the pulp (P) and the dentin (D) of a young tooth. ×135. *(B)* Higher magnification of the region outlined by rectangle *y* in *(A)*. In this region the dentinal tubules (Dt) are narrower than those at the pulpo-dentinal region. ×960. *(C)* The dentinal tubules in higher magnification of region of rectangle *x* in *(A)*. The dentinal tubules (Dt) are indicated by arrows. ×960.

WIDTH OF DENTINAL TUBULES

The dentinal tubules vary in width from the dentinoenamel to the pulpodentinal junction (Fig. 2-20). Generally, the tubules are wider at the pulpodentinal junction (approximately 5 μ) than at the dentinoenamel junction, where they narrow to about 1 μ. However, Garberoglio and Brännström (1976) have claimed that decalcification increases the diameter of the dentin tubules by removing the peritubular dentin. Their scanning electron micrograph examination of undemineralized, fractured coronal dentin revealed that, near the pulp, the tubule diameter was 2.5 μm, in the middle dentin it was 1.2 μm, and at the periphery it decreased to 0.9 μm. Under normal circumstances the odontoblastic process has been observed, both in rat dentin (Garant, 1972) and in human dentin (Brännström and Garberoglio, 1972; Tsatsas and Frank, 1972), to become attenuated at its distal end, toward the dentinoenamel junction. There, the dentinal tubule is either empty or filled with a combination of amorphous substances and thick collagen fibers (Fig. 2-21).

As the individual gets older, the dentinal tubule narrows through the deposition of peritubular dentin or the deposition of large hydroxyapa-

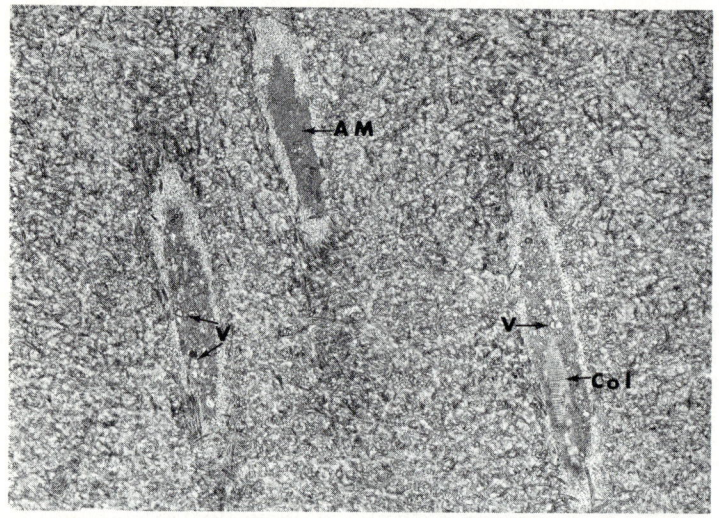

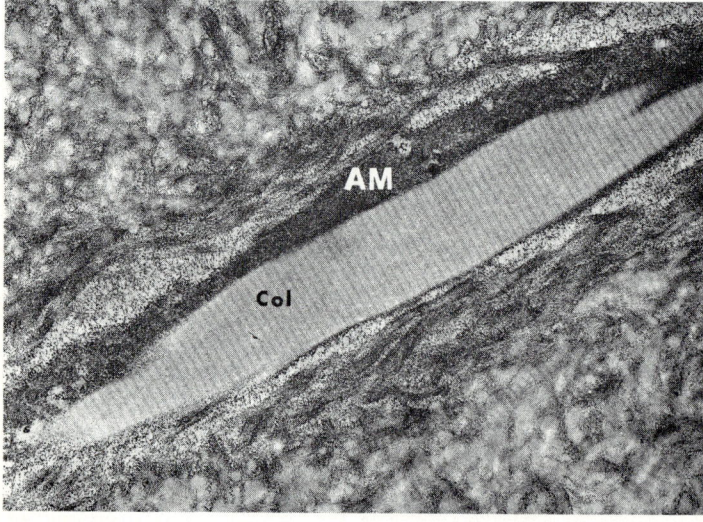

FIG. 2-21 *(Top)* Three odontoblast tubules (located about 100 μm from predentin-dentin junction) appear occluded by a dense amorphous matrix (AM), vesicular elements (V), and collagen (Col). ×8000. *(Bottom)* Thick collagen fibers (Col) and amorphous matrix (AM) occluding an odontoblast tubule. ×30,000. (Garant PR: The organization of microtubules within rat odontoblast processes revealed by perfusion fixation with glutaraldehyde. Arch Oral Biol 17:1047, 1972)

TABLE 2-1
Concentrations of the Sixteen Elements in Normal Human Enamel

GROUP	ELEMENT	NUMBER OF SAMPLES ANALYZED	MEAN CONTRIBUTION (±s.d.)
Group I	Mg	8	0.28% ± 0.01
	Na	8	0.70% ± 0.01
	Cl	8	0.32% ± 0.01
	Al	8	86.13 ppm ± 4.54
	Ca	8	37.03% ± 0.56
Group II	Cr	6	1.02 ppm ± 0.51
	Ba	7	125.11 ppm ± 23.68
	Sb	9	0.96 ppm ± 0.69
	Ag	9	0.56 ppm ± 0.29
	Zn	8	263.42 ppm ± 14.80
	Co	10	0.13 ppm ± 0.13
	Fe	9	118.27 ppm ± 71.65
Group III	Sr	7	111.19 ppm ± 9.86
Group IV	Au	7	0.11 ppm ± 0.07
	Br	8	33.79 ppm ± 5.71
	Mn	4	0.59 ppm ± 0.04

(Retief DH, Cleaton-Jones PE, Turkstra J, De Wet WJ: The quantitative analysis of 16 elements in normal human enamel and dentine by neutron activation analysis and high-resolution gamma-spectrometry. Arch Oral Biol 16:1257, 1971)

tite crystals. This is a normal aging phenomenon and may partially explain the reduction in the prevalence of dental caries in adults compared with that in children. Toward the dentinoenamel junction, the dentinal tubules send out branching processes and anastomose with each other. Close to the dentinoenamel junction, one dentinal tubule may branch into two.

METABOLIC INTERCHANGES

The enamel and the dentin are not static tissues and do not remain unchanged for the duration of an individual's life. The tubules of the dentin are constantly bathed in fluid. There is an exchange of fluid that occurs both from the pulp side outward into the dentin and from the enamel side inward toward the pulp (Pashley et al, 1981). Substances penetrate through the enamel and the dentin and into the pulp (Bartelstone, 1951).

Conversely, metabolic exchange occurs from the pulp outward through the dentinal tubules. This fluid outflow has been demonstrated by the use of systemically administered tracers. For example, when horseradish peroxidase or lanthanum nitrate are injected into the bloodstream, they pass directly from the pulp to the predentin and dentinal tubules (Tanaka, 1980; Sasaki et al, 1982). In other experiments, tagged vitamin C and tritiated glycine were found in the dentin or the pulp (Yale et al, 1959; Young and Greulich, 1963). Investigations of the ^{90}Sr content of deciduous incisors have demonstrated an accumulation of this isotope in dentin as a result of fallout from nuclear testing. The uptake of ^{90}Sr is much more intense in dentin or bone than in developing enamel (White et al, 1980). Systemically administered elements, such as fluorine and strontium, affect both matrix formation and mineralization of dentin. With some ions, the effects are indelibly recorded in the dentin as a so-called calciotraumatic response (Eisenmann and Yaeger, 1969; Meffert and Kammerer, 1973).

In recent years, systemically administered antibiotics, notably tetracyclines, were found to have been incorporated in teeth of growing children, resulting in yellowish staining of the dentin. The tetracycline, because of its affinity for calcium, is also deposited in the bones (Johnson and Mitchell, 1966). During normal bone resorption, the released tetracycline molecule can

TABLE 2-2
Concentration of the Sixteen Elements in Normal Human Dentin

GROUP	ELEMENT	NUMBER OF SAMPLES ANALYZED	MEAN CONTRIBUTION ($\pm$ S.D.)
Group I	Mg	6	$0.87\% \pm 0.03$
	Na	6	$0.55\% \pm 0.03$
	Cl	8	$0.035\% \pm 0.003$
	Al	7	68.6 ppm ± 22.5
	Ca	7	$26.24\% \pm 1.49$
Group II	Cr	8	1.99 ppm ± 0.84
	Ba	7	129.05 ppm ± 54.69
	Sb	10	0.69 ppm ± 0.41
	Ag	6	2.18 ppm ± 0.84
	Zn	9	172.81 ppm ± 11.14
	Co	10	1.11 ppm ± 0.27
	Fe	9	93.38 ppm ± 35.05
Group III	Sr	6	94.33 ppm ± 11.47
Group IV	Au	8	0.07 ppm ± 0.04
	Br	6	114.37 ppm ± 2.80
	Mn	5	0.63 ppm ± 0.05

(Retief DH, Cleaton-Jones PE, Turkstra J, De Wet WJ: The quantitative analysis of 16 elements in normal human enamel and dentine by neutron activation analysis and high-resolution gamma-spectrometry. Arch Oral Biol 16:1257, 1971)

again be incorporated into the dentin of developing teeth (Stewart, 1973).

The usefulness of fluid exchange between the pulp and the dentin is one reason for keeping the pulp alive. Through this active interchange, the dentin may be remineralized under dental caries. Also, when certain irritating substances are placed on the dentin of a tooth during operative procedures, the dentinal tubules sometimes become more mineralized. This is called sclerosis of the dentin. The mineral salts get into the tubules from the circulation of the pulp. Many other substances circulating in the bloodstream find their way to the pulp and, eventually, into the dentinal tubules and enamel.

Detection of such elements has been accomplished by various analytical procedures such as chemical analysis, direct-current spectrum excitation, spectrographic methods, x-ray emission spectrography, mass spectrometry, neutron activation analysis, and high-resolution gamma-spectrometry. The last-mentioned method was used by Retief et al (1971) to determine the concentration of 16 elements in normal human enamel and dentin (Tables 2-1 and 2-2). The concentrations of some of these elements differ depending on the individual's age and sex (Derise et al, 1974) and to their concentrations in soil (Lappalainen et al, 1981). Some of the cationic elements in dentin have a direct positive relationship with each other (Lappalainen and Knuuttila, 1982).

Dietary deficiencies, such as those of calcium and phosphorus, did not alter the tooth chemistry of experimental animals (McClure et al, 1966).

BIBLIOGRAPHY

Allred H: Histochemical observations on the lipids of carious human dentine. Nature 210:748, 1966a

Allred H: Histochemical observations on the lipids of sound human dentine. Nature 210:646, 1966b

Allred H: Investigations into the relationship between the lipid and other components of human dentine. Arch Oral Biol 13:1077, 1968

Appleton J, Morris DC: An ultrastructural investigation of the role of the odontoblast in matrix calcification using the potassium pyroantimonate osmium method for calcium localization. Arch Oral Biol 24:467, 1979

Armstrong WG: Modifications of the properties and composition of dentin matrix caused by dental caries. Adv Oral Biol 1:309, 1964

Bartelstone HJ: Radioiodine penetration through intact enamel, with uptake by bloodstream and thyroid gland. J Dent Res 30:728, 1951

Bélanger LF: Autoradiographic detection of radiosulfate incorporation by the growing enamel of rats and hamsters. J Dent Res 34:20, 1955

Bélanger LF: Autoradiographic visualization of atomic interchange in various mineralized tissues. J Nat Cancer Inst 13:288, 1958

Bergman G, Engfeldt B: Studies on mineralized dentine. Acta Odont Scand 12:99, 1955

Borggreven JMPM, Hoppenbrouwers PMM, Gorissen R: Radiochemical determination of the metabolic activity of collagen in mature dentin. J Dent Res 58:2120, 1979

Boyde A, Reith EJ: Qualitative electron probe analysis of secretory ameloblasts and odontoblasts in the rat incisor. Histochemistry 50:347, 1977

Boyde A, Reith EJ, Jones SJ: Intercellular attachments between calcified collagenous forming cells in the rat. Calc Tiss Res 191:507, 1978

Branford-White CJ: Molecular organization of heparin sulfate proteoglycan from human dentine. Arch Oral Biol 23:1141, 1978

Brännström M, Garberoglio R: The dentinal tubules and the odontoblast processes. A scanning electron microscope study. Acta Odont Scand 30:291, 1972

Butler WT, Munksgaard EC, Richardson WS, III: Dentin proteins: Chemistry, structure and biosynthesis. J Dent Res 58(B):817, 1979

Carneiro J, Leblond CP: Role of osteoblasts and odontoblasts in secreting the collagen of bone and dentine, as shown by radioautography in mice given tritium-labeled glycine. Exp Cell Res 18:291, 1959

Curley-Joseph J, Veis A: The nature and covalent complexes of phosphoproteins with collagen in the bovine dentin matrix. J Dent Res 58:1625, 1979

deBeer GR: The differentiation of neural crest cells into visceral cartilages and odontoblasts in *amblystoma*, and a re-examination of the germ-layer theory. Proc Roy Soc [Ser B], 134:377, 1947

Derise NL, Ritchey SJ, Furr AK: Mineral composition of normal human enamel and dentin and the relation of composition to dental caries: I. Macrominerals and comparison of methods of analyses. J Dent Res 53:847, 1974

Dirksen TR: Lipid Components of Sound and Carious Dentin. Publ No 62-47, School of Aerospace Medicine, USAF Aerospace Med Center, Brooks Air Force Base, Texas, Feb 1962

Dirksen TR, Marinetti GV: Lipids of bovine enamel and dentine and human bone. Calc Tiss Res 6:1, 1970

Eastoe JE: The amino acid composition of proteins from the oral tissues. II. The matrix proteins in dentine and enamel from developing human deciduous teeth. Arch Oral Biol 8:633, 1963

Eastoe JE: The chemical composition of bone and tooth. Adv Fluor Res Dent Car Prev 3:5, 1965

Eisenmann DR, Yaeger JA: Alterations in the formation of rat dentin and enamel induced by various ions. Arch Oral Biol, 14:1045, 1969

Eisenmann DR, Glick PL: Ultrastructure of initial crystal formation in dentin. J Ultrastruct Res 41:18, 1972

Embery G, Smalley JW: The influence of fluoride on the uptake of radiosulfate by rat incisor odontoblasts in vitro. Arch Oral Biol 25:659, 1980

Fiore-Donno G, Baume L-J: Etude histochimique de la dentinogènèse humaine. Helv Odont Acta 10 (Suppl 4):141, 1966

Frank RM and Nalbandian J: Comparative aspects of development of dental hard structures. J Dent Res 42:422, 1963

Grant PR: The organization of microtubules within rat odontoblast processes revealed by perfusion fixation with glutaraldehyde. Arch Oral Biol 17:1047, 1972

Garberoglio R, Brännström M: Scanning electron microscopic investigation of human dentinal tubules. Arch Oral Biol 21:355, 1976

Goldberg M, Septier D: Electron microscopic visualization of proteoglycans in rat incisor predentine and dentine with cuprolinic blue. Arch Oral Biol 28:79, 1983

Granström G, Linde A: A biochemical study of alkaline phosphatase in isolated rat incisor odontoblasts. Arch Oral Biol 17:1213, 1972

Granström G, Linde A: A comparative study of alkaline phosphatase in calcifying cartlage, odontoblasts and the enamel organ. Calc Tiss Res 22:231, 1977

Hardwick JL: Isotope studies in the penetration of glucose into normal and carious enamel and dentin. Arch Oral Biol 4:97, 1961

Hwang WSS, Tonna EA, Cronkite EP: An autoradiographic study of the mouse incisor using tritiated histidine. Arch Oral Biol 8:377, 1963

Johansen E: Microstructure of enamel and dentin. J Dent Res 43:1007, 1964

Johnson RH, Mitchell DF: The effects of tetracyclines on teeth and bones. J Dent Res 45:86, 1966

Karpishka I, Leblond CP, Carneiro J: Radioautographic investigation of the uptake of labelled methionines by the dentin and enamel matrix of growing teeth. Arch Oral Biol 1:23, 1959

Kiguel E: Fibrillar elements forming dentin and mineral seeding or crystal nucleation. Anat Rec 151:267, 1965

Kumamoto Y, Leblond CP: Visualization of C^{14} in the tooth matrix after administration of labeled hexoses. J Dent Res 37:147, 1958

Kuttler Y: Classification of dentin into primary, secondary and tertiary. Oral Surg 12:996, 1959

Läikkö I, Larmas M: Changes of phosphomonoesterase activity in human dentine during the formation of the root of the tooth. J Dent Res 59:1558, 1980

Lappalainen R, Knuuttila M: Atomic absorption spectrometric evidence of relationships between some cationic elements in human dentine. Arch Oral Biol 27:827, 1982

Lappalainen R, Knuuttila M, Salminen R: The concentrations of Zn and Mg in human enamel and dentine related to age and their concentrations in the soil. Arch Oral Biol 26:1, 1981

Larmas M: Histochemical studies on phosphatase and arylsulphatase activity in human carious dentin. Acta Odont Scand 26:357, 1968

Larmas M: A chromatographic and histochemical study of nonspecific esterases in human carious dentine. Arch Oral Biol 17:1121, 1972a

Larmas M: Alanine and aspartate aminotransferases in

sound and carious human dentine. Arch Oral Biol 17:1133, 1972b

Larmas M: Histochemical demonstration of various dehydrogenases in human carious dentine. Arch Oral Biol 17:1143, 1972c

Larsson PA, Linde A: Adrenergic vessel innervation in the rat incisor pulp. Scand J Dent Res 79:7, 1971

Leblond CP, Bélanger LF, Greulich RC: Formation of bones and teeth as visualized by radioautography. In Recent advances in the study of the structure, composition and growth of mineralized tissues. Ann NY Acad Sci 60:631, 1955

Lechner JG, Kalnitsky G: The presence of large amounts of type III collagen in bovine dental pulp and its significance with regard to the mechanism of dentinogenesis. Arch Oral Biol 26:265, 1981

Lesot H, Osman M, Ruch JV: Immunofluorescent localization of collagens, fibronectin, and laminin during terminal differentiation of odontoblasts. Develop Biol 82:371, 1981

Lester KS, Boyde A: The surface morphology of some crystalline components of dentine. In Symons NB (ed): Dentine and Pulp, pp 197–219. Baltimore, Williams and Wilkins, 1968

Llory H, Frank RM: Ultrastructure de la dentine cariée. In Prèlat J (ed): Actualites Odonto-Stomatologiques. No 88. pp 507–522. Paris, Dec 1969

McClure FJ, King CTG, Derr J, Wilk AL: Major components of the primary and secondary dentition of miniature and duroc swine fed normal vs. low phosphorus diets. Arch Oral Biol 11:253, 1966

Meffert O, Kämmerer H: The influence of fluoride on the mineralization of rat teeth. Calc Tiss Res 11:176, 1973

Miller WA, Eick JD, Neiders ME: Inorganic components of the peritubular dentin in young human permanent teeth. Caries Res 5:264, 1971

Mjör IA: Microradiography of human coronal dentine. Arch Oral Biol 11:225, 1966

Mjör IA: Human coronal dentine: Structure and reactions, Oral Surg 33:810, 1972

Mjör IA, Pindborg JJ: Histology of the Human Tooth, pp 12–13. Copenhagen, Munksgaard, 1973

Nylen MV, Scott DB: An electron microscopic study of the early stages of dentinogenesis. Washington, DC, US Government Printing Office, 1958

Odutuga AA, Prout RES: Fatty acid composition of neutral lipids and phospholipids of enamel and dentine from rat incisors and molars. Arch Oral Biol 18:689, 1973

Okamura K: Localization of serum albumin in dentin and enamel. J Dent Res 62:100, 1983

Owens PDA: Mineralization in the roots of human deciduous teeth demonstrated by tetracycline labeling. Arch Oral Biol 18:889, 1973

Pashley DH, Nelson R, Pashley EL: In-vivo fluid movement across dentine in the dog. Arch Oral Biol 26:707, 1981

Path MG, Meyer MW: Quantification of pulpal blood flow in developing teeth in dogs. J Dent Res 50:1245, 1977

Piez KA: Amino acid composition of some calcified proteins. Science 134:841, 1961

Quigley MB, Starrs JW, Zwarych PD: Demonstration of calcospherites in mature human dentin. J Dent Res 44:794, 1965

Reith EJ: The binding of calcium within the Golgi saccules of the rat odontoblast. Am J Anat 147:267, 1976

Retief DH, Cleaton-Jones PE, Turkstra J, DeWet WJ: The quantitative analysis of sixteen elements in normal human enamel and dentine by neutron activation analysis and high-resolution gamma-spectometry. Arch Oral Biol 16:1257, 1971

Rölling I, Melsen B: Dentin formation in formocresol pulpotomized primary monkey teeth studied by tetracycline and 3H-proline incorporation. Scand J Dent Res 87:403, 1979

Ruch JV, Karcher-Djuricic V, Thiebold J: Cell division and cytodifferentiation of odontoblasts. Differentiation 5:165, 1976

Sasaki T, Ishida I, Higashi S: Ultrastructure and cytochemistry on old odontoblasts in rat incisors. J Electron Micros 31:378, 1982

Scott DB: The electron microscopy of enamel and dentin. In Recent advances in the study of the structure, composition, and growth of mineralized tissues. Ann NY Acad Sci 60:575, 1955

Shackleford JM: The structure of Tomes' granular layer in dog premolar teeth. Anat Rec 170:357, 1971

Shellis RP: Structural organization of calcospherites in normal and rachitic human dentine. Arch Oral Biol 28:85, 1983

Slavkin HC, Baretta LA (eds): Developmental Aspects of Oral Biology, pp 201–242. New York, Academic Press, 1972

Slavkin HC, Tetreault C, Nimni MN, Blavetta LA: Autoradiographic and biochemical investigations of collagen biosynthesis and participation in the dentin extracellular matrix. Proc Soc Exp Biol Med 126:439, 1967

Smith AJ, Leaver AG: Distribution of the EDTA-soluble non-collagenous organic matrix components of rabbit incisor dentine. Arch Oral Biol 26:643, 1981

Smith AJ, Leaver AG: Non-collagenous components of the organic matrix of rabbit incisor dentine. Arch Oral Biol 24:449, 1979

Sognnaes RF, Wislocki GB: Histochemical observations on enamel and dentin undergoing carious destruction. Oral Surg 3:1283, 1950

Stewart DJ: The re-incorporation in calcified tissues of tetracycline released following its deposition in the bone of rats. Arch Oral Biol 18:759, 1973

Symons NBB: The cells of the odontoblast, ameloblast and internal enamel epithelial layers. Brit Dent J 98:273, 1955

Takuma S, Yanagisawa T, Sin WL: Ultrastructural and microanalytical aspects of developing dentine in rat incisors. Calc Tiss Res 24:215, 1977

Tanaka T: The origin and localization of dentinal fluid in developing rat molar teeth studied with lanthanum as a tracer. Arch Oral Biol 25:153, 1980

Ten Cate AR: A fine structural study of coronal and root dentinogenesis in the mouse: Observations on so-called 'von Korff fibres' and their contribution to mantle dentine. J Anat 125:183, 1978

Ten Cate AR, Melcher AH, Pudy G, Wagner D: The non-fibrous nature of the von Korff fibres in developing dentine. A light and electron microscope study. Anat Rec 168:491, 1970

Thomas M, Leaver AG: Identification and estimation of

plasma proteins in human dentine. Arch Oral Biol 20:217, 1975

Thomas M, Leaver AG: The less-acidic glycoproteins of the organic matrix of human dentine. Arch Oral Biol 22:545, 1977

Tiber A: The pattern of incorporation of (^{3}H)-leucine by the enamel and dentine matrices of the rhesus monkey: An autoradiographic study. Arch Oral Biol 16:1231, 1971

Tobin CE: Correlation of vascularity with mineralization in human fetal teeth. Anat Rec 174:371, 1972

Trowbridge HO, Seltzer JL: Formation of dentin and bone matrix in magnesium-deficient rats. J Periodont Res 2:147, 1967

Tsatsas BG, Frank RM: Ultrastructure of the dentinal tubular substances near the dentino-enamel junction. Calc Tiss Res 9:239, 1972

Ulmansky M, Langer M: Reaction of dental pulp to Ledermix and Calxyl. Israel J Med Sci 3:739, 1967

Warshawsky H: The presence of atypical collagen fibrils in EDTA decalcified predentine and dentine of rat incisors. Arch Oral Biol 17:1745, 1972

Weinstock A: Matrix development in mineralizing tissues as shown by radioautography: Formation of enamel and dentin. In Slavkin HC, Baretta LA (eds): Developmental Aspects of Oral Biology. pp 201–242. New York, Academic Press, 1972

Weinstock M, Leblond CP: Synthesis, migration, and release of precursor collagen by odontoblasts as visualized by radioautography after [3H] proline administration. J Cell Biol 60:92, 1974

Wennberg A, Bawden JW: Influence of the pulpal route on uptake of ^{45}Ca in enamel and dentin of developing rat molars. J Dent Res 57:313, 1978

Wennberg A, Mjör IA, Heide S: Rate of formation of regular and irregular secondary dentin in monkey teeth. Oral Surg 54:232, 1982

White BA, Deaton TG, Bawden JW: *In vivo* and *in vitro* study of ^{90}Sr in developing rat molar enamel. J Dent Res 59:2091, 1980

Yoshiki S, Kurahashi Y: A light and electron microscope study of alkaline phosphatase activity in the early stages of dentinogenesis in the young rat. Arch Oral Biol 16:1143, 1971

Young RW: Autoradiographic studies on postnatal growth of the skull in young rats injected with tritiated glycine. Anat Rec 143:1, 1962

Young RW, Greulich RC: Distinctive autoradiographic patterns of glycine incorporation in rat enamel and dentine matrices. Arch Oral Biol 8:509, 1963

Zerlotti E, Yaeger JA: Histochemistry and biophysical histology of the matrices of some mineralized tissues. Clin Orthop 51:223, 1967

3
CONNECTIVE TISSUE

Enamel is of ectodermal origin, but the other dental tissues—dentin, dental pulp, cementum, bone, and the periodontal ligament—are formed from the mesoderm, the germ layer that gives rise to all connective tissues. Connective tissues basically are the supporting tissues in the body and vary in consistency from liquid, such as the synovial fluid of joints, to hard structures like bone or dentin. The consistency of dental pulp lies between the two extremes and depends on the elements that are present in the pulp.

Connective tissue is composed of fibers and cells embedded in a ground substance or matrix that contains tissue fluid.

THE FIBERS OF CONNECTIVE TISSUE

Three types of fiber are found in connective tissue in the body: collagenous, reticular, and elastic.

COLLAGEN FIBERS

Collagen is the main protein component of all connective tissues, including the organic portion of skin, dentin, cementum, and bone.

Types

There are at least five, and perhaps as many as ten, genetically distinct types of collagen molecules in the body (Minor, 1980). The most common is Type I, designated $[\alpha 1(I)]_2 \alpha 2$. Type II and III collagens consist of three identical α chains and are designated as $[\alpha 1(II)]_3$ and $[\alpha 1(III)]_3$, respectively. Type II is found only in cartilage. Type III is seen as fine reticulin fibers. It is found in several tissues such as skin, uterus, and aorta. Type IV collagen is present in basement membranes. The molecular formula is probably $[\alpha 1(IV)]_3$. Type V collagen consists of αA and αB chains. This type tends to be localized pericellularly (Ooshima, 1981). The relative proportions of each of the different types are tissue specific.

Origin

Collagen fibers are manufactured by fibroblasts, chondroblasts, osteoblasts, cementoblasts, and odontoblasts. The fibers are not formed intracellularly but on the cell surface or extracellularly (Fitton Jackson, 1960). These fibers are embedded in ground substance and become part of the matrices of the hard tissues of the teeth. Once synthesized, deposited, and polymerized, collagen remains stable. Under normal circumstances, collagen turnover is a slow process but, in response to injury, collagen metabolism is accelerated.

Size

Collagen fibers are the most common in the body, and they give the tissue its consistency and tensile strength. The fibers are assembled in bundles or sheets several microns thick (Fig. 3-1). Tissue that contains many collagen fibers — e.g., a tendon — is dense, whereas in loose tissues there are fewer collagen fibers. The fibers may be examined by either the light microscope or the electron microscope.

The light microscope provides, through a system of optical lenses, a magnified image only of structures large enough to interrupt a beam of light (i.e., $0.2\,\mu$ or larger). The electron microscope, through a system of "lenses" composed of magnetic fields, can provide, on a fluorescent

FIG. 3-1 *(Top)* Collagen fibers. ×240. *(Bottom)* Higher magnification of collagen fiber bundles. The cells are fibroblasts. ×960.

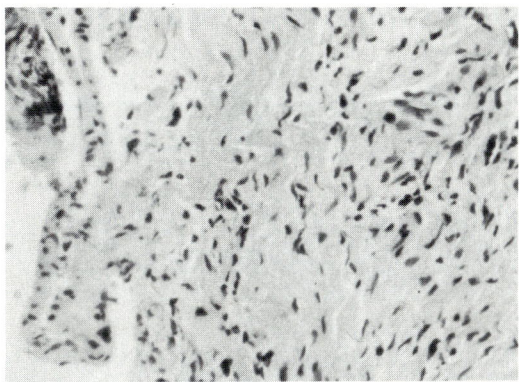

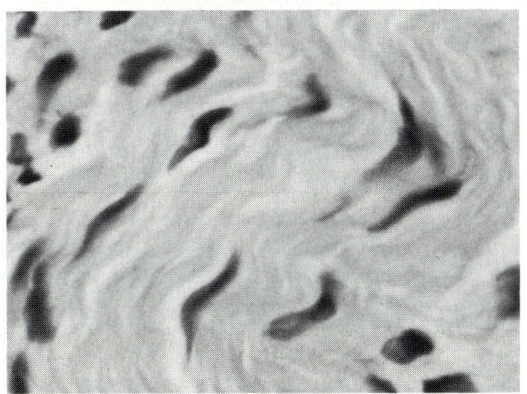

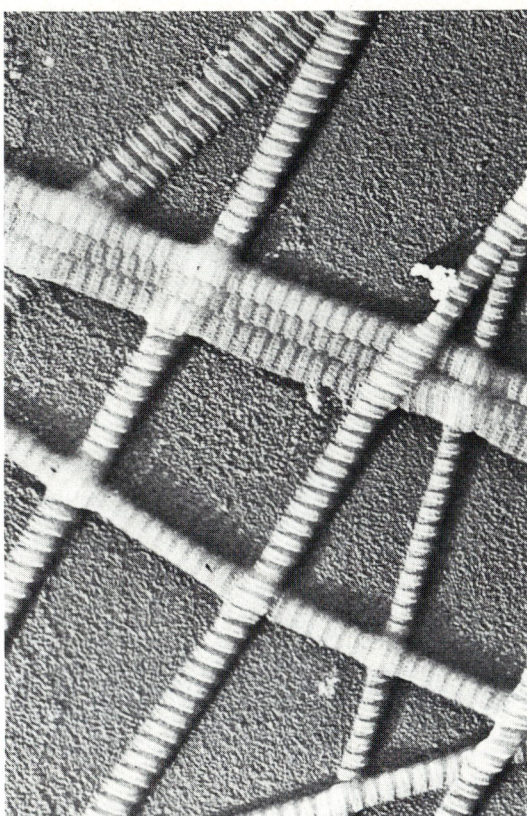

FIG. 3-2 Collagen fibrils; bands are spaced about 700 angstrom units apart. ×42,000. (Gross J: Collagen. Sci Am 204:121, 1961)

screen or a photographic plate, a magnified image of any structure capable of interrupting the electron beam.

Collagen fibers are made up of fibrils that cannot be seen at the resolution of the light microscope; at that resolution (nothing smaller than about $0.2\,\mu$) only fibers are seen. A fiber is a bundle or collection of fibrils. When examined with the electron microscope (possibly a 30 Å resolution), fibrils have a typical appearance that identifies them.

The fibrils are held or cemented together in the bundle by glycosaminoglycans and mucoproteins bound together.

The fibrils, which have a width of several thousands to less than 100 Å, are composed of well-aligned, overlapping collagen molecules of about 15 Å thickness. The fibrils exhibit bands or striations at intervals of 640 Å to 700 Å (Fig. 3-2). This periodic spacing is the "fingerprint"

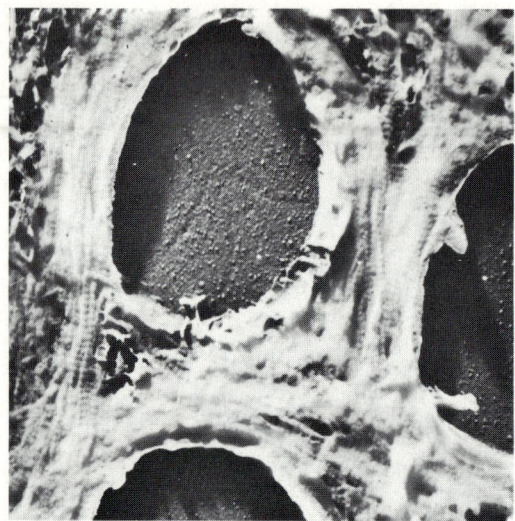

FIG. 3-3 Collagen fibrils, observed in a section of demineralized dentinal matrix. ×13,000. (Scott DB: The electron microscopy of enamel and dentin. In recent advances in the study of the structure, composition, and growth of mineralized tissues. Ann NY Acad Sci 60:575, 1955)

700 Å) to the bands seen in electron microscope studies. The collagen of dentin also has the same periodic spacing (Fig. 3-3).

The collagen molecules may be stored and secreted directly from the cisternae of the endoplasmic reticulum (Ross and Benditt, 1965; Olsen et al, 1973) or may be formed in, and stored and secreted from, the Golgi apparatus (Goldberg and Green, 1964).

Apparently, there are three forms of collagen in connective tissue: neutral-salt-soluble collagen, acid-soluble collagen or procollagen, and insoluble collagen. The strength and solubility of collagen. Collagen fibers in every part of the body are similar.

Composition

The basic collagen molecule is a group of three polypeptide chains, each made up of approximately 1000 amino acid units. Collagen molecules are synthesized by fibroblasts from a precursor, procollagen. The mechanisms are similar to those involved in the synthesis of other proteins. However, two additional steps are required prior to extracellular secretion. First, some of the prolyl and lysyl residues of the collagen polypeptide chain are hydroxylated after the chains are released from the ribosomal complexes. Subsequently, glycosylation of some of the hydroxylysyl residues of the chain takes place; the hydroxylated residues are bound in o-glycosytic linkage to glycosyl-galactosyl moieties (Wadell, 1971).

Chemically, the three main amino acid components are proline, hydroxyproline, and glycine. This has been confirmed by x-ray diffraction analysis. These fibrous proteins give the same distinctive kind of large-angle x-ray fiber diagram. Collagen gives a small-angle x-ray diagram, corresponding in period (about 640 Å to

FIG. 3-4 (Top) Collagen fibers around blood vessel (BV) in young pulp. ×96. (Bottom) Higher magnification of collagen fibers (CF) in region outlined by rectangle in upper picture. Masson's stain. ×960.

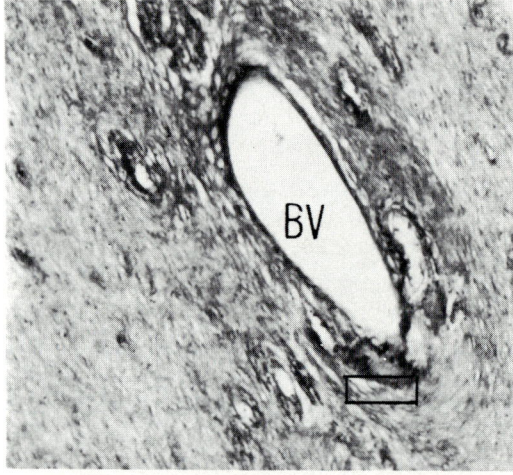

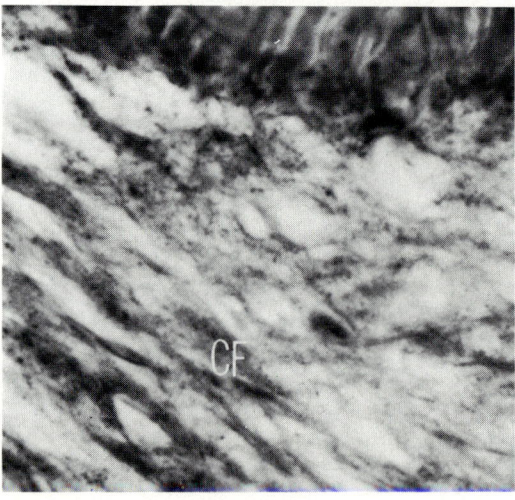

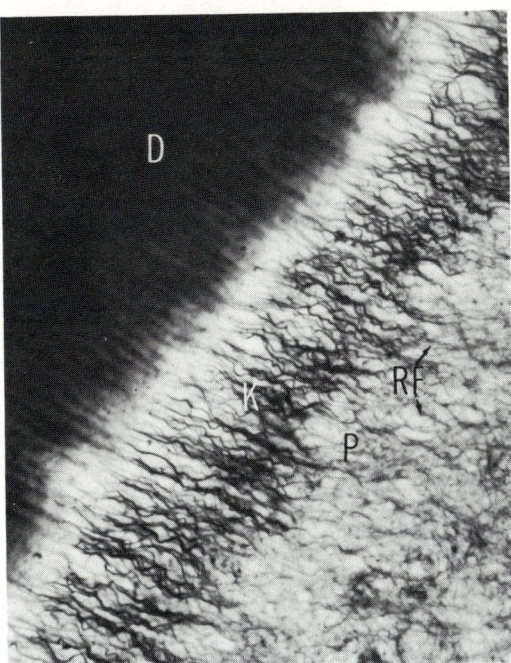 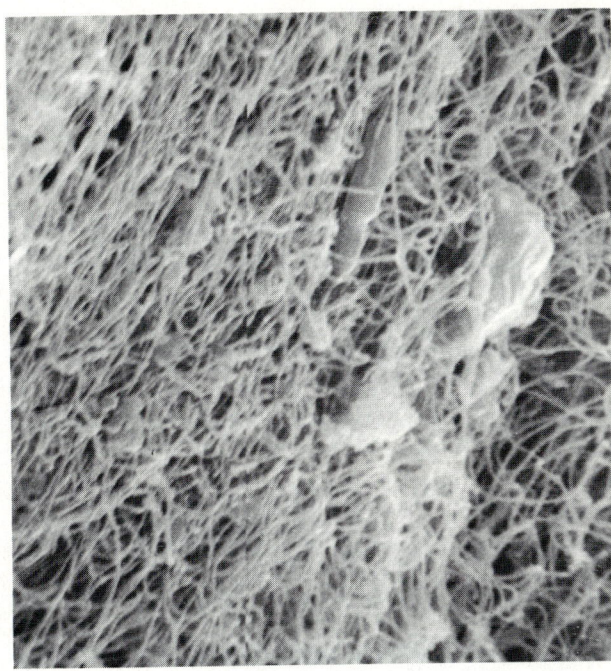

FIG. 3-5 *(Left)* Von Korff fibers (K) are reticular fibers that course from the pulp (P) through the odontoblastic layer, into the predentin. D, dentin. Other reticular fibers (RF) are present in the pulp. ×540. *(Right)* Scanning electron micrograph of pulp reticular fibers. ×5000.

of collagen fibers depends upon cross-linking of the collagen molecules (Gross, 1961). The cross links arise from certain lysines in the collagen molecule.

In histologic sections, collagen fibers are stained by most of the acid aniline dyes commonly used. In sections stained with hematoxylin and eosin they are colored pink by the eosin. Mallory's connective tissue stain colors the collagen fibers blue, owing to the aniline blue. In Masson's stain, the fibers are stained light green.

Tooth Collagen

In dentin, the matrix in which mineralization occurs is composed of collagen fibrils and glycosaminoglycans which have a tendency to attract minerals.

In young pulp, collagen fibers are found around the blood vessels as supporting elements (Fig. 3-4). As the individual gets older, more and more collagen is deposited in the pulp, with a consequent increase in collagen fibers; this is a retrogressive change that occurs normally in all pulps.

RETICULAR FIBERS

Reticular fibers are seemingly different from collagen fibers because of differences in staining. However, with the aid of the electron microscope, it has been determined that the two are similar, since they exhibit the same periodicity. Reticular fibers have an argyrophilic quality, i.e., they absorb metallic silver when treated with alkaline solutions of reducible silver salts (Fig. 3-5); a property absent in collagen fibers.

According to Melcher (1966), the argyrophilic fibers occur as two different morphologic types—reticulin, and argyrophilic young collagen. Reticular fibers are found in connective tissue early in development. They persist in adult parenchymatous organs and in the gingivae and dental pulp. Argyrophilic young collagen fibers soon appear and increase, gradually obscuring the reticulin. Eventually, the young collagen fibers mature and become nonargyrophilic.

Melcher and Eastoe (1969) have suggested that the branched argyrophilic reticulin observed in the light microscope represents silver

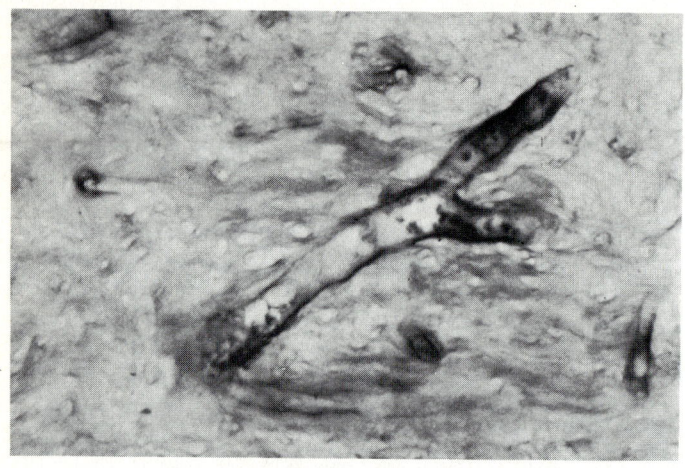

FIG. 3-6 Reticular fibers around blood vessel. ×240.

impregnation of the extracellular substance between cells. This extracellular substance is composed of fine collagen fibrils and associated ground substance.

Thus, von Korff fibers are immature collagen fibrils and ground substance found coursing from the pulp through the odontoblastic layer into the predentin (Fig. 3-5). They subsequently mature into collagen fibers and acquire the ability to attract mineral salts. As disclosed by silver stains and electron microscopy, the pulp contains many reticular fibers that form a network within its body. Practically all the tissues of the body have networks of reticular fibers wherever support is needed; for example, such fibers are found around blood vessels (Fig. 3-6). Other supporting tissues of the body also contain a network of reticular fibers, but special stains are necessary to detect them.

ELASTIC FIBERS

Elastic fibers are made by fibroblasts. The fibrous precursors may be secreted through small coated vesicles (Fahrenbach et al, 1966). The elastic fibers are composed of protein made up of two components. These consist of polypeptide chains, which differ among themselves as a result of differences in structural configuration (Hall, 1957). Elastic fibers are present in connective tissue in association with collagen fibers and ground substance. Elastic fibers are not found in the dental pulp but are present in the alveolar mucosa and submucosa. Special stains are needed to observe them.

GROUND SUBSTANCE

Chemically, the ground substance is composed of carbohydrate-containing proteins (mucoproteins and glycoproteins), which are rich in hexosamine and other carbohydrates, and of acid mucopolysaccharides, which also contain large amounts of hexosamine. It appears to be optically homogeneous.

Mucopolysaccharides are either acid or neutral. The acid mucopolysaccharides include heparin, chondroitin, hyaluronic acid, and chondroitin sulfuric acid. Hyaluronic acid is a glycosaminoglycan, a long-chain polymer composed of N-acetylglucosamine and glucuronic acid. Chondroitin sulfuric acid is composed of galactosamine and glucuronic acid, which are sulfated. Differences are discernible between the two histochemically. For example, chondroitin sulfate stains metachromatically with toluidine blue, whereas hyaluronic acid does not.

In sections of pulp tissue the glycosaminoglycans are not revealed unless special stains are employed. The periodic acid-Schiff (PAS) stain, toluidine blue and many oxidation stains are necessary.

The ground substance contains a large proportion of water bound in a colloidal state. Diffusion of electrolytes and other dissolved substances through the aqueous phase of the colloid takes place without actual movement of the interstitial fluid. The fibrils embedded in the ground substance are coated by a thin film of fluid, and this film is believed to be the avenue for movement of substances through the connective tissue.

According to Gersh and Catchpole (1949), staining reactions in frozen dried material reveal the ground substance to be more or less polymerized. The degree of polymerization varies with age, physiologic activity, and pathologic state. When the ground substance is involved in an inflammatory process, it may become depolymerized by liberated proteolytic enzymes. The ground substance has a firm, gel-like consistency when highly polymerized; it is more fluid at lower degrees of polymerization. An understanding of the ground substance is important because it reflects metabolic changes occurring in the tissues.

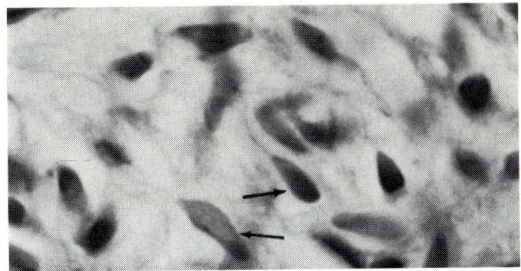

FIG. 3-7 Fibroblasts. ×960.

CELLS

The cytoplasm of cells is highly organized and contains an assortment of fibers, membrane-enclosed vesicles, and organelles. These latter include mitochondria (which manufacture adenosine triphospate (ATP), the chemical energy of the cell), ribosomes (which coordinate the synthesis of proteins), the endoplasmic reticulum, and the Golgi apparatus (which package proteins for export). In addition, there is an elaborate network of skeletal elements: microtubules, microfilaments, and intermediate filaments. These elements are involved in cell movement and maintenance of cell shape (Porter and Tucker, 1981).

Deoxyribonucleic acid (DNA) is found in the chromosomes and gives the cell its genetic character; that is, the genetic transmission from cell to cell is present in DNA. DNA normally consists of a double-strand helix. The helices proper, the "back-bones" of the molecule, are composed of an alternation of sugar (deoxyribose) and phosphate groups. Attached to each of the sugars is one of four nitrogenous "bases," generally adenine, guanine, thymine, and cytosine. Hydrogen bonds between bases link the strands. Genetic information is provided by the sequence of bases along a strand. The hereditary information, transmitted from generation to generation in the nucleic acid of the chromosomes, finds its expression in the characteristic types of proteins and enzymes.

Modern research methods, such as the use of tritium (radioactive hydrogen) enable the investigator to trace by radioautography the synthesis of DNA by the cells. When tritiated thymidine, which is used by the cells for the synthesis of DNA, is injected into animals, it appears shortly afterward in cells that are manufacturing DNA. The radioautograph locates the labeled material within the nucleus of the cell.

Cells synthesize two general classes of proteins: cytoplasmic and secreted. Cytoplasmic proteins such as ribosomal proteins, hemoglobin, or β-galactosidase are synthesized by cytoplasmic ribosomes. Proteins for secretion and export from the cell are synthesized by membrane-bound ribosomes. The genetic code in the double-chain molecule of DNA is transcribed into shorter single chains of ribonucleic acid (RNA). Since these molecules of RNA carry the genetic code to the site of protein synthesis, they are called messenger RNA. The decision for secretion is genetically controlled through messenger RNA. The information coded in the messenger RNA determines the class of ribosome to which it can attach and the fate of the protein product. Thus, attachment of messenger RNA to membrane-bound ribosomes probably determines that the protein will be secreted through the cell membrane (Redman and Sabatini, 1966).

Fibroblasts. The basic cells in all connective tissue are fibroblasts. Fibroblasts are spindle-shaped cells with oval nuclei and have cytoplasmic processes extending from the main cell body. In tissue sections stained with hematoxylin and eosin, the nucleus is usually visible, but the processes are not (Fig. 3-7). Fibroblasts are believed to elaborate the collagen fibers and ground substance. The proteins are synthesized on the ribosomes of the endoplasmic reticulum (Littlefield et al, 1955). These ribosomes are grouped into specific patterns or aggregates (Ross and Benditt, 1964; Fig. 3-8). Actively synthesizing fibroblasts have large polyribosomes that contain approximately 100 ribosomes (Kretsinger et al, 1964). The material

70 | THE DENTAL PULP

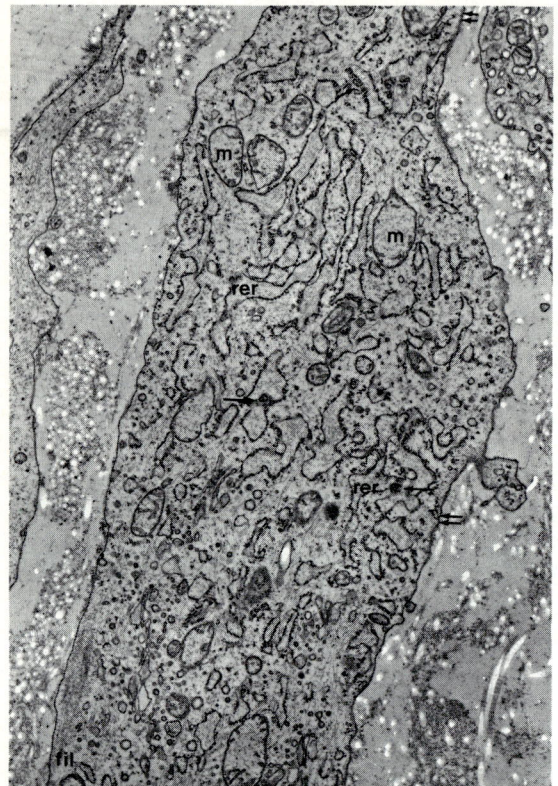

FIG. 3-8 Part of a fibroblast from a wound, 5 days old, in human skin, showing numerous profiles of rough endoplasmic reticulum (rer) and several mitochondria (m). In most areas, relatively large numbers of ribosomes are attached to the membranes of the cisternae. In zones in which the membranes are tangentially sectioned, the characteristic aggregate forms of the ribosomes (arrows) are visible. In other regions (double arrows) the cisternae of the rough endoplasmic reticulum approximate the plasma membrane of the cell. A zone of aggregates of fine filaments (fil) located in the cell periphery is characteristic of the fibroblast. Numerous individual cytoplasmic filaments are also apparent. ×17,000. (Ross R: The ultrastructure of fibrogenesis. J Dent Res 45:449, 1966. Copyright by the American Dental Association. Reproduced by permission)

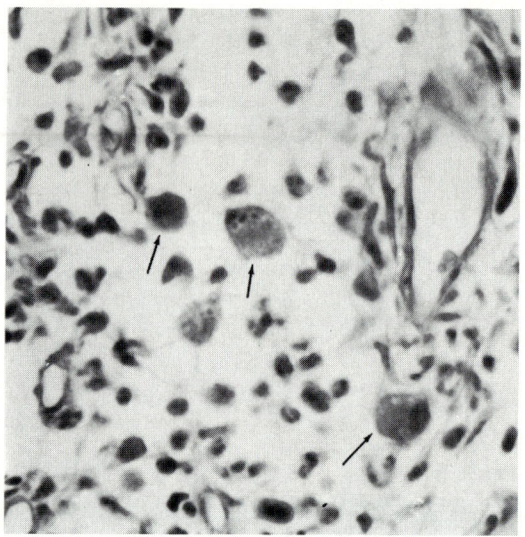

FIG. 3-9 Macrophages (arrows) that have ingested carbon particles. ×960.

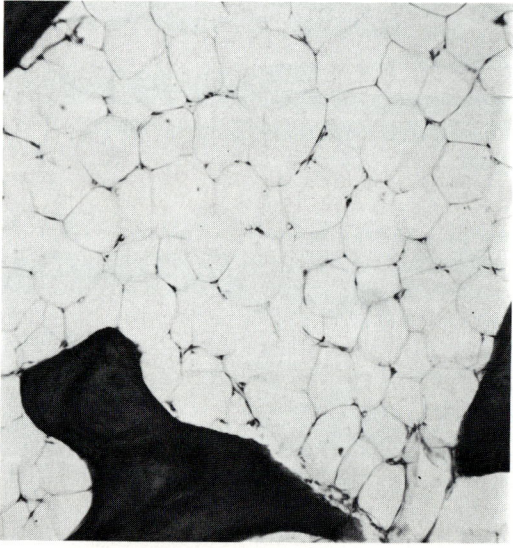

FIG. 3-10 Fat cells. ×135.

formed in the endoplasmic reticulum is transported to the Golgi apparatus where it may be altered by the addition of another substance prior to secretion extracellularly.

A fibrillar network called fibronectin may be visualized on the surface of fibroblasts. It consists of glycoprotein and is believed to function as a mediator of adhesion between cells and of cells to extracellular components (Ruoslahti et al, 1981). It is also a constituent of many basement membranes (Thesleff et al, 1981).

Macrophages, which are commonly seen, are also described in the literature as histiocytes or

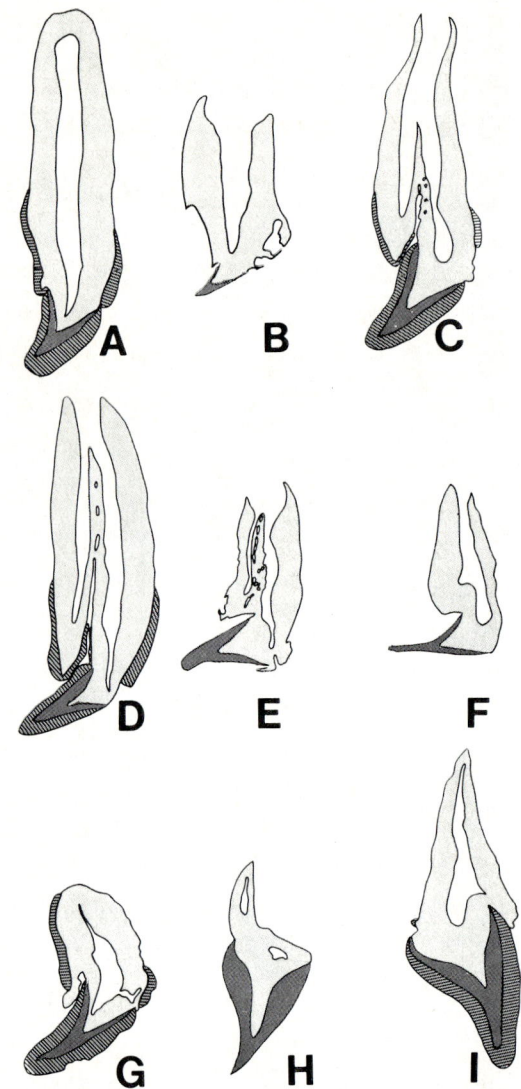

FIG. 1-23 Drawings of nine histologic specimens illustrating the relation between initial dislocation of the mineralized part of the tooth germ and later developmental disturbances. *(A)* Tooth with horizontal enamel hypoplasia. *(B to G)* Crown-dilacerated teeth. *(H and I)* Teeth with partial arrest of root formation. (Andreasen JO, Sundström B, Ravn JJ: The effect of traumatic injuries to primary teeth on their permanent successors. I. A clinical and histologic study of 117 injured permanent teeth. Scand J Dent Res 79:219, 1971)

of enamel epithelium is a prerequisite for the initiation of odontoblastic differentiation (Ruch et al, 1972, 1973; Slavkin and Bringas, 1976). The differentiation of odontoblasts is controlled by a cell-matrix type of interaction between preodontoblasts and basement membrane that separates them from the enamel epithelium (Thesleff et al, 1978). Removal of the basal lamina by enzymes results in loss of morphology and function of developing odontoblasts (Osman and Ruch, 1981). Thus, a lack of vitamin A interferes with normal dentin matrix elaboration. Inasmuch as the odontoblasts do not differentiate completely, they elaborate osteodentin instead of regular dentin. On the other hand, an excess of vitamin A has been found by Hurmerinta et al (1980) to prevent tooth morphogenesis and odontoblastic differentiation in cultured embryonic mouse molar tooth germs.

Vitamin C deficiency affects the various cells involved in tooth development, especially the odontoblasts. Vitamin C is important for the elaboration of collagen, the fibrous protein of the dentin matrix. The matrix must be elaborated before mineral salts can be attracted and precipitated into it. An abundance of mineral salts may be present in the circulation, but, if the matrix is missing, dentin or enamel cannot be formed. Vitamin C deficiencies significantly alter the development of the dentin in laboratory animals, but in the human newborn they are of little concern, since the histodifferentiation, the morphodifferentiation, and the maturation stages are not affected.

Vitamin D deficiency interferes with the mineralization process, once matrix has been elaborated. Vitamin D plays an important role in the absorption of calcium from the gastrointestinal tract. In the kidney, this vitamin causes phosphate reabsorption. In some diseases, such as celiac disease, steatorrhea and rickets, there is a disturbance in absorption of calcium from the gastrointestinal tract. The calcium becomes saponified and is excreted. Thus, there is not enough calcium for the body to absorb, and disturbances in mineralization result.

In vitamin D deficiencies, hypoplasia of enamel may occur, and dentin formation is disturbed (Messer and Guo, 1979). The teeth of rats fed on diets deficient in phosphorus and low in or normal for vitamin D exhibited increased dentinal striations and interglobular dentin. Regardless of the level of dietary calcium and phosas resting wandering cells. The macrophage differentiates from the undifferentiated cells in connective tissue, from monocytes in the bloodstream, or possibly from fibroblasts. Macrophages are phagocytes, the functions of which are the engulfment and digestion of foreign material (Fig. 3–9). During inflammatory reactions, they appear in large numbers to aid in the defense of the organism.

Fat Cells. Connective tissue also contains fat cells (Fig. 3–10). These are present in varying amounts in various connective tissues of the body. Some connective tissue, such as adipose or fatty tissue, is composed primarily of fat cells. Other subcutaneous tissues contain fewer fat cells. In the pulp, fat cells are rarely seen.

Mast cells are found in connective tissues (Fig. 3–11). They contain special granules and are believed to be involved in the production of heparin, glycosaminoglycans, serotonin, or histamine. However, their exact function is unknown.

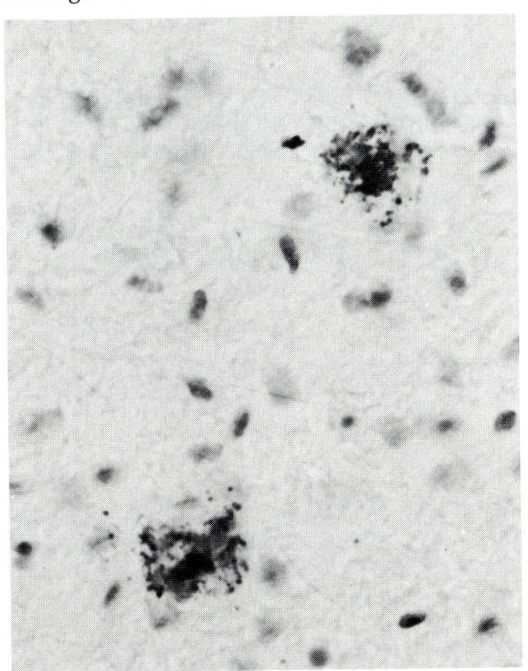

FIG. 3-11 Two mast cells in the mesentery of a rat. Note the granules. ×540.

Polymorphonuclear leukocytes, lymphocytes, plasma cells, and eosinophils, all of which are involved in inflammation, are also found in connective tissues in some instances. For example, lymphocytes are found normally in the intestinal mucosa and may be found normally in the gingival tissues. Usually, they are not found in an uninflamed pulp. Plasma cells are found in some tissues normally, but in the pulp or the periapical tissues they are found only in response to chronic inflammation. Eosinophils are present in some allergic types of inflammation. In the pulp, they are found occasionally in an inflammatory exudate.

Polymorphonuclear leukocytes are not found normally in the connective tissue. They are transported to such sites in response to injury and are then present directly in the involved tissue as well as in blood. They phagocytize foreign material.

SYSTEMIC FACTORS THAT AFFECT CONNECTIVE TISSUE

NUTRITION

When a sufficient quantity of the proper nutrients is not ingested (e.g., in starvation), important components of connective tissues—the carbohydrates and the amino acids needed for the synthesis of the glycosaminoglycans—are missing or reduced in quantity in the bloodstream. The cells of the connective tissue elaborate the ground substance and need these basic elements—the amino acids and the carbohydrates—for its manufacture.

Proteins are essential to nutrition; the amino acids contribute to a metabolic pool of "building blocks" that synthesize the various tissue proteins. If there is a protein deficiency, the amino acids—including proline, hydroxyproline, and glycine, the protein components of collagen—will not be available and, as a result, the fibrous tissue will be affected. A generalized retardation in somatic development results from protein malnutrition (Chow and Lee, 1964).

In addition, the human body may be represented as a dynamic state in which some tissue proteins are continuously being broken down and resynthesized, thereby contributing to the amino acid metabolic pool. The plasma amino acid pool, though small compared with the total body pool, is in rapid flux with extravascular and intracellular pools. Plasma amino acid concentrations are fairly constant in normal healthy subjects but are altered in patients receiving protein deficient diets (Swendseid and Kopple, 1973). Thus, such labile proteins may play an important role in resisting various stresses associated with starvation and disease (Allison, 1963).

Vitamin C. According to Wooley (1959), vitamins, hormones, and certain other substances are essential metabolites (i.e., naturally occurring compounds that are essential in living processes). Vitamin C is involved in collagen formation. A deficiency of vitamin C results in shriveling of fibroblasts. New fibroblasts do not develop fully, and, as a result, the fibrils elaborated by them are shorter, thinner, and less dense. The cells of tissues deprived of vitamin C exhibit increased permeability. Patients with scurvy have a tendency to bleed readily because the ground substance of the capillary walls either is not present or is present in inadequate concentration. This results in a leaking of fluid, with marked edema. There is also an increased fluid exchange.

It appears that saturation of crushed or injured tissue with vitamin C may encourage more rapid healing (Ringsdorf and Cheraskin; 1982). Lack of vitamin C plus protein deficiency further impedes repair.

HORMONES

Hormones are organic materials each of which has specific regulatory functions in man and animals. They do not serve as nutrients. They are made in one part of the body and function in another.

Hormones react with cells by two general patterns. In the first, illustrated by the action of epinephrine, the hormone reacts with membrane-bound nucleotide cyclase systems to stimulate the conversion of ATP to 3′5′-monophosphate (cyclic AMP). Cyclic AMP then acts as a "second messenger," reacting with cells to deliver and amplify the regulatory signal (Robison et al, 1971). In the second pattern, operative with steroid hormones, the hormone enters the cell and binds to a specific extranuclear "receptor" protein. The resulting steroid-protein complex then migrates to the nucleus, where RNA synthesis is initiated or accelerated. Such hormone-induced translocation to the nucleus, called receptor transformation by Jensen and DeSombre (1973), alters the receptor protein.

The pituitary gland is the "conductor of the endocrine symphony." With circadian periodicity (Krieger, 1970; Fig. 3–12), it releases a host of hormones that induce various endocrine glands to produce their hormones and then return messages to the pituitary that the mission is accomplished. One of the hormones liberated by the pituitary is adrenocorticotropic hormone (ACTH), which stimulates the adrenal cortex.

Glucocorticoids constitute one of the two classes of corticosteroids secreted by the cortex of the adrenal gland. They are essential to life. Among their effects is the depression of production and secretion of ACTH by the pituitary gland. Under normal circumstances, adrenal steroid levels are at a peak (approximately 20 μg/100 ml; Grollman and Grollman, 1970) in the early morning hours and progressively decline over the remainder of the 24-hour period. Normally, 15 mg to 30 mg of endogenous cortisol are manufactured daily (Little and Falace, 1980). Other hormones stimulate the gonads, the ovaries, and the thyroid. All have effects on connective tissue and may modify its response to infection (Shackelford and Feigin, 1973).

Stress. Connective tissues can be affected by the alarm reaction as described by Selye (1973). When a patient is subjected to stress (such as psychogenic stress, or that imposed by an extensive operative or surgical procedure), such information is delivered to the hypothalamus, the basal area of the brain. The hypothalamus secretes a corticotropin-releasing factor (CRF), which stimulates the pituitary to secrete ACTH. The ACTH stimulates the adrenal cortex, which elaborates cortisol or hydrocortisone. The amount of cortisol liberated depends on the stimulation of ACTH. Under stress from infection, trauma, illness, or surgery, plasma hydrocortisone secretion can approach 400 μg/100 ml (Cawson and James, 1973) or a total of 300 mg/day (Little and Falace, 1980). Even apprehension of anticipated dental procedures or minor dental surgery causes a rise in the serum 17-hydroxycorticosteroid level (Shannon et al, 1960, 1962a,b). When sufficient amounts of cortisol are in the circulation, the elaboration of ACTH is stopped.

When the body is subjected to stress (psycho-

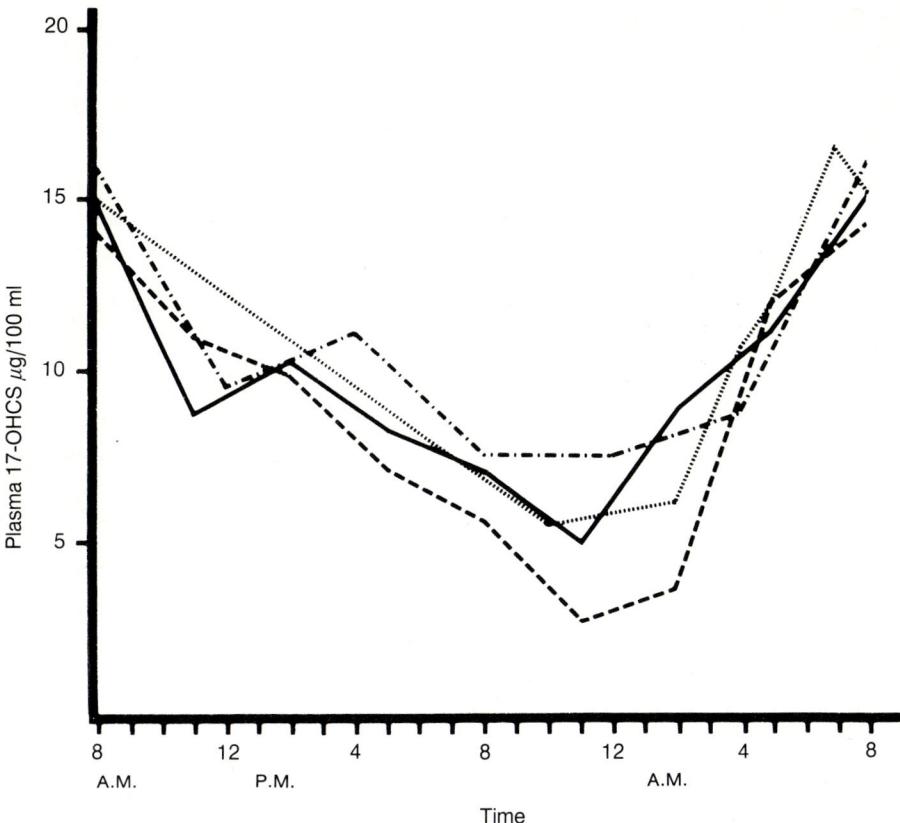

FIG. 3-12 Circadian variation of plasma 17-OHCS levels in normal human subjects (composite of present studies and those reported by other investigators). (Krieger DT: Factors influencing the circadian periodicity of adrenal steroid levels. Trans NY Acad Sci 32:316, 1970)

genic or other) the connective tissues are directly affected. Increased amounts of cortisone produce a shrinkage of the fibroblasts and reduce their number. Young fibroblasts are not developed. Thus, there is a decrease in the amount of ground substance produced, and a greater permeability of the connective tissue results. The fibers elaborated are shrunken and less dense.

Large quantities of cortisone reduce the population of mast cells in connective tissues. During the process of inflammation, there is an increased number of mast cells in certain tissues. Interference with the normal functioning of mast cells may impair the consistency and the turgidity of connective tissues.

Elevated cortisone concentrations affect host resistance to infection (Hirsch and Church, 1961). Polymorphonuclear leukocytes are phagocytic cells that destroy microorganisms or ingest dead cells, tissue debris, particles, and impurities. Although cortisone does not stop phagocytosis or the bactericidal activity of polymorphonuclear leukocytes (Glasser et al, 1977), it does interfere with their stickiness, margination, diapedesis, and migration—important events in phagocytosis (Brubaker, 1974). Thus, antibiotics usually are administered with cortisone when an infection is present.

Excessive amounts of cortisone adversely affect protein metabolism. The glucocorticoids penetrate the cell membrane and bind to receptor proteins in the nucleus, thereby influencing RNA and protein synthesis. There is an increased excretion of protein from the body during cortisone therapy. Thus, the protein components such as glycine, proline, and hydroxyproline are not present to form matrix materials and glycosaminoglycans. The end result may be alveolar osteoporosis, degeneration of the periodontal ligament fibers, and a possible increase in oral infection (Bahn, 1982).

In a patient under cortisone therapy, the cells of the adrenal cortex become atrophied because of the lack of stimulation by ACTH. Should such patients require an operation and, hence, be subjected to further stress, they may develop acute adrenal insufficiency (Kalkwarf et al, 1982) and go into shock. Under such circumstances, the body may demand a greater amount of cortisol than is being elaborated. The ACTH that is liberated has little effect on the cells, which are atrophied; hence, no cortisol is manufactured. Dosages of approximately 20 mg hydroxycortisone or its equivalent for 5 days or longer may cause adrenal suppression for as long as 2 years (Cawson and James, 1973). This condition, which can have fatal consequences (Walton and Ney, 1975), can be handled in the following way: The amount of administered cortisone is reduced gradually over a period of 2 to 3 weeks and ACTH is administered simultaneously, thereby enabling the ACTH to begin to stimulate the adrenal cortex. The atrophied cells may then regenerate and begin to liberate cortisol. When normal cortisol liberation is achieved, the stress of the operation can be met with the proper concentration of cortisol being elaborated. However, although the exact time for complete cortisol regeneration varies widely, it may take at least 1 year to regain a normal response (Malamed, 1978). In emergency operations, when there is no time for gradual reduction of cortisone therapy, a much higher dose of cortisone is administered parenterally so that the body can withstand the extra stress of the surgical procedure.

The suppressed patient who requires a stressful emergency dental procedure should be given double the daily oral dose about 8 hours before, and at, surgery (Bahn, 1982). To avoid persistent adrenal suppression, administration of dosages on alternate days appears to allow adrenal recovery in the drug-free intervals, thereby lessening side effects (Byyny, 1976). Patients on alternate-day regimens or those on chronic dosages below physiologic levels probably will not require supplementation (Bondy and Rosenberg, 1980).

Growth Hormone (GH). The anterior pituitary hormone, sometimes referred to as somatotropin, causes growth of all tissues. It increases mitosis of cells as well as their size.

Collagen formation, mast cell population, and hyaluronic acid content of tissues are increased by GH, resulting in decreased tissue permeability. Hence, there is an increase in resistance of the connective tissue to irritants, with less likelihood of spread of infection.

An overproduction of GH causes gigantism in the young because the epiphyses are not closed. In older persons acromegaly develops because the epiphyseal closure is already established.

Thyroid Stimulating Hormone (TSH). The pituitary hormone thyrotropin is concerned with the regulation of thyroid function. It controls the release of the thyroid hormone. There is an interrelationship between TSH and thyroxin through a negative feedback mechanism. This mechanism provides for a delicate balance between the responsive actions of the hypophysis and the thyroid gland. Hypophysectomy causes a drop in circulating thyroxin. On the other hand, injection of TSH increases the functioning of the thyroid gland.

Variations in secretion of TSH produce changes in thyroid activity. These changes ultimately affect protein anabolism, gluconeogenesis, and lipid metabolism.

TSH has a direct effect on the connective tissues. Histochemical studies by Asboe-Hansen (1957) and Iversen (1954) demonstrated accumulation of mast cells and mucopolysaccharides, particularly hyaluronic acid, in the retrobulbar tissue of guinea pigs with thyrotropin-induced exophthalmos. TSH also increases the volume of connective tissue.

Thyroxin. The thyroid gland elaborates the hormone thyroxin, which is essential for growth and development of tissues. The exact mechanism of its action is not known. Thyroxin may have a function in tissue differentiation and maturation, or it may be concerned with energy metabolism. It has been hypothesized that the thyroid hormone regulates all metabolic functions. The hormone supposedly increases the rate of energy exchange and oxygen consumption of all normal tissue except the thyroid gland itself.

A deficiency in thyroxin causes myxedema. In this disease there is a lower basal metabolic rate

(BMR) which can be compensated for somewhat by thyroxin administration. Clinical myxedema following thyroidectomy is caused by an accumulation of extracellular fluid that is rich in mucoprotein containing hyaluronic acid.

Parathyroid hormone is concerned primarily with calcium metabolism. It therefore affects bone, kidney, intestine, and mammary gland. Under normal conditions, parathyroid activity is regulated by the concentration of calcium ions in the blood, a calciostatic action. A decrease in the blood plasma calcium ion concentration stimulates parathyroid secretion, whereas an increase depresses secretion.

The hormone accelerates the mobilization of calcium and phosphate ions by stimulating osteocytic osteolysis. Nonionic calcium stored in bone is broken down into ionic calcium. When ionic calcium and phosphate in sufficient concentrations circulate in the *milieu interieur*, they interact with specific sites on the collagen fibrils to form small hydroxyapatite crystals, which gradually enlarge in size.

The Estrogens and the Gonadotrophic Hormones. The estrogens stimulate an increased deposition of the connective tissue ground substance by interacting with receptor proteins in connective tissue cells. They also reduce connective tissue permeability by virtue of an increase in the mast cell population. Lurie (1950) found that when tubercle bacilli were injected into rabbits that were on estrogen therapy, the likelihood of a spread of tuberculosis to the other tissues became reduced. However, when the animals were given gonadotrophic hormones, the permeability of the connective tissue was increased, and tuberculosis spread throughout the body into the rest of the organs.

INFECTION

Infection affects the connective tissues. Ordinarily, the jellylike consistency of connective tissue constitutes a mechanical barrier to the spread of pathogenic microorganisms, thereby preventing infection. According to Duran-Reynals (1933), many bacteria, particularly some strains of streptococci, liberate hyaluronidase, an enzyme that depolymerizes hyaluronic acid, one of the components of the ground substance. This explains the rapid invasion of tissues by these bacteria. Hyaluronidase affects the substrate, which is normally viscid and acts as a barrier. The viscosity of the substrate becomes close to that of water, and the bacteria are able to penetrate more readily. Hyaluronidase also affects the connective tissue cells by increasing the permeability of their membranes. Collagen fibers are frayed by hyaluronidase. Besides hyaluronidase, many other spreading factors are known.

Some bacteria do not liberate hyaluronidase; instead, they produce hyaluronic acid. These microorganisms do not have the property of invasiveness.

The fact that a bacterium can elaborate hyaluronidase does not mean it is virulent. However, it has the potential for invasiveness in certain substrates. For instance, if a particular enzyme elaborated by microorganisms is effective at a pH of 8 and the pH of the tissue is 5 or 6 (acidic), the microorganisms are not invasive, because the enzyme produced cannot function properly. However, if the pH of the environment is changed, the enzyme can operate effectively.

The connective tissues respond to infection by the protective mechanism known as inflammation. Defense cells accumulate in the tissue spaces to attack the bacteria and ingest them. The glycosaminoglycans of the ground substance, as well as reticular fibers and new fibroblasts, begin to appear in the area of injury. There is increased metachromasia. Collagen fibers develop and fill the defect with scar tissue. In chronic inflammation, the formation of fibrous tissue around the lesion tends to wall it off from the rest of the body (see Chap. 7, Inflammation and Infection).

BIBLIOGRAPHY

Allison JB: Protein malnutrition. Trans NY Acad Sci 25:293, 1963

Asboe-Hansen G: Connective Tissue in Health and Disease. New York, Philosophical Library, 1957

Avery JK, Han SS, Lee Y: Modifications of the fine structure of the incisor pulp of the guinea pig during experimental scurvy. J Dent Res 45:440, 1966

Bahn SL: Glucocorticoids in dentistry, JADA 105:476, 1982

Bondy PK, Rosenberg LE: Metabolic Control and Disease, 8th ed, pp 1429–1450. Philadelphia, WB Saunders Co, 1980

Bowness JM: Present concepts of the role of ground substance in calcification. Clin Orthop 59:233, 1968

Brubaker LH: Unsticky neutrophils. New Engl J Med 29:674, 1974

Byyny, RL: Withdrawal from glucocorticoid therapy. N Engl J Med 295:30, 1976

Cawson RA, James J: Adrenal crisis in a dental patient having systemic corticosteroids. Brit J Oral Surg 10:305, 1973

Chow BF, Lee C: Effect of dietary restriction of pregnant rats on body weight gain in the offspring. J Nutr 82:10, 1964

Duran-Reynals F: Studies on certain spreading factors existing in bacteria and its significance for bacterial invasiveness. J Exp Med 58:161, 1933

Duran-Reynals F: The ground substance of the mesenchyme and hyaluronidase. Ann NY Acad Sci 52:943, 1950

Fahrenbach WH, Sandberg LB, Cleary EG: Ultrastructural studies on early elastogenesis. Anat Rec 155:563, 1966

Fitton Jackson S: Fibrogenesis and the formation of matrix. In Rodahl K, Nicholson JT, Brown EM (eds): Bone As A Tissue, pp 165–185. New York, McGraw-Hill, 1960

Gersh I, Catchpole HR: The organization of ground substance and basement membrane and its significance in tissue injury, disease and growth. Am J Anat 85:451, 1949

Glasser L, Huestis DW, Jones JF: Functional capabilities of steroid-recruited neutrophiles harvested for clinical transfusion. New Engl J Med 297:1033, 1977

Goldberg B, Green H: An analysis of collagen secretion by established mouse fibroblast lines. J Cell Biol 22:227, 1964

Grollman A, Grollman EF: Pharmacology and Therapeutics, 7th ed, pp 758–776. Philadelphia, Lea and Febiger, 1970

Gross J: Studies on the fibrogenesis of collagen. Some properties of neutral extracts of connective tissue. In Tunbridge RE (ed): Connective Tissue, a Symposium, p 45. Springfield, Ill, Charles C Thomas, 1957

Gross J: Collagen. Sci Am 204:121, 1961

Hall DA: Chemical and enzymatic studies on elastin. In Tunbridge RE (ed): Connective Tissue, a Symposium, p 238. Springfield, Ill, Charles C Thomas, 1957

Ham AW: Histology, 7th ed. Philadelphia, JB Lippincott, 1974

Hirsch JG, Church AB: Adrenal steroids and infection: The effect of cortisone administration on polymorphonuclear leukocyte function and on serum opsonins and bactericidins. J Clin Invest 40:794, 1961

Iversen K: Hormonal influence. In Asboe-Hansen G (ed): Connective Tissue in Health and Disease. Copenhagen, Munksgaard, 1954

Jensen EV, DeSombre ER: Estrogen-receptor interaction. Science 182:126, 1973

Kalkwarf KL, Hinrichs JE, Shaw DH: Management of the dental patient receiving corticosteroid medications. Oral Surg 54:396, 1982

Kretsinger RH, Manner G, Gould BS, Rick A: Synthesis of collagen on polyribosomes. Nature (London) 202:438, 1964

Krieger DT: Factors influencing the circadian periodicity of adrenal steroid levels. Trans NY Acad Sci 32:316, 1970

Linke KW: Elektronenmikroskopische untersuchung über die differenzierung der interzellularsubstanz der menschlichen lederhaut. Z Zellforsch 42:331, 1955

Little JW, Falace DA: Dental Management of the Medically Compromised Patient, p 145. St. Louis, CV Mosby Co, 1980

Littlefield JW, Keller EB, Gross J, Zamecnik PC: Studies on cytoplasmic ribonucleoprotein particles from the liver of the rat. J Biol Chem 217:111, 1955

Lurie MB: Mechanisms affecting spread in tuberculosis. In The ground substance of the mesenchyme and hyaluronidase. Ann NY Acad Sci 52:1074, 1950

Malamed SF: Medical Emergencies in the Dental Office. St. Louis, CV Mosby, 1978

Martin GR: Recent progress in collagen research. J Dent Res 50:268, 1971

Melcher AH: Gingival reticulin: Identification and role in histogenesis of collagen fibers. J Dent Res 45:426, 1966

Melcher AH, Eastoe JE: The connective tissues of the periodontium. In Melcher AH, Bowen WH (eds): The Biology of the Periodontium, pp 176–343. London, Academic Press, 1969

Minor RR: Collagen metabolism. Am J Path 98:227, 1980

Obrink B: A study of the interactions between monomeric tropocollagen and glycosaminoglycans. Eur J Biochem 33:387, 1973

Olsen BR, Berg RA, Kishida Y, Prockop DJ: Collagen synthesis: Localization of prolyl hydroxylase in tendon cells detected with ferritin-labeled antibodies. Science 182:825, 1973

Ooshima A: Collagen αB chain: Increased proportion in human atherosclerosis. Science 213:666, 1981

Porter KR, Tucker JB: The ground substance of the living cell. Sci Amer 244(5):57, March, 1981

Redman CM, Sabatini DD: Vectorial discharge of peptides released by puromycin from attached ribosomes. Proc Nat Acad Sci 56:608, 1966

Ringsdorf WM, Jr, Cheraskin E: Vitamin C and human wound healing. Oral Surg 53:231, 1982

Robison GA, Butcher RW, Sutherland EW: Cyclic AMP. New York, Academic Press, 1971

Ross R, Benditt EP: Wound healing and collagen formation. IV. Distortion of ribosomal patterns of fibroblasts in scurvy. J Cell Biol 22:365, 1964

Ross R, Benditt EP: Wound healing and collagen formation. V. Quantitative electron microscope radiographic observations of proline H^3 utilization by fibroblasts. J Cell Biol 27:83, 1965

Ruoslahti E, Engvall E, Hayman E: Fibronectin: Current concepts of its structure and functions. Collagen Res 1:95, 1981

Selye H: The evolution of the stress concept. Am Scient 61:690, 1973

Shackelford PG, Feigin RD: Periodicity of susceptibility to pneumococcal infection: influence of light and adrenocortical secretions. Science 182:285, 1973

Shannon IL, Prigmore JR, Hester WR, McCall CM, Isbell GM: Stress patterns in dental patients. Local anesthesia and simple exodontia. Pamphlet No 61-23, School of Aviation Medicine, USAF Aerospace Med Ctr (ATC), Brooks Air Force Base, Texas, Dec 1960

Shannon IL, Isbell GM, Prigmore JR, Hester WR: Stress in dental patients. The serum free 17-hydroxycorticosteroid response in routinely appointed patients undergoing simple exodontia. Pamphlet No 62-27, School of Aerospace Medicine, USAF Aerospace Med Ctr, Brooks Air Force Base, Texas, Jan, 1962a

Shannon IL, Szmyd L, Prigmore JR: Stress in dental patients. Serum and urine 17-hydroxycorticosteroid responses in impaction patients. Pamphlet No 62-59, School of Aerospace Medicine, USAF Aerospace Medical Division (AFSC), Brooks Air Force Base, Texas, April, 1962b

Swendseid ME, Kopple JD: Nitrogen balance, plasma amino acid levels, and amino acid requirements. Trans NY Acad Sci 35:471, 1973

Ten Cate AR, Melcher AH, Pudy G, Wagner D: The non-fibrous nature of the von Korff fibres in developing dentine. A light and electron microscope study. Anat Rec 168:491, 1970

Thesleff I, Barrach HJ, Foidart JM, Vaheri A, Pratt RM, Martin GR: Changes in the distribution of type IV collagen, laminin, proteoglycan, and fibronectin during mouse tooth development. Devl Biol 81:182, 1981

Tunbridge RE: Connective tissue, a Symposium. Springfield Ill, Charles C Thomas, 1957

Wadell MCL: Alteration of protein synthesis in cartilage by a synthetic double-stranded polyribonucleotide. J Dent Res 50:1072, 1971

Walton J, Ney RL: Current concepts of corticosteroids—uses and abuses. Disease A Month 1–35, June 1975

Wooley DW: Antimetabolites. Science 129:615, 1959

4
THE PULP AS CONNECTIVE TISSUE

The dental pulp is a connective tissue system composed of cells, ground substance, and fibers. The cells manufacture a fundamental matrix, which then acts as site and precursor for the fiber complex—the principal and relatively stable end-product of the system. The fiber complex is composed of collagen and reticulin.

THE CELLS OF THE PULP

FIBROBLASTS

The basic cells of the pulp are fibroblasts, which are similar to connective tissue fibroblasts found elsewhere in the body (Fig. 4–1). In the scanning electron microscope, it can be seen that they form a syncytium of spindle-shaped cells (Fig. 4–2). In the young pulp there is a great preponderance of fibroblasts, as compared with collagen fibers.

Electron micrograph studies suggest that the fibroblasts are active in collagen synthesis. The fibroblasts of guinea pig and human pulps reveal well-developed organelles with extensive, dense, rough-surfaced endoplasmic reticulum in the form of dilated cisternae. These cisternae contain an amorphous, irregularly beaded, electron-dense substance with occasional filaments. Rows and clusters of ribosomes are present (see Fig. 3–8). The Golgi apparatus has an extensively developed stack and a large number of vesicles and vacuoles. The mitochondria are large, with straight cristae running transversely across the matrix. A dense cytoplasmic ground substance contains varying numbers of intracellular fibrils. A cilium is frequently found near the nucleus and an additional centriole may be located perpendicular to the long axis of the cilium (Han et al, 1965; Avery et al, 1966; Griffin and Harris, 1966). Collagen fibers are present on the cell body and its processes.

Dental pulp fibroblasts in tissue culture have been shown to synthesize at least six glycoproteins, the major one being fibronectin. According to Shuttleworth et al (1982), the association of fibronectin with Type III pulpal collagen may give rise to the reticulin fibers of the dental pulp.

Pulp fibroblasts also synthesize and secrete chondroitin sulfate as the major sulfated glycosaminoglycan. In addition, they manufacture heparin and dermatan sulfates (Shuttleworth et al, 1982) and possess the potential for resorbing extracellular collagen (Ten Cate et al, 1976; Torneck, 1981).

The fibroblasts exhibit faint metachromasia, and phosphatase and adenosine triphosphate (ATP) activity (Severson, 1968). Sudanophilic

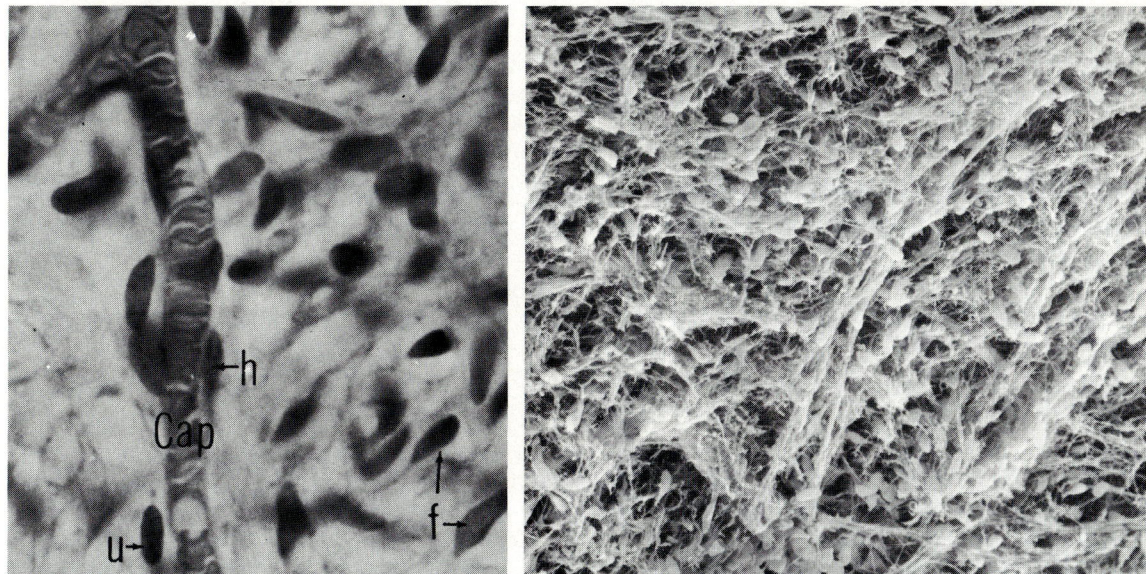

FIG. 4-1 *(Left)* Cells of the pulp. Histiocyte (h) near a capillary (Cap). An undifferentiated mesenchymal cell (u) is also seen. Most of the pulp cells are fibroblasts (f). ×960. *(Right)* Scanning electron micrograph showing fibroblasts and fibers of the coronal dental pulp. ×400. (Seltzer S, Rainey E, Gluskin AH: Correlation of scanning electron microscope and light microscope findings in uninflamed and pathologically involved human pulps. Oral Surg 43:910, 1977)

(lipid) particles are present in their cytoplasm. Most of the known neutral lipids and phospholipids, such as cholesterol and phosphatidylcholine, are present in the dental pulp (Rabinowitz and Rossman, 1979; Rabinowitz, 1980). The cells of the pulp have a considerable anaerobic glycolytic capacity (Pejrone, 1965). As the individual gets older, glycogen and other periodic acid-Schiff (PAS)-positive materials increase, a finding compatible with that of an anaerobic environment (Russell, 1967). In older tissues, the cellular elements begin to decrease. There are more fibers and fewer cells (Fig. 4-3) and the fibers apparently become wider. The increase in the width of the collagen fibers is associated with increasing amounts of dermatan sulfate and decreased amounts of chondroitin sulfate (Shuttleworth et al, 1982). This fiber increase and cell reduction has clinical implications, in that a more fibrous pulp is less able to defend itself against irritants than is a young, highly cellular pulp. The fibroblasts of the pulp are responsible for the increase in size of denticles, inasmuch as dentinoid material elaborated around the denticles comes from the fibroblasts, not from the odontoblasts.

Both fibroblasts and odontoblasts are derived from the mesenchyme, but odontoblasts are more highly differentiated cells than are fibroblasts.

Differentiation may be explained as follows. In the process of maturation, cells assume special and characteristic shapes, sizes, and functions. Thus, some immature mesenchymal cells develop in such a way that they become fibroblasts—cells capable of producing collagen. Some cells become more highly differentiated than others. For example, nerve cells are much more highly differentiated than are fibroblasts. When a highly differentiated cell dies, it cannot be replaced. The less advanced the stage of differentiation, the more easily the cell can be replaced.

By analogy, the general population in the United States numbers approximately 230 million. Of these, about 135,000 people have differentiated into dentists. A further stage of differentiation among this 135,000 would produce 5000 or 6000 specialists. Obviously, such specialists are much more difficult to replace than are less differentiated members of the population.

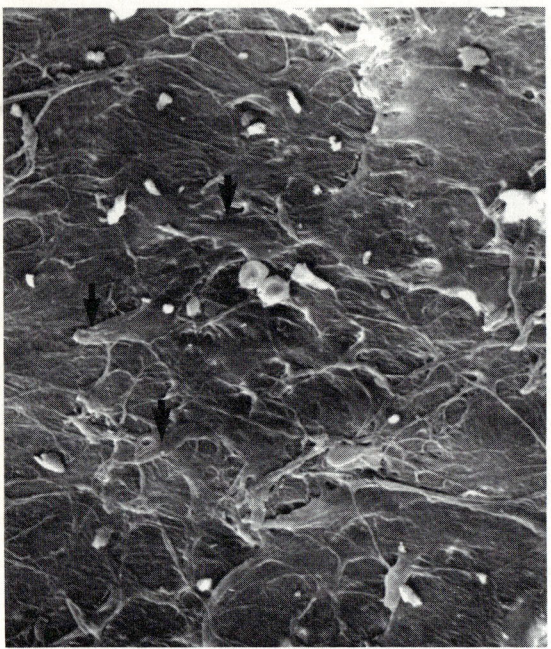

FIG. 4-2 Scanning electron micrograph of pulp fibroblasts (arrows), forming syncytium. Two erythrocytes are in center. ×1000. (Mizrahi SJ, Tucker JW, Seltzer S: A scanning electron microscope study of the efficacy of various endodontic instruments. J Endodont 1:10, 1975)

ODONTOBLASTS

The odontoblast is a highly differentiated cell in the pulp. Efforts directed toward the growth of odontoblasts in tissue culture are meeting with increasing success (Glasstone, 1973; Kisby and Douglas, 1983), and more will be learned of the behavior of these cells, in time. The main function of the odontoblasts is the production of dentin. Morphologic variations occur in the odontoblasts, ranging from the tall columnar cells in the crown of the tooth to a low columnar type in the middle of the root. In the root portion of the tooth, the odontoblasts are shorter and are more or less cuboidal. Toward the apex, they are flattened and look more like fibroblasts.

In the coronal portion of the pulp, where odontoblasts are more columnar, they elaborate regular dentin with regular dentinal tubules (Fig. 4-4 *left*). In the midportion, the tubules are fewer and less regular (Fig. 4-5). The odontoblasts in the apical portion appear less differentiated and elaborate less tubular, more amorphous dentin (Fig. 4-4, *right*).

In tissue sections, the appearance of the odontoblasts varies, depending in part on fixation, staining, and plane of sectioning. Occasionally, only the cell nuclei are visible. They may appear either uniformly stained hyperchromatic, without evidence of nucleoli or chromatin material, or with discrete chromatin threads dispersed throughout the nucleus (Fig. 4-6). In the latter case, nucleoli may be visible. The cytoplasm of the cell may or may not be evident.

Electron Microscope Findings

In scanning electron micrographs, odontoblasts appear as large, closely aligned, multilayered, sweet potato–shaped cells. They average 3 to 4 μm in width and 8 to 10 μm in length (Fig. 4-7). Transmission electron micrographs of odontoblasts have revealed fine structures that indicate that these cells engage in protein production.

Nucleus. The nucleus of a typical odontoblast is ellipsoidal and contains chromatin and nucleoli. The nucleus is surrounded by two thin membranes, each about 50 Å in thickness. The inner membrane appears to be continuous, but the outer one is interrupted at points by openings ranging from 600 Å to 1000 Å in length. Granules with an average diameter of 150 Å are attached to the outer nuclear membrane (Scott, 1955; Fig. 4-8).

Nucleolus. In electron microscope examinations of human teeth, Iványi (1972) found that differentiated odontoblasts contained one to four nucleoli. The nucleoli from fully developed teeth were ring-shaped, which is typical for the reversibly inhibited, or low, rate of synthesis of ribonucleic acid (RNA). In less developed teeth, compact nucleoli, representative of types active in RNA production, were found.

Cytoplasm. According to Jesson (1967), Garant et al (1968), Reith (1968), and Takuma and Nagai (1971), most of the cytoplasm is occupied by an extensive rough-surfaced endoplasmic reticulum (rER) and by numerous transitional vesicles of the rER.

Contact between tubules and vesicles of the endoplasmic reticulum with the nuclear membrane has been noted by Garant et al (1968). A

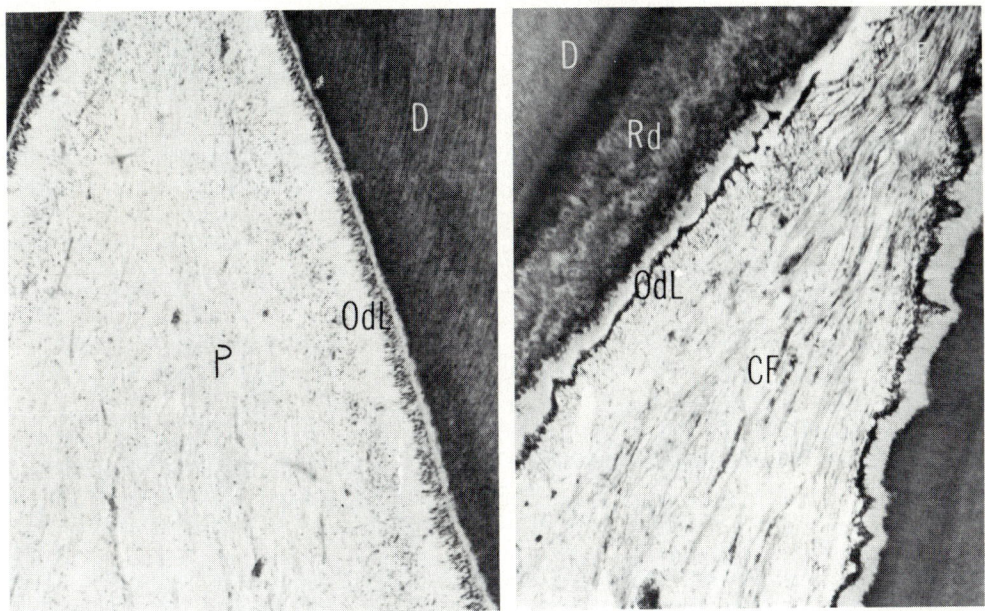

FIG. 4-3   Aging of dental pulp. *(Left)* Physiologically young pulp (P) of an upper cuspid. It is highly cellular and has few collagen fibers. The odontoblastic layer (OdL) is 6 to 8 cells in depth. D, dentin. ×96. *(Right)* Aged pulp of an upper cuspid. The pulp space has been reduced by the deposition of reparative dentin (Rd). The odontoblastic layer (OdL) is thinned. Collagen fibers (CF) are present in abundance. D, dentin. ×96.

FIG. 4-4   *(Left)* Scanning electron micrograph of regular dentinal tubules in coronal portion of tooth. ×1800. *(Right)* Scanning electron micrograph of amorphous dentin in apical region of tooth. ×600.

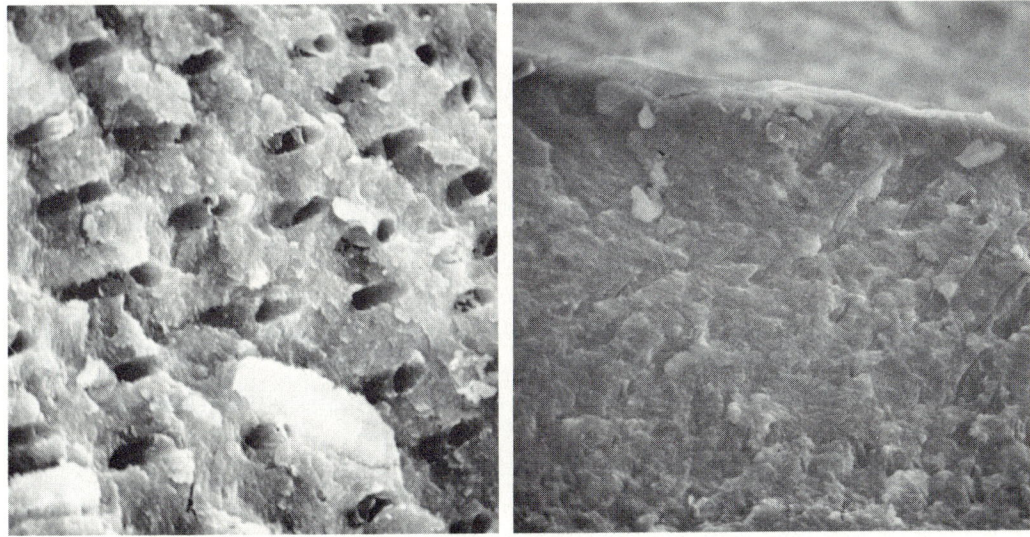

82 | THE DENTAL PULP

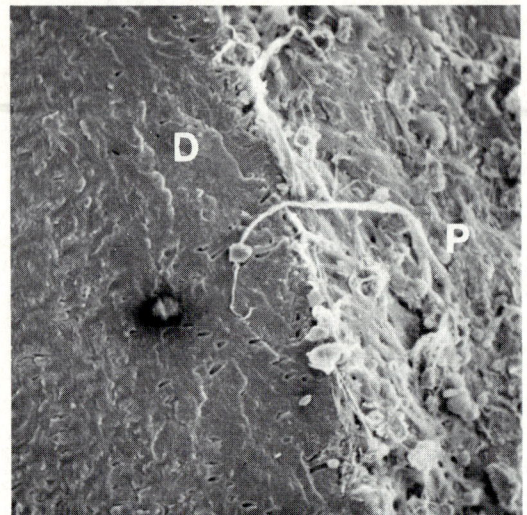

FIG. 4-5 Scanning electron micrograph of dentin (D) and pulp (P) from midportion of tooth. The surfaces of collagen fibers and fibroblasts are shown. Fibroblasts are represented by elevations. A nerve fiber has been torn and is folded over the dentin.

mation along the predentin border (Fig. 4-10; see also Fig. 4-13). Generally, the odontoblastic layer is about six to eight cells deep. The cells are parallel and in continuous contact, possibly due to the presence of fibronectin (Linde et al, 1982), and they branch dichotomously toward the enamel. The organelles, which are situated in the cell body, extend as far as the level of the modified terminal bar apparatus, which is part of the junctional complexes (described below), whereby odontoblasts contact their neighbors

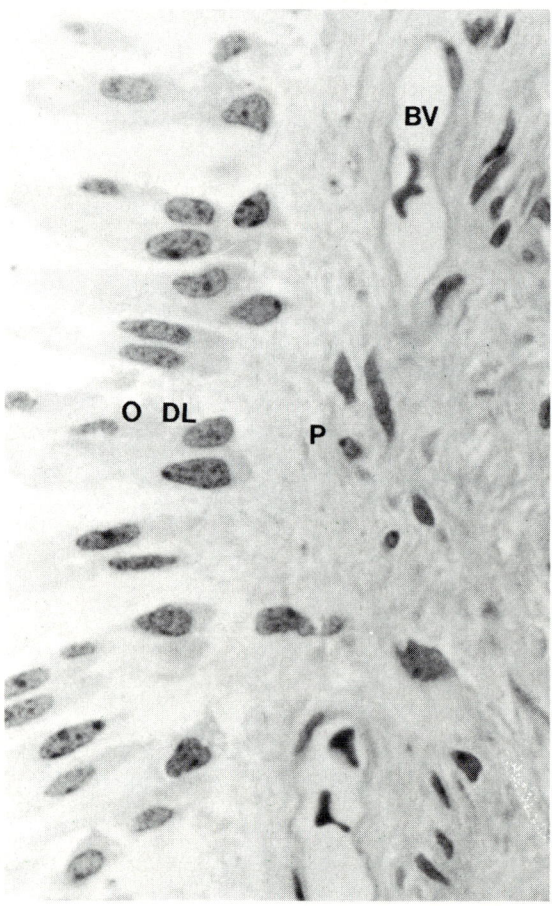

FIG. 4-6 Light micrograph of peripheral zone of dental pulp (P). The odontoblastic layer (ODL) consists of palisading cells with oval, vesicular nuclei and prominent nucleoli. Chromatin threads are dispersed throughout the nucleus. BV, Blood vessel lined with a flattened endothelial cell nucleus. ×850. (Courtesy of Dr. Calvin Leifer, Temple University School of Dentistry, Philadelphia)

fine fibrillar material is present within the cisternae of the rER. The central portion of the odontoblast is occupied by a large Golgi apparatus. Vesicles, containing fibrillar material similar to that found within the cisternae of the rER, are concentrated near each immature face of the Golgi apparatus. Other small coated vesicles devoid of electron-dense material are also present in the cytoplasm. Membrane-bound granules of varying sizes and shapes, possibly lysosomes, containing a highly dense material are found in the cytoplasm (Fig. 4-9). Secretory granules containing mineral deposits (abacus bodies) are present in the area of the Golgi complex (see Fig. 4-8). Mitochondria are evenly distributed throughout most of the cell body, usually closely associated with cisternal elements of the rER. Centrioles are present throughout the region of the Golgi complex. Arising from one of the pair of centrioles, a rudimentary cilium is frequently seen. Filaments of approximately a 50-Å diameter are abundantly present within the cytoplasm (Fig. 4-9). Large numbers of microtubules, 200 Å to 250 Å in diameter but of undetermined length, are also present (Fig. 4-15).

The odontoblasts are lined up in palisade for-

(Fig. 4–9; Reith, 1968). Distal to the level of this apparatus is the material that constitutes the odontoblastic process.

The Odontoblastic Process. Each odontoblastic process traverses the predentin, and then occupies a canaliculus in the dentin (Fig. 4–11), predominately filling the lumen of the dentinal tubule (Fig. 4–12). The odontoblastic processes (called dentinal fibers, or Tomes' fibers; Fig. 4–13) are cytoplasmic tubular projections (Fig. 4–14).

The odontoblastic processes are usually devoid of major cytoplasmic organelles. According to Jesson (1967) and to Garant et al (1968), numerous coated vesicles are present. The coated vesicles at the secretion front most likely are pinocytotic, enabling the odontoblasts to ingest material from the predentin (Reith, 1968; Sasaki, Ishida, and Higashi, 1982). Many vesicles are continuous with the cell membrane in the region of the predentin. The number of coated vesicles decreases within the portion of the process that extends into the mineralized zone. Dense (secretory) granules and lysosome-like bodies are also present. Numerous filaments are oriented parallel to the cell membrane (see Fig. 1–7). According to Reith (1968), these fine filaments are the most characteristic feature of the odontoblastic process and its branches. They are the only components that are always seen in the branches. Microtubules are the next most prevalent cytoplasmic component. They are seen in virtually every portion of the process. They are oriented longitudinally to the long axis (Fig. 4–15). Groups of microvesicles, similar to those seen in the Golgi apparatus, are situated near the plasma membrane.

Intercellular Junctions. Small regions of the plasma membranes between cells (intercellular junctions), are visible only by electron microscopy. There are three types of intercellular junctions: (1) impermeable, (2) adhering, and (3) communicating.

IMPERMEABLE JUNCTIONS, also known as *tight* junctions, help the cell maintain a distinct internal environment. In these junctions, the plasma membranes of adjacent cells appear to fuse and afford a tight seal between the cells.

ADHERING JUNCTIONS are maintained by desmosomes, which are the intercellular bridges seen in light microscopy. There are three types of

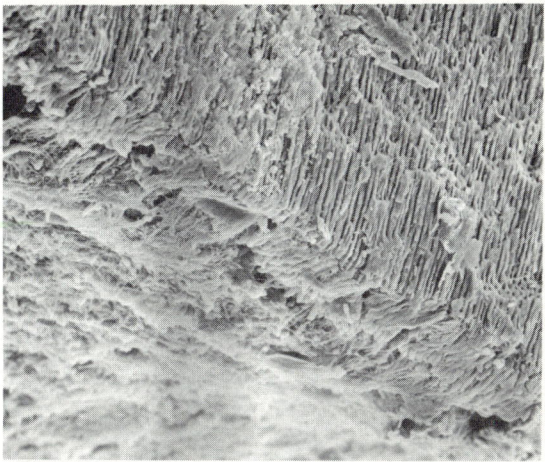
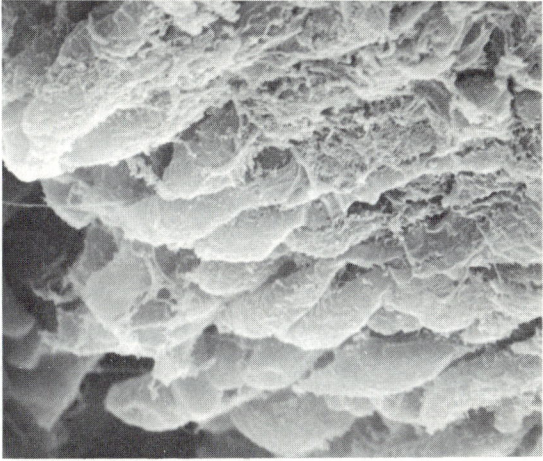

FIG. 4-7 *(Top)* Border of dentin and pulp in region of pulp horn. ×200. *(Bottom)* Higher magnification of odontoblasts lining predentin. ×2000. (Seltzer S, Rainey E, Gluskin AH: Correlation of scanning electron microscope and light microscope findings in uninflamed and pathologically involved human pulps. Oral Surg 43:910, 1977)

desmosomes; belt, spot, and hemidesmosomes. Adhering junctions promote adhesion between cells.

COMMUNICATING JUNCTIONS, also known as gap junctions, are structures that mediate direct transfer of chemical messages between cells. They enable cells to exchange nutrients and signal molecules for coordination of function. All three types are present in the odontoblastic layer.

(Text continued on p. 86)

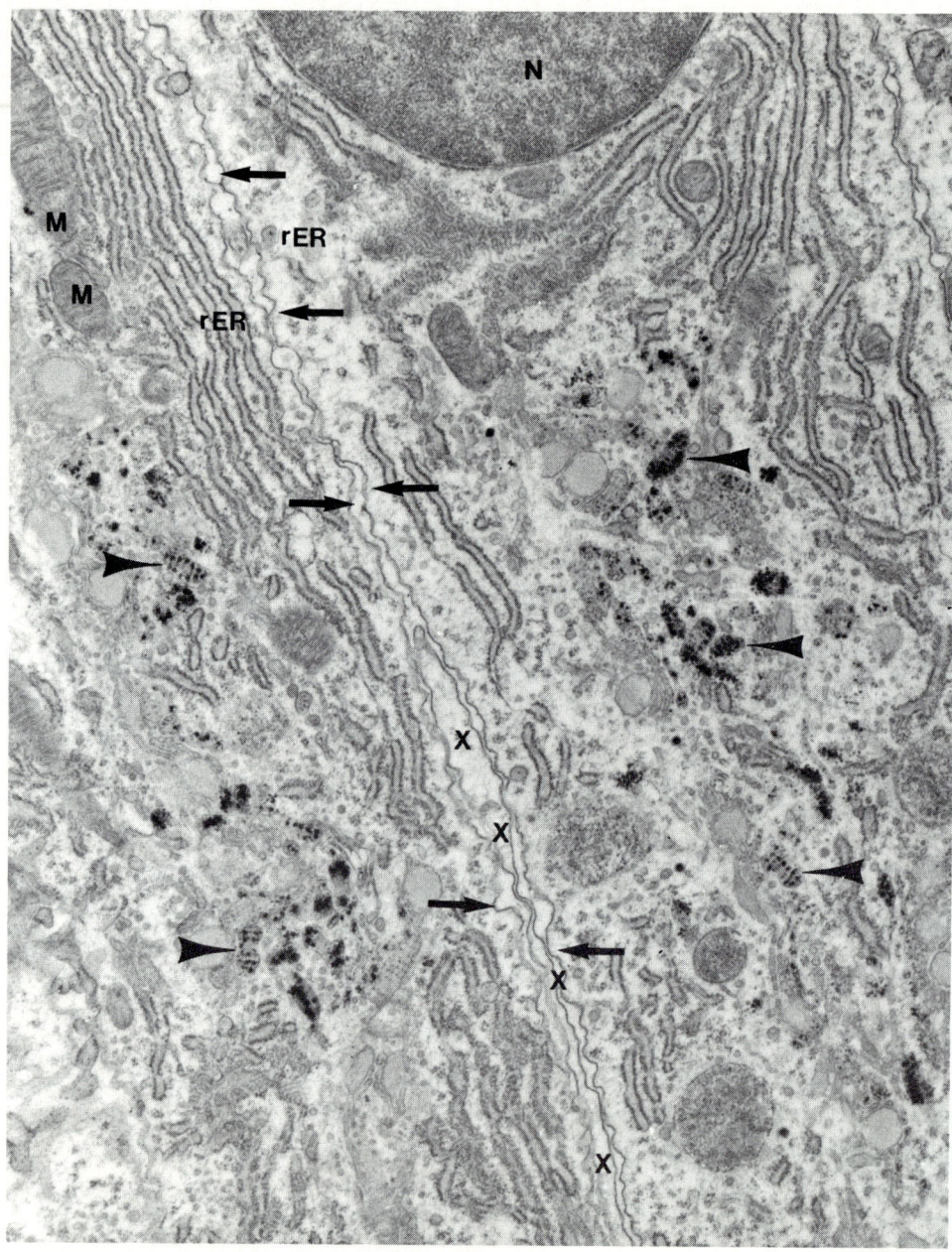

FIG. 4-8 Parts of two neighboring odontoblasts. The arrows point to the plasma membranes of the cells. At top, the nucleus (N) is bounded by a paired membrane. In the lower part of the illustration, a small portion of a third cell appears (X). The abacus bodies of the Golgi apparatus (arrowheads) have been stained with pyroantimonate. N, nucleus; rER, rough endoplasmic reticulum; M, mitochondria. ×5600. (Courtesy of Dr. E. J. Reith, Temple University, Philadelphia)

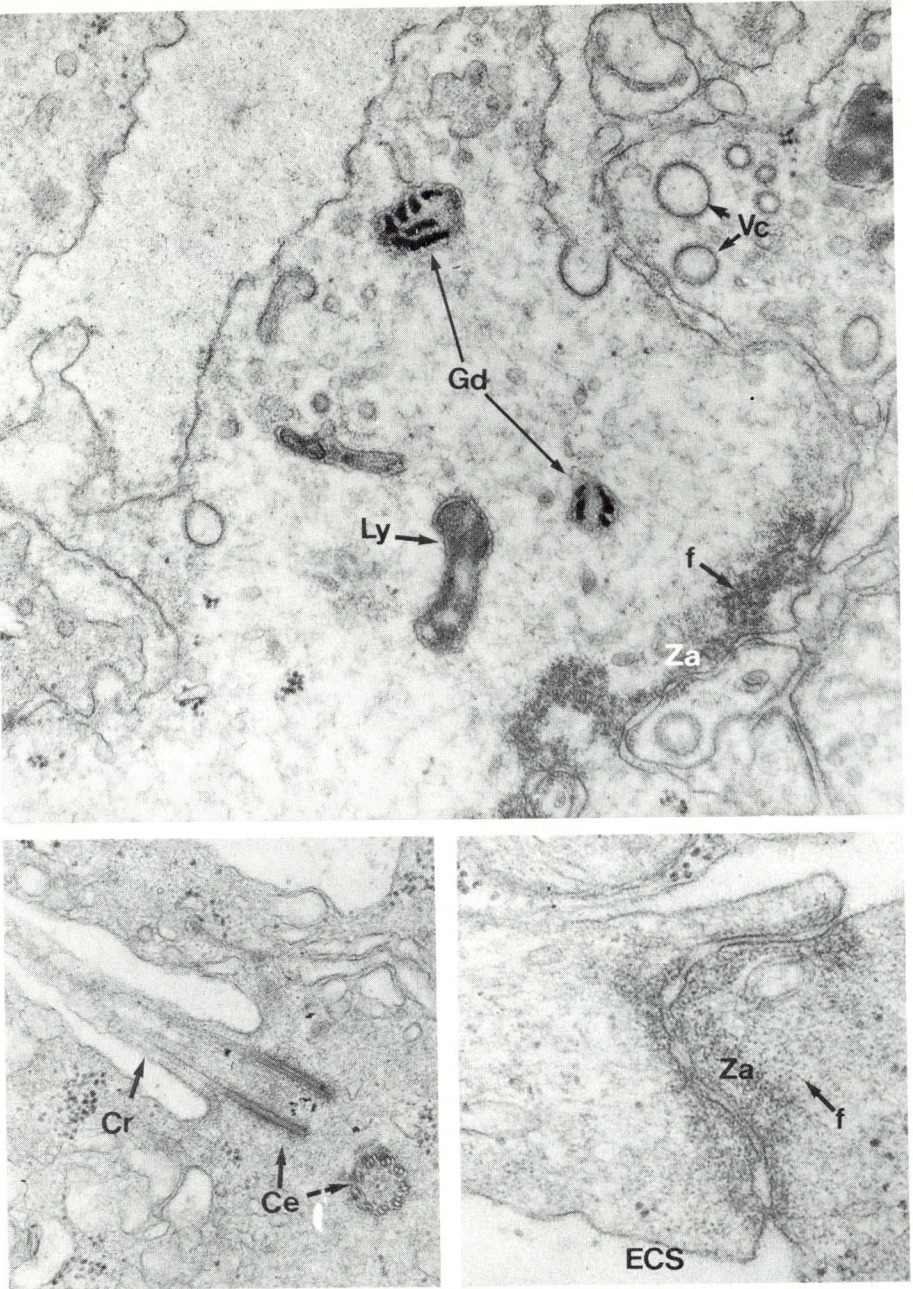

FIG. 4-9 *(Top)* Region of the odontoblastic process just proximal to the terminal web. Fine cytoplasmic filaments (f) condensed near the cell membrane form part of the attachment apparatus, the zonula adherens (Za). Several coated vesicles (Vc), dense granules (Gd), and lysosomelike bodies (ly) are present. The cell membrane is continuous with the membrane of a coated vesicle. ×36,000. *(Bottom, left)* Cytoplasmic area adjacent to the Golgi complex, showing a rudimentary cilium (Cr) apparently formed from one of the centrioles (Ce). ×24,000. *(Bottom, right)* Enlarged view of a zonula adherens (Za). Note the concentration of fine filaments (f), cut in cross section, adjacent to the opposed cell membranes. ECS, extracellular space. ×54,000. (Garant PR, Szabo G, Nalbandian J: The fine structure of the mouse odontoblast. Arch Oral Biol 13:857, 1968)

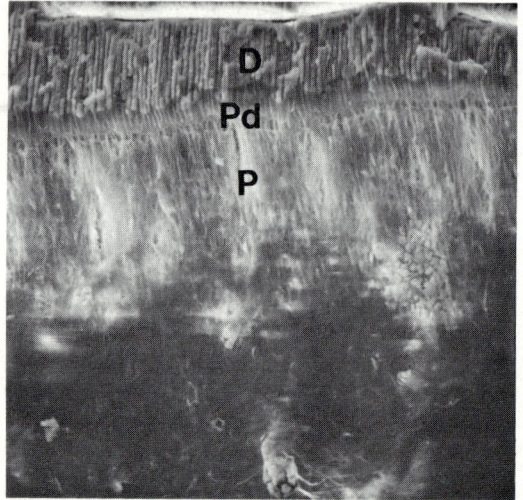
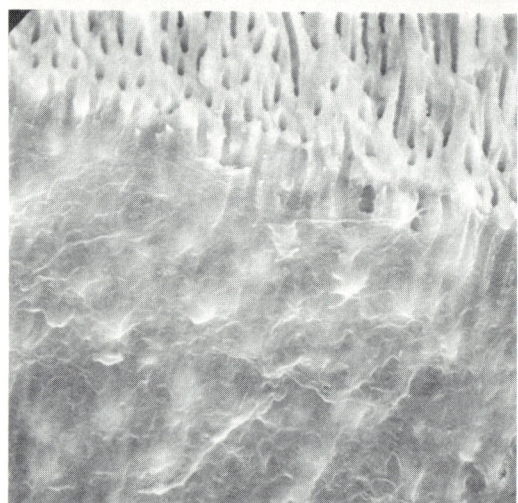
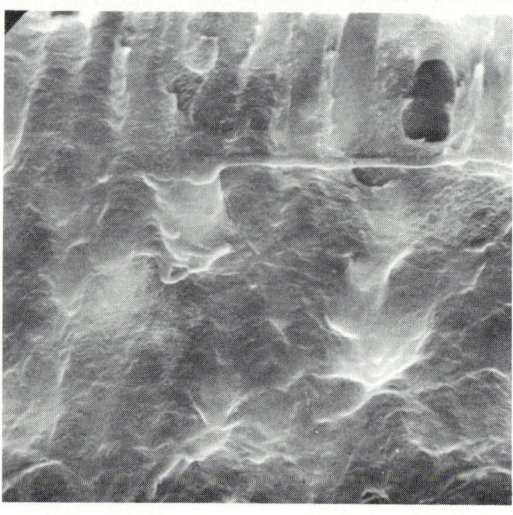

FIG. 4-10 *(Top)* Scanning electron micrograph of pulp-dentin border. D, dentin; Pd, predentin; P, pulp. ×300. *(Center)* Higher magnification of odontoblastic layer at pulp-predentin border. ×1000. *(Bottom)* Higher magnification of middle figure. The surface of the odontoblasts are visible as elevations. ×3000.

Odontoblastic Junctional Complexes. It has long been known from studies with the light microscope that surface epithelial cells possess terminal bars at their apical extremities. In the electron microscope, the terminal bars are seen to consist of several components, designated as junctional complexes. These components are a zonula occludens (tight junction), a zonula adherens, and sometimes a macula adherens.

In the border region between odontoblastic processes and cell bodies, neighboring odontoblasts are in close contact with each other and with other pulp cells (Holland, 1977; Sasaki et al, 1982). These regions contain terminal bar and terminal web structures and they were formerly called tight junctions (Garant et al, 1968; Fig. 4-16). At higher magnification, these structures are seen to be small gap junctions, tight junctions, and desmosomelike junctions (Sasaki et al, 1982; Fig. 4-17). Freeze-fracture replicas of kitten odontoblasts revealed further details of the three types of intercellular junctions between odontoblasts (Fig. 4-18). Such junctions permit the passage of small substances between cells. Thus, the junctional complex present at the apical end of the odontoblast may not be entirely similar to that seen at the apical ends of epithelial cells. In the odontoblast, the junctional complex does not completely encircle the cell, since collagen and nerve fibers are permitted to pass through the cellular junctions.

Tight adhesion occurs between odontoblasts, and they are not easily separated. According to Boyde et al (1978), experimental conditions that cause shrinkage and separation of cementoblasts and osteoblasts also produce shrinkage but fail to cause separation of the odontoblasts at the region of the junctional complex.

Nerve Endings. Although the presence of nerves in the dentinal tubules is controversial, nerve endings in juxtaposition to the odontoblastic processes have been reported (see Chap. 6, The Nerve Supply of the Pulp and Pain Perception).

(Text continues on p. 90)

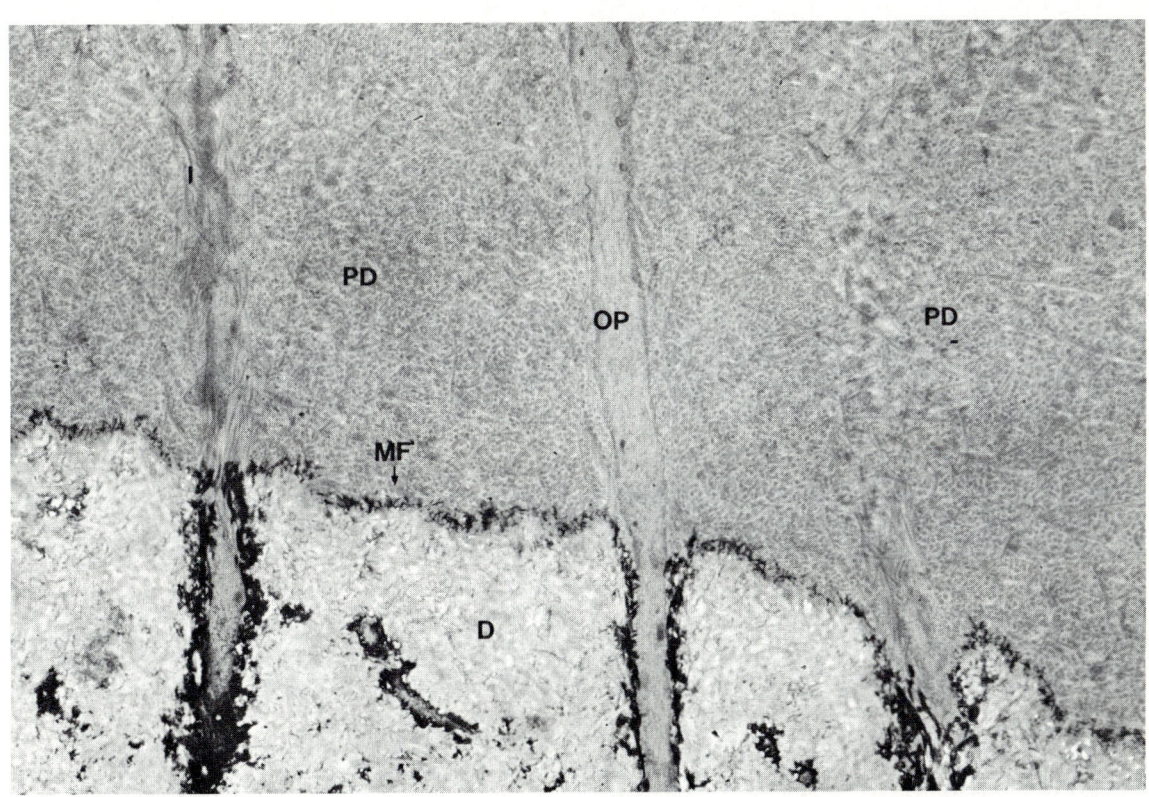

FIG. 4-11 Boundary between predentin (PD) and dentin (D). An odontoblastic process (OP) extends from predentin to dentin without any apparent alteration in its ultrastructure. The mineral has been lost from the dentin, but some is retained at the mineralization front (MF) and at the edges of the dentinal tubules. ×14,000. (Courtesy of Dr. E. J. Reith, Temple University, Philadelphia)

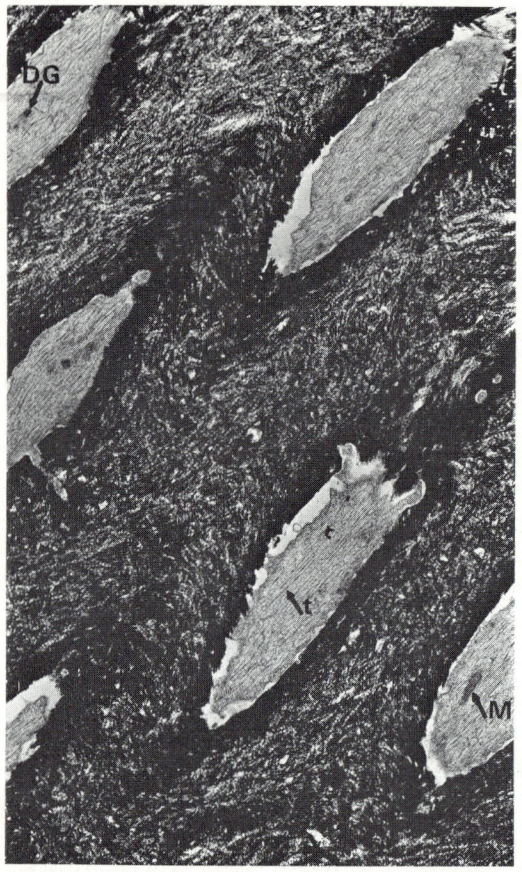

FIG. 4-12 Tangential section through fully mineralized dentin. Odontoblast processes, although slightly shrunken, appear well preserved, as evidenced by the presence of numerous microtubules (t). Mitochondria (M) and dense granules (DG) are present deep within the processes. ×10,000. (Garant PR: The organization of microtubules within rat odontoblast processes revealed by perfusion fixation with glutaraldehyde. Arch Oral Biol 17:1047, 1972)

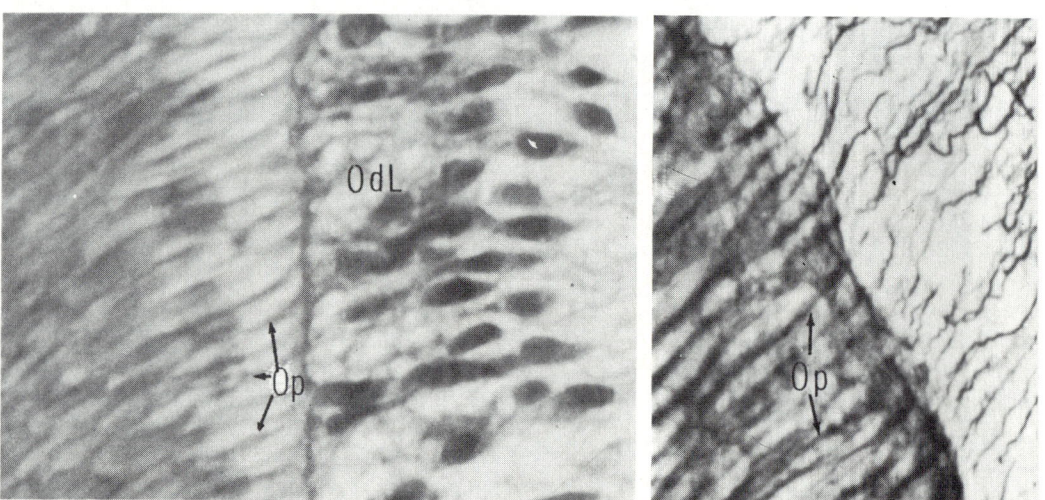

FIG. 4-13 Tomes' fibers (Op) of the odontoblasts (OdL), entering dentinal tubules. *(Left)* Hematoxylin and eosin. ×960. *(Right)* Silver stain. ×960.

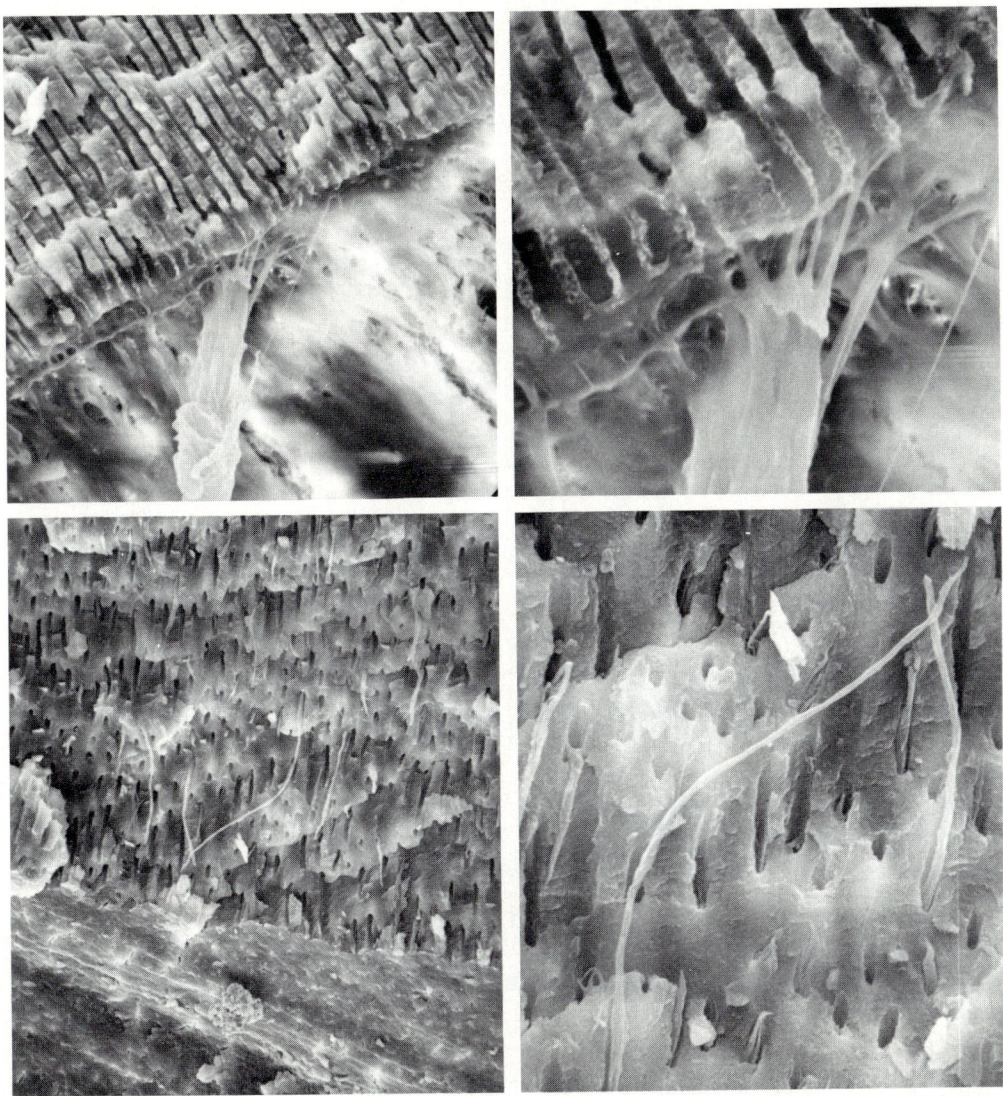

FIG. 4-14 *(Top, left)* Scanning electron micrograph of odontoblastic layer. The odontoblasts are bunched together as a result of being torn from the dentin when the tooth was cracked open. ×600. *(Top, right)* Higher magnification of photograph at left, showing the odontoblastic processes entering the dentinal tubules. ×1800. *(Bottom, left)* Surface of dentin with pulp removed. ×600. *(Bottom, right)* Higher magnification of figure at *bottom left*, showing some remaining odontoblastic processes emerging from dentinal tubules. ×1800.

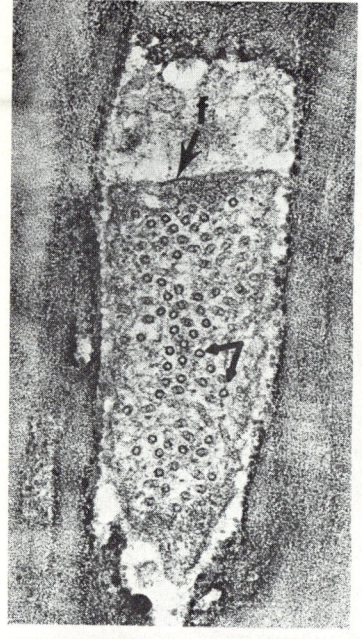
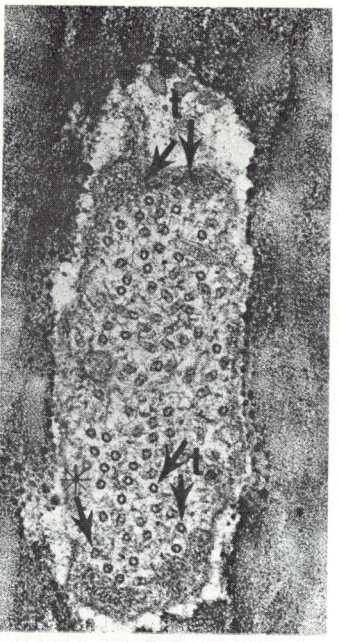
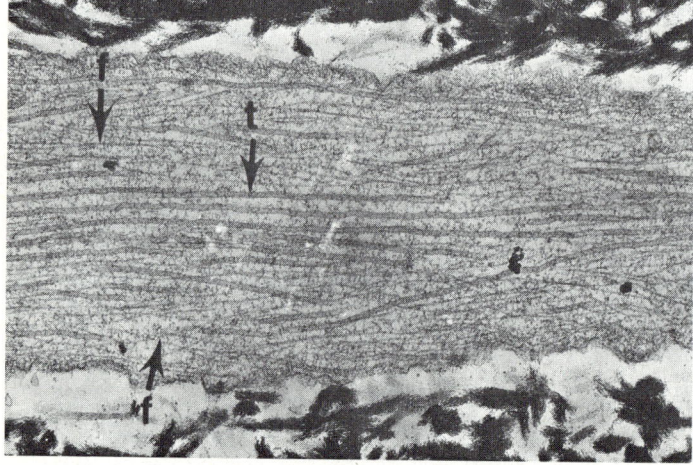

FIG. 4-15 *(Top, left and right)* Cross-sectioned odontoblast processes situated deep within demineralized dentin. Closely packed microtubules (t) are the major structural feature. Dense aggregation of filaments are seen in the cortical regions of the processes (f). (asterisk), Microtubules containing a central electron-dense dot. ×60,000. *(Bottom)* Longitudinal section of odontoblast process, illustrating the characteristic parallel alignment of microtubules (t) and cytoplasmic filaments (f). The microtubules appear to be spaced equidistantly over several microns, suggesting the presence of some intertubular stabilizing structure. ×40,000. (Garant PR: The organization of microtubules within rat odontoblast processes revealed by perfusion fixation with glutaraldehyde. Arch Oral Biol 17:1047, 1972)

Odontoblastic Communications

The odontoblastic nuclei always remain at the inner border of the dentin, and, unlike the osteoblasts, they do not become buried unless they are pathologically involved (Fig. 4–19). The odontoblastic processes are in contact with adjacent processes through an extensive lateral branch system (Kaye and Herold, 1966; Fig. 4–20). The odontoblasts also contact cells more centrally located in the pulp through fine protoplasmic processes, possibly owing to the presence of fibronectin, a mediator of cell-to-cell adhesion (Linde et al, 1982). Thus, the odontoblasts may be regarded as part of a mesenchymal syncytium (Fig. 4–21). This cellular contact is significant because, if an odontoblast is injured, other odontoblasts are affected. The cells on either side are affected by the breakdown products of the injured odontoblasts. When the dentin is injured through operative procedures, the normal palisade arrangement of

(Text continues on p. 94)

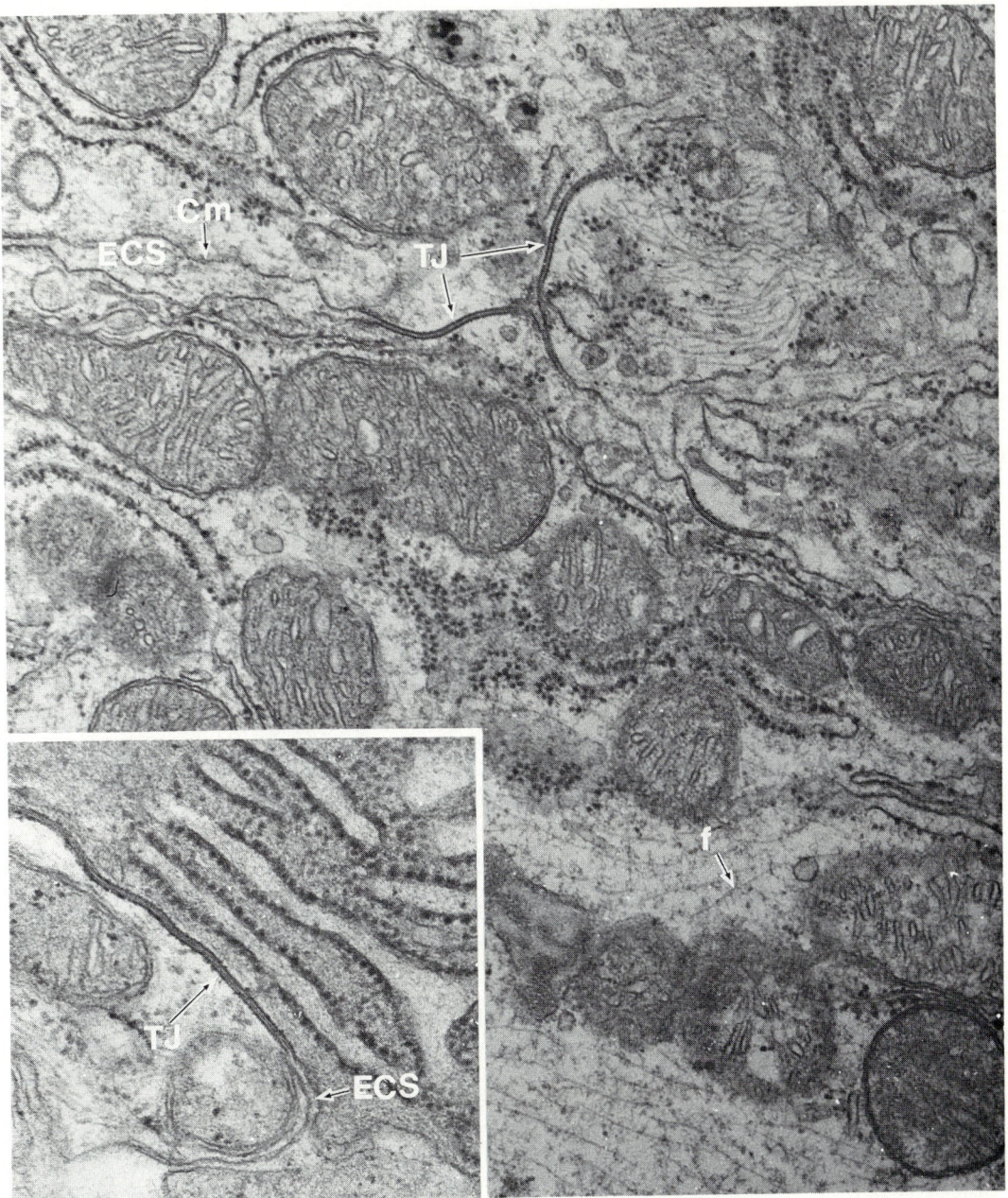

FIG. 4-16 Portions of several adjacent odontoblasts, showing regions of close apposition (TJ) of opposing cell membranes (Cm). Note presence of fine filaments (f) within the cytoplasm. ECS, extracellular space. ×35,400. (Inset) Close apposition of adjacent cell membranes of two odontoblasts forming a tight junction (TJ). Note the intermediate dense line which is believed to be formed by fusion of the opposing outer leaflets of the cell membranes, with consequent obliteration of the extracellular space (ECS). ×48,000. (Garant PR, Szabo G, Nalbandian J: The fine structure of the mouse odontoblast. Arch Oral Biol 13:857, 1968) Author's note: the structures labeled tight junctions (TJ) are now believed to be gap junctions.

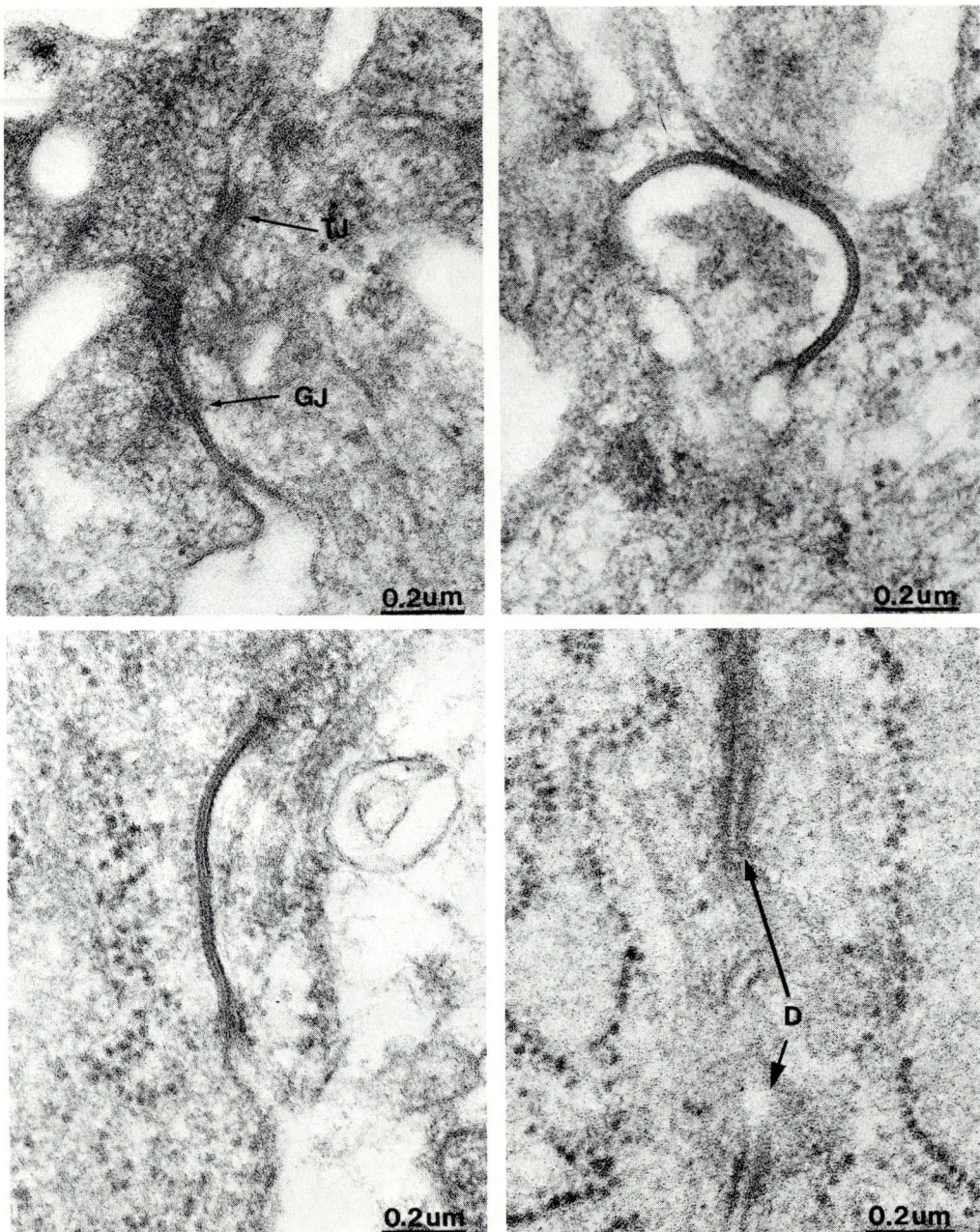

FIG. 4-17 Three types of intracellular junctions between odontoblasts. *(Top, left)* High-power view of a distal terminal bar composed of a small gap junction (GJ) and a tight junction (TJ). ×80,000. *(Top, right)* Gap junction between adjacent odontoblasts, a five-layered structure between two neighboring cell membranes. ×80,000. *(Bottom, left)* Gap junction between odontoblast and pulp cell in the subodontoblast layer. ×80,000. *(Bottom, right)* Desmosomelike junctions (D) between adjacent odontoblasts identified as a pair of cell-membrane electron-dense plaques with a few associated cytoplasmic filaments. ×80,000. (Sasaki T, Nakagawa K, Higashi S: Ultrastructure of odontoblasts in kitten tooth germs as revealed by freeze-fracture. Arch Oral Biol 27:897, 1982)

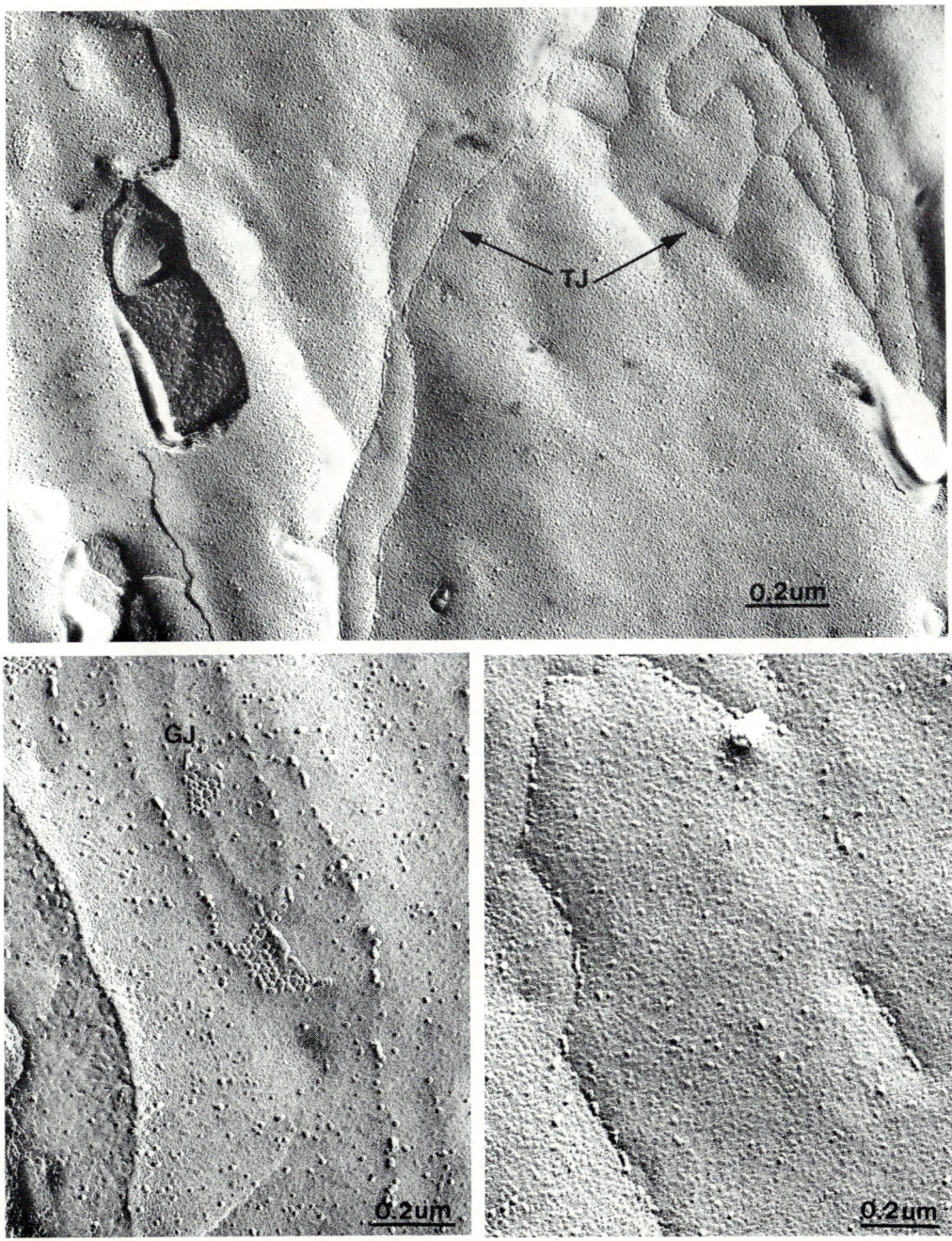

FIG. 4-18 *(Top)* Freeze-fracture replica of distal portion of odontoblast. The distal junctional complex is formed mainly from macular tight junctions (TJ). ×50,000. *(Bottom, left)* High-power view of a distal junctional complex composed of both gap junctions (GJ) and a tight junction representing linear assemblies of particles on the cell-membrane P-face. ×100,000. *(Bottom, right)* Tight junctions as continuous and discontinuous rows of particles along shallow grooves on cell membrane E-face. ×100,000. (Sasaki T, Nakagawa K, Higashi S: Ultrastructure of odontoblasts in kitten tooth germs are revealed by freeze-fracture. Arch Oral Biol 27:897, 1982)

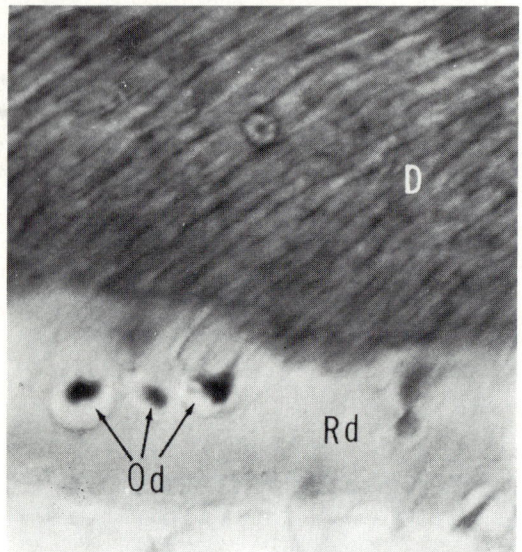

FIG. 4-19 A high magnification of several odontoblasts (Od) that have been encased by reparative dentin (Rd). D, dentin. When the new dentin becomes mineralized, the odontoblastic nuclei no longer will be visible in histologic sections. ×960.

the odontoblasts is altered, resulting in disruption of the continuity of these cells (Fig. 4-22). Thus, injury to the dentin of the tooth creates a reaction within the pulp.

The cytoplasm of the odontoblasts contains a basophilic stippling attributable to the presence of RNA. Minute sudanophilic (probably lipid; Stewart et al, 1965) granules and vacuoles are scattered throughout the cytoplasm and the dentinal fibers. The cytoplasm also stains intensely for alkaline phosphatase and moderately for adenosine triphosphatase (ATPase). Acid phosphatase activity and nonspecific esterases are also present in the odontoblastic and subodontoblastic zones (Goggins and Fullmer, 1967). Staining by methylene blue, toluidine blue, and the PAS method suggests the presence of a carbohydrate-protein complex.

Other histochemical studies (Goggins and Fullmer, 1966; Linde and Ljunggren, 1970) have revealed the presence of various dehydrogenases in the odontoblasts and the cells of the subodontoblastic cell-rich zone. These findings suggest that these cells are capable of glycolysis and fatty acid metabolism plus a functional citric acid cycle and pentose shunt.

Esterases of various types have been detected histochemically and electrophoretically in the odontoblasts and subodontoblastic layers of the pulp and in pulp homogenates, indicating intracellular anabolic or digestive functions (Strachan et al, 1967).

The function of odontoblasts is the secretion of ground substance and collagen. When dentin is being formed, granules and droplets accumulate between the nucleus of the cell and the predentin. A Golgi apparatus in the same region becomes more open-meshed and disperses in the direction of the predentin. The organic matrix of dentin develops in the extracellular space around the formative ends of the odontoblasts. Tomes' fibers contain a lipid element demonstrable by sudan black; small amounts of alkaline phosphatase are demonstrable also. In response to caries, abrasion, attrition, and other processes involving the dentin, an age change or metamorphosis takes place in the dentinal fibers. The end-product of this change is referred to as transparent or sclerotic dentin.

FIG. 4-20 Scanning electron micrograph of odontoblastic processes in contact with processes in other dentinal tubules. ×1800. (Mizrahi SJ, Tucker J, Seltzer S: A scanning electron microscopic study of the efficacy of various endodontic instruments. J Endodont 1:10, 1975)

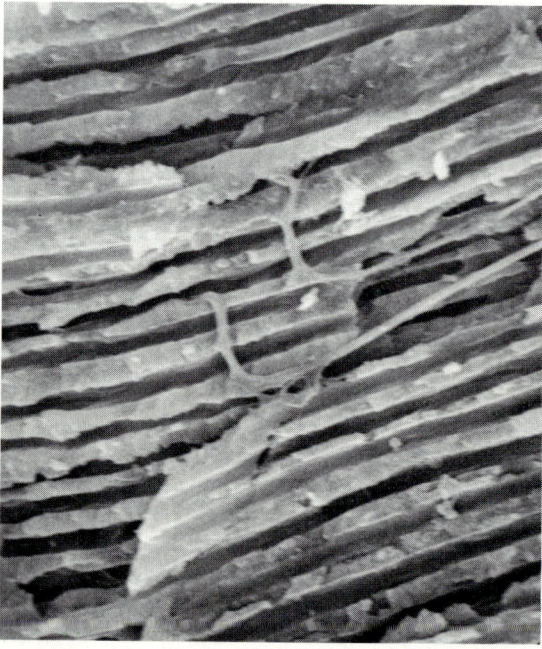

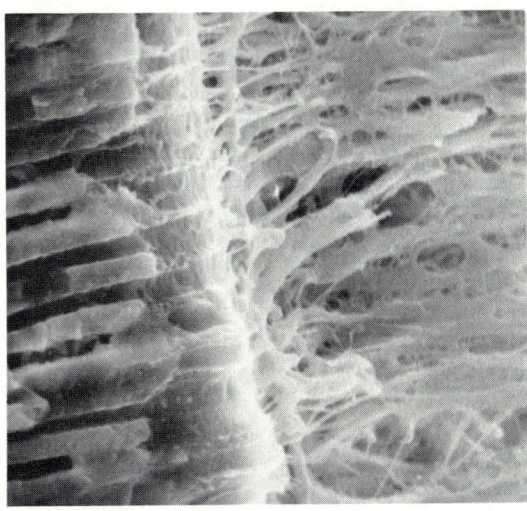 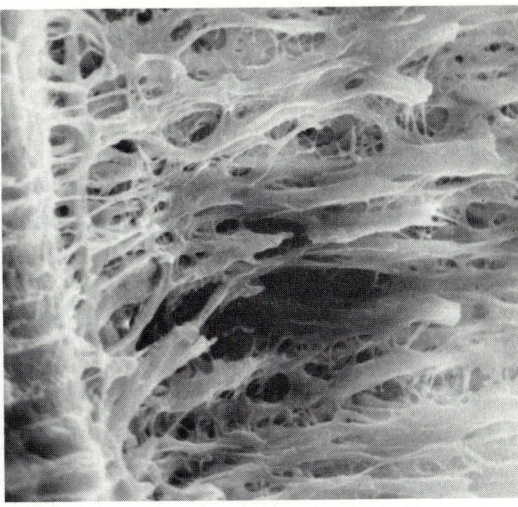

FIG. 4-21 *(Left)* Scanning electron micrograph of odontoblastic layer, demonstrating intercommunication between odontoblasts. ×1800. *(Right)* Toward deeper pulp tissue, communications are seen between cells. ×1800.

Under the layer of odontoblasts in the coronal portion of the tooth, there is a cell-free zone (the layer of Weil) that contains nerve elements. In the middle or apical portions, cell-free zones are not observed (Gotjamanos, 1969).

Beneath the zone of Weil is the cell-rich zone. This zone contains fibroblasts and undifferentiated mesenchyme cells, the reservoir from which odontoblastlike cells are supplied following injury. Stanley (1962) has reported the presence of mitotic figures in differentiating pulp cells under a region of injury.

DEFENSE AND OTHER CELLS

Some of the cells in the pulp are defense cells. Histiocytes, or resting wandering cells, are usually found near the blood vessels. They have long, slender, branching processes and are able to withdraw these processes and change quickly into macrophages when the need arises (see Fig. 4-1).

Undifferentiated mesenchymal cells are present in the pulp, as they are in all connective tissue. They are capable of becoming macrophages during injury. They also may become fibroblasts, odontoblasts, or osteoclasts. Undifferentiated mesenchymal cells constitute a reservoir of cells upon which the body can call to assume functions that are not ordinarily needed. In the pulp, they are usually found outside the

FIG. 4-22 Disruption of the odontoblastic layer (OdL), caused by an operative procedure. The palisaded arrangement is disordered and the odontoblasts are no longer parallel. Pd, predentin; D, dentin. ×960.

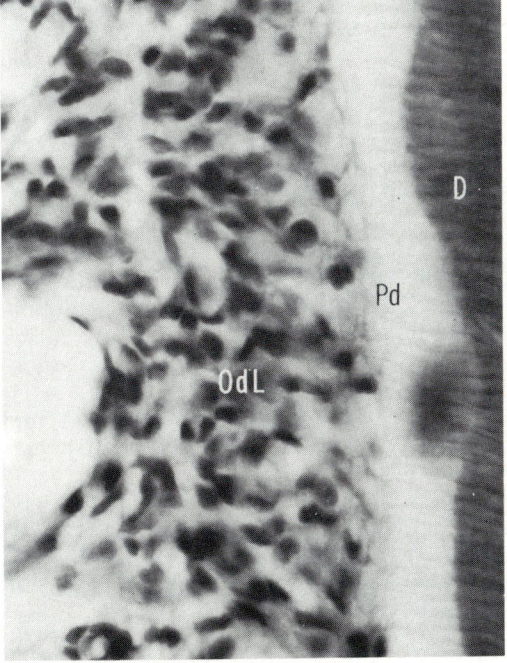

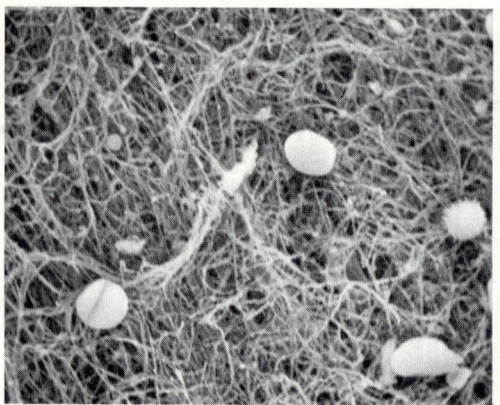 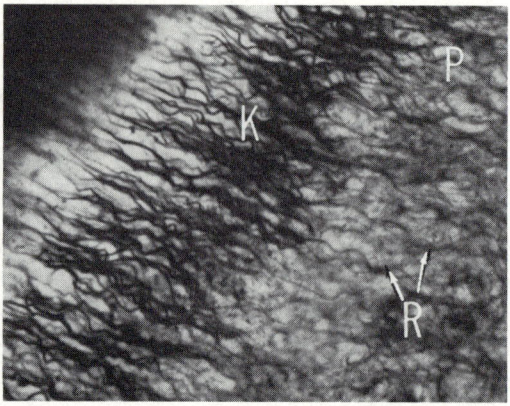

FIG. 4-23 *(Left)* Scanning electron micrograph of reticular fibers in pulp. ×1800. *(Right)* Reticular fibers (R) of the pulp (P), stained with silver salts. Von Korff fibers (K) pass between the odontoblasts and into the predentin. Cells are not visible. ×240.

vessel walls. Before injury, they appear elongated; following injury, they differentiate into macrophages and, as such, can ingest foreign material. Characteristically, a macrophage has numerous vesicles, vacuoles, and membrane-bound bodies, known as lysosomes. The lysosomes contain various hydrolytic enzymes that aid in the breakdown of the ingested material. Stability or lability of the lysosomal membrane of pulp cells is affected by multiple factors, including drugs, infections, and immunologic phenomena (Spott and Rosett, 1973).

Other transitional cell forms in the pulp include ameboid cells of various types and lymphoid wandering cells.

Fat cells are not ordinarily found in the pulp. The presence of mast cells in the human dental pulp has been reported in one tooth (Anneroth and Brännström, 1964). Mast cells have been found in the pulp of a monkey tooth (Wislocki and Sognnaes, 1950) and have been described in the normal gingivae of monkeys and humans.

Lymphocytes are not found usually in the uninflamed pulp, but transitional forms that may develop into mature lymphocytes may be found.

Plasma cells and eosinophils are not found in the uninflamed pulp but are found there following injury.

Pericytes are found in the walls of the precapillaries and metarterioles (see Fig. 5-7). Formerly, they were believed to be concerned with the contraction of the blood vessel walls. Avery (1973) has pointed out that pericytes have prominent Golgi apparatus, abundant endoplasmic reticulum, and associated ribosomes — features of cells that synthesize and secrete proteins. It is possible therefore that the function of pericytes is to manufacture the connective tissue of the precapillary region. They may be muscle-type cells, but their exact function is unknown.

FIBERS

The fibers of the pulp are the same as those of other connective tissues. Reticular (argyrophylic) fibers are found around blood vessels and around the odontoblasts in the pulp. The intercellular spaces contain a fine network of reticular fibers (Fig. 4-23, *left*) which may become transformed into collagen.

Collagen fibers are synthesized by the pulpal fibroblasts. Griffin and Harris (1966) noted that collagen precursors were formed in the dilated cisternae of the rER. The precursors were then transported to the exterior of the cell by secretory vesicles derived from the Golgi apparatus (Breyan and Schilder, 1977). After secretion from the cell, the procollagen molecule is cleaved with procollagen peptidase. The collagen molecules are then cross-linked to form fibrous collagen (Shuttleworth et al, 1980).

Once extruded, the young fibril is electron dense as a result of association with a specialized mucopolysaccharide cementing material. With maturity, collagen fibers, of approximately 750

Å diameter, develop. Type III collagen constitutes 28% to 45% of the pulp collagen (Shuttleworth et al, 1978, 1980; Lechner and Kalnitsky, 1981; van Amerongen, 1983), but some Type I collagen is also present (Takagi et al, 1975). It is possible that Type III collagen may be identified, histologically as reticulin. As the pulp matures, the mucopolysaccharide cementing substance between fibrils apparently diminishes. In addition to the fibrils, Griffin and Harris noted two types of filaments in the extracellular milieu. One type had a relatively straight contour and was approximately 200 Å in diameter and exhibited a 200 Å periodicity. The other type was coiled, branched, and irregularly beaded and was 100 Å in diameter. The first type was associated with the collagen fibrils more often than the second.

Fine argyrophilic fibers, arising in the pulp, form spirally twisted bundles that pass between the odontoblasts and fan out into the unmineralized dentin or predentin in a delicate meshwork. These fibers, called von Korff fibers, form the fibrillar framework of the dentin (Fig. 4–23, *right*). They stain in much the same way as do the fibers of bone and connective tissue and are buried in a jellylike organic ground substance prior to mineralization. It is presumed that this ground substance is secreted by the odontoblasts. The fibrillar organic framework is collagenous, as confirmed by electron microscopic examination of thin sections of dentin (Nylen and Scott, 1960) as well as by histochemical techniques.

There are two prominent patterns of collagen deposition in dental pulp: diffuse, in which the collagenous fibers lack definite orientation, and bundle type (Fig. 4–24), in which large, coarse bundles run parallel to nerves or independently (Stanley and Ranney, 1962). Coronal pulp tissue has more bundle collagen than diffuse collagen. In young pulps, few collagen fibers are found. As the pulp gets older, more and more collagen is elaborated (Fig. 4–25; Uitto and Ranta, 1973), and this increase is mostly in Type III collagen (Takagi et al, 1975; Hayakawa et al, 1981). However, Stanley and Ranney found that there was little correlation between the chronologic age of the patient and the quantity of collagen present in the coronal pulp tissue.

Pulp collagen fiber turnover is fairly high, compared with that of other dental tissues (Orlowski, 1977a,b).

Regardless of age, the apical portion of the

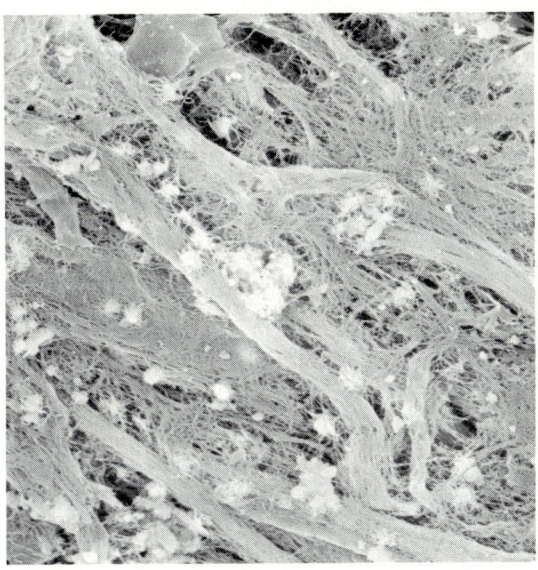

FIG. 4–24 Scanning electron micrograph of collagen bundles in the coronal dental pulp. ×3000.

pulp is usually more fibrous than the coronal portion (van Amerongen et al, 1983). Perhaps the Type III collagen and proteoglycans act as an incompressible cushion to protect the arterial plexus and the odontoblastic layer from pressure, as Hayakawa et al (1981) have pointed out. Clinically, the apical pulp tissue has a whitish appearance due to the preponderance of collagen fibers.

Extirpation of a young, cellular pulp with a broach is rather difficult because of the pulp's resiliency. An aged pulp that is fibrous and mineralized has an appearance similar to that of an absorbent paper point when extirpated.

GROUND SUBSTANCE

The ground substance of the pulp is part of the system of ground substances in the body. It influences the spread of infection, metabolic changes in cells, stability of crystalloids, and the effects of hormones, vitamins, and other metabolic substances.

The ground substance of the pulp is similar to that of connective tissue elsewhere in the body; it is composed of protein associated with glycoproteins and acid mucopolysaccharides. As demonstrated by histochemistry, electrophoresis, and autoradiography (Linde, 1973; Embery,

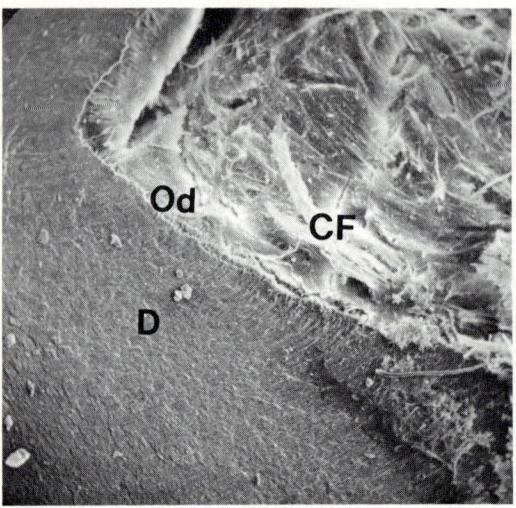 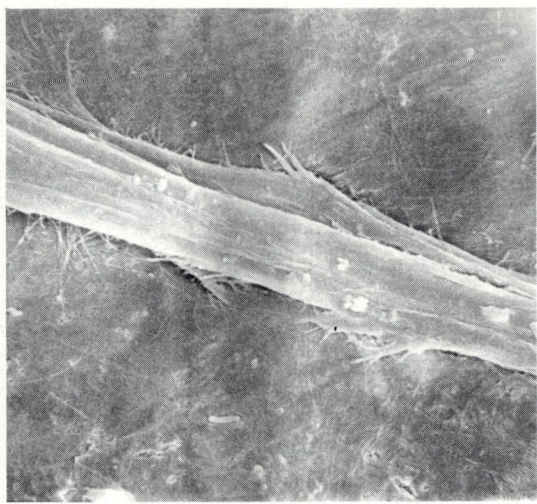

FIG. 4-25 *(Left)* Scanning electron micrograph of collagen fibers in older coronal pulp. D, dentin; Od, Odontoblastic layer; Cf, collagen fibers. ×60. *(Right)* Scanning electron micrograph of collagen fiber lying on dentin wall. ×1800.

1974), the acid mucopolysaccharides are glycosaminoglycans of the hyaluronic acid type, dermatan sulfate, and chondroitin sulfates (Engfeldt and Hjerpe, 1972). Orlowski (1974) has estimated that 20% of the pulpal carbohydrate is in glycosaminoglycans. In the pulps of eruped human teeth, dermatan sulfate is the major glycosaminoglycan (Embery, 1976).

The following properties have been attributed to glycosaminoglycans: water retention, ion-binding and electrolyte distribution during mineralization (Bowness, 1968), and influence on collagen fibrillogenesis (Obrink, 1973).

The pulps of growing teeth stain metachromatically, but this property is diminished or absent in fully formed teeth (Wislocki and Sognnaes, 1950). Also, endogenous pulp oxygen consumption is higher during dentinogenesis than after dentin formation has been completed (Fisher et al, 1959). The metabolism of the cells and the fibers of the pulp is mediated through the ground substance. The ground substance, a viscid fluid, is described by Engel (1958) as the *milieu interieur* through which metabolites pass fom the circulation to the cells and through which breakdown products from the cells come back to the venous circulation. There is no way for nutrients to get from the blood supply to the cells other than through the ground substance. In order to be transported from the blood vessels to the cells, nutrients must be dissolved in the ground substance. In a similar manner, substances excreted by the cell must go through the ground substance to get into the efferent circulation. Thus, hyaluronic acid regulates metabolite transport (Laurent et al, 1969), and the metabolic role of the ground substance influences the vitality of the pulp. The enzyme hyaluronidase degrades hyaluronic acid. Hyaluronidase activity has been detected in rabbit dental pulp, indicating that this enzyme functions to degrade the glycosaminoglycans (Sakamoto et al, 1981).

The pressure of the pulp interstitial tissue fluid depends directly on capillary pressure. The pulp tissue pressure has been used as a monitor of the pulp intracapillary pressure. Measurements of pulp tissue hydrostatic pressure, through an analysis of dentinal pulp fluid, have indicated that the pressure rises an average of 15 mm Hg in the early stages of inflammation. It gradually returns to normal values (Bender, 1978).

Depolymerization by enzymes elaborated by microorganisms found in pulp inflammation may change the ground substance of the pulp. For example, microorganisms that elaborate hyaluronidase have the ability to depolymerize the hyaluronic acid, which is a component of the ground substance. Likewise, microorganisms elaborate chondroitin sulfatase and other enzymes that can affect the polymerization of the ground substance. In fact, mucopolysaccharidase activity has been detected, by histochemical techniques, within the pulps of resorbing deciduous teeth. According to Alexander et al (1980), these enzymes are capable of degrading the ground substance of the pulp and dentin by disrupting the glycosaminoglycan-collagen linkage. Thus, the ground substance plays a significant role in health and disease of the pulp and dentin.

SYSTEMIC FACTORS THAT AFFECT THE PULP

Certain systemic conditions affect the cells, fibers, and ground substance of the connective tissue of the pulp.

VITAMIN DEFICIENCY

Deficiency of certain vitamins, notably vitamin C, affects fibroblasts generally and specifically affects the fibroblasts in the dental pulp. Studies in animals show that the odontoblasts are affected demonstrably when there is a deficiency of ascorbic acid. The cells either degenerate or lose their morphology and become indistinguishable from other pulp cells (Denmark, 1966). In electron microscopic examinations, the fibroblasts of scorbutic guinea pigs appear smaller and contain a diminished number of intracellular organelles. Many cells are devoid of endoplasmic reticulum (ER). If present, the ER is dilated and contains a decreased number of ribosomes. The number of intra- and intercellular fibrils are increased (Avery et al, 1966; Ross, 1966; Fig. 4–26).

Such changes have been described by Westin (1925) and by Dalldorf (1935) in humans suffering from scurvy.

Hunt and Paynter (1959) found that guinea pigs on a diet deficient in ascorbic acid had severely affected periodontal tissues. The collagen fibers were especially affected. The defects were due to lack of fiber synthesis rather than fiber destruction.

HORMONES AND HORMONAL IMBALANCE

Steroids. Systemic administration of high doses of corticosteroids to rabbits inhibits collagen synthesis in the dental pulps, resembling the anti-anabolic effect of starvation (Uitto and Manthorpe, 1983). Long-term systemic steroid therapy delays bone and wound healing and affects the odontoblasts, thereby inhibiting dentinogenesis.

Glickman and Shklar (1954) premedicated rats with daily doses of cortisone for periods up to 40 days and then observed the effects on their teeth. They found that, in both the molar and the incisor teeth, the odontoblastic layer was severely disrupted, with disintegration and necrosis of the cells. However, the continuously growing incisors were more sensitive to the effects of cortisone than were the molars. There was a reduction in the number of fibroblasts, the capillary walls were disturbed, and there was marked tissue degeneration.

Lisanti and Hill (1955) premedicated dogs for a period of 2 weeks or 1 month with cortisone and then drilled cavities in their teeth. The dentin was then cauterized by heat from 200°F to 600°F. The animals were sacrificed after varying periods of time. There was marked impairment of healing in the cortisone-treated animals as compared with the controls. In other animals, which were given cortisone postoperatively, there was no interference with healing. This demonstrated the effect of systemic influences on local reactions.

Glucocorticoids have been used on the dentin of prepared cavities prior to restoration to reduce pulpal inflammation (Fry et al, 1960; Mosteller, 1962; Dachi et al, 1964). They have been recommended also for pulp capping. However, the benefits of steroid therapy are extremely questionable, since interference with the process of inflammation permits the uninhibited growth of microorganisms and may lead to pulpal degeneration. Also, since steroids diminish the height, number, and tinctorial properties of the odontoblasts, they inhibit reparative dentinogenesis—an effect that is clearly detrimental (Ulmansky and Langer, 1957). Antibiotics, antiseptics, and dentin-stimulating agents such as calcium hydroxide have been added to counteract the deleterious effects of the steroids—a questionable form of treatment, that illustrates the futility of this type of therapy.

Diabetes. Diabetics tend to age more quickly because of obliterative endarteritis. There is impairment of nutrition and metabolic processes. Tissue repair is interfered with in diabetics.

With respect to the pulp, a rise in plasma glucose levels produces a correlative rise in glucose concentrations in the dentinal pulp fluid (Haldi and John, 1965).

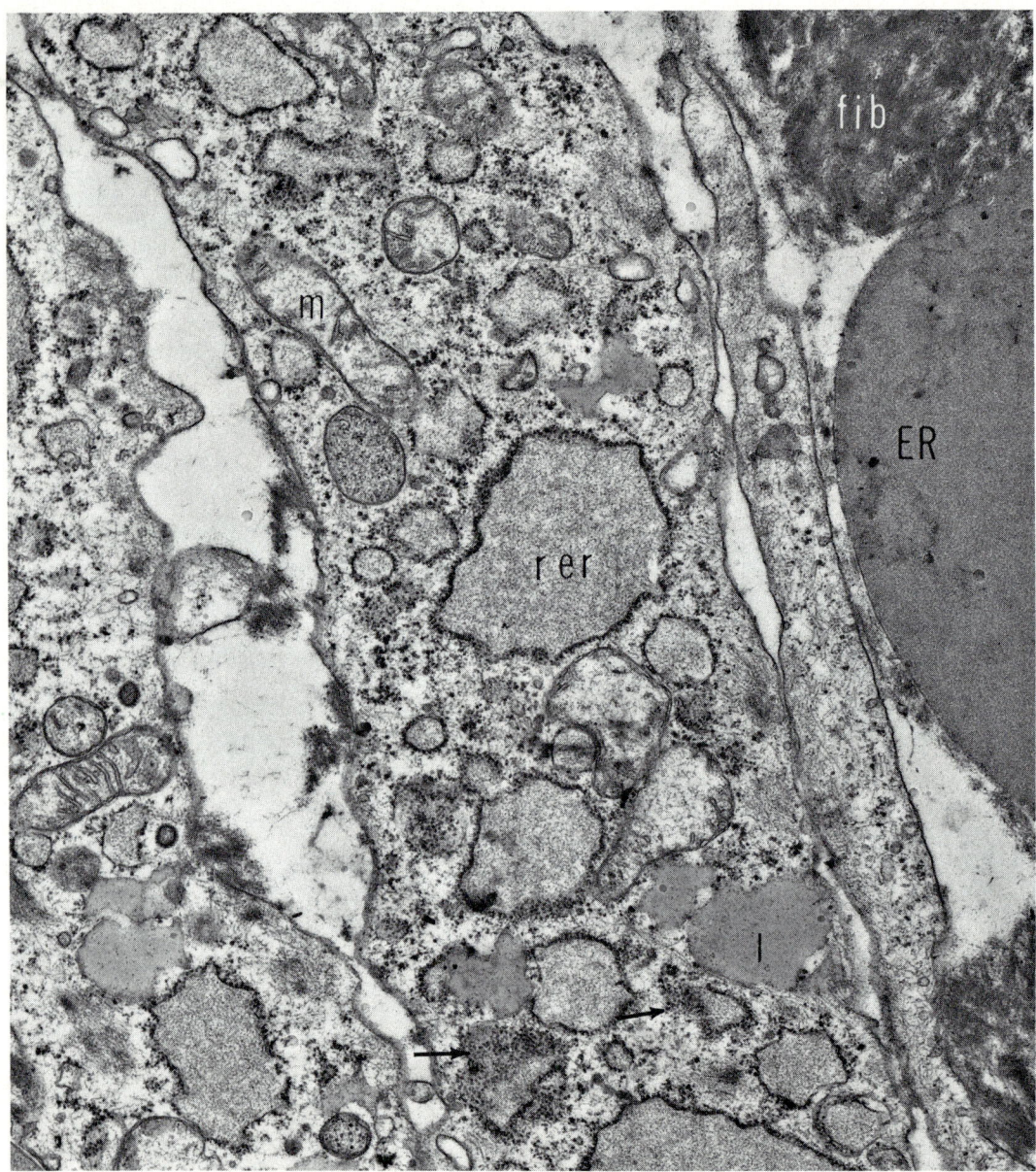

FIG. 4-26 Electron micrograph showing parts of several fibroblasts from a 14-day-old wound in the skin of a scorbutic guinea pig. The cisternae of the rough endoplasmic reticulum (rer) appear dilated and vacuolar, and they contain dense material and display no apparent loss of ribosomes. In zones where the membranes are tangentially sectioned (arrows), the loss of the characteristic arrangement of the aggregate of attached ribosomes is apparent. Lipid deposits (l), mitochondria (m) and fine cytoplasmic filaments can be seen. In the extracellular regions, part of an erythrocyte (ER) and the fibrillar material (fib) seen in scurvy are apparent. ×22,500. (Ross R: The ultrastructure of fibrogenesis. J Dent Res 45:449, 1966. Copyright by the American Dental Association. Reproduced by permission)

Diabetes produces degenerative and inflammatory changes in the pulp, and dentinogenesis is consequently affected.

In studying the dental structures of Chinese hamsters with spontaneous hereditary diabetes, Cohen et al (1963), found degenerative changes in the periodontal and the pulpal tissues. The pulps of noncarious teeth were atrophic, with degenerative changes in the odontoblasts, the fibroblasts, the ground substance, and the dentin. In carious teeth, the pulps were acutely inflamed. Even in the absence of pulp exposure, abscesses, as well as large quantities of reparative dentin, were present.

Glickman and Shklar (1954) induced alloxan diabetes in experimental animals. The predentin of these animals was wider than normal, and there was interference in mineralization.

Thyroid Deficiency. Baume and associates (1954) showed that animals subjected to thyroidectomy displayed a marked reduction in vascularity of the pulp, with a hypermineralization of bone and dentin. There was rapid deposition of dentin, which narrowed the lumen of the pulp, and all tissues showed a decreased amount of cellular elements.

PROTEIN DEFICIENCY

Dietary proteins are essential for the formation and maintenance of tissue structure; they constitute the main sources of amino acids and nitrogen, which are needed for the synthesis of body proteins. Dietary proteins may also serve as energy sources (Enwonwu, 1973).

Glickman and Shklar (1954), in their study of rats that had been deprived of protein for 4 to 9 weeks, did not notice any changes in the pulps. However, whether interference with dentinal repair would occur following irritation of the pulp was not determined. In comparable studies, Stahl et al (1958) found that protein-deprived rats developed larger regions of periapical rarefaction around teeth subjected to occlusal interference after the pulps were exposed. Around the teeth of rats that were not deprived of protein, the regions of rarefaction were smaller. Osteogenic activity and localization of inflammation were interfered with in the protein-deprived animals. Stahl (1966) has also shown that protein deficiency results in degeneration of connective tissue fibers of the periodontium, osteoporosis of the alveolar bone, and retardation of cementum deposition.

SYSTEMIC VIRUS INFECTION

In experimental animals, systemic virus infections have been demonstrated to have an effect on the dental pulp. In investigations by Kreshover and Hancock (1956) on lymphocytic choriomeningitis and by Fleming (1958) on Shope papilloma virus, the odontoblasts were found to be injured. The pulps of mice infected with polyoma virus exhibited degenerative changes that increased in severity with the onset of carious lesions. The eventual result was pulp necrosis (Cohen and Shklar, 1965).

Conversely, it has been shown that infection of the dental pulps of experimental animals with viruses resulted in systemic manifestations. Benda et al (1972) inoculated herpes simplex viruses into the exposed pulps of rabbits. The resulting infection was found to travel centripetally along the trigeminal nerve to the Gasserian ganglion and eventually, after 5 days, to the brain stem.

HEREDITARY DISEASES

A number of diseases have been reported to affect the dental pulp. These include diseases of the blood (sickle-cell anemia, Witkop, 1973, Andrews and England, 1983); leukemia (Stern and Cole, 1973); disorders of the reticuloendothelial system (Hand-Schüller-Christian disease, Gamble and Stanley, 1964); neurologic diseases, such as Sturge-Weber disease (Baer et al, 1961); metachromatic leukodystrophy (Gardner and Zeman, 1965); Krabbe's leukodystrophy (Witkop, 1973); Fabry's disease (Desnick et al, 1972); and Niemann-Pick disease (Stewart, 1970). Pulp biopsy has been suggested as a means of confirming the diagnoses of these diseases (Gardner, 1967; Stewart, 1970; Desnick et al, 1972).

TUMOR TRANSPLANTATION

Reports of tumor metastases to the dental pulp are sparse, possibly because the dental pulps are usually not studied postmortem. However, epitheliomas, sarcomas, and Burkitt's lymphomas have been found in human dental pulps (Stanley, 1973). Experimentally, Tawa ascites tumor has been transplanted successfully by Sakaki et al (1971) into the pulp of the lower incisor of rats. The pulp cells and odontoblasts underwent atrophic changes and were replaced by tumor cells. The ameloblasts were unaffected.

BIBLIOGRAPHY

Alexander SA, Swerdloff M, Caputo L: Dental pulp mucopolysaccharidase: Identification and role in tooth resorption. J Dent Res 59:1404, 1980

Andrews CH, England MC, Jr: Sickle cell anemia: An etiological factor in pulpal necrosis. J Endodont 9:249, 1983

Anneroth G, Brännström M: Auto-fluorescent granular cells and mast cells in the human gingiva and dental pulp. Odont Revy 15:10, 1964

Avery JK: Structural elements of the young normal human pulp. In Siskin M (ed): The Biology of the Human Dental Pulp, pp 3–15. St. Louis, CV Mosby, 1973

Avery JK, Han SS, Lee Y: Modifications of the fine structure of the incisor pulp of the guinea pig during experimental scurvy. J Dent Res 45:440, 1966

Baer PN, Stanwich L, Alloy J, Merritt AD, Lewis JR: Gingival hemangioma associated with Sturge-Weber Syndrome. Report of a case. Oral Surg 14:1383, 1961

Baume LS, Becks H, Ray JC, Evans HM: Hormonal control of tooth eruption. I. The effect of thyroidectomy on the upper rat incisor. J Dent Res 33:80, 1954

Benda R, Petrovič Š, Rychterová V: Transmission of herpes virus along the trigeminal nerve in rabbits. Acta Virol 16:459, 1972

Boyde A, Reith EJ: The pattern of mineralization of rat molar dentine. Z Zellforsch 94:479, 1969

Boyde A, Reith EJ, Jones SJ: Intercellular attachments between calcified collagenous tissue forming cells in the rat. Cell Tiss Res 191:507, 1978

Breyan D, Schilder H: An electron microscopic study of collagen formation in the dental pulp of the human premolar and rat incisor. Oral Surg 44:437, 1977

Cohen MM, Shklar G: Pulpal pathosis in mice infected with polyoma virus. Oral Surg 20:245, 1965

Cohen MM, Shklar G, Yerganian G: Pulpal and periodontal disease in a strain of Chinese hamsters with hereditary diabetes mellitus. Oral Surg 16:104, 1963

Dachi SF, Ross A, Stigers RW: Effects of prednisolone on the thermal sensitivity and pulpal reactions of amalgam-restored teeth. JADA, 69:565, 1964

Dalldorf G: The pathology of vitamin C deficiency. JAMA 111:1376, 1935

Denmark SJ: Ascorbic acid staining of scorbutic guinea pig incisors. J Dent Res 45:762, 1966

Desnick SJ, Witkop CJ, Jr, Krivit W, Thies JK, Desnick RJ: Fabry's disease (ceramide trihexosidase deficiency): diagnostic confirmation by analysis of dental pulp. Arch Oral Biol 17:1473, 1972

Embery G: Glycosaminoglycans of human dental pulp. J Biol Buccale 4:229, 1976

Embery G: The isolation of chondroitin 4-[35S] sulfate from the molar teeth of young rats receiving sodium [35S] sulfate. Calc Tiss Res 14:59, 1974

Engel MB: Integrated behavior in connective tissues. Oral Surg 11:724, 1958

Engfeldt B, Hjerpe A: Glycosaminoglycans of dentin and predentine. Calc Tiss Res 10:152, 1972

Enwonwu CO: Elements of dietetics for the general practitioner. Int Dent J 23:317, 1973

Fisher AK, Belding JH, Opinsky JS, Spinella DJ: The influence of the stage of tooth development on the oxygen quotient of normal bovine dental pulp. J Dent Res 38:208, 1959

Fleming HS: Shope papilloma virus and tooth germ transplants. Oral Surg 11:549, 1958

Frank RM: Etude au microscope electronique de l'odontoblaste et du canalicule dentinaire humain. Arch Oral Biol 11:179, 1966

Fry AE, Watkins RF, Photak NM: Topical use of corticosteroids for the relief of pain sensitivity of dentine and pulp. Oral Surg 13:594, 1960

Gamble JW, Stanley HR: Hand-Schüller-Christian disease with involvement of the dental pulp. Oral Surg 18:272, 1964

Garant PR, Szabo G, Nalbandian J: The fine structure of the mouse odontoblast. Arch Oral Biol 13:857, 1968

Gardner DG: Pulpectomy as a diagnostic procedure in metachromatic leukodystrophy. Oral Surg 23:379, 1967

Gardner DG, Zeman W: Biopsy of the dental pulp in the diagnosis of metachromatic leucodystrophy. Develop Med Child Neurol 7:620, 1965

Glasstone S: The development of teeth and jaws in tissue culture. J Dent Assn S Afr 28:328, 1973

Glickman I, Shklar G: The effects of systemic disturbances on the pulp of experimental animals. Oral Surg 7:550, 1954

Goggins JF, Fullmer HM: Dehydrogenase histochemistry of the rat molar pulp. Arch Oral Biol 11:1365, 1966

Goggins JF: Hydrolytic enzyme histochemistry of the rat molar pulp. Arch Oral Biol 12:639, 1967

Gotjamanos T: Cellular organization in the subodontoblastic zone of the dental pulp. 1. A study of cell-free and cell-rich layers in pulps of adult rat and deciduous monkey teeth. Arch Oral Biol 14:1007, 1969

Griffin CJ, Harris R: Ultrastructure of collagen fibrils and fibroblasts of the developing human dental pulp. Arch Oral Biol 11:659, 1966

Haldi J, John K: Correlative rise and fall of glucose in blood plasma and dental pulp fluid. J Dent Res 44:10, 1965

Han SS, Avery JK, Hale LE: The fine structure of differentiating fibroblasts in the incisor pulp of the guinea pig. Anat Rec 153:187, 1965

Hayakawa T, Iijima D, Hashimoto Y, Myokei Y, Takei T, Matsui T: Developmental changes in the collagens and some collagenolytic activities in bovine dental pulps. Arch Oral Biol 26:1057, 1981

Holland GR: Structural relationships in the odontoblast layer. In Anderson DJ, Matthews B (eds): Pain in the Trigeminal Region, pp 25–35. Elsevier/North-Holland Biomedical Press, 1977

Hunt AM, Paynter KJ: The effects of ascorbic acid deficiency on the teeth and periodontal tissues of guinea pigs. J Dent Res 38:232, 1959

Iványi D: Nucleoli of human odontoblasts. Arch Oral Biol 17:931, 1972

Jessen H: The ultrastructure of odontoblasts in perfusion fixed, demineralized incisors of adult rats. Acta Odont Scand 25:491, 1967

Kawasaki K, Tanaka S, Ishikawa T: On the daily incremental lines in human dentine. Arch Oral Biol 24:939, 1980

Kaye H, Herold RC: Structure of human dentine. 1. Phase contrast, polarization, interference and brightfield microscopic observations on the lateral branch system. Arch Oral Biol 11:355, 1966

Kisby LE, Douglas WHJ: Isolation, culture, and characterization of bovine odontoblasts. AADR Abstr 9, J Dent Res 62:170, 1983

Kreshover SJ, Hancock JA: The effect of lymphocytic choriomeningitis on pregnancy and dental tissues in mice. J Dent Res 35:467, 1956

Laurent TC, Wasteson Å, Öbrink B: Macromolecular properties of glycosaminoglycans (mucopolysaccharides) and proteoglycans. In Ageing of Connective and Skeletal Tissue. Stockholm, Nordiska Bokhandelns Förlag, 1969

Lechner JH, Kalnitsky G: The presence of large amounts of type III collagen in bovine dental pulp and its significance with regard to the mechanism of dentinogenesis. Arch Oral Biol 26:265, 1981

Linde A, Johansson S, Jonsson R, Jontell M: Localization of fibronectin during dentinogenesis in rat incisor. Arch Oral Biol 27:1069, 1982

Linde A, Ljunggren A: Lactate dehydrogenase isoenzyme patterns of human dental pulp. J Dent Res 49:1469, 1970

Lisanti VF, Hill RG: The effect of imbalance of adrenal hormones on pulp reactions and dentin deposition. J Dent Res 34:761, 1955

Mosteller JH: Use of prednisolone in the elimination of postoperative thermal sensitivity. A clinical study. J Pros Dent 12:1176, 1962

Nylen MV, Scott DB: Electron microscopic studies of odontogenesis. J Ind D A 39:406, 1960

Orlowski WA: Analysis of collagen, glycoproteins and acid mucopolysaccharides in the bovine and porcine dental pulp. Arch Oral Biol 19:255, 1974

Orlowski WA: The turnover of collagen in the dental pulp of rat incisors. J Dent Res 56:437, 1977a

Orlowski WA: A potential for high collagen turnover in the molar pulp independent of eruption. J Dent Res 56:1488, 1977b

Pejrone CA: Anaerobic glycolysis in dental pulp. J Dent Res 44:521, 1965

Rabinowitz JL, Rossman S: Lipid composition of human dental pulp. Arch Oral Biol 24:477, 1979

Reith EJ: Collagen formation in developing molar teeth of rats. J Ultrastruct Res 21:383, 1968

Ross R: The ultrastructure of fibrogenesis. J Dent Res 45:449, 1966

Russell DL: The distribution of glycogen in bovine dental pulp. J Dent Res 46:1182, 1967

Sakaki T, Tsurumi N, Kawakatsu K, Kawahata K: Experimental studies on the intrapulpal transplantation of Tawa sarcoma in the rat. Gann 62:21, 1971

Sakamoto N, Nakajima T, Ikunaga K, Shidahara H, Okamoto H, Okuda K: Identification of hyaluronidase activity in rabbit dental pulp. J Dent Res 60:650, 1981

Sasaki T, Ishida I, Higashi S: Ultrastructure and cytochemistry on old odontoblasts in rat incisors. J Electron Microsc 31:378, 1982

Sasaki T, Nakagawa K, Higashi S: Ultrastructure of odontoblasts in kitten tooth germs as revealed by freeze-fracture. Arch Oral Biol 27:897, 1982

Schour I: Noyes' Histology and Embryology, 8th ed, Philadelphia, Lea & Febiger, 1960

Severson AR: Histochemical demonstration of adenosine triphosphatase in dental tissue. J Dent Res 47:1201, 1968

Shuttleworth CA, Berry L, Bloxsome C, Wilson NHF: Synthesis of sulfated glycosaminoglycans by rabbit dental pulp fibroblasts in culture. Arch Oral Biol 27:729, 1982

Shuttleworth CA, Berry L, Wilson NHF: Biosynthesis of glycoproteins of rabbit dental pulp fibroblasts in culture. Arch Oral Biol 27:645, 1982

Shuttleworth CA, Berry L, Wilson N: Collagen synthesis in rabbit dental pulp fibroblast cultures. Arch Oral Biol 25:201, 1980

Shuttleworth CA, Ward JL, Hirschmann PN: The presence of type III collagen in the developing tooth. Biochim Biophys Acta 535:348, 1978

Spott RJ, Rosett T: Lysosomes and the dental pulp. Oral Surg 36:569, 1973

Stahl SS: Response of the periodontium to protein-calorie malnutrition. J Oral Med 21:146, 1966

Stahl SS, Miller SC, Goldsmith ED: The influence of occlusal trauma and protein deprivation on the response of periapical tissue following pulp exposure in rats. Oral Surg 11:536, 1958

Stanley HR: The effect of systemic diseases on the human pulp. In Siskin M (ed): The Biology of the Human Dental Pulp, pp 606–648. St. Louis, CV Mosby, 1973

Stanley HR, Ranney RR: Age changes in the human dental pulp. I. The quantity of collagen. Oral Surg 15:1396, 1962

Stern MH, Cole WL: Radiographic changes in the mandible associated with leukemic cell infiltration in a case of acute myelogenous leukemia. Oral Surg 36:343, 1973

Stewart JM, Clairbourne EA, Luikart GA: A histologic and histochemical study of lipids in human odontoblasts. J Dent Res 44:608, 1965

Stewart RE: Dental pulp biopsy in the diagnosis of neurological disorders in childhood. J Hosp Dent Pract 4:13, 1970

Strachan DS, Rapp R, Avery JK: Demonstration of multiple esterases of the human dental pulp after electrophoresis in starch and acrylamide gels. J Dent Res 46:1471, 1967

Takagi T, Saito S, Kuboki Y, Sasaki S: Age-related changes of the collagen of periodontium, gingiva and dental pulp. Jap J Oral Biol 17:432, 1975

Takuma S, Nagai N: Ultrastructure of rat odontoblasts in various stages of their development and maturation. Arch Oral Biol 16:993, 1971

Tanaka T: The origin and localization of dentinal fluid in developing rat molar teeth studied with lanthanum as a tracer. Arch Oral Biol 25:153, 1980

Ten Cate AR, Deporter DA, Freeman E: The role of fibroblasts in the remodeling of periodontal ligament during physiologic tooth movement. Am J Ortho 69:155, 1976

Torneck CD: 1. A report of studies into changes in the fine structure of the dental pulp in human caries pulpitis. J Endodont 7:8, 1981

Uitto V-J, Manthorpe R: Selective inhibition of collagen

biosynthesis in the dental pulps of glucocorticoid-treated rabbits. Arch Oral Biol 28:241, 1983

Uitto V-J, Ranta R: Procollagen proline hydroxylase activity in human dental pulp at various stages of development. Proc Finn Dent Soc 69:254, 1973

Ulmansky M, Langer M: Reaction of dental pulp to Ledermix and Calxyl. Israel J Med Sci 3:739, 1967

Van Amerongen JP, Lemmens IG, Tonino GJM: The concentration, extractability and characterization of collagen in human dental pulp. Arch Oral Biol 28:339, 1983

Van Hassel HJ: Physiology of the human dental pulp. In Siskin M (ed): The Biology of the Human Dental Pulp, pp 16–24. St. Louis, CV Mosby, 1973

Westin G: Scorbutic changes in the teeth and gums in man. D Cosmos 67:868, 1925

Wislocki GB, Sognnaes RF: Histochemical reactions of normal teeth. Am J Anat 87:239, 1950

Witkop CJ, Jr: Manifestations of genetic diseases in the human pulp. In Siskin M (ed): The Biology of the Human Dental Pulp, pp 54–59. St. Louis, CV Mosby, 1973

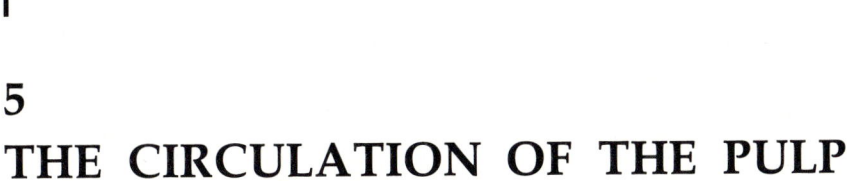

5
THE CIRCULATION OF THE PULP

The circulation of the blood is the transportation system by means of which the various cells of the body are supplied with nutrients and the waste products from the cells are removed for elimination from the body.

SYSTEMIC CIRCULATION

From the venae cavae the blood passes into the right atrium, and from there it is pumped through the right ventricle and into the lungs by way of the pulmonary artery. The blood is oxygenated in the lungs and returns to the heart, by way of the pulmonary vein, to the left atrium and is pumped through the left ventricle to the aorta. The aorta gives off blood vessels (arteries) that divide into smaller and smaller branches; the smallest arteries are called arterioles.

The arterial supply to the pulps of the teeth originates from the posterior superior alveolar, the infraorbital, and the inferior alveolar branches of the internal maxillary artery (Fig. 5–1). A single artery or several smaller arteries enter the pulps through the apical foramen or foramina. In addition, numerous smaller vessels enter through lateral and accessory foramina.

Blood is returned to the heart by the venous system. The pulpal veins, together with other venous tributaries, form the pterygoid plexus located posterior to the maxillary tuberosity. The pterygoid plexus drains into the internal maxillary vein, which joins with the superficial temporal vein to form the retromolar mandibular vein. The blood is then returned, through the external or the internal jugular vein, to the superior vena cava. The right atrium receives the blood from the superior vena cava and the cardiopulmonary circulatory cycle is repeated. (Fig. 5–2).

The development of the vascular system structurally and functionally is related directly to the needs of the tissues. The blood vessels and the connective tissue form a single functioning system.

MICROCIRCULATION

The primary function of microcirculation is to transport nutrients to, and to remove metabolic waste products from, the tissues. Thus, the physiology of the tissue depends on the circulatory transport process, which is governed by many

(This chapter was prepared with the generous assistance of Dr. Syngcuk Kim, School of Dental and Oral Surgery, Columbia University, New York.)

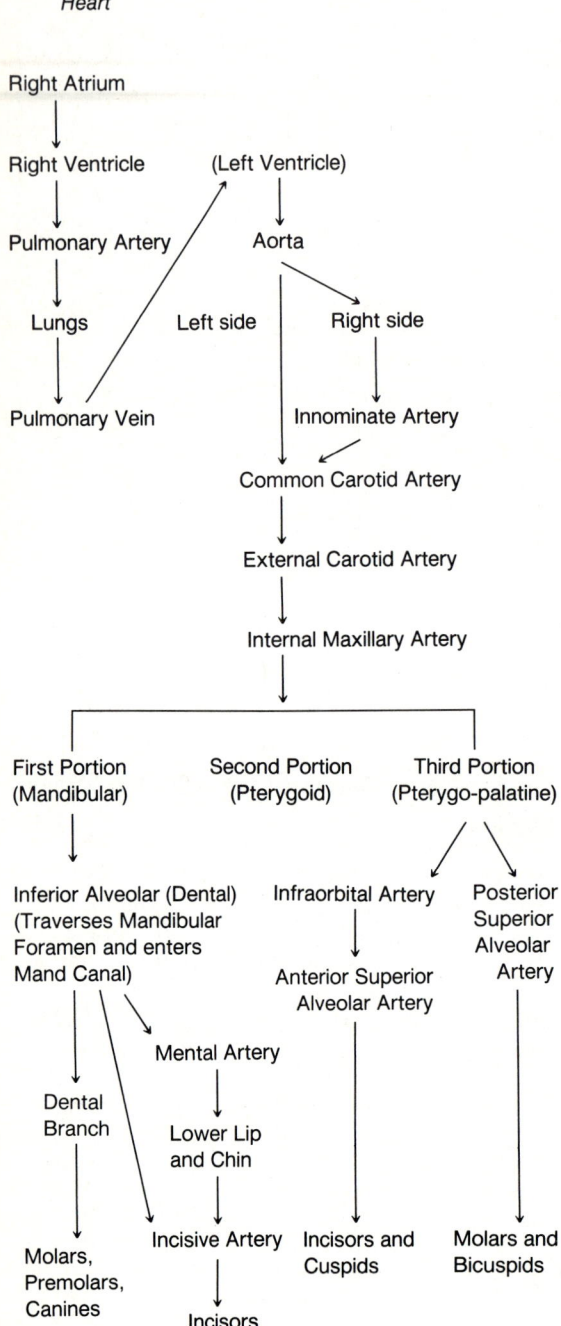

FIG. 5-1 Arterial blood supply to the teeth.

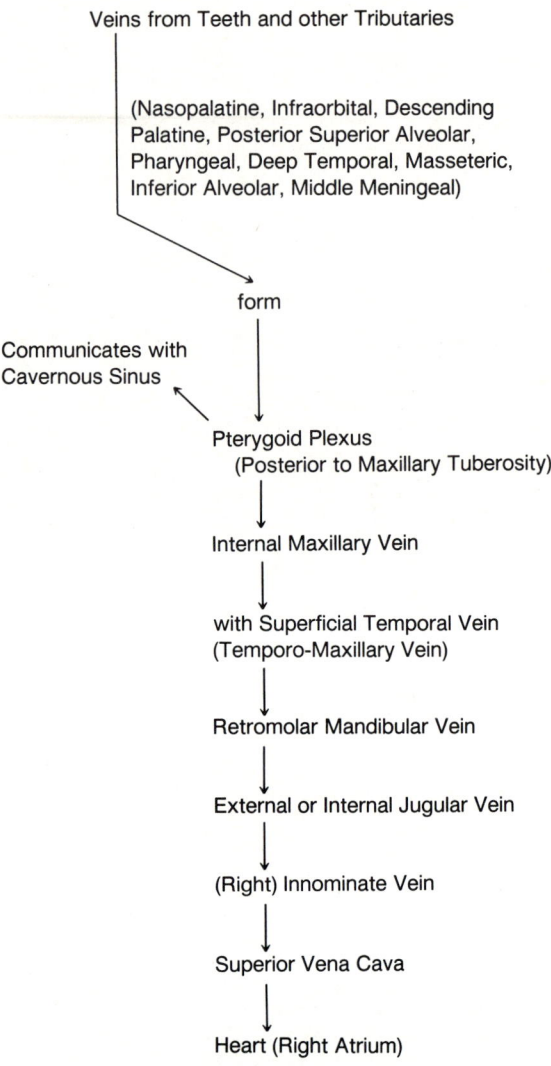

FIG. 5-2 Venous drainage from the teeth.

functional parameters of the microcirculation. Knowledge of the microcirculation is prerequisite for an understanding of the pathophysiologic processes of tissue disorders. Alterations in microcirculatory functions contribute to pathologic processes in the tissues, and microcirculatory adjustments may occur in connective tissue disorders as compensatory and homeostatic mechanisms.

Architecture of the Microvascular Network

The major microcirculatory vessels are the arterioles, the capillaries, and the venules. At the arteriole subdivision, true microcirculation

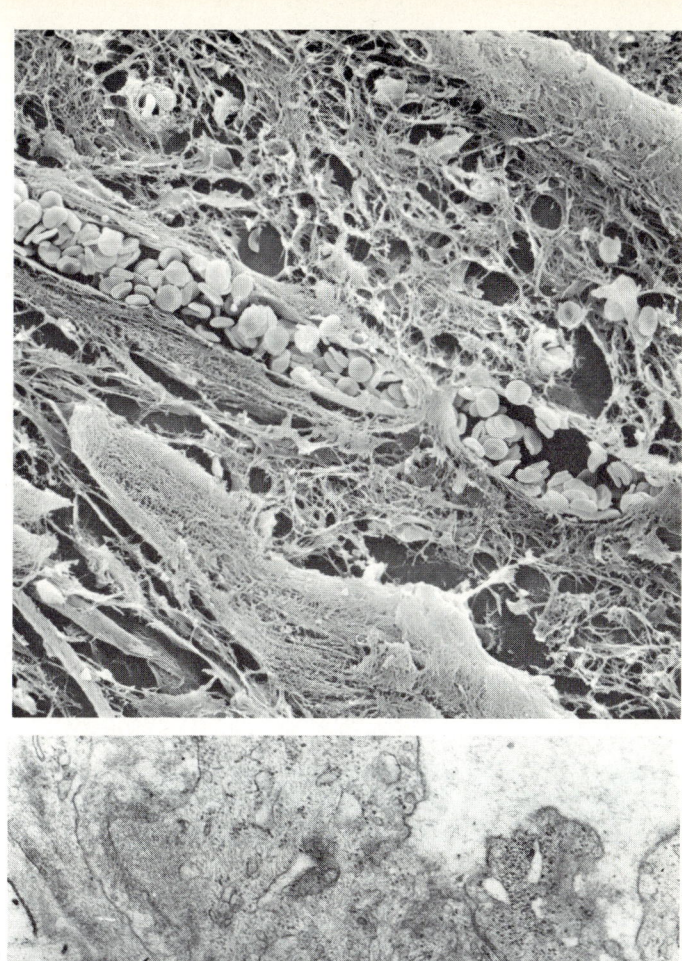
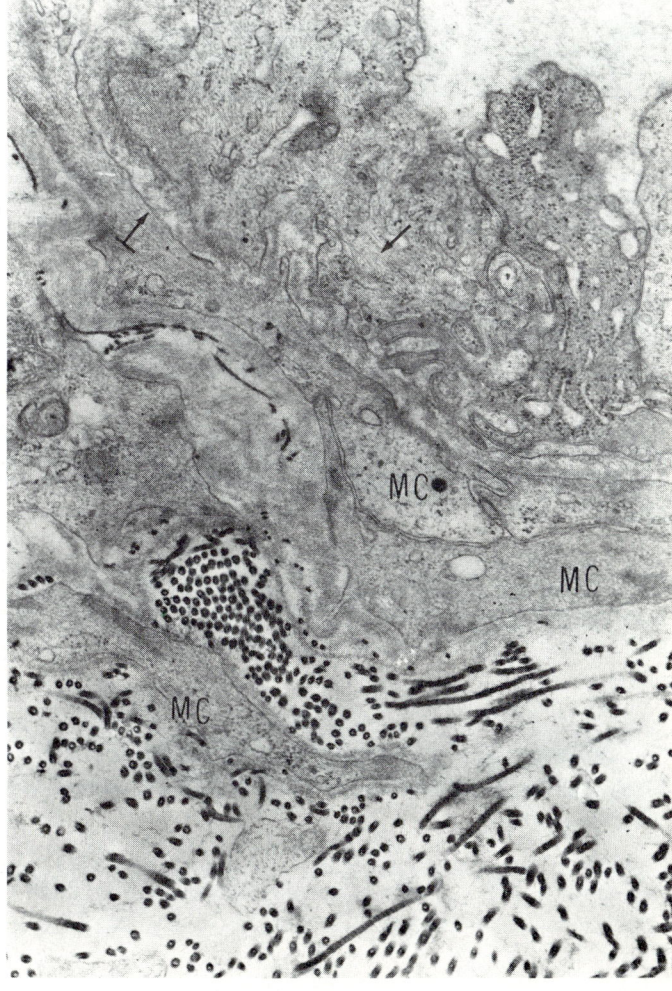

FIG. 5-3 *(Top)* Scanning electron micrograph of arteriole. ×5000. *(Bottom)* Arteriole of calf dental pulp. Endothelium contains small bundles of fine filaments (→). Tunica media is composed of 2 or 3 layers of smooth muscle cells (MC) with fine bundles of myofilaments in the cytoplasm (↦). ×25,000. (Kukletová M: Submicroscopic structure of blood vessels in the calf dental pulp. Scripta Medica 43:109, 1970)

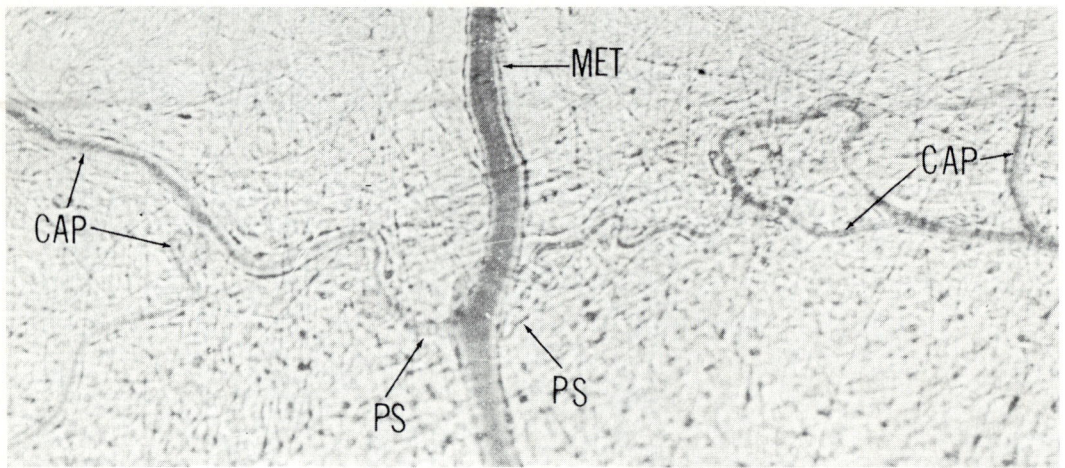

FIG. 5-4 Capillaries in the mesentery of the rat. The larger vessel is a metarteriole (MET). Two side branches with sphincters (PS) at the point of exit, followed by a network of true capillaries (CAP), are shown. ×150. (Courtesy of B. W. Zweifach, New York University School of Medicine, New York)

begins. The arterioles are resistance vessels measuring approximately 50 μm in diameter and have several layers of smooth muscle, which provide for control of vascular geometry. Just prior to feeding into the capillaries, arterioles are called terminal arterioles.

The terminal segment of the arteriole is a vessel of capillary dimensions, furnished with scattered smooth muscle cells lying at various distances from one another. The muscle cells form spiral twists on the surface of the endothelial tube (Fig. 5-3). They divide into smaller vessels called metarterioles or precapillaries, which have incomplete musculature. Metarterioles give off capillaries, which are about 8 μ in diameter (Fig. 5-4). The precapillaries drain into venules, which join to form veins, and the largest veins empty into the venae cavae (Fig. 5-5).

The arterioles, the capillaries, and the venules are, to some extent, able to respond to the variations in the requirements of the functioning tissues. Small aggregates of muscle elements are found at the points of branching of visceral arterioles and capillaries. These are sphincterlike in structure and have abundant innervation (Fig. 5-6). The arterioles regulate the blood supply to specific tissue areas by means of their sphincterlike mechanisms. The venules in a given area can return the blood to the local circulation, thereby prolonging the duration of contact with the surrounding tissue.

FIG. 5-5 An idealized diagram of the vessels in the microcirculation. Dark protrusions represent smooth muscle coating. AVA, arteriovenous anastomosis. (Courtesy of Dr. S. Kim, Columbia University, New York)

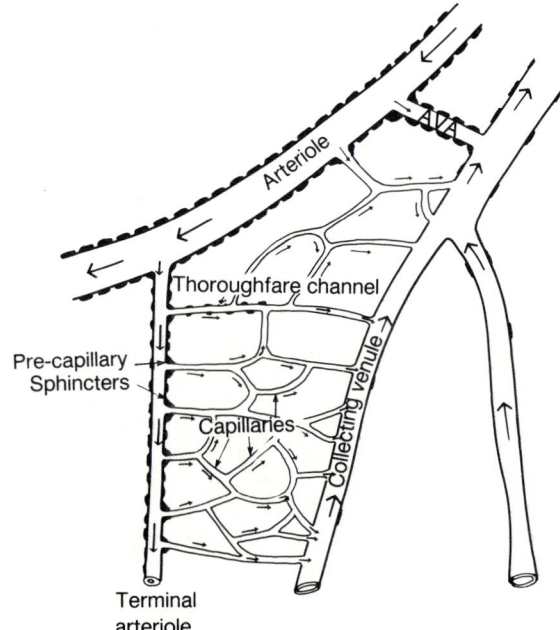

CAPILLARIES

Capillaries have an average diameter of 8 μm to 10 μm. They are the exchange vessels responsible for the transport of materials between blood and tissues. They possess only a single layer of endothelium and a basement membrane (Fig. 5–7). Capillaries are surrounded by a loose group of reticular and collagenous fibers. The basement membrane is composed of fine reticular filaments embedded in a homogeneous mucopolysaccharide matrix (Fig. 5–8). The wall of a capillary is not more than 0.5 μ in thickness and is a semipermeable membrane that permits the exchange of fluid.

The main morphologic characteristic of the capillaries is the general absence of smooth muscle cells. Only a few precapillary sphincters are found in the microcirculation (see Fig. 5–4). These regulate blood flow to capillaries,

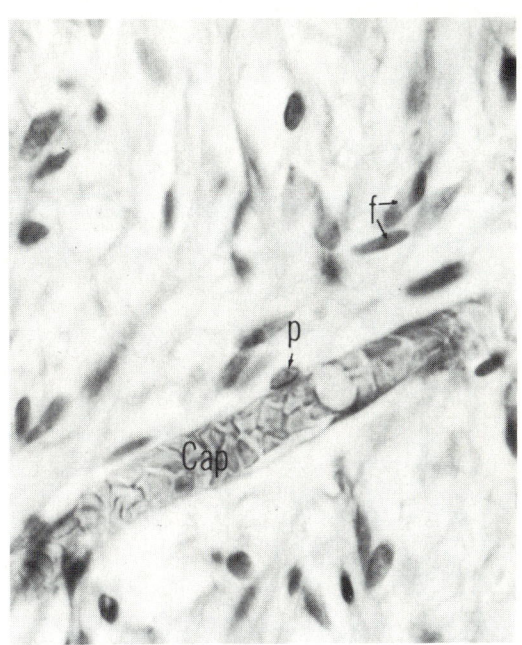

FIG. 5–7 A pericyte (p) in the wall of a capillary (Cap) in the pulp. Nearby are fibroblasts (f). ×960.

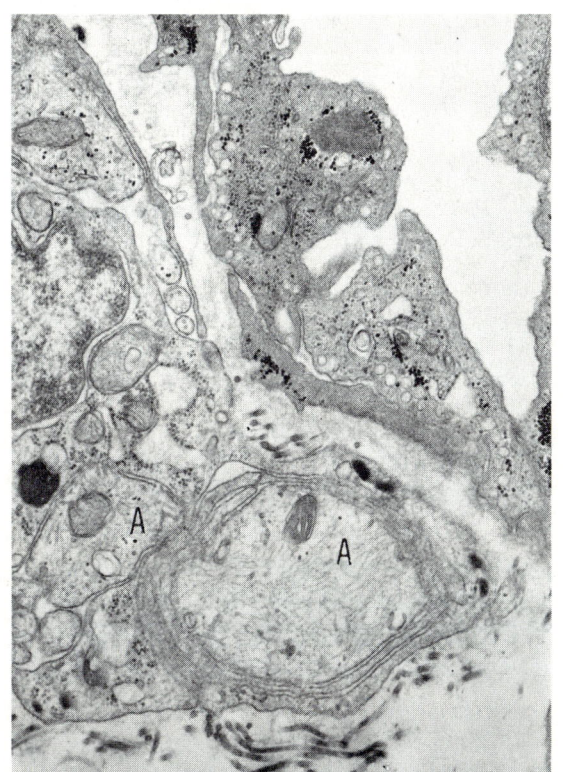

FIG. 5–6 Nonmedullated nerve fiber near a blood vessel. The axons (A) are still enclosed in Schwann-cell cytoplasm. ×30,000. (Kukletová, M: Submicroscopic structure of blood vessels in the calf dental pulp. Scripta Medica 43:109, 1970)

and thus participate in the transcapillary exchange process. The sphincter closes or dilates as a result of chemical stimulation. The sphincter acts like a floodgate: when blood is needed in an area, it opens; when blood is no longer needed, it constricts. In some vascular beds, arterioles and venules are connected by thoroughfare channels, which measure 10 μm to 15 μm in diameter and have smooth muscles covering their arteriolar ends (see Fig. 5–5).

The luminal surface of the endothelial cells is lined by a thin layer of glycoprotein, and the tissue side is covered by the basement membrane (see Fig. 5–8). Probably, the glycoprotein and the basement membrane play a role in controlling capillary permeability.

Types of Capillaries

Depending on its morphologic features, the capillary endothelium can be classified into three basic types: continuous, fenestrated, and discontinuous.

Continuous endothelium is devoid of fenestrations. The intercellular space contains gap junctions, which are localized narrowings with a width of 50 Å to 100 Å. The basement membrane is contiguous with a continuous endothe-

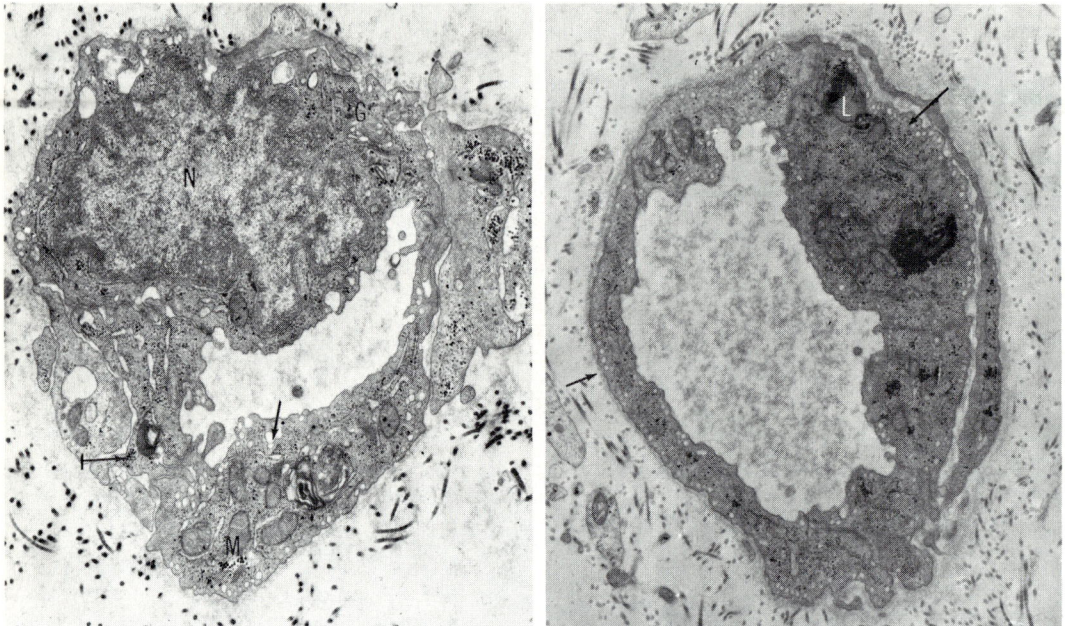

FIG. 5-8 *(Left)* Capillary in calf dental pulp. N, lobulated nucleus; M, small mitochondria; G, Golgi complex. These are numerous pinocytotic vesicles (→), β granules of glycogen (↦), and a continuous basement membrane. ×30,000 *(Right)* Capillary with an incomplete pericyte sheath. Pinocytotic vesicles are aligned into chains (→). Beta granules of glycogen (↦) and a secondary lysosome (L) are labeled. Note the continuous basement membrane. ×25,000. (Kukletová M: Submicroscopic structure of blood vessels in the calf dental pulp. Scripta Medica 43:109, 1970)

lium similar to that found in lungs, muscle, the central nervous system, and the dental pulp. Fenestrated endothelium has regional thinning (fenestrations) of the capillary walls. Some of the fenestrations are completely open, whereas others are covered by a thin, closed diaphragm. Fenestrated capillaries exist in the renal glomerulus, in the intestinal mucosa, in the sulcular gingiva, and in the pulp among odontoblasts near the predentin (Corpron et al, 1973). Discontinuous endothelium has wide, intercellular spaces, approximately 500 Å to 100 Å in width. The basement membrane is discontinuous. Discontinuous endothelium is found in the spleen, liver, and bone marrow.

An important ultrastructural feature of the capillary endothelium is the presence of pinocytotic vesicles (see Fig. 5-8). These vesicles, which measure approximately 700 Å in diameter, are formed by invagination of the plasmalemmal membrane of the endothelial cell. Some of the vesicles are attached to the plasmalemmal membrane on both the blood front and tissue front, whereas others exist as free bodies in the cytoplasm. Transendothelial channels are formed by the simultaneous attachment of one venule to both fronts, or by a chain of two or more vesicles attached to one another as well as to the plasmalemmal membrane.

In the venous system, capillaries coalesce into postcapillary venules. A smooth muscle coat begins to appear in the medium-sized venules, measuring approximately 50 μ or larger in diameter. An idealized diagram of the vessels in the microcirculation is shown in Figure 5-5.

Transcapillary Exchange

Nutritional material moves from the blood vessel to the cells according to the laws of hydrostatic and osmotic pressures. The distance between cells and capillaries is not more than 50 μm—the limit at which cells can be supplied from the capillaries with various nutrients (Zweifach, 1961).

Transcapillary exchange is the major function of the microcirculation, which includes transporting nutrients and oxygen to, and removing waste products from, the tissues.

Transcapillary exchange occurs by diffusion, filtration-absorption, and micropinocytosis. The driving force behind diffusion is a concentration gradient; i.e., the direction of flux is from the high to the low concentration. The endothelial cell membrane is lipoid, and thus substances with a high lipid solubility, e.g., O_2 and CO_2, have a high diffusion coefficient through the entire endothelial cell membrane. Water-soluble substances do not diffuse readily through the membrane; the degree of their diffusion depends on the geometry of the capillaries, such as the size of channels and the pore system. Physiologic regulation of transcapillary diffusion is achieved mainly by controlling the available capillary surface area. As shown in Figure 5–9, the fluid filtered in transcapillary exchange by filtration and absorption across a capillary membrane is proportional to the net filtration pressure resulting from the fluid mechanical pressure (hydrostatic pressure; P_c and P_t) and the colloidal osmotic pressure (πc and πt). Normally, the higher pressure in the arteriolar capillaries favors filtration, whereas the lower pressure in the venular capillaries causes fluid absorption. During inflammation, vasodilation results in an increase in intravascular pressure (P_c) and capillary permeability, favoring filtration and thus causing edema.

Micropinocytosis involves a slow but active transport of proteins. The bidirectional nature of the process has also been confirmed.

The capillary bed is extensive. If all the capillaries in the body were put end to end, they would extend about 60,000 miles. In some forms of shock, the capillaries are dilated and the blood retreats to the capillary bed, reducing the amount in the general circulation. It is only when the blood returns from the capillary bed to the circulation that the symptoms are relieved.

The number of capillaries in a given area depends on the number of cells in that area. For example, more capillaries are observed in muscle tissue than in any of the secretory glands.

CONTROL OF BLOOD FLOW

The blood supply to any given area is controlled by nerve impulses and humoral agents. Arteries and arterioles are innervated; hence, impulses produce contraction of the muscle in the vessel wall. The lumen of the vessels is thereby increased or decreased to control the amount of circulating blood in the area. The regulation of blood flow is mediated by smooth muscles situated in the walls of arterioles and venules.

A hormonal mechanism also is involved in the control of blood flow. Epinephrine, which is liberated from the adrenal medulla, causes vasoconstriction (i.e., the muscles of the blood vessels are constricted), thereby limiting the flow of blood. For dilation of the vessels, the parasympathetic (cholinergic) nerves liberate acetylcholine.

STUDIES OF PULPAL VESSELS

Pulpal and periodontal blood vessels have been studied by a variety of techniques including cinematography and optical, electron, and x-ray microscopy (Fig. 5–10). For visualization, blood vessels have been studied histochemically or injected with dyes, gelatins, latex, radiopaque substances, and plastic microspheres (Fig. 5–11). The foreign materials are usually injected under pressure or perfused through the arterial circulation in vivo (Russel and Kramer, 1956; Saunders, 1957; Kramer, 1960). Takaha-

FIG. 5-9 Factors determining fluid exchange in capillaries. (Courtesy of Dr. S. Kim, Columbia University, New York)

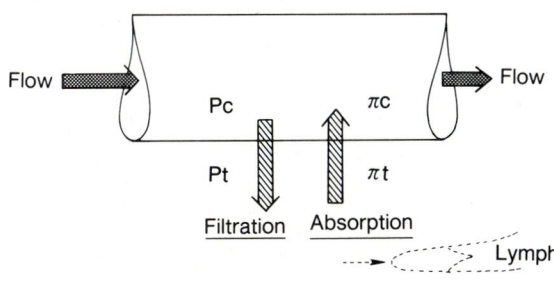

P_c = Capillary hydrostatic pressure
P_t = Tissue hydrostatic pressure
πc = Intravascular osmotic pressure
πt = Tissue osmotic pressure
▶ Blood flow
▷ Fluid movement

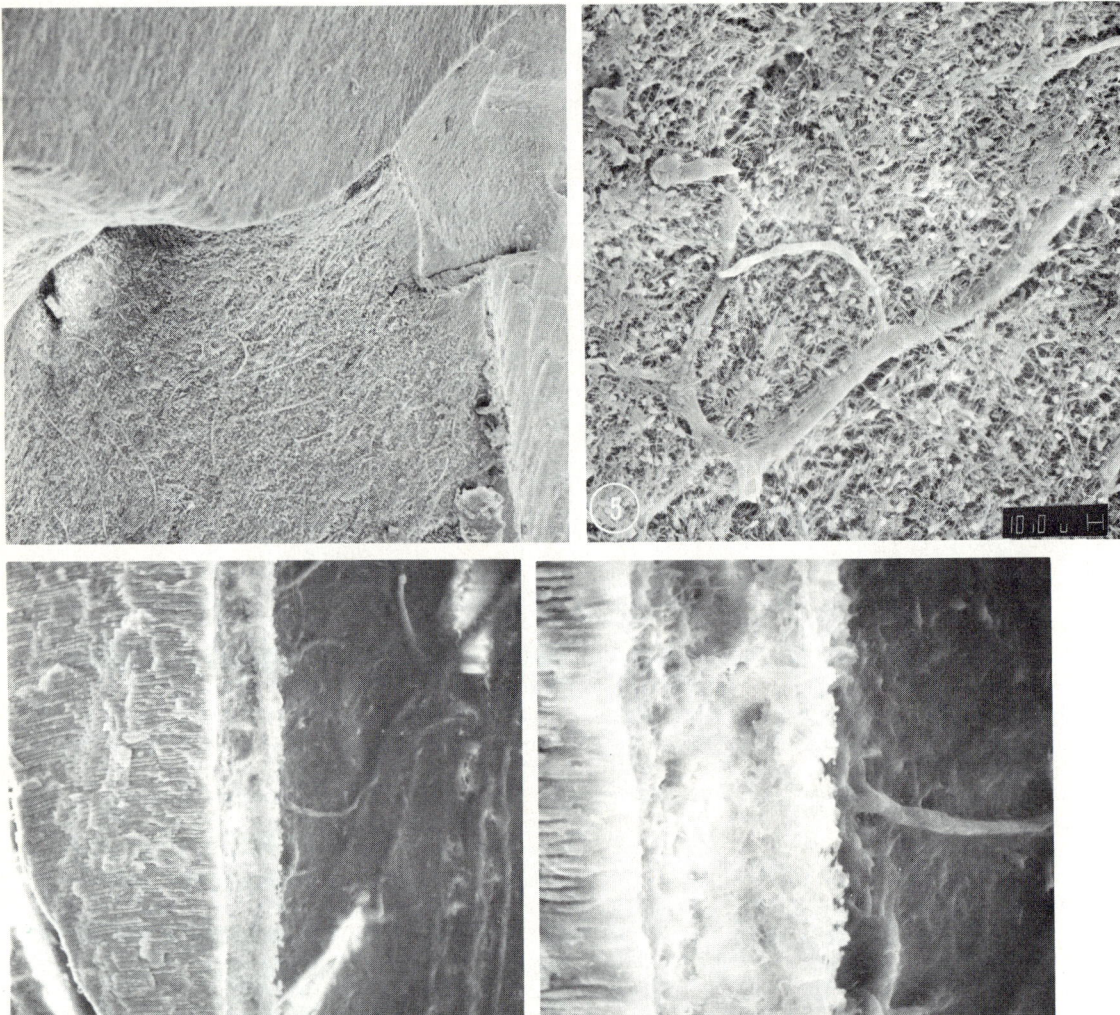

FIG. 5-10 *(Top, left)* Scanning electron micrograph of coronal portion of pulp. ×40. *(Top, right)* Higher magnification of left photograph showing pulpal blood vessels. ×400. *(Bottom, left)* Scanning electron micrograph of capillaries in subodontoblastic plexus. ×180. *(Bottom, right)* Higher magnification of capillary supplying odontoblasts. ×600.

shi et al (1982), using a low-viscosity synthetic resin, made vascular casts of dog pulps for stereoscopic examination under the scanning electron miscroscope (Fig. 5-12). The casts showed that the main feeding arterioles entered the root canal through the apical foramina and traversed the central portions to reach the coronal portion of the pulp (Fig. 5-13). Some arterioles looped in a U-turn configuration (Fig. 5-14); others coursed toward the dentin and sent out many fine subdentinal branches. Pulp chamber arterioles could be separated into two groups: one advanced coronally toward the pulp horn, branching and forming a dense terminal capillary network toward the dentin (Fig. 5-15). The other ran between the floor and the roof of the pulp chamber, also branching into a dense terminal capillary network. The terminal capillary network beneath the dentin, i.e., the subodontoblastic capillary plexus, was almost

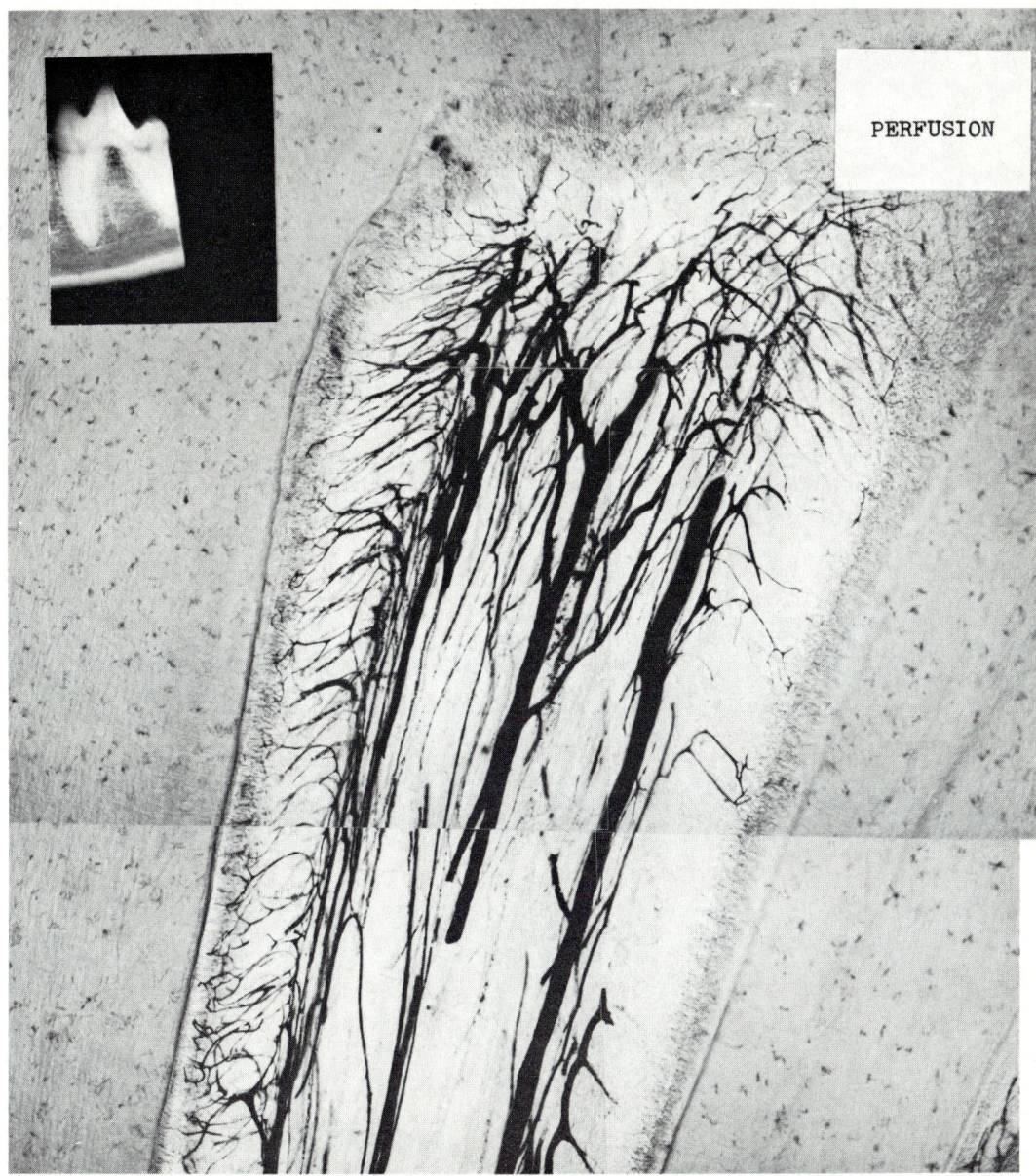

FIG. 5-11 The pulp of a lower molar of a dog *(inset)* perfused with India ink. The central vessels give off numerous branches that course toward the odontoblastic layer. A rich subodontoblastic capillary network is present. ×54.

perpendicular to the main trunk vessels (Fig. 5-16). The average capillary luminal diameter was less than 10 μm. The terminal capillaries drained into the venules beneath the dentin, and merged to form the primary venules. These joined, thereby increasing their luminal diameter as they advanced toward and through the apical foramina. Arteriovenous and veno-venous anastomoses and U-turn loops appeared to be unique features of the pulpal vessels, but their

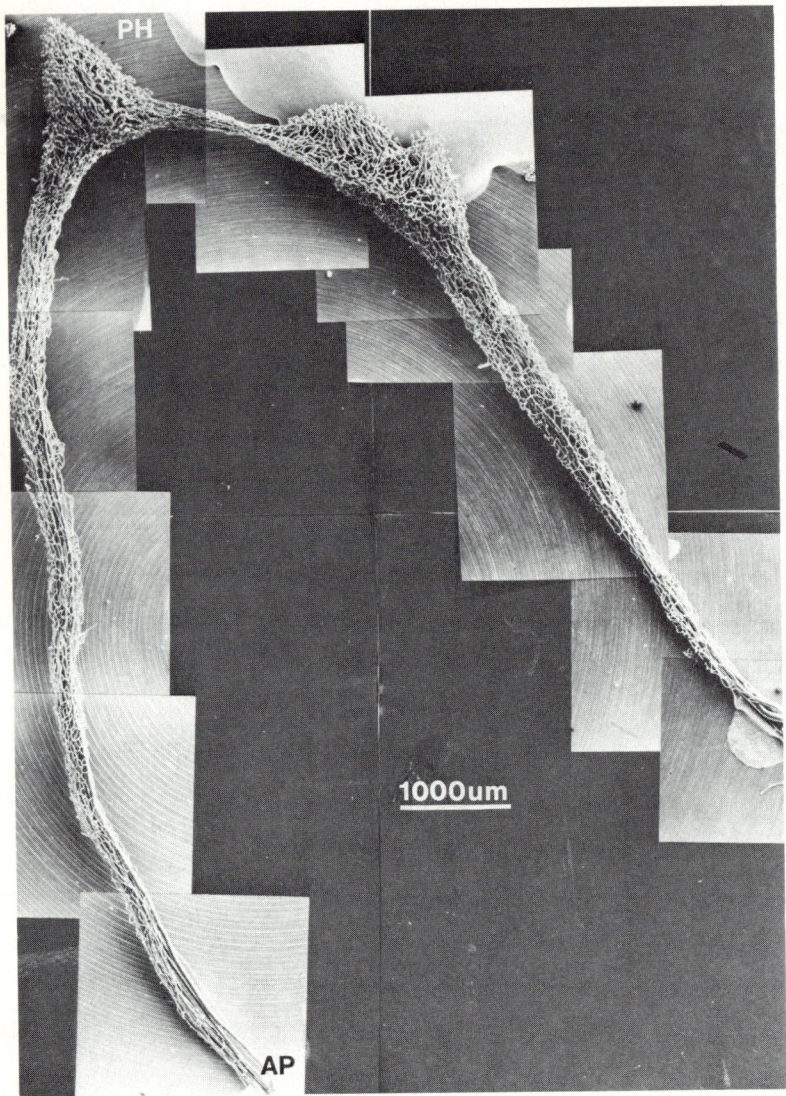

FIG. 5-12 Composite photomicrograph of the vasculature of the dog dental pulp. AF, root apex; PH, pulp horn. (Courtesy of Dr. K. Takahashi, Kanagawa Dental College, Kanagawa, Japan)

exact functional roles remain to be elucidated. Such direct connections between arterial and venous systems have previously been demonstrated in the dental pulp by Provenza (1958) and by Kramer (1960).

Ultrastructure of the Pulp Capillary

The ultrastructure of the pulp capillaries has been studied by Han and Avery (1963), Kukletová (1970), Harris and Griffin (1971), Corpron et al (1973), Dahl and Mjör (1973), and Rapp et al (1977). They found that the cytoplasm of the endothelial cells contained rough endoplasmic reticulum (rER), a small Golgi complex, occasional mitochondria, and filaments (Fig. 5-17). The trilamellar cell membrane connected with the endoplasmic reticulum through infoldings. The presence of frequent pinocytotic vesicles suggested that they may play a role in the transcapillary exchange. Furthermore, Corpron et al and Rapp et al observed fenestrations in the subodontoblastic capillaries (Fig. 5-18). They postulated that these fenestrations provide rapid transport of metabolites from the capillaries to the adjacent odontoblasts.

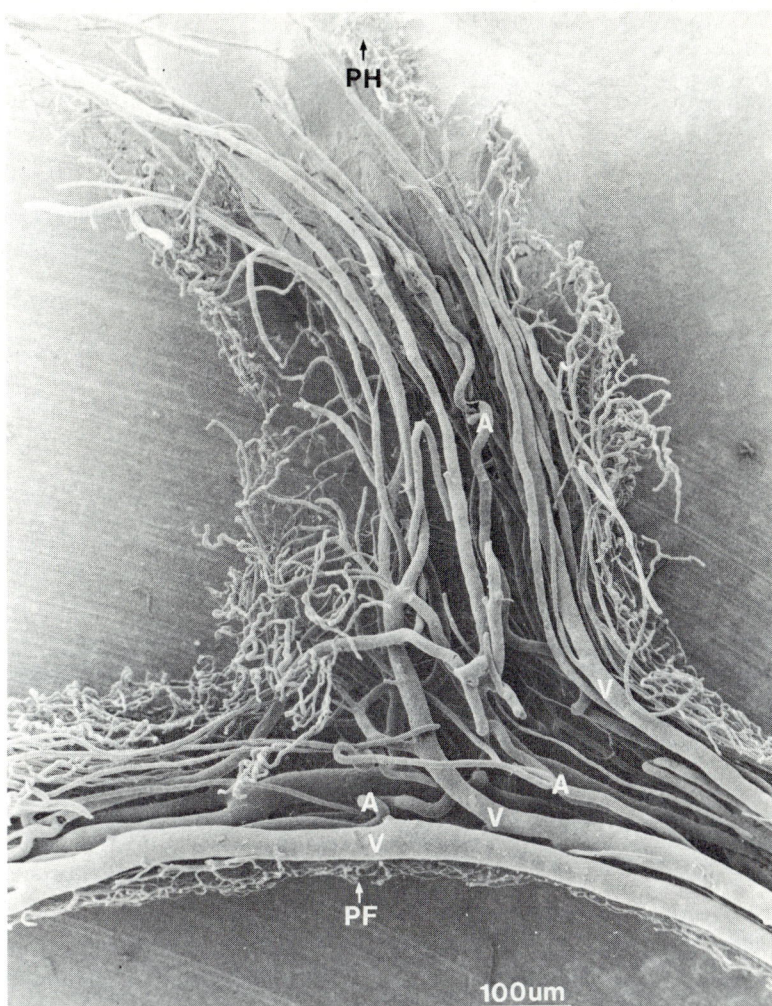

FIG. 5-13 Main arterioles that enter the pulp chamber are separated into two groups; one advances coronally toward pulp horn, and the other runs between the floor and the roof of the pulp chamber. PH, pulp horn; PF, pulp floor; A, arteriole; V, main venule. Scale bar = 100 μm. (Takahashi K, Kishi Y, Kim S: A scanning electron microscope study of the blood vessels of dog pulp using corrosion casts. J Endodont 3:131, 1982)

REGULATION OF PULPAL HEMODYNAMICS

Chemical Regulation

Nerves help to regulate the blood supply to the dental pulp (Kim et al, 1980). Sympathetic (adrenergic) nerve fibers liberate norepinephrine, which constricts the vessels. Parasympathetic (cholinergic) nerves liberate acetylcholine, which dilates the vessels.

The catecholamines, such as epinephrine or norepinephrine, exert their physiologic effects on receptors in the blood vessels, called adrenoreceptors. There are two types of adrenoreceptors, alpha (α) and beta (β). The blood vessels of the pulp contain both α and β adrenoreceptors. The α receptors are responsible for contraction of the vascular musculature and produce vasoconstriction. Stimulation of β receptors causes a relaxation of the vascular musculature. Apparently, the pulpal blood vessels contain β adrenoreceptors (Kim and Chien, 1983) but are poorly equipped with them (Tønder and Naess, 1978).

Circulating catecholamines such as adrenaline or noradrenaline exert less of a vasoconstrictor effect than local sympathetic nerve activation. Humoral agents, such as acetylcholine, histamine, or bradykinin, when infused intra-arterially, may inhibit a sympathetic vasoconstrictor response to stimulation (Edwall, 1980). At least in the pulps of dogs and cats, cholinergic

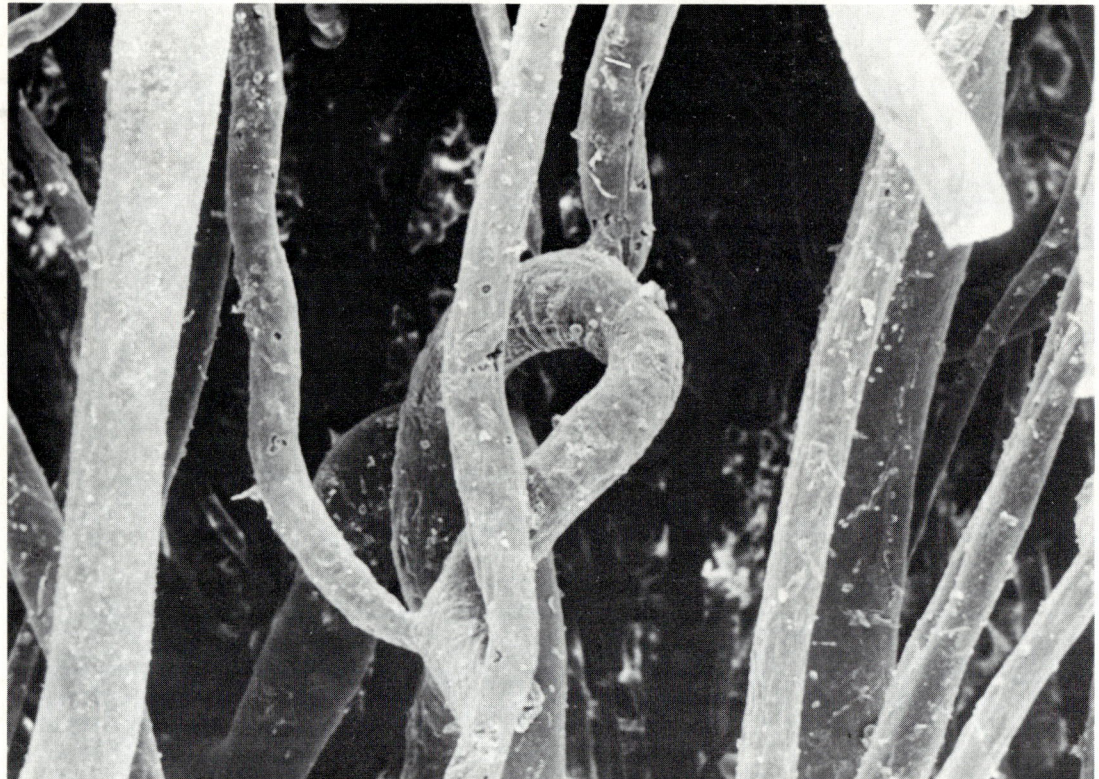

FIG. 5-14 Arteriolar U-turn. (Courtesy of Dr. K. Takahashi, Kanagawa Dental College, Kanagawa, Japan)

vasodilating fibers are absent (Tønder and Naess, 1978).

Ongoing studies indicate that there are subtypes of α and β receptors called α_1 and α_2, and β_1 and β_2. Their role in the control of blood flow to the pulp has not yet been clearly elucidated.

Vasoconstriction

Intra-arterial administration of norepinephrine in the dog, the cat, and the rat decreases pulpal blood flow (Edwall and Kindlovà, 1971; Tønder, 1975; Kim, 1981). The flow reduction was blocked by the α-adrenergic antagonist phenoxybenzamine (PBZ), indicating the presence of an α-adrenergic system that was responsible for the decrease in pulpal blood flow (Kim, 1981).

Various studies indicate that the sympathetic adrenergic vasoconstrictor system causes variations in systemic hemodynamics, which, in turn, influence pulpal hemodynamics. At the resting stage, the pulpal vessels are not under the tonic influence of sympathetic nerve discharge. However, electrical stimulation of the cervical sympathetic trunk causes a severe reduction of pulp blood flow in the dog, the cat, and the rat (Edwall and Kindlovà, 1971; Tønder, 1975; Scott et al, 1972; Kim, 1981), owing to activation of α adrenoreceptors (Ahlberg and Edwall, 1977; Tønder and Naess, 1978). The intra-arterial injection of the α blocker PBZ markedly reversed the reduction of pulpal blood flow induced by such electrical stimulation (Kim, 1981). Reflex excitation of the sympathetic nervous system by experimental hypotension (nitroprusside infusion and hemorrhage) or decrease in systemic oxygen transport (extreme hemodilution and hemoconcentration) causes pulpal vasoconstriction and a reduction of pulpal blood flow (Kim et al, 1980; Kim, 1981). Induction of experimental hypotension in dogs subjected to cervical sympathectomy and adrenalectomy causes less pulpal vasoconstriction and less flow reduction than in normal dogs.

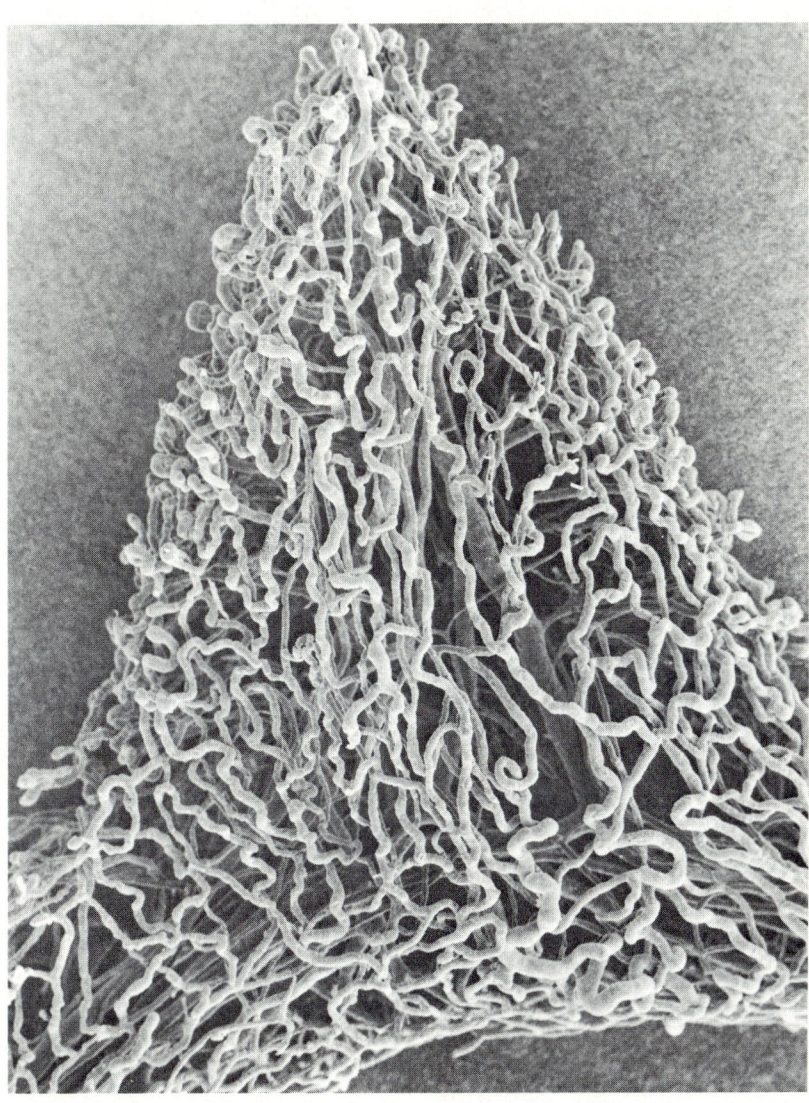

FIG. 5-15 Pulp horn exhibiting dense terminal capillary network below odontoblastic layer. (Courtesy of Dr. K. Takahashi, Kanawaga Dental College, Kanagawa, Japan)

Histochemical investigations have also been performed to substantiate the physiologic findings. Numerous investigators have reported the presence of autonomic adrenergic constrictor fibers in the pulps of several mammalian species (Fig. 5-19; Waterson, 1967; Kukletova et al, 1968; Larsson and Linde, 1971; Pohto and Antila, 1972).

In addition to the sympathetic adrenergic system, other chemical mediators cause vasoconstriction. The intra-arterial injection of an inflammatory mediator, serotonin (5-hydroxytryptamine), caused a decrease in pulpal blood flow in dogs (Kim et al, 1983). The functional significance of such flow reduction remains to be elucidated.

Vasodilation

Pulpal vessels are apparently equipped with β-adrenergic receptors. Activation of β-receptors by intra-arterial injection of isoproterenol (ISO) caused a paradoxical reduction of pulpal blood flow in dogs (Tønder, 1976; Kim, 1981). Tønder (1976) proposed that the flow reduction following intra-arterial ISO infusion resulted from "stealing" of blood flow by the adjacent tissues, which have a much greater vasodilator response to ISO. Kim (1981) found that the flow response

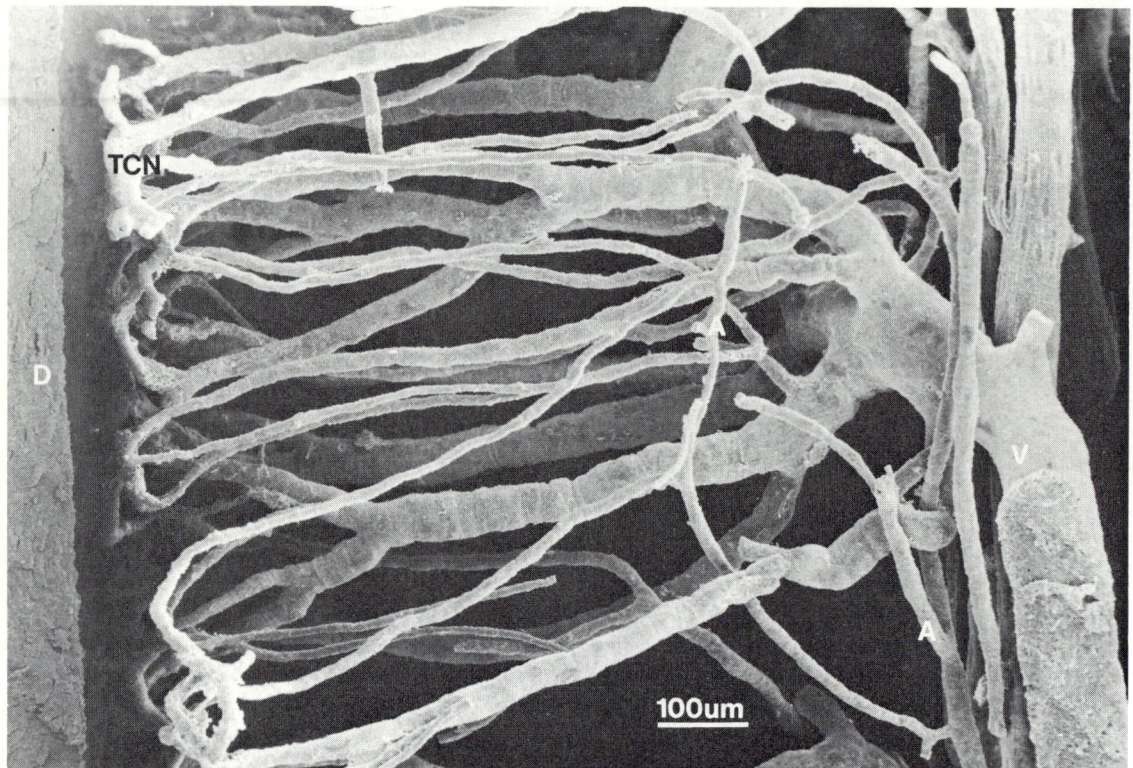

FIG. 5-16 Subodontoblastic capillary plexus is positioned almost perpendicular to main trunk vessels. Capillaries form continuous round connections between arterioles and draining venules. D, dentin; TCN, terminal capillary network beneath dentin; A, terminal arteriole; V, venule. (Takahashi K, Kishi Y, Kim S: A scanning electron microscope study of the blood vessels of dog pulp using corrosion casts. J Endodont 3:131, 1982)

to ISO was blocked by the β-antagonist propranolol; propranolol alone caused no flow changes in the pulp. Moreover, in the rat microcirculation, ISO caused a transient increase in flow, followed by a reduction; the arteriolar dilation was accompanied by a venular constriction. These microcirculatory responses to ISO were blocked by propranolol. Thus, the paradoxical response of pulpal blood flow to ISO may be related to the low compliance environment. In such an environment, the passive compression of venules could result from active dilation of arterioles with an attendant rise in extravascular pressure.

Effects of various humoral substances and biogenic amines on pulp blood flow have been studied, with conflicting results. Bradykinin *increased* pulp blood flow in the cat only when the vascular tone was high after sympathetic stimulation (Edwall and Olgart, 1972). Using the microsphere injection method, Kim et al (1982) found that pulp blood flow *decreased* following intra-arterial bradykinin injection. A biphasic flow response, i.e., an initial increase, was followed by a drastic decrease. The flow reduction following vasodilation is related to the low compliance environment of the tooth, in which an active dilation of arterioles results in an increase in tissue pressure and a passive compression of the venules. The passive compression could increase the flow resistance and thereby cause a reduction in pulp blood flow.

Substance P (SP), an undecapeptide, when released from peripheral sensory neurons, causes vasodilation (Skrabanek and Powell, 1977). Intra-arterial injections of SP in cats caused an increase in pulpal blood flow (Gazelius et al, 1977). Antidromic pulp stimulations caused vasodilation (Gazelius and Olgart, 1980), suggesting a role for SP, released from

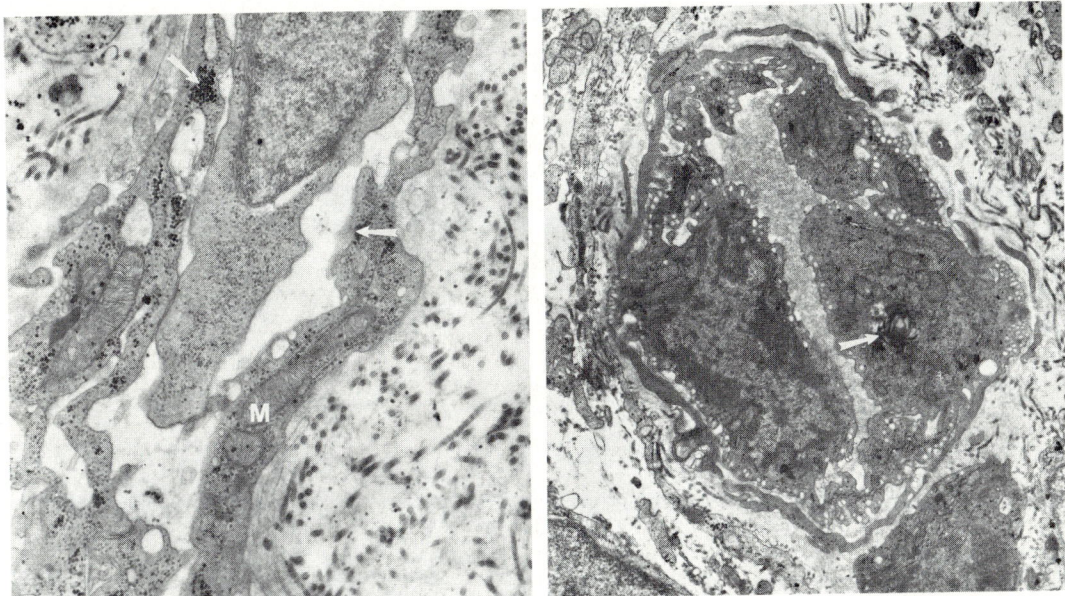

FIG. 5-17 *(Left)* Longitudinal section through a capillary. Mitochondria (M); glycogen (arrows). ×30,000. *(Right)* Capillary within pericyte sheath. There are numerous pinocytotic vesicles and a basement membrane. Glycogen (arrow). ×25,000. (Kukletová M: Submicroscopic structure of blood vessels in the calf dental pulp. Scripta Medica 43:109, 1970)

FIG. 5-18 *(Left)* Capillary (lower right) located among odontoblasts (OD) near predentin (PD). ×8000. *(Right)* Fenestrations (arrows) in thin section of endothelial cell (EC). Continuous basal lamina separates capillary wall from adjacent odontoblast. RBC, red blood cell. ×32,000. (Corpron RE, Avery JK, Lee SD: Ultrastructure of capillaries in the odontoblastic layer. J Dent Res 52:393, 1973. Copyright by the American Dental Association. Reproduced by permission)

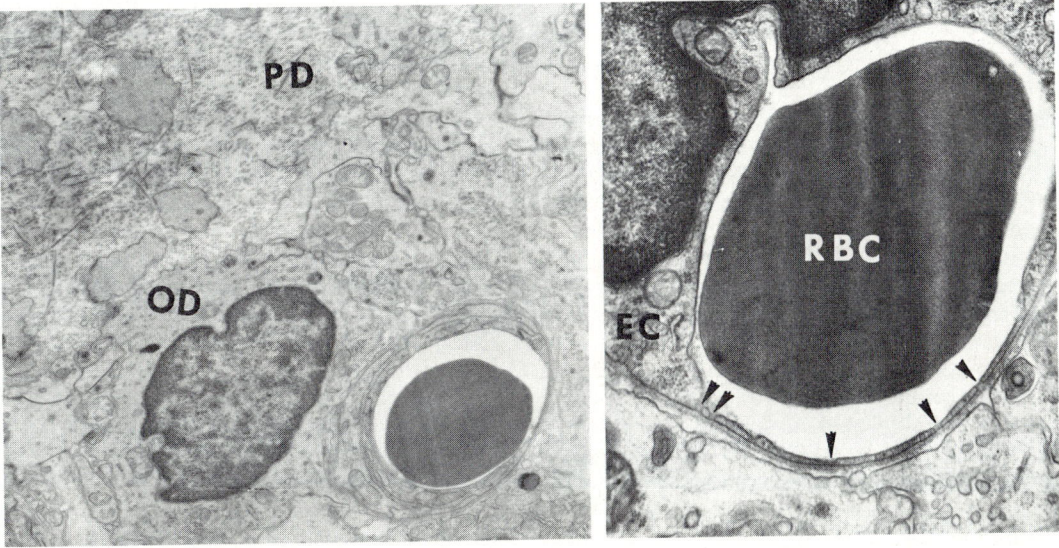

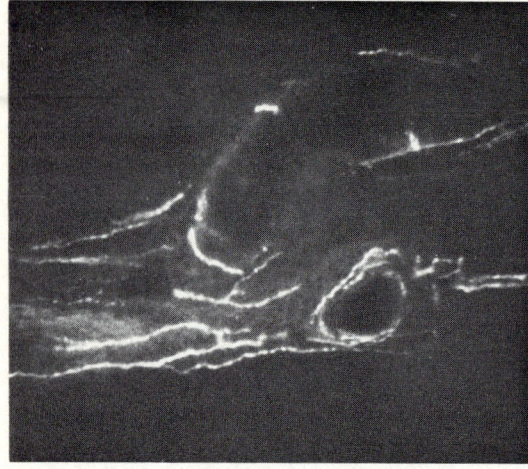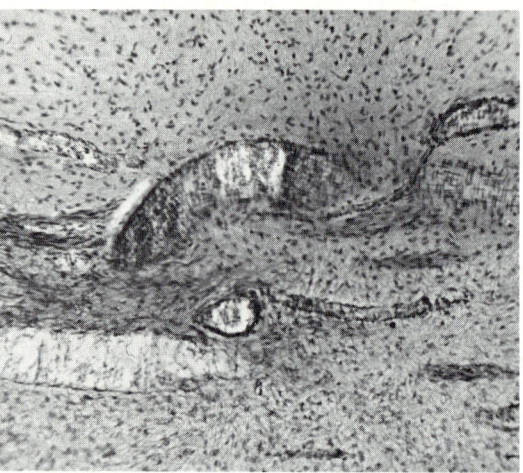

FIG. 5-19 *(Left)* Oblique section frame of the pulp from the upper first molar of a monkey. The bright lines are fluorescent adrenergic fibers running along blood vessels. ×225. *(Right)* The coverslip has been removed and the section in the left frame has been stained with light green and iron hematoxylin, revealing the morphology of blood vessels. ×170. (Pohto P, Antila R: Innervation of blood vessels in the dental pulp. Int Dent J 22:228, 1972)

pulpal neurons, in regulating local pulpal blood flow (Brodin et al, 1981).

Although conclusive evidence for cholinergic terminals in the pulp is still lacking, the presence of acetylcholinesterase (AChE) in the pulp has been shown by Pohto and Antila (1972) and Avery et al (1974). Results of the effects of AChE on pulp blood flow have been conflicting, leaving this area of pulp blood flow poorly understood.

Rates of Pulpal Blood Flow

As reviewed by Meyer and Path (1979), Meyer (1980), and Kim et al (1980), pulp blood flow has been measured in the teeth of experimental animals with tracer disappearance methods using ^{42}K, ^{86}Rb, ^{131}I, H_2 gas, and ^{133}Xe; electrical impedance; plethysmography; and the radioactive microsphere technique. Of these, the ^{42}K, the ^{86}Rb, the ^{133}Xe, and the microsphere methods yielded the highest and most similar blood flow values—approximately 40 to 50 ml/min/100 g pulp tissue. Blood flow values for various oral and visceral tissues at a hematocrit of 45% were compared (Fig. 5-20). It can be seen that blood flow in the pulp is relatively high, compared to that of other oral tissues and skeletal muscle. However, blood flow per unit weight of kidney, spleen, and other vital organs was substantially higher. Thus, blood flow seems to reflect the functional capacity of an organ.

Structural and Functional Heterogeneity in Pulpal Circulation

The anatomic heterogeneity of the vascular network within the pulp is closely related to the heterogeneous regional flow distribution (Meyer and Path, 1979; Kim, 1981). The highest capillary density occurs in the peripheral layer of the coronal region. The core of the apical region has the lowest density. Blood flow of the coronal half of the pulp is about twice as much as that of the apical half. The average peripheral blood flow in the coronal region is 70 ml/min/100 g pulp flow, whereas the average flow in the core of the apical region measures 15 ml/min/100 g. Comparisons among flow values, measured with 8 μ, 9 μ, and 15 μ microspheres, indicate considerable shunting of 8 μ and 9 μ spheres in the pulp, most of the shunting occurring in the apical half (Meyer and Path, 1979; Kim, 1981). The shunting is facilitated by numerous shunts and U-turn loops in the apical half of the pulp (Takahashi et al, 1982).

Intravital Microscopic Study

Many investigators (Taylor, 1950; Pohto and Scheinin, 1958; Kozam and Bennett, 1959; Scott et al, 1972) have observed the living pulp circulation directly. Using essentially the same tooth preparation, but adding state of the art microcirculatory methods, Kim et al (1983)

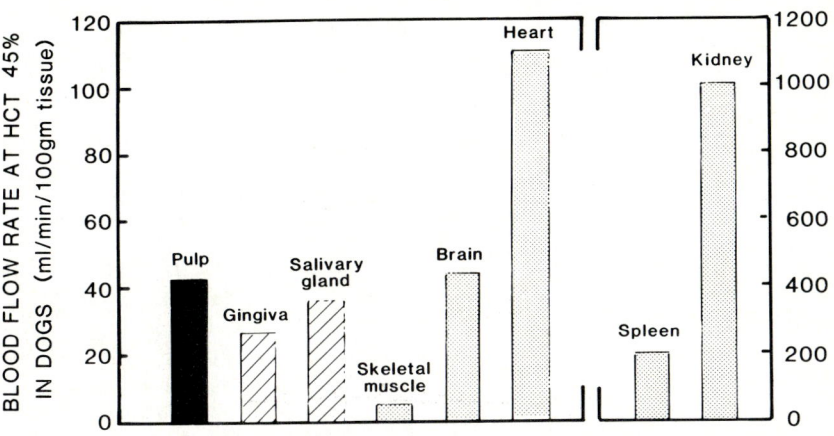

FIG. 5-20 Blood flow rate per 100 g tissue weight for various organs and tissues at hematocrit of 45%. (Courtesy of Dr. S. Kim, Columbia University, New York)

studied microcirculatory dynamics of the pulp in the rat incisor tooth. Vascular dimensions were accurately measured with an electronic video image shearing technique (Intaglietta and Tomkins, 1973). The flow velocity was determined using the modified "two-slit" photometric method with an analogue self-tracking correlator (Wayland and Johnson, 1967; Tompkins et al, 1974). Kim et al found that the fastest mean intravascular flow velocity in a 42 μm arteriole was 2.1 mm/sec; the slowest mean intravascular flow velocity (0.11 mm/sec) was measured in an 11 μm postcapillary venule. Mean flow velocity sharply decreased with decreasing vessel diameter on the arterial side. On the venous side, a gradual upturning of the velocity curve was observed in 24 μm to 72 μm diameter vessels. The fastest mean velocity obtained in the venous side was 0.7 mm/sec in a 61 μm venule, which was substantially slower than the fastest mean velocity of a comparable arteriolar vessel.

LYMPHATICS

The lymphatic system is a second circulatory system whose primary function is to recirculate the interstitial fluid to the bloodstream. The lymphatic system also serves as a transport system for the products of cells into the blood circulation. In the tissues, the lymphatic system arises from a fine mesh of small, thin-walled lymph capillaries. Interstitial fluid diffuses through the walls of these capillaries to become lymph, a colorless or pale yellow liquid. The composition of lymph is similar to that of the interstitial fluid and to that of blood plasma. The lymphatic capillaries converge to form larger vessels that resemble veins. These larger vessels are equipped with valves to prevent backflow. An extensive network of lymphatic vessels and ducts carries the tissue fluid back into the vascular system. Before reaching the bloodstream, the fluid is filtered through lymph nodes and glands that are distributed along the larger lymphatics. The filtering action of the lymph nodes protects the body against the invasion of microorganisms and other foreign matter. The resident white blood cells in the nodes ingest and destroy the noxious material. Lymph nodes also are the centers for proliferation and storage of lymphocytes and other antibody-manufacturing cells produced in the thymus gland.

Lymph and fluid from the teeth and subcutaneous tissues drain into the submaxillary and submental glands and eventually to superficial and deep cervical glands that are distributed along the external and internal jugular veins. On the left side of the body the fluid is then drained into the thoracic duct; on the right side it is collected by the jugular duct. From these ducts the fluid is returned to the bloodstream at the junctions of the left and the right internal jugular and subclavian veins (Fig. 5-21).

LYMPHATICS IN THE DENTAL PULP

The presence of lymphatic vessels in the dental pulp has been the subject of controversy, because of the close morphologic resemblance of lymphatic vessels and veins or capillaries (Sulz-

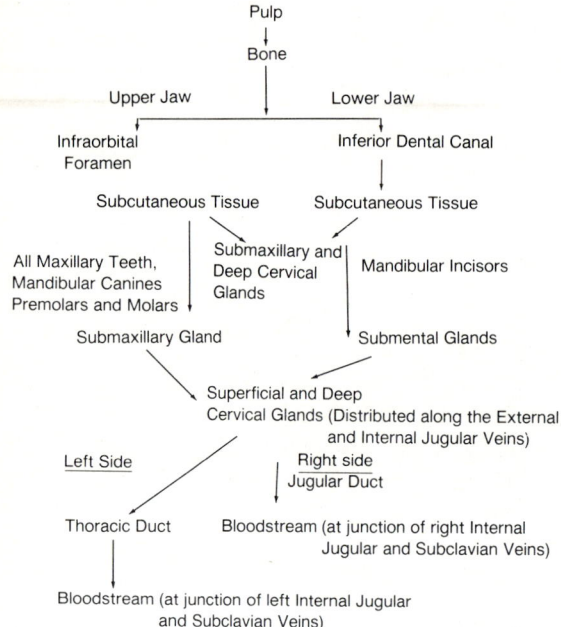

FIG. 5-21 Schema of lymphatics and lymphatic drainage of the oral structures.

mann, 1965). The main structural differences between the lymphatic vessels and capillaries are the lack of a basement membrane and the absence of fenestration in the endothelial cells. Observations with the light (Ruben et al, 1971) and the electron microscope (Kukletová, 1970; Dahl and Mjör, 1973) point to the probability that the pulp does contain lymphatics (Fig. 5-22). In addition, Brown et al (1969) have claimed that a recording of osmotic pressure in the pulp is indirect evidence that pulpal lymphatics do exist.

In tracking the lymphatic circulation of dog and human pulps, Bernick and Patek (1969), and Bernick (1977) showed that lymph capillaries originated as blind openings near the zone of Weil and the odontoblastic layer. They drained into small thin-walled collecting vessels that frequently communicated with each other. The collecting vessels then passed apically in the pulp, accompanying blood vessels and nerves. Lateral lymph capillaries also emptied into the collecting vessels that coursed toward the apex (Fig. 5-23). The large caliber lymphatic vessels contained valves, which are not present in similar-sized veins. Multiple collecting lymph vessels exited through the apical foramen to drain into large lymph vessels in the periodontal ligament. However, Takada (1973), employing electronmicroscopy with an intra-arterial dye injection method, did not find lymphatic vessels in the pulp of any of the experimental animal species. The presence of lymphatic vessels in the pulp is therefore still a matter of controversy.

Intrapulpal Pressure

Leakage of blood proteins and other substances through the walls of the capillaries into the tissue spaces produces interstitial fluid. Lymphatic drainage returns the fluid and proteins to the bloodstream. The pressure of such fluid in the

FIG. 5-22 A section through what may be a lymphatic vessel, showing endothelial projections and a polymorph within the lumen (L). Note the absence of a basal lamina. Note also the thinness of the endothelium and the communication (arrow) between the vessel lumen and the surrounding tissue. Glutaraldehyde-osmium. ×15,000. (Kukletová M: An electron-microscopic study of the lymphatic vessels in the dental pulp in the calf. Arch Oral Biol 15:1117, 1970)

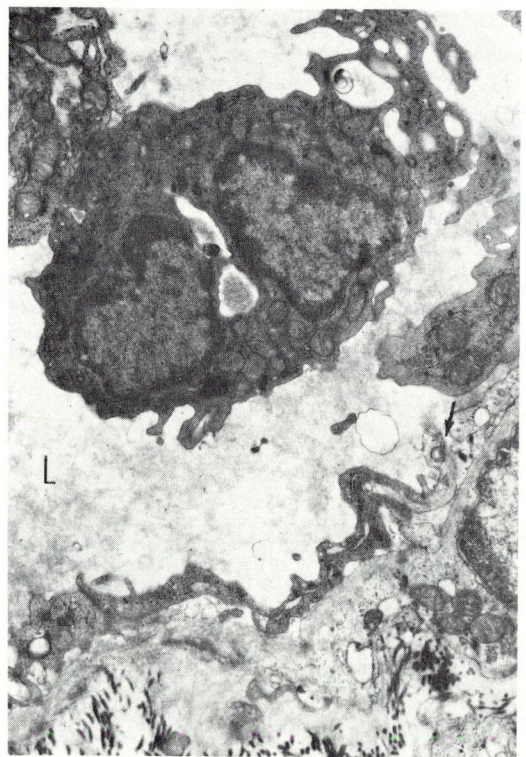

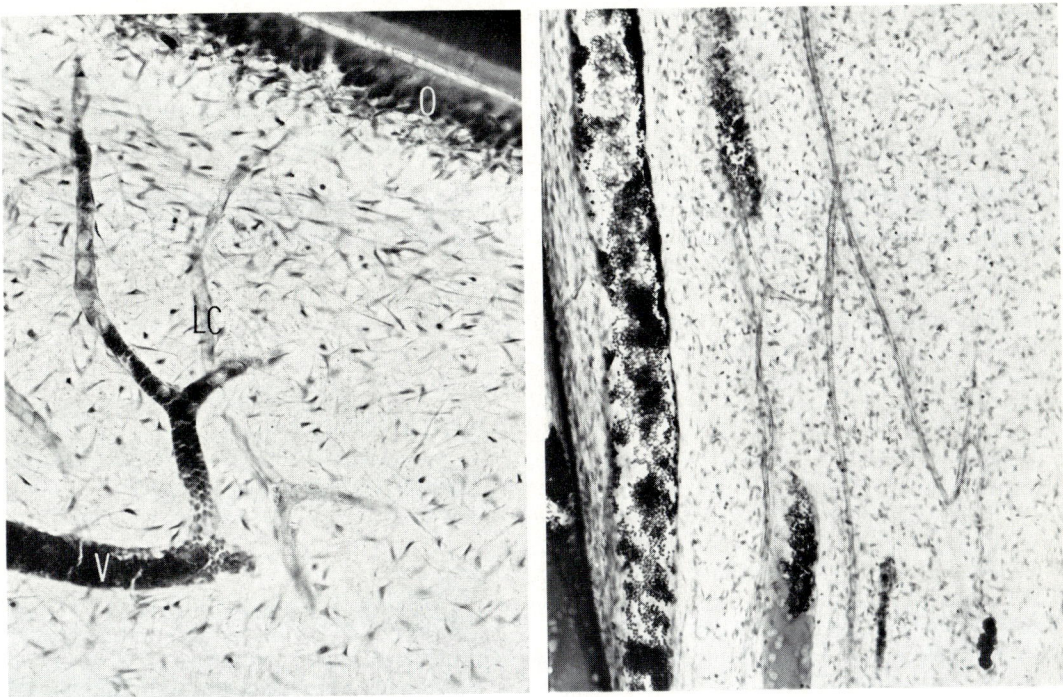

FIG. 5-23 *(Left)* Section of the lateral surface of the pulp of an incisor. The lymph capillary appears adjacent to the odontoblastic layer. Note its relation to the accompanying vein. O, odontoblastic layer; LC, lymph capillary; V, vein. Verhoeff's iron hematoxylin stain. ×250 *(Right)* Section of pulp from a canine tooth. The area shown is at lower border of the coronal portion. The parallel lymph vessels form a communication around a vein. Verhoeff's iron hematoxylin stain. ×150. (Bernick S, Patek PR: Lymphatic vessels of the dental pulp in dogs. J Dent Res 48:959, 1969. Copyright by the American Dental Association. Reproduced by permission)

pulp, variably designated as pulp blood pressure, dental pulp fluid pressure, or pulp tissue pressure, has been the subject of investigations. The tissue pressure or interstitial fluid pressure is directly related to the capillary blood pressure. Since the capillary pressure cannot be measured, a number of methods have been devised for measuring the tissue pressure of the dental pulp in dogs. Among these are photoelectric methods (Upthegrove et al, 1968), pressure transducer systems (Brown and Yankowitz, 1964), tonometric measurements (Christiansen et al, 1977), and micropuncture techniques (Tønder and Kvinnsland, 1983). Experiments by Moist and Yanov (1965) and Brown and Beveridge (1966) indicate that the tooth pulp pressure can be measured by sealing a polyethylene tube into a tap made through the enamel and dentin. In Brown and Beveridge's experiments the tubing was connected to a pressure transducer and a microsyringe, and the system was filled with Ringer's solution. Measurement of the fluid pressure was then correlated with measurements of systemic arterial blood pressure, monitored by a catheter implanted into the left internal thoracic artery.

The results indicated that the tooth pulp pressure was pulsatile, with the number of pulses per minute corresponding to the dog's heart rate. However, the pressure was less than that of the systemic arterial pulse.

Pulp pressure measurements have been reported in a wide range from less than 1 to 100 mm Hg (Brown and Yankowitz, 1964; Kawamura et al, 1967; Tønder and Kvinnsland, 1983).

The intrapulpal pressure can apparently be modified by changes in arterial blood pressure, by increased venous pressure (Tønder and Kvinnsland, 1983), and by other factors over short intervals. However, other mechanisms may isolate the pulp from arterial pressure changes.

Reduction in intrapulpal blood pressure can occur when sympathetic efferent nerves are electrically stimulated, yet pressure in the branches of the maxillary artery remain unaffected (Weiss et al, 1970). The pulpal blood vessel response is due to activation of α adrenoreceptors (Ahlberg and Edwall, 1977; Tønder and Naess, 1978).

Increased tissue pressure apparently occurs in response to pulp inflammation. Tønder (1983) used glass micropipettes connected to a servo-controlled counter-pressure system to measure the pulp tissue pressure of cats' teeth. Control pulpal tissue pressure was 5.5 mm Hg, versus 16.3 mm Hg in the experimentally inflamed pulp. Pulpal tissue pressure a millimeter or two away from the inflamed site was 7.0 mm Hg.

According to Stenvik et al (1972), pulp pressure increases up to 50 mm Hg when pulps are exposed. Such exposure is usually coincidental with a rapid increase of interstitial fluid. The pressure drops dramatically to between 5 and 15 mm Hg when the pulp tissue at the exposure site becomes necrotic.

CLINICAL CORRELATIONS

LOCAL ANESTHETICS

Vasoconstrictors are added to a local anesthetic agent for the purpose of prolonging the anesthetic state and for obtaining a deeper anesthesia by confining the anesthetic to the injection site. The most commonly used vasoconstrictor in dental local anesthetic is epinephrine. Blood flow in the pulp is reduced following infiltration of local anesthetics that contain epinephrine (Olgart and Gazelius, 1977). When dogs' teeth were infiltrated with lidocaine and 5 μg to 20 μg of epinephrine, the blood flow to the pulps was decreased by about 30% (Meyer et al, 1964). Even greater flow reduction was determined by using the 15 μ microsphere injection method (Kim, 1981). The induced vasoconstriction produced by epinephrine is due to stimulation of α-adrenergic receptors located in the pulpal blood vessels. At doses of epinephrine exceeding 10^{-8} M, the pulpal vessels collapse and total ischemia of the pulp results (Simard-Savoie et al, 1979). In addition, Van Hassel (1973) and Simard-Savoie et al found that the pulp tissue pressure is depressed by deposition of local anesthetics with high concentrations of vasoconstrictors near the pulpal blood vessels. However, Langeland's investigations (1962) demonstrated that the human dental pulp is not damaged seriously or permanently by injection of local anesthetics; similar pulp morphology was observed in teeth extracted under general anesthesia. By way of confirmation, Röckert and Örtendal (1980) found that respiratory activity of rat pulps after 2 to 5 hours of anoxia was not significantly different from that of control pulps. They concluded that the anaerobic respiratory activity of the dental pulp would enable it to survive the vasoconstrictor activity of the local anesthetic. In clinical usage, the vasoconstrictor effect of epinephrine may be reduced by some local anesthetics, such as lidocaine, which possesses a vasodilator effect (Lemay-Laliberte, 1972).

Ligamental Injection

Recently, the ligamental injection technique has become popular. Neither carbocaine nor saline solutions anesthetize the pulp when injected ligamentally. The anesthetic must contain epinephrine if the ligamental injection is to be effective. These results raise questions about the effectiveness of the extrapulpal pressure injection. Pulpal blood flow in dogs' teeth decreased by 85% compared to that of controls following the ligamental injection using 2% lidocaine plus 1:100,000 epinephrine (Kim, 1982). Furthermore, there was wide-spreading of the anesthetic solution into the adjacent tissues from the site of injection when a dyed anesthetic solution, or other dyes, was injected. Cardiovascular changes may follow the injection of an epinephrine-containing anesthetic agent. Thus, the wisdom of using the ligamental injection technique is open to question.

Intrapulpal anesthesia is often obtained by injecting the anesthetic into the pulp tissue under pressure when infiltration or conduction anesthesia fails. The resultant anesthesia is supposedly attributed to the pharmacologic action of the anesthetic on the nerve cell membrane. However, a similar anesthetic effect was obtained by injecting normal saline solution into the pulp (Birchfield and Rosenberg, 1975). Whether this anesthesia is due to circulatory interference from the mechanical pressure of the injection is open to conjecture. However, some support for this concept has been offered by Edwall and Scott (1971). They found a strong relationship between dentinal excitability and the capillary circulation of the pulp. When the pulp microcirculation was decreased, nerve excitability transiently increased. This increase was followed by a rapid decrease almost to zero. Under clinical conditions, Van Hassel found a similar relationship (Bender, 1978). An immediate pain response occurred when cold was applied to the tooth. With continued maintenance of the stimulus, the pain diminished and then disappeared. Apparently the temperature drop produced a vasoconstriction of the pulpal capillaries, thereby reducing the blood flow.

GENERAL ANESTHETICS

General anesthetics apparently do have an effect on the velocity of blood flow in the pulp. Scott et al (1972) found that in rats increasing the level of general anesthesia reduced the resting flow velocity and enhanced the effect of sympathetic nerve stimulation so that flow velocity fell to zero in the first 30 seconds. The effects gradually disappeared over a period of an hour. Whether or not such blood flow interferences would adversely affect the pulp remains conjectural.

TEMPERATURE CHANGES AND DRUGS

Temperature changes and drugs applied to the dentin affect the microcirculation of the dental pulp.

Temperature Elevation

A 10°C to 15°C increase in pulp temperature, induced by a heating wire wrapped around the tooth, caused arteriolar dilation and a linear increase in intrapulpal pressure of 2.5 mm Hg per degree centigrade. The pressure gradually returned to normal as the tooth cooled. Irreversible changes occurred when vasodilation was sustained by heating the pulp to 45°C for prolonged periods, resulting in persistent increased pulp pressure (Van Hassel and Brown, 1969).

Heat generated by tooth preparation may cause pulpal inflammation and thereby affect pulpal blood flow. The microcirculation in rat incisor teeth, prepared with and without water spray, was observed under intravital microscopy. Tooth preparation with copious water spray to the dentin from all angles resulted in insignificant changes in pulpal blood flow. However, tooth preparation without water spray caused considerable reduction in pulpal blood flow. This reduction remained low even 1 hour after the preparation, indicating permanent damage to the circulatory system (Kim et al, 1983). There was an increase in flow through the apically positioned arteriovenous anastamoses and a redistribution of flow from the drilled side to the opposite side. The initiation of pulpal damage probably resulted from the alteration of the microvasculature. Moreover, histopathologic changes in response to tooth preparation indicated that a burn lesion developed in the pulp when the tooth was prepared to within 1 mm of the remaining dentin layer.

Temperature Reduction

Intermittent application of subfreezing temperatures to extracted human teeth (Augsburger and Peters, 1981) and to the maxillary canines of dogs produces a transient fall in intrapulpal blood pressure. At temperatures lower than $-2°C$, the pulp tissues exhibit immediate pulpal pathology, such as vascular engorgement and necrosis (Frank et al, 1972). Substances such as hydrogen peroxide and carbon dioxide produce gas emboli in the capillaries of the odontoblastic layer and reduce the blood flow (Pohto and Scheinin, 1961, 1967; Edwall and Olgart, 1972).

A systematic determination of changes in microcirculatory dynamics following various dental procedures and materials currently used in dentistry should help to elucidate the pathophysiologic mechanisms of pulpal disorders. In addition, results of such studies should provide methods for procedures that will cause minimal harmful effect to the pulp.

ENDODONTIC THERAPY

During endodontic therapy, if only part of the pulp is extirpated, profuse hemorrhage occurs, because of the increased diameters of the vessels in the central part of the pulp. From a clinical standpoint, there would be less hemorrhage if the pulp were extirpated closer to the apex of the tooth. Excessive bleeding during instrumentation of the canal may indicate that some pulp tissue has remained in the apical third of the root canal (Fig. 5–24).

During tooth development, there is great cellular activity coronally in areas of active dentin formation; hence, blood vessel density is increased. Apically, there is not as great a need for a concentrated blood supply; thus, near the apex of the developing tooth bud the connective tissue is relatively avascular. After eruption, the subodontoblastic capillary plexus is larger than during tooth development. In the floor of the pulp chamber, there is a rich blood supply.

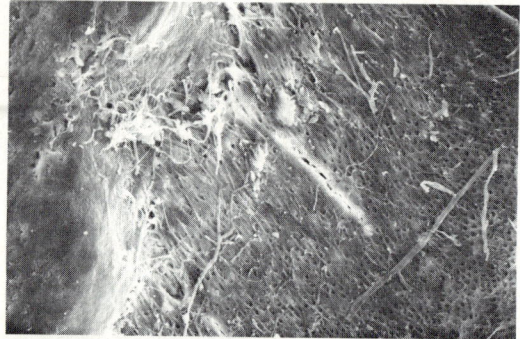
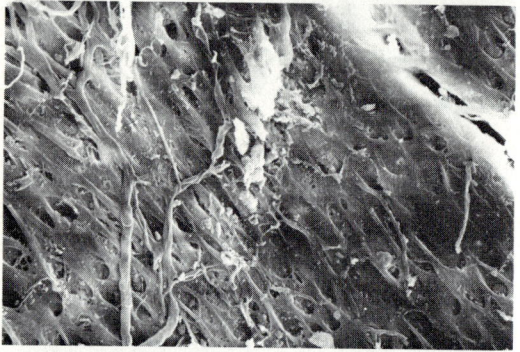
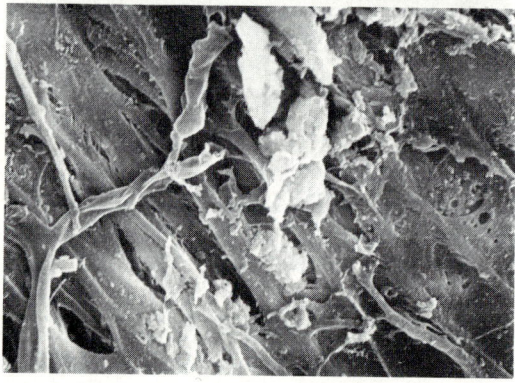

FIG. 5-24 *(Top)* Scanning electron micrograph of apical portion of root canal after pulp extirpation and instrumentation. ×300. *(Middle)* Higher magnification of wall of canal. Network of blood vessels is visible. ×1000. *(Bottom)* Higher magnification of middle figure, showing blood vessels remaining on dentinal wall. ×3000.

AGING

In older pulps, circulation is decreased. Atherosclerotic changes take place in the blood vessels, which narrow and become increasingly calcified (Fig. 5-25). Finally, circulation becomes impaired; consequently, cells atrophy and die, and fibrosis increases.

PERIODONTAL DISEASE

Periodontal disease also causes reduction of the circulation in the dental pulp. As a consequence, degenerative pulp changes may take place (Fig. 5-26). Reparative processes in older fibrotic pulps are diminished as a result of a reduction in the blood supply; hence, reactions to severe operative injuries are more likely to result in pulp necrosis.

Excessive irradiation also produces a marked degree of arteriosclerosis and arteriolosclerosis, resulting in pulp necrosis.

Many pulps have a collateral circulation, which can be seen by an examination of serial sections of extracted teeth. The pulps are supplied with blood not only by vessels that enter the apical foramina but also through some vessels that enter along the lateral aspects of the roots and the interradicular regions. Consequently, inflammatory pulp changes do not cause self-strangulation of the pulp, as had been believed heretofore. Thus, resolution of pulp inflammation can and does occur.

ANTERIOR OSTEOTOMY

Occlusal abnormalities may be corrected by maxillary or mandibular segmental osteoto-

FIG. 5-25 Calcification (Ca) of the wall of a blood vessel (BV) in the pulp (P). The tooth was periodontally involved. D, dentin. ×96.

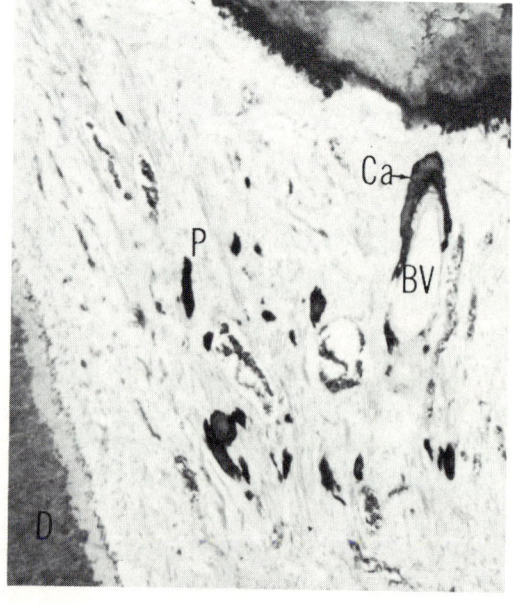

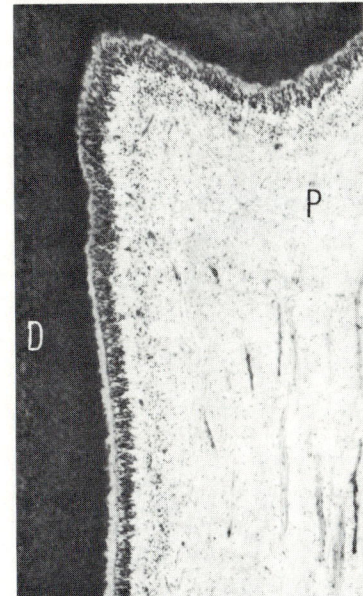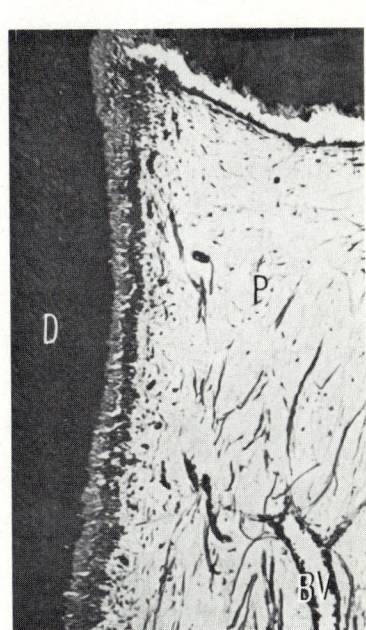

FIG. 5-26 Atrophic changes due to periodontal disease. *(Left)* A bicuspid not involved periodontally. The pulp (P) is highly cellular. Blood vessels are not dilated. D, dentin. ×96. *(Right)* A bicuspid, periodontally involved. The cell content of the pulp (P) is decreased. A central blood vessel (BV) is dilated. D, dentin. ×96. (Seltzer S, Bender IB, Ziontz M: The dynamics of pulp inflammation: correlations between diagnostic data and actual histologic findings in the pulp, Oral Surg 16:846, 1963)

mies. Attempts have been made to determine the effects of such procedures on the blood flow to the oral mucosa, bone, and dental pulp. Techniques that have been used for this purpose include microangiography (Bell, 1975), isotope fractionization and particle distribution (Meyer and Cavanaugh, 1976), and the hydrogen washout technique (Indresano and Lundell, 1983). The results indicate that, of all the tissues, pulpal blood flow was most severely decreased (by 82%) immediately after surgery (Indresano and Lundell, 1983). However, blood flow is apparently reestablished, since clinical reports have claimed that pulp responses to thermal and electrical stimuli return to normal in more than 90% of cases (Pepersack, 1973; Theisen and Guernsey, 1976).

CHANGES DUE TO INFLAMMATION

In acute inflammation, chemical mediators released from injured cells excite sensory nerve fibers, which then act on the muscular elements of the blood vessels and cause dilation of the vessels. The permeability of the capillaries, which do not have muscle cells, is increased by the action of similar substances in the ground substance of the capillary walls. Other substances, which depolymerize the ground substance, and thus cause increased permeability, also may be involved in inflammation. The increased permeability of the vessels permits the escape of plasma proteins and leukocytes from the capillaries into the inflamed area to carry out neutralization, dilution, and phagocytosis of the irritant.

During chronic inflammation, pulp tissue pressure is elevated, although reduced from the high pressures resulting from acute inflammation (Van Hassel, 1973; Tønder and Kvinnsland, 1983). The muscular elements in the microcirculation reestablish control over capillary pressure. Capillary permeability is gradually decreased as repair occurs.

During inflammation, the effects of infiltration anesthesia are diluted, which results in a diminution of anesthesia.

Pashley (1979) has pointed out that a vasoconstrictor in a local anesthetic may reduce the rate of removal or inactivation of toxic bacterial products that permeate through carious dentin into the pulp. The accumulation of toxic products in an inflamed area may lead to an elevation of toxin concentration in pulp interstitial fluid. Increased capillary permeability, arteriolar dilatation, and increased pulp tissue pressure may follow. A vicious circle of further reduction in blood flow leading to a further elevation of interstitial fluid toxin concentration may then ensue.

In severe inflammation, the lymphatic vessels

are closed, resulting in persistently increased fluid and pulp pressure. The end result may be pulp necrosis (Bernick, 1977).

BIBLIOGRAPHY

Ahlberg KF, Edwall L: Influence of local insults on sympathetic vasoconstrictor control in the feline dental pulp. Acta Odont Scand 35:103, 1977

Augsburger RA, Peters DD: In vitro effects of ice, skin refrigerant, and CO_2 snow on intrapulpal temperature. J Endodont 7:110, 1981

Avery JK, Cox CF, Corpron RE, Trefz BR: Distribution of adrenergic and cholinergic nerve endings in mouse molars utilizing morphological and cytochemical analysis. J Dent Res 53: Special Issue 74, 1974

Bell WH: Bone healing and revascularization after total maxillary osteotomy. J Oral Surg 33:253, 1975

Bender IB: Pulp biology conference: A discussion. J Endodontol 4:37, 1978

Bernick S: Age changes in the blood supply to molar teeth of rats. Anat Rec 144:265, 1962

Bernick S: Lymphatic vessels of the human dental pulp. J Dent Res 56:70, 1977

Bernick S: Morphological changes to lymphatic vessels in pulpal inflammation. J Dent Res 56:841, 1977

Bernick S: Vascular supply to the developing teeth of rats. Anat Rec 137:141, 1960

Bernick S, Patek, PR: Lymphatic vessels of the dental pulp in dogs. J Dent Res 48:959, 1969

Birchfield J, Rosenberg, PA: Role of the anesthetic solution in intrapulpal anesthesia. J Endodontol 1:26, 1975

Brodin E, Gazelius B, Olgart L, Nilsson G: Tissue concentration and release of substance P-like immuno-reactivity in the dental pulp. Acta Physiol Scand 111:141, 1981

Brown AC, Beveridge EE: The relation between tooth pulp pressure and systemic arterial pressure. Arch Oral Biol 11:1181, 1966

Brown AC, Barrow BL, Gadd GN, Van Hassel HJ: Tooth pulp transcapillary osmotic pressure in the dog. Arch Oral Biol 14:491, 1969

Brown AC, Yankowitz D: Tooth pulp pressure and hydraulic permeability. Circ Res 15:42, 1964

Christiansen RL, Meyer MW, Visscher MB: Tonometric measurement of dental pulpal and mandibular marrow blood pressures. J Dent Res 56:635, 1977

Corpron RE, Avery JK, Lee SD: Ultrastructure of capillaries in the odontoblastic layer. J Dent Res 52:393, 1973

Dahl E, Mjör IA: The fine structure of the vessels in the human dental pulp. Acta Odont Scand 31:228, 1973

Edwall L: 4. Regulation of pulpal blood flow. J Endodont 6:434, 1980

Edwall L, Kindlovà M: The effect of sympathetic nerve stimulation on the rate of disappearance of tracers from various oral tissues. Acta Odont Scand 29:397, 1971

Edwall L, Olgart LB: Influence of cavity washing agents on pulpal microcirculation in the cat. Acta Odont Scand 30:39, 1972

Frank U, Freundlich J, Tansy MF, Chaffee RB, Jr, Weiss RC, Kendall FM: Vascular and cellular responses of teeth after localized controlled cooling. Cryobiology 9:526, 1972

Gazelius B, Olgart L: Vasodilation in the dental pulp produced by electrical stimulation of the inferior alveolar nerve in the cat. Acta Physiol Scand 108:181, 1980

Gazelius B, Olgart L, Edwall L, Trowbridge HO: Effects of substance P on sensory nerves and blood flow in the feline dental pulp. In Anderson DJ, Matthews B (eds): Pain in the Trigeminal Region. Amsterdam, Elsevier/North Holland Biomedical Press, 1977

Han SS, Avery JK: The ultrastructure of capillaries and arterioles of the hamster dental pulp. Anat Rec 145:549, 1963

Harris R, Griffin CJ: The ultrastructure of small blood vessels of the normal human dental pulp. Austral Dent J 16:220, 1971

Indresano AT, Lundell MI: Blood flow changes in the rabbit maxilla following an anterior osteotomy. J Dent Res 62:743, 1983

Intaglietta M, Tompkins W: Microvascular measurements by video shearing and splitting. Microvasc Res 5:309, 1973

Kawamura Y, Kato Y, Kato I: Studies on the dental pulp pressure. J Osaka Univ Dent Sch 7:7, 1967

Kim S: Presentation at the 39th annual meeting of the Association of Endodontics, 1982

Kim S: Regulation of Blood Flow of the Dental Pulp Macrocirculation and Microcirculation Studies, Ph.D. dissertation, Columbia University, 1981

Kim S, Chien S: Effects of β-agonist isoproterenol on pulpal hemodynamics. AADR Abstr 280, J Dent Res 62:200, 1983

Kim S, Fan FC, Chen RYZ, et al: Effects of changes in systemic hemodynamic parameters on pulpal hemodynamics. J Endod 6:392, 1980

Kim S, Fan F-C, Chen RYZ, Simchon S, Schuessler GB, Chien S: 3. Effects of changes in systemic hemodynamic parameters on pulpal hemodynamics. J Endodont, 6:394, 1980

Kim S, Grayson A, Kim B, Schacter W: Effects of dental procedures on pulpal blood flow in dogs. J Dent Res 62:268, 1983

Kim S, Trowbridge H, Kim B, Chien S: Effects of bradykinin on pulpal blood flow in dogs. J Dent Res 61 (Program and Abstracts of Papers): 293, 1982

Kim S, Lipowsky H, Usami S, Chien S: Arteriovenous distribution of hemodynamic parameters in the rat dental pulp. Microvas Res 27:28, 1984

Kindlova M, Matena V: Blood circulation in the rodent teeth of the rat. Acta Anat Basel 37:163, 1959

Kozam G, Bennett, BW: Blood circulation in the dental pulp. JADA 59:458, 1959

Kramer IRH: A technique for the injection of blood vessels in the dental pulp using extracted teeth. Anat Rec 11:91, 1951

Kramer IRH: Vascular architecture of the human dental pulp. Arch Oral Biol 2:177, 1960

Kukletová M: An electron-microscopic study of the lymphatic vessels in the dental pulp in the calf. Arch Oral Biol 15:1117, 1970

Kukletová M: Submicroscopic structure of blood vessels in the calf dental pulp. Scripta Medica, 43:109, 1970

Kukletová M, Zahrádka J, Lukas Z: Monaminergic and

cholinergic nerve fibres in the human dental pulp. Histochemie 16:154, 1968
Langeland K: Effects of local anesthetics on pulp tissue. Dent Prog 3:13, 1962
Larsson P-A, Linde A: Adrenergic vessel innervation in the rat incisor pulp. Scand J Dent Res 79:7, 1971
Lemay-Laliberte H: Etude Physiopharmacologique du Tissu Pulpaire chez le Chien. Master's thesis, Université de Montreal, Canada, 1972
Liebman FM, Consenza F: Study of blood flow in the dental pulp by an electrical impedance technique. Phys Med Biol 7:167, 1962
Meyer M, Weiner D, Grim E: Blood flow in the dental pulp of the dog. Proc Soc Exp Biol Med 116:1038, 1964
Meyer MW: Distribution of cardiac output to the oral tissues in dogs. J Dent Res 49:787, 1970
Meyer MW: 5. Methodologies for studying pulpal hemodynamics. J Endodont 6:466, 1980
Meyer MW, Cavanaugh GD: Blood flow changes after orthognathic surgery. Maxillary and mandibular subapical osteotomies. J Oral Surg 34:495, 1976
Meyer MW, Path MG: Blood flow in the dental pulp of dogs determined by hydrogen polarography and radioactive microsphere methods. Arch Oral Biol 24:601, 1979
Moist RR, Yanov HM: Measurement of pulpal blood pressure. J Dent Res 44:570, 1965
Mori K: Identification of lymphatic vessels after intraarterial injection of dyes and other substances. Microvascular Res 1:268, 1969
Olgart L, Gazelius B: Effects of adrenaline and felypressin (octapressin) on blood flow and sensory nerve activity in the tooth. Acta Odont Scand 35:69, 1977
Pashley DH: 2. The influence of dentin permeability and pulpal blood flow on pulpal solute concentrations. J Endodont 5:355, 1979
Path MG, Meyer MW: Heterogeneity of blood flow in the canine tooth in the dog. Arch Oral Biol 25:83, 1980
Pepersack WJ: Tooth vitality after alveolar segmental osteotomy. J Maxillofac Surg 1:85, 1973
Pohto M, Scheinin A: Microscopic observations on living dental pulp. I. Method for intravital study of circulation in rat incisor pulp. Int Dent J 22:228, 1958
Pohto M, Scheinin A: Microskopiska undersökningar av levande tandpulpa. Odont Tidskr 69:86, 1961
Pohto M, Scheinin A: Vital microscopy of the pulp in the rat incisor. VII. Reactions to silicate cements. Suom Hammaslaak Toim 63:178, 1967
Pohto P, Antila R: Innervation of blood vessels in the dental pulp. Int Dent J 22:228, 1972
Provenza DV: The blood vascular supply of the dental pulp with emphasis on capillary circulation. Circ Res 6:213, 1958
Rapp R, El-Labban NB, Kramer IRH, Wood D: Ultrastructure of fenestrated capillaries in human dental pulps. Arch Oral Biol 22:317, 1977
Röckert HOE, Örtendal T: Recovery of aerobic respiratory activity of the dental pulp after anoxic periods of two to five hours. IRCS Med Sci: Biochemistry; Cell and Membrane Biology; Dental and Oral Biology. Pathology 8:99, 1980
Ruben MP, Prieto-Hernandez JR, Gott FK, Kramer GM, Bloom AA: Visualization of lymphatic microcirculation of oral tissues. II. Retrograde lymphography. J Periodont 42:774, 1971
Russel LH, Kramer IRH: Observations on the vascular architecture of the dental pulp. J Dent Res 37:957, 1956
Saunders RL de CH: Microradiographic studies of human adult and fetal dental pulp vessels. In X-ray Microscopy and Microradiography, p 561. New York, Academic Press, 1957
Scott D, Jr, Scheinin A, Karjalainen S, Edwall L: Influence of sympathetic nerve stimulation on flow velocity in pulpal vessels. Acta Odont Scand 30:277, 1972
Simard-Savoie S, Lemay H, Taleb L: The effect of epinephrine on pulpal microcirculation. J Dent Res 58:2074, 1979
Skrabanek P, Powell D: Substance P. Ann Res Rev Vol 1. London, Churchill Livingstone, 1977
Stenvik A, Iverson J, Mjör IA: Tissue pressure and histology of normal and inflamed tooth pulps in macaque monkeys. Arch Oral Biol 17:1501, 1972
Sulzmann R: Zur frage des lymphabflusses innerhalb der zahnpulpa. Deutsche Zahnärztl Zeitschr 20:353, 1965
Takahashi K, Kishi Y, Kim S: A scanning electron microscope study of the blood vessels of dog pulp using corrosion resin casts. J Endodont 8:131, 1982
Taylor AC: Microscopic observation of the living tooth pulp. Science 111:40, 1950
Theisen FC, Guernsey LH: Postoperative sequelae after anterior segmental osteotomies. Oral Surg 41:139, 1976
Tompkins WR, Monti R, Intaglietta M: Velocity measurements of self-tracking correlator. Rev Sci Instrum 45:647, 1974
Tønder KH: The effects of variations in arterial blood pressure and baroreceptor reflexes on pulpal blood flow in dogs. Arch Oral Biol 20:345, 1975
Tønder KH: Effect of vasodilating drugs on external carotid and pulpal blood flow in dogs: "Stealing" of dental perfusion pressure. Acta Physiol Scand 97:75, 1976
Tønder KJH, Kvinnsland I: Micropuncture measurements of interstitial fluid pressure in normal and inflamed dental pulp in cats. J Endodont 9:105, 1983
Tønder KJH, Naess G: Nervous control of blood flow in the dental pulp in dogs. Acta Physiol Scand 104:13, 1978
Upthegrove DD, Bishop JG, Dorman HL: Indirect determination of the blood pressure in the dental pulp. Arch Oral Biol 13:929, 1968
Van Hassel HJ: Physiology of the human dental pulp. In Siskin M (ed): The Biology of the Human Dental Pulp, pp 16–24. St. Louis, CV Mosby, 1973
Van Hassel HJ, Brown AC: Effect of temperature changes on intrapulpal pressure and hydraulic permeability in dogs. Arch Oral Biol 14:301, 1969
Waterson A: Fluorescent structures in the rabbit dental pulp. Aust J Exp Biol Med Sci 45:309, 1967
Wayland H, Johnson P: Erythrocyte velocity measurement in microvessels by a two split photometric method. J Appl Physiol 22:333, 1967
Weiss RC, Tansy MF, Chaffee RB, Jr: Functional control of intrapulpal vasculature. I. Relationship of tooth pulp and lateral nasal artery pressures. J Dent Res 49:1407, 1970
Weiss RC, Tansy MF, Chaffee RB, Kendall FM: Func-

tional control of intrapulpal vasculature. II. Physiologic evidence of a sympathetic cholinergic vasoactive system. J Dent Res 51:1350, 1972

Wiederhielm CA, Woodbury JW, Kirk S, Rushmer RF: Pulsatile pressures in the microcirculation of frog's mesentery. Am J Physiol 207:173, 1964

Wynn W, Haldi J, Hopf MA, John K: Pressure within the pulp chamber of the dog's tooth relative to arterial blood pressure. J Dent Res 42:1169, 1963

Zweifach BW: Functional Behavior of the Microcirculation, p 4. Springfield, Ill, Charles C Thomas, 1961

6
THE NERVE SUPPLY OF THE PULP AND PAIN PERCEPTION

PHYSIOLOGY OF NEURAL CONDUCTION

The neuron is the basic cell of the nervous system. Like other cells, each neuron has a nucleus and surrounding cytoplasm. The cell membrane of the neuron is composed of a biomolecular layer of lipid between two layers of protein. The neuron has one relatively long branch (the axon) and numerous fine branches (dendrites). The axon transmits brief electrical waves called nerve impulses; the dendrites receive nerve impulses from other cells.

Electron microscopic examinations reveal that the neuron contains organelles, such as mitochondria, Golgi apparatus, and endoplasmic reticulum. The endoplasmic reticulum manufactures protein that flows down the axon, replenishing its cellular material. The organelles are involved in the structural changes in ribonucleic acid (RNA).

The physiology of neural conduction is related to changes in the cell membrane. Various drugs such as aspirin (Barker and Levitan, 1971) and biologic amines (De Robertis, 1971) can alter the membrane potential of the neuron, causing changes in membrane permeability. The resting potential of the neuron depends on the selective permeability of the cell membrane and on the sodium pump of the cell. Selective permeability and the sodium pump produce a separation of positive and negative ions across the cell membrane.

Stimulation of a neuron causes it to depolarize in the region of the stimulus. Subsequently, adjacent areas of the cell membrane are also depolarized. Such depolarization during the passage of excitation along the neuron constitutes the action potential, or nerve impulse.

In myelinated nerve fibers, the resting and action potentials generate at the nodes of Ranvier. When a fiber is depolarized, the nodes become active. If one of the nodes is active and the adjacent node is inactive, the local circuit current between the nodes depolarizes the adjacent inactive node. This continuous internodal hopping or excitation of the impulse from one node to the next is known as saltatory conduction (Ruch et al, 1965).

The cell information, in the form of the action potential, is transduced into a chemical message. During excitation, there is a rapid increase of sodium ions in the cell. To a lesser degree, potassium ions flow out. The flow of negative ions is apparently not involved.

(This chapter was prepared with the generous assistance of Dr. Syngcuk Kim, School of Dental and Oral Surgery, Columbia University, New York)

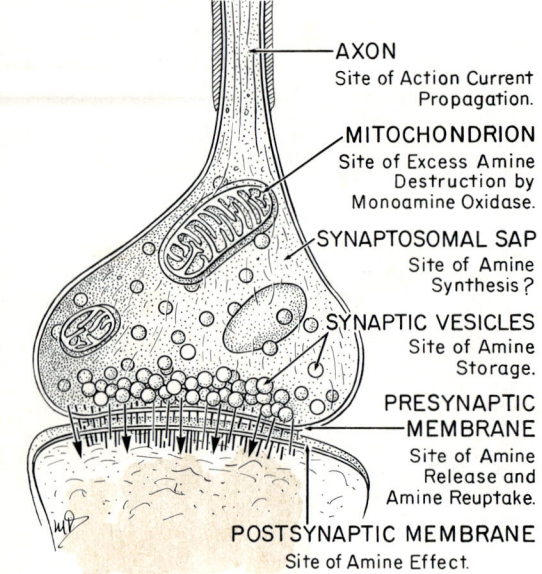

FIG. 6-1 Schematic section of amine synapse. (McGeer PL: The chemistry of mind. Am Sci 59:221, 1971)

Within approximately one millisecond of the firing of a nerve impulse, the sodium-potassium resting level is restored and the cell membrane is repolarized or "cocked" for the next firing. This high metabolic activity renders nerve tissue highly sensitive to lack of oxygen.

THE SYNAPSE

The axonal electrical impulse ceases abruptly when it reaches the point where the axon's terminal fibers make contact with another nerve cell. These junction points are knoblike structures called synapses. Thus, neurons are physiologically connected through a synapse.

Between the synaptic knob and the synaptic membrane of the adjoining nerve cell is a uniform space of about 20 millimicrons, called the synaptic cleft.

To continue beyond the synapse, the nerve impulse must be regenerated on the other side. The presynaptic information is transferred to the synapse in the form of the action potential. The postsynaptic cell develops its action potential from the chemical information elicited from the action potential of the presynaptic cell. Acetylcholine (ACh) is one of the chemical mediators or transmission messengers of neural transmission. ACh is associated with protein molecules stored in vesicles, tiny sacs or packets, in the terminals of the presynaptic cell (McGeer, 1971; Fig. 6-1). When the action potential stimulus reaches the packets, the protein-acetylcholine bond is broken and ACh is released. ACh diffuses across the synaptic cleft and becomes attached to the specific receptor sites on the postsynaptic cell membrane.

Presumably, the receptor sites are associated with fine channels in the cell membrane; these channels are opened up by the attachment of the transmitter substance to the receptor sites. The opening of the channels alters the permeability of the postsynaptic cell membrane to sodium and potassium ions; sodium ions pass out. The intense ionic flux changes the electrical potentials of the postsynaptic cell. Depolarization also depends on the presence of calcium ions in the surrounding extracellular fluid. According to Katz (1971), depolarization opens up specific "calcium gates" in the terminal axon membrane, leading to an influx of calcium ions. Thus, increased calcium uptake results from depolarization (Blaustein, 1971). The calcium ions, on reaching the internal surface of the axon membrane, cause discharge of the vesicles into the synaptic cleft. An action potential is thus elicited in the postsynaptic cell.

A second type of synapse—an electrical synapse—has been found in the central nervous system. The electrical synapse does not utilize a chemical transmitter; there is a direct flow of current from the presynaptic to the postsynaptic cell (Kandel, 1970).

THE INHIBITORY SYNAPSE

Synapses that inhibit the firing of a nerve cell have been identified in the nervous system. Such inhibition may occur even though the nerve cell may be receiving a volley of excitatory impulses. The inhibitory synapse makes the cell's internal voltage more negative than it normally is—a voltage opposite to that needed for generating an action potential. Eccles (1965) found that the inhibitory transmitter substance opens the cell membrane to the flow of potassium ions but not to that of sodium ions. During synaptic inhibition, the outflow of potassium ions renders the inside potential of the membrane more negative than it is in the resting state. Thus, the fundamental difference between synaptic excitation and synaptic inhibition is that, in the former, the membrane passes sodium ions freely; in the latter, sodium ions are largely excluded.

NERVE FIBERS

The terms medullated and myelinated, which are used in reference to nerve fibers, are synonymous. Myelinated fibers have a sheath of myelin, a substance composed largely of fatty substances, or lipids (Figs. 6–2 and 6–3, *right*). The myelin sheath, which functions as an insulator, has concentric alternate layers of lipid and of protein, with the molecules of one layer stacked at right angles to the molecules of the other (Korn, 1966). Myelin appears to be an internal proliferation of the plasma membrane of the Schwann cell. Unmyelinated (or nonmedullated) nerve fibers are surrounded by a single layer of the Schwann cell plasma membrane (Fig. 6–3). Unmyelinated nerves are usually found in the autonomic nervous system; they accompany the blood vessels. Such nerve fibers come into contact with those elements of the capillary bed known as arterioles, metarterioles, arteriovenous bridges, or precapillary sphincters. True capillaries have no nerve supply (see Chap. 5, The Circulation of the Pulp.)

PAIN FIBER TYPES

Pain receptors transmit their messages to the central nervous system at different rates, depending on the sizes and coating of the nerves. Group A α and β fibers are myelinated and have a diameter that varies between 4 μ and 20 μ. A fibers are present in somatic and visceral nerves; they carry touch, pressure, and proprioceptive impulses at a speed that may reach 80 m/sec. A δ fibers are the smallest group of myelinated fibers. Their diameters vary between 1.0 and 5.0 μ and they carry pain impulses at a velocity of 12 to 20 m/sec.

The C fibers are unmyelinated and have a smaller diameter, i.e., 0.3 μ to 1.0 μ. They carry pain sensations at a lower speed, approximately 0.6 to 1.0 m/sec.

Pain sensation is also mediated by the autonomic nervous system. The neurons of this system are similar, anatomically, to the somatic afferent neurons (sensory nerves); the cell bodies of the sympathetic and parasympathetic nerves lie in dorsal root ganglia. The central processes enter the posterior roots of the spinal cord. The afferent peripheral processes go to visceral receptors. Some of these afferent fibers

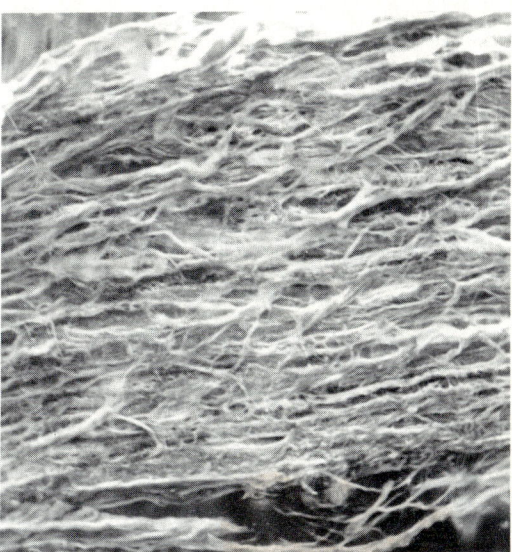

FIG. 6-2 Scanning electron micrograph of mandibular (myelinated) nerve of dog. ×600.

have been defined as B fibers, being intermediate to A and C fibers in size and speed of conduction.

Dental pain may be induced by stimulation of segments of the autonomic nervous system. For example, faradic stimulation of the superior cervical ganglion produces pain behind the ear and in the teeth of the lower jaw. The sympathetic vasoconstrictor fibers from the cervical ganglion are nonmyelinated.

PAIN RECEPTORS

The sensory receptors for pain (nociceptors), primarily Aδ and C fibers, are free nerve endings. Almost all areas of the body are innervated with pain receptors; they are present in the skin, in the adventitia of blood vessels, in the aponeurotic sheaths, in the vicinity of the pulp-dentin border, and in deep somatic and visceral structures. Some structures have more pain receptors than others. All free nerve endings are small, unmyelinated axons that overlap without fusing. However, myelinated nerve fibers are also pain receptors.

Action potentials are elicited in the pain receptors by any noxious agent that causes destruction of cells or injures tissue. These stimuli may be classified as mechanical, chemical, thermal, and electrical. Thus, pain may be elicited by visceral distention, visceral inflammation,

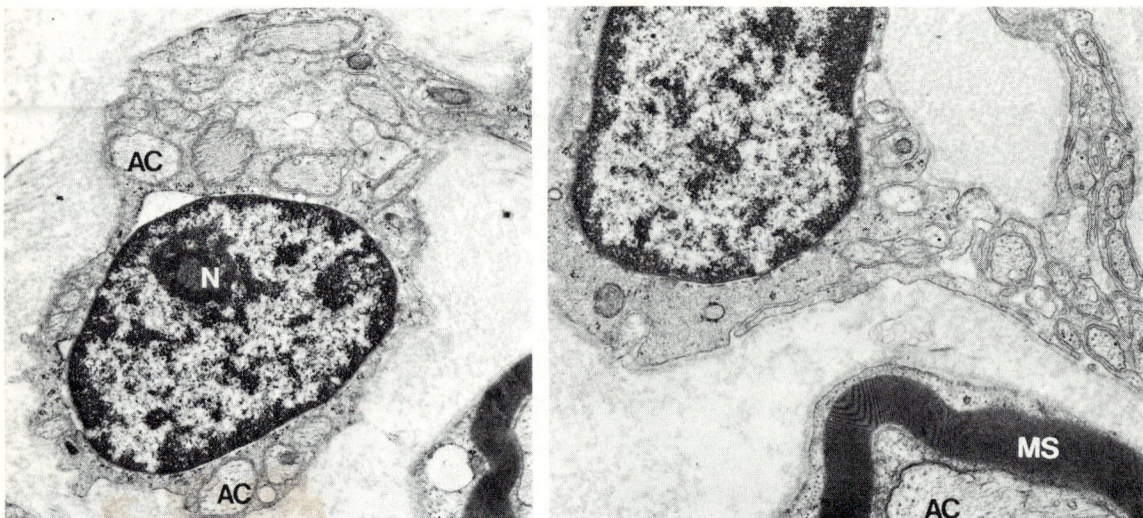

FIG. 6-3 *(Left)* Electron micrograph showing a Schwann cell of the dental pulp. Section is cut through the cell body, demonstrating the nucleus (N). Processes of the neural connective tissue cell (Schwann cell) surround nonmyelinated axon cylinders (AC). ×27,500. *(Right)* Electron micrograph. Schwann cell of the dental pulp similar to that shown in left frame. In the lower portion of the electron micrograph is a myelinated nerve fiber. Note the concentric membranes of the myelin sheath (MS) surrounding the axon cylinder (AC). ×27,500. (Courtesy of Dr. Calvin Leifer, Temple University School of Dentistry, Philadelphia)

vasoconstriction, vasodilation, radiant heat, and other factors.

Adrenergic Fibers

Epinephrine and norepinephrine are liberated at the ends of sympathetic nerve fibers, where they serve as chemical mediators for carrying the nerve impulses to effector organs.

Chemically, the two compounds differ only slightly. They have similar pharmacologic actions that resemble the effects of stimulation of the sympathetic nervous system. They are classified as sympathomimetic agents. The sympathetic nerves contain predominantly norepinephrine; norepinephrine is released at most postganglionic sympathetic terminals.

Cholinergic Fibers

Cholinergic nerves are primarily the so-called parasympathetic nerves at whose endings ACh is released. On stimulation, ACh is released from an inactive, bound form and is rapidly converted to less active free choline and acetate by the enzyme cholinesterase. In the subsequent recovery period, the choline is recombined with acetate and once more incorporated into the structure of the nerve.

INNERVATION OF THE TEETH

The teeth are supplied by the second and third divisions of the fifth cranial (trigeminal) nerve (Fig. 6-4).

The trigeminal spinal tract nucleus consists of the interpolaris, oralis, and caudalis subtracts. Nociceptive afferent fibers in the ophthalmic, maxillary, and mandibular divisions of the trigeminal (V) nerve pass by way of the trigeminal ganglion to the brainstem. Pulpal pain excites all nuclei in the trigeminal spinal tract nucleus. Pulp afferent inputs project to the subnucleus caudalis, which is specifically involved in pain and temperature transmission. Afferents also project to other nuclei at more rostral levels, including the subnucleus oralis, which has been associated with tactile sensation (Fig. 6-5). Such nerve impulse projections raise the question whether dental sensations register exclusively as pain. Thus, dental nerves may contain receptors associated with other sensory modalities, such as temperature and touch (Mumford, 1969). Both medullated and nonmedullated nerve fibers leave the alveolar nerve as a common dental nerve. This nerve divides into multiple branches as it traverses the bone. At the

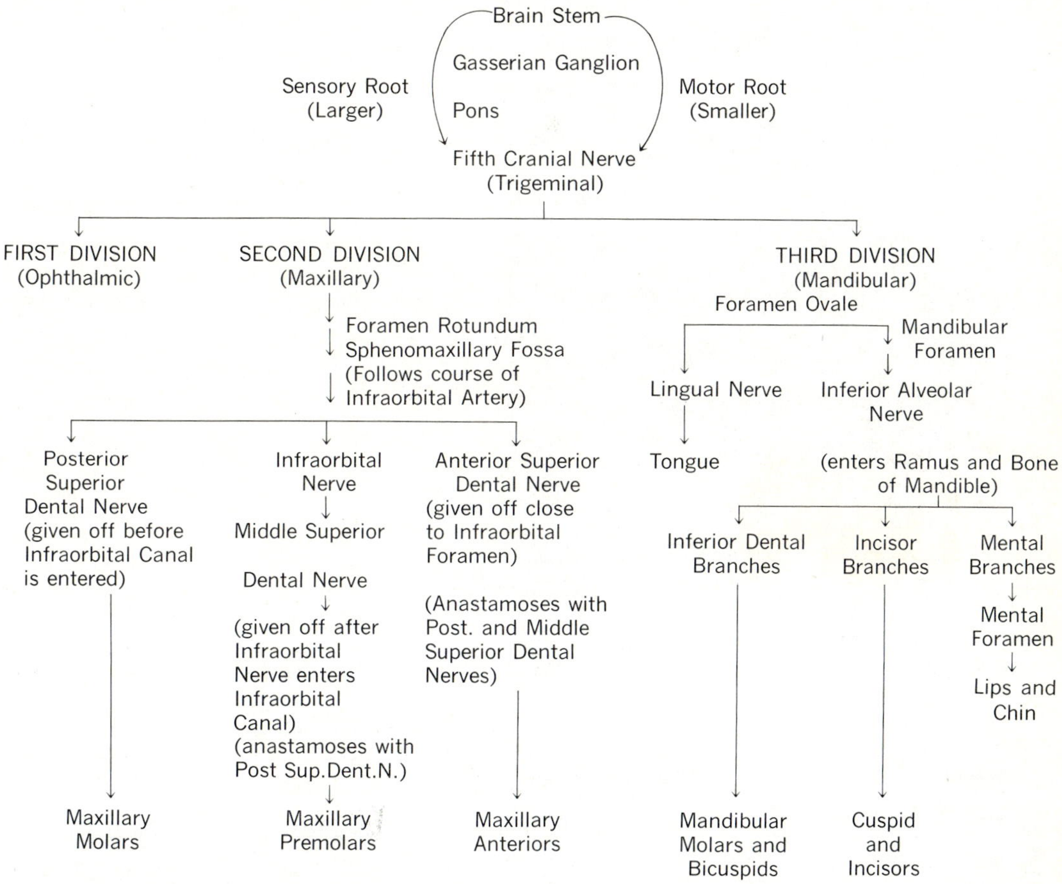

```
                        ┌─ Brain Stem ─┐
                        │ Gasserian Ganglion │
  Sensory Root          │                    │   Motor Root
   (Larger)             │       Pons         │   (Smaller)
                        │                    │
                        └ Fifth Cranial Nerve ┘
                             (Trigeminal)
```

| FIRST DIVISION (Ophthalmic) | SECOND DIVISION (Maxillary) | THIRD DIVISION (Mandibular) Foramen Ovale |

SECOND DIVISION (Maxillary):
- Foramen Rotundum
- Sphenomaxillary Fossa
- (Follows course of Infraorbital Artery)

Posterior Superior Dental Nerve (given off before Infraorbital Canal is entered)	Infraorbital Nerve → Middle Superior Dental Nerve (given off after Infraorbital Nerve enters Infraorbital Canal) (anastamoses with Post Sup.Dent.N.)	Anterior Superior Dental Nerve (given off close to Infraorbital Foramen) (Anastamoses with Post. and Middle Superior Dental Nerves)
Maxillary Molars	Maxillary Premolars	Maxillary Anteriors

THIRD DIVISION (Mandibular):
- Lingual Nerve → Tongue
- Inferior Alveolar Nerve (enters Ramus and Bone of Mandible) via Mandibular Foramen

Inferior Dental Branches	Incisor Branches	Mental Branches → Mental Foramen → Lips and Chin
Mandibular Molars and Bicuspids	Cuspid and Incisors	

FIG. 6-4 Nerve supply to the teeth.

FIG. 6-5 Nociceptive pathway to the trigeminal spinal tract nucleus. RF, reticular formation. (Courtesy of Dr. S. Kim, Columbia University, New York)

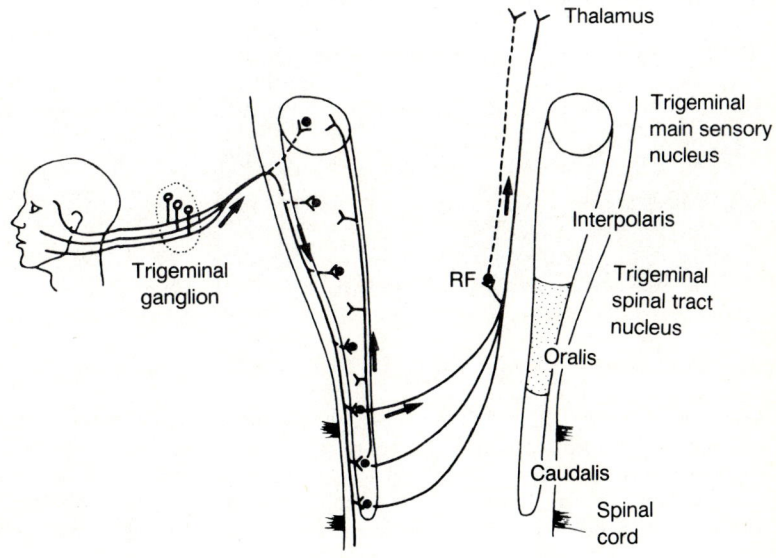

136 | THE DENTAL PULP

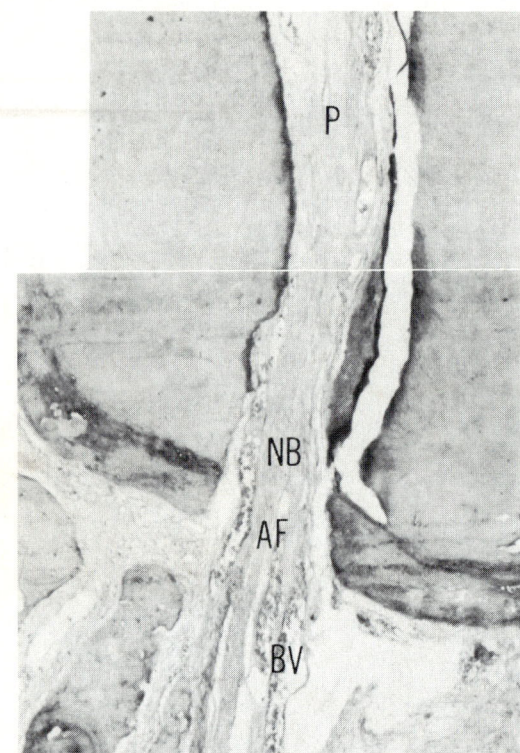
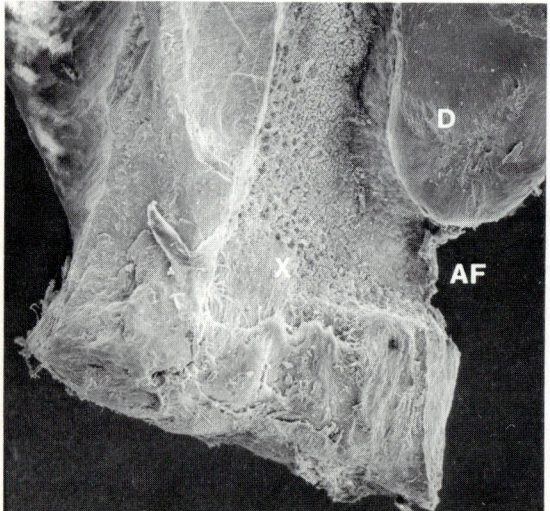
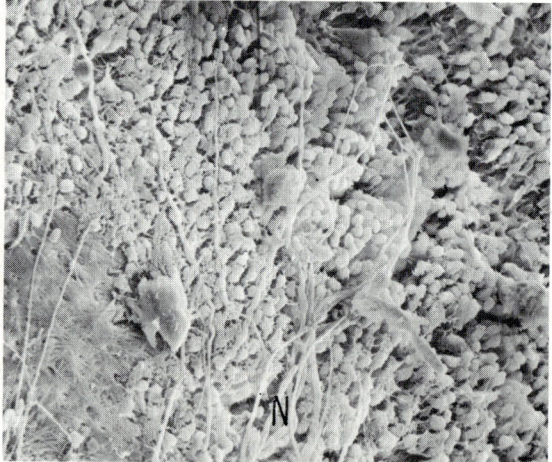

FIG. 6-6 *(Top)* Medullated nerve bundle (NB), entering the apical foramen (AF) together with blood vessels (BV). P, radicular pulp tissue. ×54. *(Bottom, left)* Scanning electron micrograph of apical region of human molar. AF, apical foramen; D, dentin. ×40. *(Bottom, right)* Higher magnification of region depicted by X on left figure showing nerves (N) entering pulp. ×1000.

apical alveolar plate, the branches, probably Aδ and C axons, enter the periodontal ligament in each of the four tooth surfaces. The nerves enter the apical foramina and unite to form a common pulpal nerve (Fig. 6-6).

The nerve trunks enter the root with the afferent blood vessels either as accompanying individual units or as intimately associated nerve sheaths (neuroadventitia; Provenza, 1968).

Some of the mature nerve trunks may be as large as 5 μm to 13 μm in diameter and may contain as many as 1200 neurofibrils (Avery, 1981). The predominant innervation of the pulp is of the Aδ to C fiber range (Beasley and Hol-

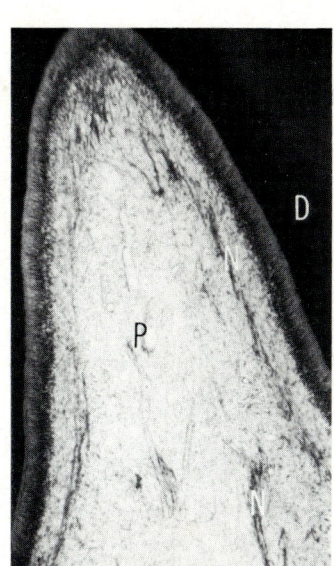
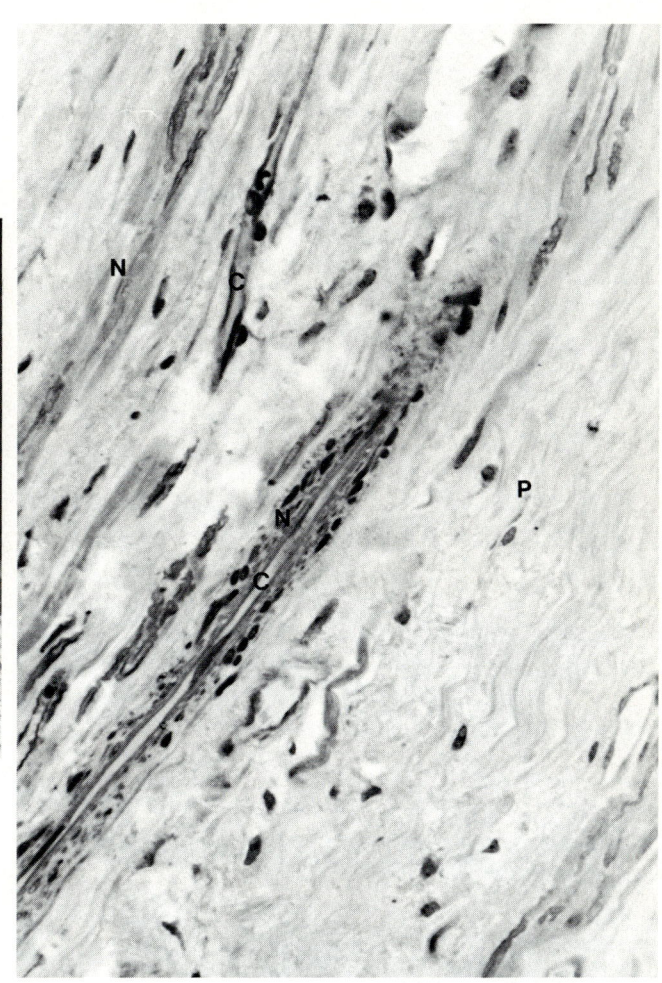

FIG. 6-7 *(Left)* Nerve trunks (N), proceeding toward the odontoblastic layer of pulp (P). D, dentin. ×54. *(Right)* Higher magnification of nerve trunks in the coronal pulp (P). Nerves (N) surround capillaries (C). ×960.

land, 1978). Few unmyelinated axons are found near the apex of the tooth. According to Holland (1980), such axons number less than 400.

The pulpal nerve proceeds coronally, together with the afferent blood vessels (Fig. 6-7). When it reaches the coronal portion of the tooth, the pulpal nerve divides into cuspal nerves (Bernick, 1968; Fig. 6-8). Older studies have claimed that most of the pulp nerve fibers are myelinated and consist of Schwann-cell cytoplasm, myelin sheath, and axon (Graf and Björlin, 1951; Miyoshi et al, 1966). Several more recent studies have found that the number of unmyelinated axons in the pulps of teeth is greater than the number of myelinated axons. Johnsen and Johns (1978) found 2240 unmyelinated axons, as compared to 361 myelinated axons in dogs' teeth. In cats' teeth, 34.9% unmyelinated C fibers and 65.1% myelinated and unmyelinated Aδ fibers were found by Nähri et al (1982). On approaching the cell-free zone, the cuspal nerves, a mixture of myelinated and unmyelinated axons, most of which no longer have a myelin sheath and have incomplete Schwann cell sheaths, branch repeatedly and give rise to an overlapping network of nerves, called the plexus of Raschkow by Mummery (1919; Fig. 6-9). These nerve twigs either end among the stroma of the pulp or terminate among the odontoblasts. Holland (1977) has estimated the number of nerve endings in the periphery of the pulp to be about 1000/mm². A few fibers enter the predentin or dentin (Fig. 6-10).

The nonmedullated nerve twigs in the odontoblastic layer are approximately 1.0 μ or less in

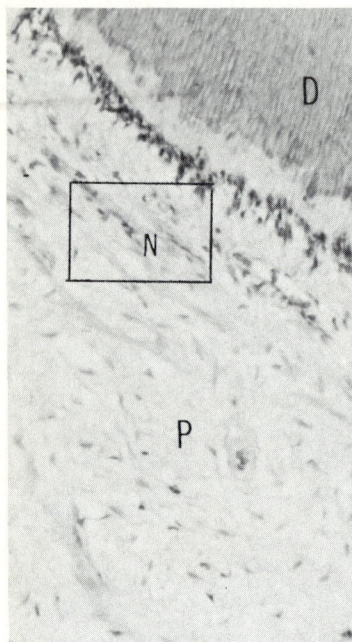
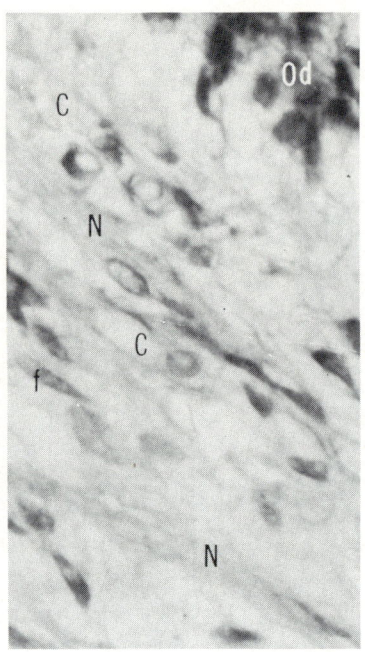

FIG. 6-8 *(Left)* Arborization of nerve fibers (N) in the coronal portion of the pulp (P). D, dentin. ×240. *(Right)* Higher magnification of region outlined by rectangle at *left*, showing network of nerve fibers (N) and capillaries (C). Od, odontoblasts; f, fibroblast. ×960.

FIG. 6-9 Scanning electron micrograph of remnants of the plexus of Raschkow remaining on the dentinal wall after pulp extirpation and root canal instrumentation. ×6000.

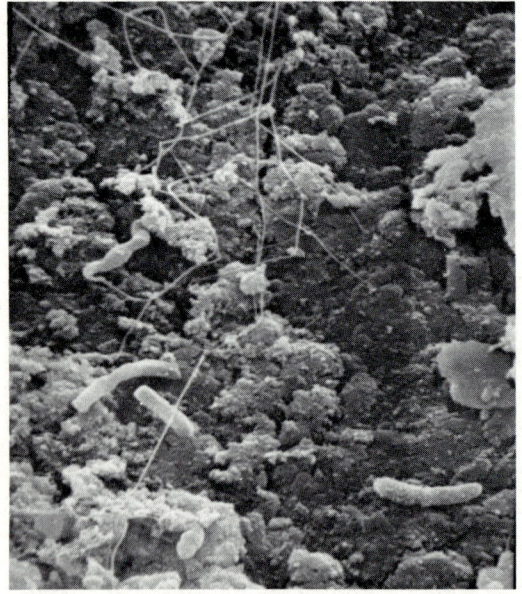

diameter. A few axons are still ensheathed by a thin Schwann-cell covering and have a beaded appearance (Arwill, 1967; Avery, 1973; Byers, 1979). When they pass into the dentin or predentin, they may form a loop and return to the odontoblastic region. However, such "loops" may be artifacts. They have not been detected by autoradiography (Byers, 1980). In primary teeth and developing permanent teeth, there are no nerves in the predentin or dentin (Rapp et al, 1967). In young permanent teeth the odontoblasts recede during dentinogenesis. The nerves may be trapped in newly formed dentin. However, this concept has not been completely accepted by Berger and Byers (1983), whose experiments have shown that cut or crushed nerves can regenerate and reenter the dentinal tubules. Possibly, both nerve entrapment and regrowth can account for the presence of nerves in dentin. The nerves attempt to maintain their relationship with the odontoblasts.

Identification of Nerve Pathways by Labeling

Cytolabeling methods, using anterograde and retrograde intra-axonal transport proteins, have been used to identify sensory and autonomic nerve pathways and to demonstrate their origins and peripheral distribution.

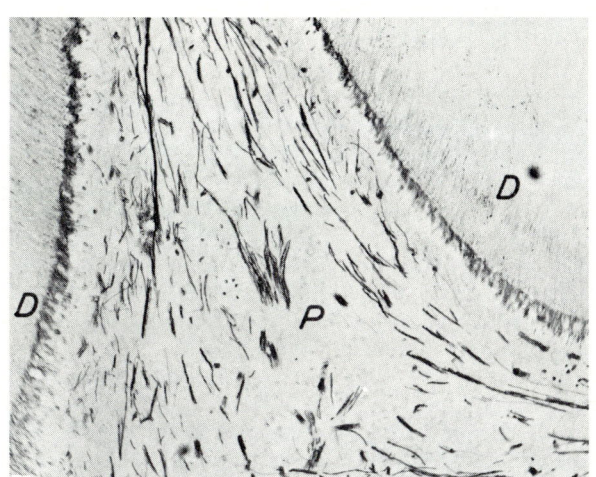

FIG. 6-10 *(Top)* A longitudinal section from a human premolar tooth; a portion of the coronal pulp (P), showing nerve fibers. D, dentin. ×60. *(Bottom, left)* A section of pulp and dentin in situ from a human canine tooth. Nonmyelinated nerve fibers, passing between the odontoblasts (O) into the dentin (D). PD, predentin. ×600. *(Bottom, right)* The same section and field as at *left*. Counterstained with Harris's hematoxylin to contrast the nuclear structures. (Rowles, SL, Brain EB: Arch Oral Biol 2:64, 1960)

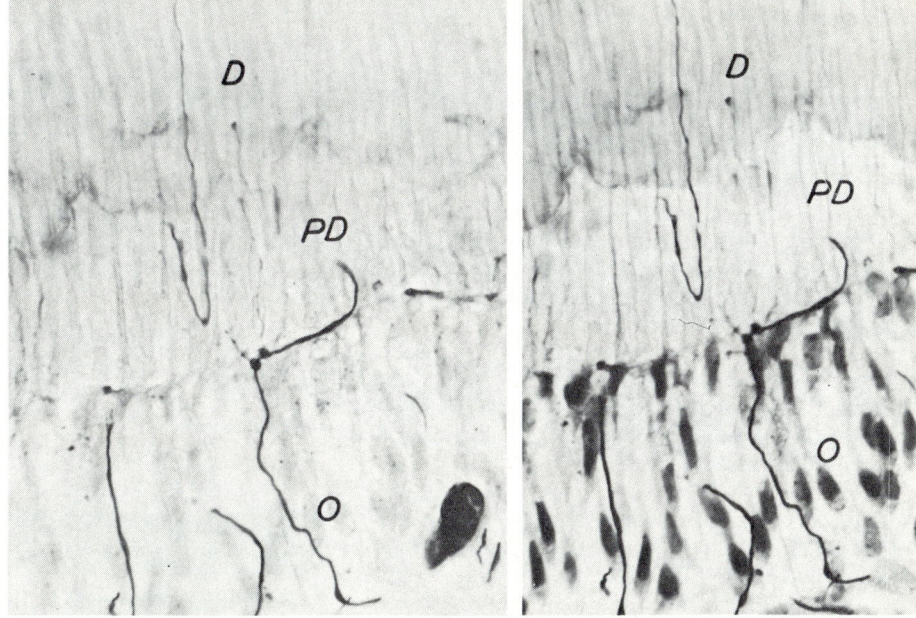

Anterograde transport systems using ^{3}H-leucine (Droz and Leblond, 1963; Menke, 1973), and ^{3}H-proline (Fink et al, 1975), have been demonstrated by radioautography. Droz and Leblond (1963) injected ^{3}H-leucine intraperitoneally. They found the labeled protein in the cell bodies of the brain, spinal cord, and Gasserian (trigeminal) ganglia. Menke (1973) and Fink et al, (1975) injected the trigeminal ganglion of experimental animals with ^{3}H-leucine or ^{3}H-proline; radioautographs showed that the protein was transported from the cell body to the peripheral axon terminations. The label was found in the subodontoblastic region, the predentin, and the inner and middle dentin, but not in the pulp, the odontoblastic layer, or the outer regions of the dentin.

A retrograde rapid axonal transport method has been developed to amplify the radioautographic tracing of the peripheral nerve distribution. This method traces peripheral neuronal pathways from their terminal nerve endings to the cells of origin. To map this neuronal distribution, labeled horseradish peroxidase (^{3}H-HRP) is used for intra-axonal retrograde tracing (LaVail and LaVail, 1972; LaVail et al, 1973).

HRP is an exogenous protein marker used to trace both sensory and autonomic nerves. These include motor, sympathetic, and pre- and postganglionic neurons. The movement of HRP is primarily retrograde; the marker travels from the terminal nerve endings to their cell bodies. The protein is not transported from one neuron to another and does not jump the synaptic gap. Furstman et al (1975) have shown that injection of ^{3}H-HRP into the pulp of a rat molar resulted in labeling of the associated first-order neuronal cell bodies in the ipsilateral trigeminal ganglion.

Extensive studies (Chiego et al, 1980) have shown that, following injection of the ^{3}H-HRP into pulps of posterior monkey teeth, labeled cells were present in the ipsilateral trigeminal, superior cervical, and otic ganglia. Labeled cells were also found in the ipsilateral but not contralateral mesencephalic nucleus of the trigeminal nerve. However, in another study, when the pulps of the right side, including the central and lateral incisors, were injected with ^{3}H-HRP, positive labeling was found in both right and left trigeminal ganglia. Positive labeling was found only ipsilaterally in the right superior cervical ganglia and mesencephalic nucleus. These observations indicate that sympathetic nerve fibers do not cross over the midline. However, there is a crossover of sensory nerves in the central incisor teeth, confirming previous reports of transmedian innervation of central and lateral incisors (Anderson and Pearl, 1974; Maderio et al, 1978).

Labeled cell bodies were present in the mesencephalic nucleus ipsilaterally in all animals after injecting ^{3}H-HRP. Injection of ^{3}H-leucine into the mesencephalic nucleus demonstrated the presence of labeling in the pulp (Chiego et al, 1979).

Labeling in both the mesencephalic nucleus and the pulp following anterograde and retrograde axoplasmic transport of the radioactive proteins appears to indicate the presence of a sensory modality, other than pain, in the dental pulp.

Neurovascular Relationships

The muscular elements of the afferent pulpal blood vessels are innervated. Beaded nerve terminals are found in intimate association with the muscle fibers of arterioles, metarterioles, and precapillaries, but capillaries are not innervated. The perivascular nerve endings are adrenergic postganglionic fibers concerned with neurovascular reflexes, primarily vasoconstriction. Such sympathetic nerve fibers are concentrated on the arterioles (Ogilvie et al, 1966; Pohto and Antila, 1968a,b).

There is an intricate relationship between sensory nerve activity and pulp blood flow. Edwall and Scott (1971) found that tooth warming during sympathetic stimulation slowly and gradually increased both blood flow and sensory nerve activity. Tooth cooling resulted in a gradual decrease in blood flow and sympathetic nerve activity. Measurements of sensory nerve activity and pulpal blood flow have been made simultaneously by Edwall and Scott. Electrodes were placed in contact with the dentin of prepared dental cavities to measure nerve reactions. Pulpal blood flow was measured in the same tooth by the ^{125}I desaturation method. Both blood flow and sensory nerve activity decreased in response to sympathetic stimulation. Tooth warming caused an increase in both parameters. This suggests that the excitability of sensory units in the tooth is strongly modulated by changes in pulpal microcirculation induced by stimulation of nonmyelinated sympathetic vasoconstrictor fibers. In addition, there are large and small cholinergic sensory neurons and small substance P sensory axons, both of which terminate on pulpal blood vessels (Byers, 1983).

THEORIES OF TOOTH PAIN PERCEPTION

When teeth are drilled or when exposed dentin is subjected to touch, to hot or cold liquids, to food or air, or to sweet or sour fluids, a painful reaction is experienced. Moreover, dentin may be extremely sensitive despite pulp inflammation, which may cause the destruction of dentinal nerve endings (Lilja et al, 1982). The mechanisms whereby thermal, chemical, electrical, or tactile stimuli are transmitted through the dentin are not completely understood. Whether the dentin is innervated or the odontoblasts are transducers for nerve impulses is controversial. In addition, the traditional view that irritation of the dentin stimulates only pain receptors has now been questioned; the possibility that there are separate receptors in the dentin for cold, heat, and pressure has been advanced (Pimenidis and Hinds, 1977; Avery, 1981).

There is no clear-cut explanation of how a stimulus applied to dentin can influence nerve fibers that apparently do not penetrate all of the dentinal tubules (Byers, 1979), or even the bulk of the dentin. Several hypotheses for dentinal sensitivity have been proposed. The three most prevalent theories are dentinal nerve stimulation, the dentinal receptor theory, and the hydrodynamic theory.

DENTINAL NERVE STIMULATION

Innervation of Dentin

Whether dentin is actually innervated has been the subject of controversy. Studies of the innervation of the teeth, based on chemical staining of the nervous elements, are somewhat misleading. Traditionally, silver salts have been used to disclose the distribution of nerve fibers because nerve tissue has an affinity for silver. However, the demonstration of nerves by staining with silver salts may be an artifact inasmuch as other structures, such as reticular and collagen fibers, are also stained. Thus, blackened collagen fibers may be mistaken for nerves.

Light Microscopic Studies. At the light microscopic level, variable penetration of dentin by a limited number of nerve fibers has been demonstrated (Bernick, 1968; Langeland and Yagi, 1972).

Others have claimed that the nerve fibers terminate about the cell bodies of the odontoblasts (Rapp et al, 1957).

Electron Microscopic Studies. Several electron microsocpic studies have differed with respect to the findings on dentin innervation. Part of the problem has been that, in the dentin, unmyelinated nerve fibers are difficult to identify positively with the electron microscope because cellular extensions of the odontoblasts have similar ultrastructural components.

Fearnhead (1968) could find no synaptic or other special form of connection between odontoblasts and nerves, although he did notice an intimate contact between axons and odontoblasts over quite large distances in many places.

The cytoplasmic content of intradentinal nerve fibers is variable. Sometimes the nerve cytoplasm is more dense than that of the odontoblast process, but not always (Roane et al, 1973).

According to the investigations of Arwill (1968), Frank (1969), and Corpron and Avery (1973), the ultrastructure of nerve endings and the odontoblastic processes are different in the dentinal tubules. The nerves that enter the dentin rarely have an associated Schwann cell. In contrast, the ultrastructure of odontoblastic processes rarely shows organelles other than microtubules and microfilaments. Arwill (1967) and Frank (1968, 1969) have pointed out that the nerve fibers contain numerous mitochondria, whereas the odontoblast process has a scarcity of mitochondria (Fig. 6–11). Arwill (1967) found nerve fibers in the predentin and called

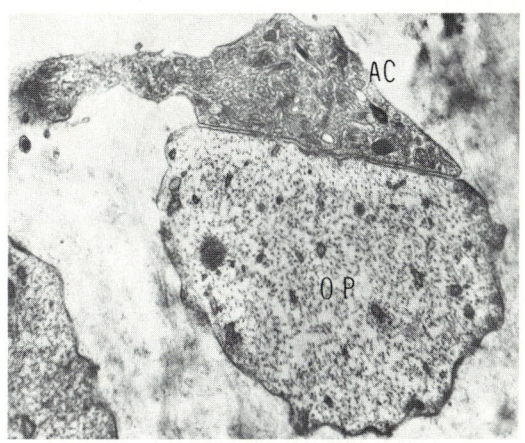

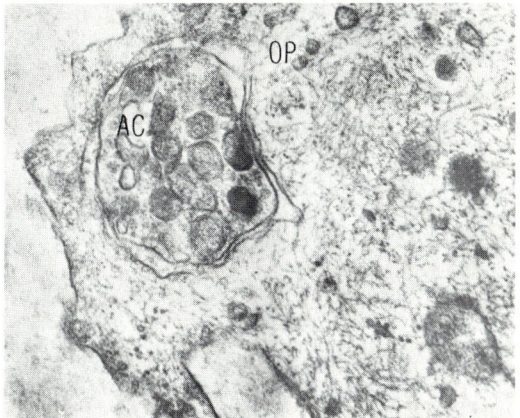

FIG. 6-11 *(Top)* "Associated cell" (AC) seemingly penetrating the predentinal matrix, adjoins an odontoblastic process (OP). Note the vesicular content of the associated cell and the gap between the two cells, resembling a synaptic cleft. ×28,000. *(Bottom)* Associated cell (AC) totally surrounded by an odontoblastic process (OP). The associated cell is very rich in mitochondria and differs in morphology from the odontoblastic process. ×47,600. (Arwill T: Studies on the ultrastructure of dental tissues. II. Odontologisk Revy 18:191, 1967)

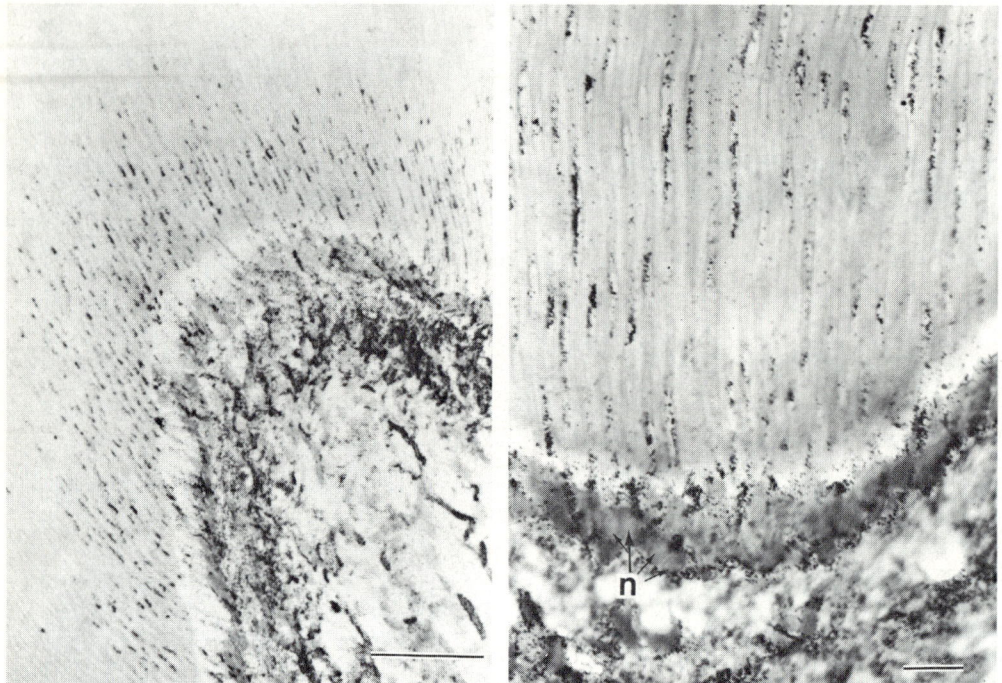

FIG. 6-12 Horizontal sections near tip of cusp of second upper right molar fixed 7 days postinjection. *(Left)* Low magnification showing silver grains concentrated over subondontoblast plexus and inner dentin. Scale bar = 50 μm. *(Right)* High magnification showing silver grains in discontinuous linear arrays over dentinal tubules. Odontoblast nuclei (n) are not labeled. Scale bar = 10 μm. (Byers MR, Kish SJ: Delineation of somatic nerve endings in rat teeth by radioautography of axon-transported protein. J Dent Res 55:419, 1976)

them associated cells, but neither he nor Thomas and Payne (1983) were able to find them in the dentin (Fig. 6-11). Arwill questioned the nervous origin of the associated cells. On the other hand, Fink et al (1975), Byers and Kish (1976), Pimenidis and Hinds (1977), Byers and Matthews (1981), and Byers and Dong (1983) found that, following injection of ^{3}H-proline or ^{3}H-leucine into the trigeminal ganglion of rats, cats, and monkeys, labeled sensory nerves were found in the molar pulps. Silver grains were also found extending along the dentinal tubules to approximately 75 μm to 150 μm (one third to one half the thickness) of dentin (Fig. 6-12). The label was confined almost exclusively to nerve axons and endings; the odontoblastic cell bodies and processes were not significantly labeled (Fig. 6-13). Occasionally, two axons, separated by a narrow cleft, were found adjacent to each other in the dentin (Byers et al, 1982; Fig. 6-14).

A scanning electron microscope study by Tidmarsh (1981) revealed beaded structures, possibly nerves, in the dentin as far as halfway between the pulp and the dentinoenamel junction. Frank (1966) demonstrated that in the predentin and inner dentin the nerve fiber followed a straight course along the odontoblast process and was in close contact with it. A small submicroscopic space separated both plasma membranes. The nerve was located in a concavity of the surface of the odontoblast (a sort of groove or gutter) (Fig. 6-15). At the periphery of the inner dentin, and in lateral canal branchings, the inside of the nerve fiber became twisted around the odontoblast process. These "corkscrew" fibers had complex infoldings into the odontoblastic process, suggesting a functional relationship. However, the plasma membranes separated the nerve fibers from the odontoblasts. Similar findings were reported by Byers and Kish (1976).

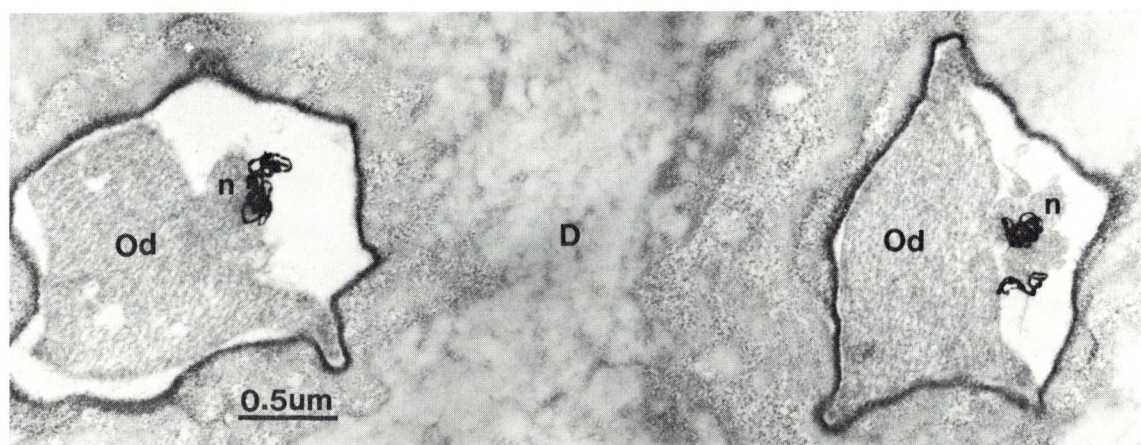

FIG. 6-13 EM autoradiographs from a mandibular molar cusp. Note that the silver grains occur over or next to the small nervelike processes (n) and do not label the odontoblasts (Od) or dentin (D). The axons-nerve endings often occur in clusters. ×25,000. (Byers MR, Dong WK: Autoradiographic location of sensory nerve endings in dentin of monkey teeth. Anat Rec 205:441, 1983)

Between the nerve endings and the odontoblastic process, electron-dense thickenings of the plasma membranes of both structures were visible. The distance between both plasmalemmas was 200 to 400 Å.

Gap junctions between nerve endings or terminal axons and other cells in rat molar pulps were not detected by Byers (1977, 1979). However, other electron microscope studies have shown the presence of gap junctions in the odontoblastic layer between nerve-like cell processes and odontoblasts as well as between nerve cell processes with each other (Matthews and Holland, 1975; Holland, 1975, 1976). However, it is not possible to distinguish between odontoblastic processes and pulpal axons in the gap junctions on the basis of their microtubule and microfilament populations (Holland, 1980). It is likely that the gap junctions seen in the odontoblastic layer only connect odontoblasts to each other or to fibroblasts (Byers et al, 1982).

DENTINAL RECEPTOR THEORY

The odontoblasts and their processes are perceived to act as dentinal receptor mechanisms, whereby they participate in the initiation and transmission of sensory stimuli in dentin.

As discussed above, numerous investigations have provided structural evidence for the presence of nerve fiberlike structures adjacent to the odontoblastic processes in the dentinal tubules

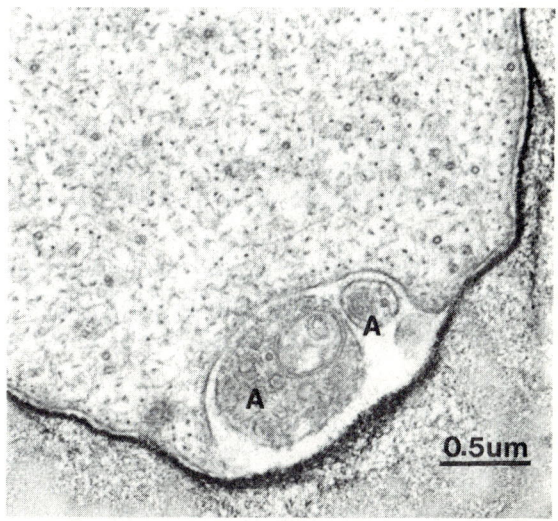

FIG. 6-14 Typical example of dentinal axon morphology. Two axons (A), separated by a narrow (5 nm–10 nm) cleft, are adjacent. Scale bar = 0.5 μm. ×45,900. (Byers MR, Neuhaus SJ, Gehrig JD: Dental sensory receptor structure in human teeth. Pain 13:221, 1982)

close to the pulp-dentin junction. Because of their proximity, it is tempting to hypothesize a close functional relationship between these associated cells and the odontoblastic process. However, synaptic junctions, which are essen-

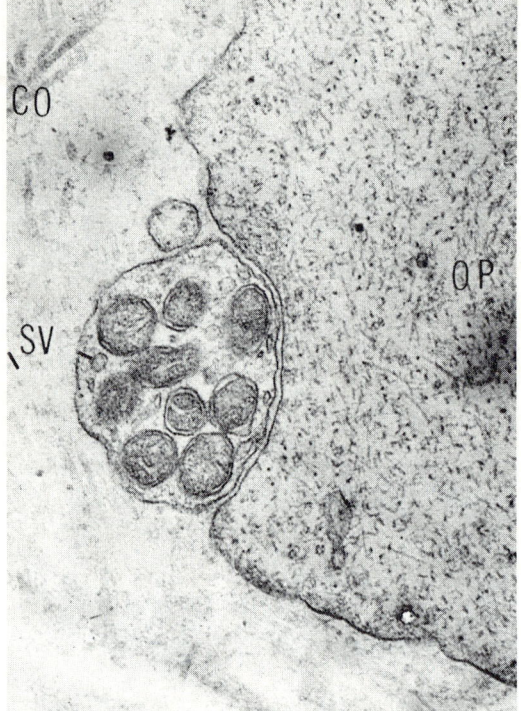

FIG. 6-15 Transverse section through an odontoblastic process (OP) in the predentin layer. A transverse section of an unmyelinated nerve fiber can be seen in close association to the process. The axoplasm contains numerous mitochondria and some synaptic-vesiclelike structures (SV). CO, noncalcified collagenous matrix of predentin. ×67,000. (Frank RM: Ultrastructure of human dentine. Third Europ Symp Calc Tiss 17:259, 1966)

tial for nerve conduction between the associated cells and odontoblastic process, have not been definitely found. Therefore, the histologic evidence for such structures is inconclusive.

Recording of Electrical Activity From Dental Nerve Fibers

Physiologic evidence supporting the theory is based on recordings of electrical activity from dentinal cavities of experimental animals (Scott and Tempel, 1965; Scott, 1966, 1968; Yamada, 1969; Matthews, 1970; Haegerstam, 1976a; Edwall and Scott, 1971; Olgart and Gazelius, 1977; Ahlberg, 1978). The recording procedures by Scott and Tempel (1965) were as follows: After cavity preparation, a recording electrode was placed in contact with the floor of the dentin cavity. Various stimuli, such as thermal changes, touch, and chemical agents, evoked electrical potentials. Scott and Tempel postulated that the electrical activity originated in single receptor units in the dentin and that a terminal segment of the afferent neuron was located among the odontoblast cells or distributed within the lumen of the dentinal tubule. Their results, supported somewhat by the findings of Mumford (1965), suggested that the dentin may contain separate receptors for heat, cold, and touch.

Investigations similar to those of Scott and Tempel (1965) and Scott and Stewart (1965) were conducted by Matthews (1970) on the canine teeth of cats. The results of those investigations cast doubt on the presumption that electrical activity recorded from dentin originates from receptor terminals in the dentin. Matthews found that the response to thermal stimulation recorded directly from an intact pulp was similar to that recorded from the overlying dentin. Furthermore, impulses could be recorded with an electrode placed on the floor of a cavity from electrically stimulated radial nerve fibers placed in the pulp chambers after the original pulps had been removed. Such findings indicated that recordings of electrical activity from the dentin do not necessarily originate from nerves in the dentin but probably originate from nerves in the pulp.

According to Haegerstam (1976b) and Lisney (1979), in most of the investigations mentioned above, the action potentials of fast-conducting nerves have been recorded. The types of nerve fibers that responded to dentin stimulation were not identified. Nähri et al (1982a) exposed and dissected the inferior alveolar nerve in dogs. The exposed dentin surface at the tip of the tooth crown was then stimulated both electrically and mechanically. The individual fibers that responded to electrical stimulation were thus identified. Subsequently, the pulp nerve units were tested by irritating the dentin by scraping with a probe, repeated air blasts, and applying dry, absorbent cotton and 4.9 mol/l $CaCl_2$ solution. They found that all of the responding units were fast conducting. On the other hand, Nähri et al (1982b) found that application of heat caused a dull, poorly localized pain, induced by activity in slowly conducting fibers. A considerable number of the slow conductors belong to the C-fiber group.

Few measurement studies of intradental sensory nerve activity in man have been reported. Edwall and Olgart (1977) used basically the same sensory recording technique as that used for cats. They applied various stimuli, such as cold, heat, and air blasts, to the dentin. The subjects' reactions were then measured in two ways: pinching the hand of the experimenter when pain was felt, and measuring the length of finger span. They found that nerve impulse activity evoked by the different stimuli was consistently associated with pain reaction. As the temperature of the tooth was raised, there was a concomitant increase both in sensory nerve activity and in finger span, indicating elicitation of pain (Fig. 6–16).

Thermal changes have been implicated in altering the response of nerves in or near the dentin. However, they have not been found to alter the reaction time of dentin uniformly. Naylor (1963) found the threshold temperature to cold stimulation of human dentin to be approximately 30°C. He later (1968) reported that the reaction time to thermal stimulation of dentin was lengthened by cutting the dentin with an uncooled bur. Such cutting caused damage to the odontoblasts.

Drugs, pressure, and osmotic changes have also been reported to alter dentinal pain responses. Topical application of aspirin to the dentin promptly inhibited both steady-state discharge and response to a brief heat stimulus (Scott, 1968). However, damaging drugs, such as silver nitrate, zinc chloride, and strontium chloride, did not reduce dentin sensitivity, according to Anderson (1963).

Pain-inducing substances such as potassium chloride, ACh, 5-hydroxytryptamine, and histamine, have consistently failed to evoke pain when applied to the dentin (Anderson, 1968, Brännström, 1962). Sugar solutions and calcium chloride solutions with osmotic pressures up to 2800 atmospheres did produce pain in dentin (Anderson et al. 1958; Anderson and Ronning, 1962). However, as Anderson has pointed out, the latter findings do not prove that a receptor mechanism is present in the dentin; instead, the nerves in the pulp may have been stimulated.

Transducer Mechanism

In effect, the postulation of the dentinal receptor mechanism carries the implication that the odontoblast has a special sensory function and that the odontoblastic process–nerve-ending junctional complex in or near the odontoblastic layer functions as an excitatory synapse. Furthermore, it implies that a mechanism similar to

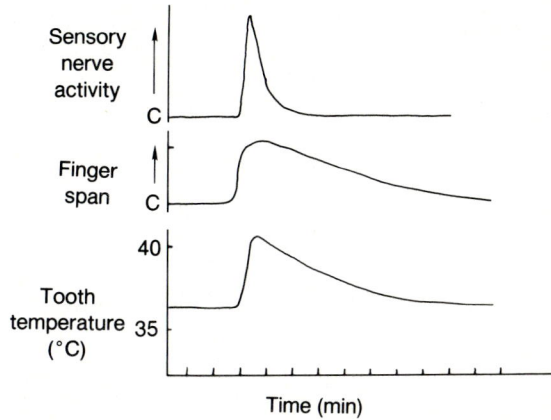

FIG. 6–16 An idealized diagram of a typical experiment with a human in response to warming the teeth. Sensory nerve activity and finger span were simultaneously recorded. (Courtesy of Dr. L. Edwall, Stockholm, Sweden)

the inhibitory synapse found in other nerve cells must be present.

Frank (1969) estimated that a cavity preparation of 1 mm² would involve about 60,000 dentinal tubules. Should there be one nerve fiber for each 2000 dentinal tubules, at least 30 nerve endings would be stimulated; if there were one nerve fiber for each 200 tubules, 300 nerve endings would be irritated in a cavity preparation 1 mm².

The numbers of innervated dentinal tubules in human teeth may actually be much greater. Byers et al (1982) found frequent "clusters" of coronal dentin with innervation in three to ten adjacent tubules (Fig. 6–17).

Frank concluded that the intradentinal receptor presents a unique type of neurosensitive complex in which intimate connections exist between the odontoblast process and a sensory fiber.

The odontoblast and its process has been perceived as a transducer mechanism. Rapp and co-workers (1968) believed that the transformation of the action potential into a chemical message could be inferred from the demonstration of acetylcholinesterase activity in the dentin.

Cholinergic Nerves in Dentin

ACH and acetylcholinesterase (AChE) play an essential role in the transmission of nerve impulses. Both substances are present in all cholinergic neurons (Tewari and Bourne, 1960).

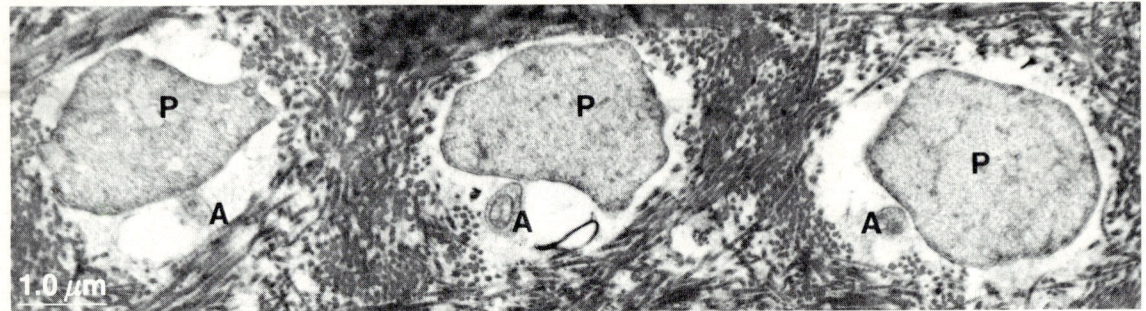

FIG. 6-17 A cluster of adjacent dentinal tubules at the predentin-dentin border. Each tubule contains an axon (A) and an odontoblast process (P). Decalcified sample. ×10,350 (Byers MR, Neuhaus SJ, Gehrig JD: Dental sensory receptor structure in human teeth. Pain 13:221, 1982)

On stimulation of the nerves, ACh is released from an inactive, bound form and is rapidly converted to less active free choline and acetate by the enzyme AChE. AChE terminates the passage of nerve impulses by its inactivation of ACh. Thus, the localization of AChE in tissue indicates the presence of ACh (Koelle, 1962).

The presence of AChE has been demonstrated in the dentin and pulp of human teeth by histochemical (Avery and Rapp, 1959), microdiver and radiometric (Pavlin and Vidmar, 1979), and electrophoretic (Rapp et al, 1968) techniques.

In the pulp and odontoblasts, cholinesterase was found by Rapp and Avery (1967), Arwill and Lilja (1971), and Pavlin and Vidmar (1979). According to Avery (1981), the presence of cholinergic nerves in the pulp may indicate either a sensory (post-ganglionic) or a parasympathetic function, or both. In the dentin, AChE staining has been found throughout the length of the odontoblastic processes and their branches and in the predentin (Rapp et al, 1968).

However, Ten Cate and Shelton (1966) and Pohto and Antila (1968b), found no cholinergic activity in the odontoblasts or their processes.

Adrenergic Nerves in Dentin

Although dentin innervation is almost entirely sensory, some adrenergic nerve endings have been found in the walls of the pulpal blood vessels (Nakano et al, 1970; Larsson and Linde, 1971; Pohto and Antila, 1972) and in the odontoblastic layer and the predentin (Avery, 1975).

HYDRODYNAMIC THEORY

Brannström (1963) hypothesized that dentin pain and odontoblastic displacement were related. Injury to the odontoblasts (e.g., by cavity preparation, pressure, or thermal changes) caused displacement of the contents of the dentinal tubules. The intimate relationship of the odontoblasts with nerve fibers at the pulpodentinal border would result in mechanical stimulation of those fibers. Subsequently, Brännström and Åström (1964) found that pain was elicited when freshly exposed dentin was touched with a dry, absorbent paper point. When dentin was exposed to saliva for 1 week, however, it was no longer sensitive to absorbent paper, although scraping with a probe still evoked pain. They concluded that the odontoblasts, which had degenerated, had little or nothing to do with the transmission of pain stimuli through the dentin, an observation previously made by Kramer (1955). Kramer had been unable to find a correlation between displacement of odontoblasts after cavity preparation and cavity filling and pain.

Brännström and co-workers (1966, 1967, 1969, 1972) and Lilja (1980) have postulated a hydrodynamic mechanism underlying dentin sensitivity. The dentinal pulp fluid expands and contracts in response to the application of stimuli. Inasmuch as the fluids have a coefficient of expansion greater than that of solid dentin, the contents of the dentinal tubules move pulpward or externally in response to a given stimulus. A rapid outward flow of dentinal pulp fluid by capillary attraction occurs through exposed dentinal tubule apertures. Thus, thermal stimuli, scraping, drilling, and sugar applications all cause outward movement of dentinal fluid. The fluid movement stimulates the nerves in the pulp (Trowbridge et al, 1980; Nähri et al, 1982a). Although it is difficult to understand why minor pressure such as probing on the dentin causes pain, the force exerted on dentin by light pressure from an explorer may be high. Thus, compression of fluid or mechanical distortion of tubule orifices by a probe tip can cause fluid displacement and pulpal sensory nerve excitation.

Acid etching of dentin, which opens dentinal tubules, is also capable of increasing fluid flow, resulting in increased dentin sensitivity (Brännström et al, 1979; Lilja, 1980). Greenhill and Pashley (1981) found that fluid flow from citric acid-treated dentin disks was reduced by treatment with various clinical desensitizing agents. According to Pashley et al (1982), the fluid flow in the dentinal tubules may be reduced, consequently lessening dentinal sensitivity, by several possible mechanisms: (1) occlusion of the tubules by large numbers of bacteria from plaque or saliva, (2) mineralized deposits within the dentinal tubules from exposure of dentin to saliva, and (3) adsorption of salivary or plasma proteins onto the dentinal tubules. Pashley et al found that treating dentin disks with plasma caused a large decrease in hydraulic conductance. Less dramatic results were obtained with serum (plasma less platelets and fibrinogen).

Impregnation of the dentin surface with resin has also been found to abolish dentinal hypersensitivity (Brännström et al, 1979; Nordenvall and Brännström, 1980; Nähri et al, 1982a).

Some confirmation of the hydrodynamic hypothesis may be found in the investigations of Mumford and Newton (1969) and Horiuchi and Matthews (1973). The application of hydrostatic pressure to the dentin of freshly extracted human teeth resulted in an electric potential across the dentin. The development of these electric potentials could excite sensory receptors in the pulp, according to Mumford and Newton. However, the experiments of Greenwood et al (1972) raise doubts that the current flowing through dentin would be sufficient to excite nerve receptors.

According to Matthews (1977), heat stimulation in the form of hot saline solution applied to dentin activates pulp axons. Thus, as Horiuchi and Matthews (1973) and Anderson et al (1970) have pointed out, although fluid flow through dentin can cause pain, some stimuli may cause pain by other mechanisms.

Pulpal Tissue Pressure and Pain

Heating of the tooth and pulpitis cause tissue pressure to increase significantly. Conversely, cold causes the intrapulpal pressure to drop (Beveridge and Brown, 1965; Van Hassel and Brown, 1969; Stenvik et al, 1972). The pulsation of the heart beat and the throbbing of a toothache have been found to be synchronized (Mumford, 1976). These findings suggest that there is a close relationship between the changes in blood flow, pulpal tissue pressure, and dental pain. Following pulpitis, changes in pulpal tissue pressure are a local phenomenon (Van Hassel, 1971; Nähri, 1978; Tønder and Kvinnsland, 1983). Why then does the pressure change cause pain? Nähri (1978) found that elevated hydrostatic pressure activated the pulp nerve fibers. Furthermore, in some of the recorded pulp nerve fibers, suction stimulation caused nerve activation, similar to that produced by pressure elevation. Such studies strongly support the hypothesis that the deformation of the tissue, caused by the local pressure differences, is responsible for the activation of the sensory nerve fibers; the tissue pressure change in itself is not the cause. Thus, the conclusion that the pulp is a mechanoreceptor for the transmission of pain seems reasonable.

MODULATION OF NERVE IMPULSES BY POLYPEPTIDES OR OTHER NEUROTRANSMITTERS

A number of polypeptides have been implicated as regulators of neural transmission. Of these, plasma kinins (kallidins or bradykinins) and substance P have been postulated by Kroeger (1968) as modulators of nerve impulses in the pulp.

Plasma kinins are polypeptides having vasopressor activity; they are formed from the interaction of certain enzymes of body secretions (kallikreins) with certain plasma proteins that are related to the blood-clotting and clot-lysis mechanisms. Kallikreins may be of glandular or of plasma origin. Plasma kinins, when applied to dentin, fail to produce pain (Anderson and Naylor, 1962).

Substance P is an undecapeptide similar to the plasma kinins but differing in physiologic activities.

Kroeger postulated that plasma kinins and substance P selectively alter the permeability of the odontoblastic cell membrane and that the pulp neurons are more prone to fire upon receipt of subsequent stimuli. He believed that plasma kinins were formed in the pulp when kallikreins, released as a result of nerve stimulation, acted on interstitial fluid (lymph or plasma). Under normal circumstances, pulp tissue contains enzymes capable of inactivating plasma kinins. Substance P, present in a preformed but bound state in certain peripheral nerves, is also released upon the arrival of nerve impulses (Brodin et al, 1981a). Numerous small axons, immunoreactive to substance P, have been found in the teeth of the dog, the cat, and man by Olgart et al (1977) and Brodin et al (1981b). The dental pulp appeared to be one of the SP-richest organs outside the central nervous system. These axons were found along blood vessels throughout the pulp and most appeared to terminate in the plexus of Raschkow. Substance P causes vasodilation and increases capillary permeability, which according to Pashley et al (1982) would permit increased concentrations of plasma proteins to leak into the dentinal fluid. Pashley et al hypothesized that blockage of the dentinal tubules by the proteins could account for decreasing dentin sensitivity.

Prostaglandins (PGs) are chemical mediators synthesized from long-chain C_{20} polyunsaturated fatty acids, such as arachidonic acid. They are potent inflammatory agents. Rat pulp tissue contains an appreciable amount of prostaglandins (Hirafuji et al, 1980). In uninflamed rat dental pulp, the production of prostaglandin E_2 is possibly stimulated by serotonin, which can increase the availability of free arachidonic acid from cellular phospholipid stores (Hirafuji et al, 1982). The prostaglandins sensitize the pain receptors to stimulation by histamine, bradykinin, substance P, and other pain mediators.

Other neurotransmitters, including **histamine** (Olgart, 1974), **serotonin** (Olgart, 1979), and **vasoactive intestinal peptide** (Olgart et al, 1981) have been detected in the dental pulp and may have an effect on dentin sensitivity. Thus, the polypeptides may act as modulators, not as transmitters, of nerve impulses in the pulp.

BIBLIOGRAPHY

Ahlberg KF: Influence of local noxious heat stimulation on sensory nerve activity in feline dental pulp. Acta Physiol Scand 103:71, 1978
Anderson DJ (ed): Sensory mechanisms in dentine: Proceedings of A Symposium Held at the Royal Society of Medicine, London, September 24th, 1962. New York, Macmillan, 1963
Anderson DJ: The pulp as a sensory organ. In Finn SB (ed): Biology of the Dental Pulp Organ, pp 273–280. Birmingham, University of Alabama Press, 1968
Anderson DJ, Curwen MP, Howard LV: The sensitivity of human dentin. J Dent Res 37:669, 1958
Anderson DJ, Hannam AG, Matthews B: Sensory mechanisms in mammalian teeth and their supporting structures. Physiol Rev 50:171, 1970
Anderson DJ, Matthews B: An investigation into the reputed desensitizing effect of applying silver nitrate and strontium chloride to human dentine. Arch Oral Biol 11:1129, 1966
Anderson DJ, Naylor MN: Chemical excitants of pain in human dentine and dental pulp. Arch Oral Biol 7:413, 1962
Anderson DJ, Ronning GA: Dye diffusion in human dentine. Arch Oral Biol 7:505, 1962a
Anderson DJ, Ronning GA: Osmotic excitants of pain in human dentine. Arch Oral Biol 7:513, 1962b
Anderson KV, Pearl GS: Transmedian innervation of canine tooth pulp in cat. Exp Neurol 44:35, 1974
Armstrong D, Dry R, Keele C, Markham J: Observations on chemical excitations of cutaneous pain in man. J Physiol 120:326, 1953
Arwill T: Some morphological aspects of the dentinal innervation. In Anderson DJ (ed): Sensory Mechanisms in Dentine, pp 3–14. Oxford, Pergamon Press, 1963
Arwill T: Studies on the ultrastructure of dental tissues. II. The predentine pulpal border zone. Odont Rev 18:191, 1967
Arwill T: The ultrastructure of the pulpo-dentinal border zone. In Symons NBB (ed): Dentine and Pulp, pp 147–167. Baltimore, Williams and Wilkins, 1968
Arwill T, Lilja J: Ultrastructural localization of cholinesterase activity in the dental pulp. In Emelin N, Zotterman Y (eds). Oral Physiology, Procedures of International Symposium. Stockholm, Pergamon Press, 1971
Avery JK: Repair potential of the pulp. J Endodont 7:205, 1981
Avery JK: A possible mechanism of pain conduction in teeth. Ann Histochim 8:59, 1963
Avery JK: Response of the pulp and dentin to contact with filling materials. J Dent Res 54 (Special Issue B):188, 1975
Avery JK, Rapp R: An investigation of the mechanism of neural impulse transmission in human teeth. Oral Surg 12:190, 1959
Avery JK, Rapp R: Pain conduction in human dental tissues. In Agnew RG (ed): Problems of Oral and Facial Pain, pp 489–500. Dent Clin North Am. Philadelphia, WB Saunders, 1959
Barker JL, Levitan H: Salicylate: Effect on membrane permeability of molluscan neurons. Science 172:1245, 1971
Beasley WL, Holland GR: A quantitative analysis of the innervation of the pulp of the cat's canine tooth. J Comp Neurol 178:487, 1978
Bernick S: Innervation of the human tooth. Anat Rec 101:81, 1948
Bernick S: Innervation of the teeth and periodontium of the rat. Anat Rec 125:185, 1957
Bernick S: Innervation of teeth and periodontium after enzymatic removal of collagenous elements. Oral Surg 10:323, 1957
Bernick S: Innervation of the teeth and periodontium. In Agnew RG (ed): Problems of Oral and Facial Pain, pp 503–513. Dent Clin North Am. Philadelphia, WB Saunders, 1959

Bernick S: Differences in nerve distribution between erupted and non-erupted human teeth. J Dent Res 43:406, 1964
Blaustein MP: Preganglionic stimulation increases calcium uptake by sympathetic ganglia. Science 172:391, 1971
Bock O: Über die innervation des dentins. Deutsch Zahnärztl 15:838, 889, 1960
Brännström M: Dentinal and pulpal response. I. Application of reduced pressure to exposed dentine. II. Application of an air stream to exposed dentine. Acta Odont Scand 18:1, 17, 1960
Brännström M: Dentinal and pulpal response. V. Application of pressure to exposed dentin. J Dent Res 40:960, 1961
Brännström M: Dentin sensitivity and aspiration of odontoblasts. JADA 66:366, 1963
Brännström M: The elicitation of pain in human dentine and pulp by chemical stimuli. Arch Oral Biol 7:59, 1962
Brännström M: A hydrodynamic mechanism in the transmission of pain-producing stimuli through the dentine. In Anderson DJ (ed) Sensory Mechanisms in Dentine, p 73. Oxford, Pergamon Press, 1963
Brännström M: The hydrodynamics of the dentine; its possible relationship to dentinal pain. Internat Dent J 22:219, 1972
Brännström M: Physiopathological aspects of dentinal and pulpal response to irritants. In Symons NBB (ed) Dentine and Pulp: their Structure and Reactions, p 231. London, Livingstone, 1968
Brännström M: Sensitivity of dentine. Oral Surg 21:517, 1966
Brännström M, Åström A: A study of the mechanism of pain elicited from the dentin. J Dent Res 43:619, 1964
Brännström M, Johnson G, Linden LÅ: Fluid flow and pain response in the dentin produced by hydrostatic pressure. Odont Rev 20:15, 1969
Brännström M, Johnson G, Nordenvall K-J: Transmission control of dentinal pain: resin impregnation for the desensitization of dentin. JADA 99:612, 1979
Brännström M, Linden LÅ, Åström A: The hydrodynamics of the dental tubule and of pulp fluid; a discussion of its significance in relation to dentinal sensitivity. Caries Res 1:310, 1967
Brashear AD: Innervation of teeth. JADA 23:662, 1936
Brodin E, Gazelius B, Lundberg JM, Olgart L: Substance P in trigeminal nerve endings. Occurrence and release. Acta Physiol Scand 111:501, 1981a
Brodin E, Gazelius B, Olgart L, Nilsson G: Tissue concentration of substance P-like immunoreactivity in the dental pulp. Acta Physiol Scand 111:141, 1981
Byers MR: The development of sensory innervation in dentin. J Comp Neurol 191:413, 1980
Byers MR: Fine structure of trigeminal receptors in rat molars. In Anderson DJ, Matthews B (eds): Pain in the Trigeminal Region, pp 13–24. Elsevier/North Holland Biomedical Press, 1977
Byers MR: Large and small trigeminal nerve endings and their associations with odontoblasts in rat molar dentin and pulp. In: Bonica JJ (ed) Advances in Pain Research and Therapy, Vol 3, pp 265–270, New York, Raven Press, 1979
Byers MR, Dong WK: Autoradiographic location of sensory nerve endings in dentin of monkey teeth. Anat Rec 205:441, 1983
Byers MR, Kish SJ: Delineation of somatic nerve endings in rat teeth by radioautography of axon-transported protein. J Dent Res 55:419, 1976
Byers MR, Matthews B: Autoradiographic demonstration of ipsilateral and contralateral sensory nerve endings in cat dentin, pulp, and periodontium. Anat Rec 201:249, 1981
Byers MR, Neuhaus SJ, Gehrig JD: Dental sensory receptor structure in human teeth. Pain 13:221, 1982
Chiego DJ, Bradley BE, Cox CF, Avery JK: Anterograde axoplasmic transport of H3-leucine after injection into the mesencephalic nucleus of the trigeminal nerve. Anat Rec 193:504, 1979
Chiego DJ, Cox CF, Avery JK: H^3-HRP analysis of the nerve supply of primate teeth. J Dent Res 59:736, 1980
Corpron RE, Avery JK: The ultrastructure of intradentinal nerves in developing mouse molars. Anat Rec 175:585, 1973
DeRobertis E: Molecular biology of synaptic receptors. Science 171:963, 1971
Droz B, Leblond CP: Axonal migration of proteins in the central nervous system and peripheral nerves as shown by radioautography. J Comp Neurol 121:325, 1963
Eccles J: The synapse. Sci Am 212:56, 1965
Edwall L, Olgart L: A new technique for recording of intradental sensory nerve activity in man. Pain 3:121, 1977
Edwall L, Scott D, Jr: Influence of changes in microcirculation on the excitability on the sensory unit in the tooth of the cat. Acta Physiol Scand 31:289, 1971
Engström H, Öhman A: Studies on the innervation of human teeth. J Dent Res 39:799, 1960
Fearnhead RW: The histological demonstration of nerve fibres in human dentine. In Anderson DJ (ed): Sensory Mechanisms in Dentin, pp 15–26. Oxford, Pergamon Press, 1963
Fearnhead RW: Innervation of dental tissues. In Miles AEW (ed): Structural and Chemical Organization of Teeth, Vol I, pp 247–281. New York, Academic Press, 1968
Fink BR, Kish SJ, Byers M: Rapid axonal transport in trigeminal nerve of rat. Brain Res 90:85, 1975
Frank RM: Étude au microscope électronique de l'odontoblaste et du canaliculé dentaire humain. Arch Oral Biol 11:179, 1966
Frank RM: Attachment sites between the odontoblast process and the intradentinal nerve fiber. Arch Oral Biol 13:833, 1968
Frank RM: Ultrastructural relationship between the odontoblast, its process and the nerve fibre. In Symons NBB (ed): Dentine and Pulp: Their Structure and Reactions, pp 115–145. London E & S Livingstone, 1968
Frank RM: Dentinal sclerosis and ultrastructural basis of dentinal sensitivity. Paradont 1:11, 1969
Furstman L, Saporta S, Kruger L: Retrograde axonal transport of horseradish peroxidase in sensory nerves and ganglion cells of the rat. Brain Res 84:320, 1975
Gasser HS: Les Prix Nobel en 1940–1944, p 128. Stockholm, PE Norstedt, 1946
Graf W, Björlin G: Diameters of nerve fibers in human tooth pulps. JADA 43:186, 1951
Gray EG, Guillery RW: Synaptic morphology in the nor-

mal and degenerating nervous system. In Bourne GH, Danielli JF (eds): International Review of Cytology, pp 111–182. New York, Academic Press, 1966

Greenhill JD, Pashley DH: The effects of desensitizing agents on the hydraulic conductance of human dentin in vitro. J Dent Res 60:686, 1981

Greenwood LF, Horiuchi H, Matthews B: Electrophysiological evidence on the types of nerve fibers excited by electrical stimulation of teeth with a pulp tester. Arch Oral Biol 17:701, 1972

Haegerstam G: The effect of veratrine and aconite on the excitability of sensory units in the tooth of the cat. Acta Physiol Scand 98:1, 1976a

Haegerstam G: The origin of impulses recorded from dentinal cavities in the tooth of the cat. Acta Physiol Scand 97:121, 1976b

Held AJ, Baud CA: The innervation of the dental organ. Oral Surg 18:1262, 1955

Hirafuji M, Satoh S, and Ogura Y: Prostaglandins in rat pulp tissue. J Dent Res 59:1535, 1980

Hirafugi M, Terashima K, Satoh S, Ogura Y; Stimulation of prostaglandin E_2 biosynthesis in rat dental pulp explants *in vitro* by 5-hydroxytryptamine. Arch Oral Biol 27:961, 1982

Holland GR: Lanthanum hydroxide labelling of gap junctions in the odontoblast layer. Ant Rec 186:121, 1976

Holland GR: Membrane junctions on cat odontoblasts. Arch Oral Biol 20:551, 1975

Holland GR: Microtubule and microfilament populations of cell processes in the dental pulp. Anat Rec 198:421, 1980

Holland GR: Structural relationships in the odontoblast layer. In Anderson DJ, Mathews B (eds): Pain in the Trigeminal Region, pp 25–35. Elsevier/North-Holland Biomedical Press, 1977

Horiuchi H, Matthews B: In-vitro observations on fluid flow through human dentine caused by pain-producing stimuli. Arch Oral Biol 18:275, 1973

Johnsen D, Johns S: Quantitation of nerve fibers in the primary and permanent canine and incisor teeth in man. Arch Oral Biol 23:825, 1978

Katz B: Quantal mechanism of neural transmitter release. Science 173:123, 1971

Kandel ER: Nerve cells and behavior. Sci Am 223:57, 1970

Kim S: Regulation of blood flow of the dental pulp of dogs: Macrocirculation and microcirculation studies. Thesis, Columbia University, 1981

Koelle GB: A new general concept of the neurohumoral functions of acetylcholine and acetylcholinesterase. J Pharm Pharmacol 14:65, 1962

Korn ED: Structure of biological membranes. Science 153:1491, 1966

Kramer IRH: Relationship between dentine sensitivity and movements in contents of the dentinal tubules. Brit Dent J 98:391, 1955

Kroeger DC: Possible role of neurohumoral substances in the pulp. In Finn SB (ed): Biology of the Dental Pulp Organ: A Symposium, pp 334–346. Birmingham, University of Alabama Press, 1968

Langeland K, Yagi T: Investigations on the innervation of teeth. Int Dent J 22:240, 1972

Larrson P-A, Linde A: Adrenergic vessel innervation in the rat incisor pulp. Scand J Dent Res, 79:7, 1971

LaVail JH, LaVail MM: Retrograde axonal transport in the central nervous system. Science 176:1416, 1972

LaVail JH, Winston KR, Tish A: A method based on retrograde intraaxonal transport of protein for identification of cell bodies of origin of axons terminating within the CNS. Brain Res 58:470, 1973

Lilja J, Nordenvall KJ, and Brännström M: Dentine sensitivity, odontoblasts and nerves under dessicated or infected experimental cavities. Swed Dent J, 6:93, 1982

Lisney SJW: Evidence for primary afferent depolarization of single tooth-pulp afferents in the cat. J Physiol 288:437, 1979

McGeer PL: The chemistry of mind. Am Scientist 59:221, 1971

Maderio MC, Percinoto C, Silva MG: Clinical significance of supplementary innervation of the lower incisor teeth: A dissection study of the mylohyoid nerve. Oral Surg 46:608, 1978

Matthews B: Nerve impulses recorded from dentine in the cat. Arch Oral Biol 15:523, 1970

Matthews B: Responses of intradental nerves to electrical and thermal stimulation of teeth in dogs. J Physiol 264:641, 1979

Matthews B, Holland GR: Coupling between nerves in teeth. Brain Res 98:354, 1975

Matthews JL, Dorman HL, Bishop JC: Fine structures of the dental pulp. J Dent Res 38:940, 1959

Menke RA: An autoradiographic demonstration of trigeminal nerve terminations in the tooth. Master's thesis, Loyola University, 1973

Miyoshi S, Nishijima S, Imanishi I: Electron microscopy of myelinated and unmyelinated nerve fibers in human dental pulp. Arch Oral Biol 11:845, 1966

Mumford JM: Pain perception threshold and adaptation of normal human teeth. Arch Oral Biol 10:957, 1965

Mumford JM: Toothache and Orofacial Pain. Edinburgh, Churchill-Livingstone, 1976

Mumford JM, Newton AV: Transduction of hydrostatic pressure to electric potential in human dentin. J Dent Res 48:226, 1969

Mummery JH: The Microscopic Anatomy of the Teeth, p 212. London, Oxford University Press, 1919

Nachmansohn D: Transmission of nervous influx in central nervous system; presence of cholinesterase and role of acetylcholine. C R Soc Biol 126:783, 1937

Nachmansohn D: Cholinesterase in nerve fibers. C R Soc Biol 128:516, 1938

Nachmansohn D: Cholinesterase in tissue of nervous system. C R Soc Biol 127:894, 1938

Nachmansohn D: Chemical mechanism of nerve activity. Ann NY Acad Sci 47:395, 1946

Nachmansohn D: Role of acetylcholine in conduction. Bull John Hopkins Hosp 83:463, 1948

Nähri M: Activation of dental pulp nerves of the cat and the dog with hydrostatic pressure. Proceedings of the Finnish Dental Society 74:Suppl V, 1978

Nähri M, Jyväsjärvi E, Hirvonen T, Huopaniemi T: Activation of heat-sensitive nerve fibers in the dental pulp of the cat. Pain 14:317, 1982b

Nähri M, Virtanen A, Huopaniemi T, Hirvonen T: Conduction velocities of single pulp nerve fibre units in the cat. Acta Physiol Scand 116:209, 1982

Nähri MVO, Hirvonen TJ, Hakumäki MOK: Activation of

intradental nerves in the dog to some stimuli applied to the dentine. Arch Oral Biol 27:1053, 1982a

Naylor MN: Studies on the mechanism of sensation to cold stimulation of human dentine. In Anderson, DJ (ed): Sensory Mechanisms in Dentine, pp 80–87. Oxford, Pergamon Press, 1963

Naylor MN: The effect of silver nitrate and the uncooled high-speed bur on dentine sensitivity. In Symons, NBB (ed): Dentine and Pulp, pp 247–253. Baltimore, Williams & Wilkins, 1968

Nakano G, Kuzuya H, and Nagatsu T: Catecholamines in the dental pulp. J Dent Res, 49:1549, 1970

Nordenvall K-J, Brännström M: In vivo resin impregnation of dentinal tubules. J Prosth Dent 44:630, 1980

Ogilvie RW, Gillilan LA, Knapp DE: Physiologic evidence for the presence of vasoconstrictor fibers in the dental pulp. J Dent Res 45:979, 1966

Olgart L: Excitation of intradental sensory units by pharmacological agents. Acta Physiol Scand 92:48, 1974

Olgart L: Local mechanisms in dental pain. In Beers RF, Jr, Bassett EG (eds). Mechanisms of Pain and Analgesia Compounds, pp 285–294. New York, Raven Press, 1979

Olgart L, Gazelius B: Effects of adrenaline and felypressin (octapressin) on blood flow and sensory nerve activity in the tooth. Acta Odont Scand 35:69, 1977

Olgart L, Hökfelt T, Nilsson, G, Pernow B: Localization of substance P-like immunoreactivity in nerves of the tooth pulp. Pain 4:153, 1977

Olgart L, Lundberg JM, Gazelius B: Localization and vasodilator effects of substance P (SP) and vasoactive intestinal polypeptide (VIP) in the cat dental pulp. J Dent Res 60(B) Abstr 68:1260, 1981

Pashley DH, Nelson R, Kepler EE: The effects of plasma and salivary constituents on dentin permeability. J Dent Res 61:978, 1982

Pavlin R, Vidmar V: Cholinesterases and choline acetylase in isolated human and rat odontoblasts. Arch Oral Biol 24:217, 1979

Pimenidis MZ, Hinds JW: An autoradiographic study of the sensory innervation of the teeth. II. Dental pulp and periodontium. J Dent Res 566:835, 1977

Pohto P, Antila R: Demonstration of adrenergic nerve fibres in human dental pulp by histochemical fluorescence method. Acta Odont Scand 26:137, 1968a

Pohto P, Antila R: Acetylcholinesterase and noradrenaline in the nerves of mammalian dental pulps. Acta Odont Scand 26:641, 1968b

Pohto P, Antila R: Innervation of blood vessels in the dental pulp. Int Dent J, 22:228, 1972

Provenza DV: Comparative morphology of the pulp vascular system. In Finn SB (ed): Biology of the Dental Pulp Organ: A Symposium, pp 353–363. Birmingham, University of Alabama Press, 1968

Rapp R, Avery JK, Rector R: A study of the distribution of nerves in human teeth. J Canad D A 23:447, 1957

Rapp R, Avery JK, Strachan DS: The distribution of nerves in human primary teeth. Anat Rec 159:89, 1967

Rapp R, Avery JK, Strachan DS: Possible role of acetylcholinesterase in neural conduction within the dental pulp. In Finn SB (ed): Biology of the Dental Pulp Organ: A Symposium. pp 309–325. Birmingham, University of Alabama Press, 1968

Roane JB, Foreman DW, Melfi RC, Marshall FJ: An ultrastructural study of dentinal innervation in the adult human tooth. Oral Surg 35:94, 1973

Ruch TC, Patton HD, Woodbury JW, Towe AL: Neurophysiology, 2nd ed, p 47. Philadelphia, WB Saunders, 1965

Scott D, Jr: Excitation of the dentinal receptor in the tooth of the cat. In DeReuek AVS, Knight J (ed): Clba Foundation Exposium on Touch, Heat and Pain, pp 261–273. London, J&A Churchill, 1966

Scott D, Jr: Aspirin: action on receptor in the tooth. Science 161:180, 1968

Scott D, Jr, Stewart GG: Excitation of the dentinal receptor of the cat by heat and chemical agents. Oral Surg 20:784, 1965

Scott D, Jr, Tempel TR: A study in the excitation of dental pulp nerve fibres. In Anderson DJ (ed): Sensory Mechanisms in Dentine, p 27. Oxford, Pergamon Press, 1963

Scott D, Jr, Tempel TR: Neurophysiological response of single receptor units in the tooth of the cat. J Dent Res 44:20, 1965

Seltzer S: Hypothetic mechanisms for dentine sensitivity. Oral Surg 31:388, 1971

Stenvik A, Iverson J, Mjör IA: Tissue pressure and histology of normal and inflamed tooth pulps in macaque monkeys. Arch Oral Biol 17:1501, 1972

Ten Cate AR, Shelton L: Cholinesterase activity in human teeth. Arch Oral Biol 11:423, 1966

Tewari HB, Bourne GH: Histochemical localization of specific and nonspecific cholinesterases and simple esterases in myelinated nerves. Exp Cell Res 21:245, 1960

Thomas HF, and Payne RC: The ultrastructure of dentinal tubules from erupted human premolar teeth. J Dent Res 62:532, 1983

Tidmarsh BG: Contents of human dentinal tubules. Int Endo J 14:191, 1981

Tiegs DW: Further remarks on the terminations of the fibers in human teeth. J Anat 72:234, 1938

Tønder KH, Kvinnsland I: Micropuncture measurements of interstitial fluid pressure in normal and inflamed dental pulp in cats. J Endodont 9:105, 1983

Trowbridge HO, Franks M, Korostoff E, Emling R: Sensory response to thermal stimulation in human teeth. J Endodont 6:405, 1980

Van Hassel HJ: Physiology of the human dental pulp. Oral Surg 32:126, 1971

Van Hassel HJ, Brown AC: Effect of temperature changes on intrapulpal pressure and hydraulic permeability in dogs. Arch Oral Biol 14:301, 1969

Winter HF, Bishop JG, Dorman HL: Transmembrane potentials of odontoblasts. J Dent Res 42:594, 1963

Yamada M: Recording of nerve potential. Internat Dent J 19:239, 1969

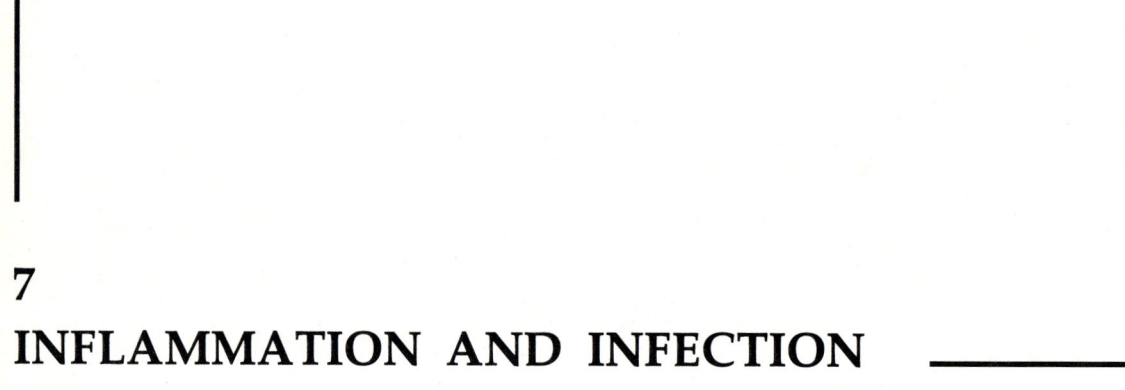

7
INFLAMMATION AND INFECTION

Inflammation involves complex vascular and lymphatic reactions, as well as local tissue reactions. It is the tissues' reaction to injury as well as its mechanism for repair. All of the components of the connective tissue—cells, fibers, and ground substance—are involved and are affected by the products that are liberated during the process of inflammation.

The inflammatory response ranges from a simple, transient increase in capillary permeability to severe tissue breakdown and necrosis. Recent observations indicate that various types of inflammatory reactions are caused by different mechanisms, many of which are exceedingly complex. For convenience, inflammation is described under two general headings—acute and chronic.

ACUTE INFLAMMATION

MORPHOLOGIC AND PHYSIOLOGIC CHANGES

The morphologic and physiologic changes that take place during the process of inflammation can be illustrated by scratching one's forearm with a fingernail. Shortly, a number of alterations can be seen. First, there is a blanching of the scratched surface. Then a red streak appears.

Inasmuch as tissue was injured by the rubbing of the epithelium, the observed phenomena are an indication of the initiation of an inflammatory process. Initially, there was a contraction of the blood vessels, resulting in the blanching. Soon afterward, the redness occurred because the blood vessels dilated. A series of further changes takes place, depending on the severity of the injury. There is a slowing of the bloodstream in this area. Eventually, if the inflammation is severe, stasis results, with clumping of the red blood cells within the blood vessels (Fig. 7–1).

Changes in the Endothelial Lining. The endothelial lining of the vessels begins to undergo certain changes. The endothelial cells swell, and the lining becomes leaky.

Various substances, called chemical mediators, are responsible for the leakiness of the vascular endothelium and for other inflammatory events, such as chemotaxis, described below. The chemical mediators involved in increasing capillary permeability are derived either from cells or from plasma.

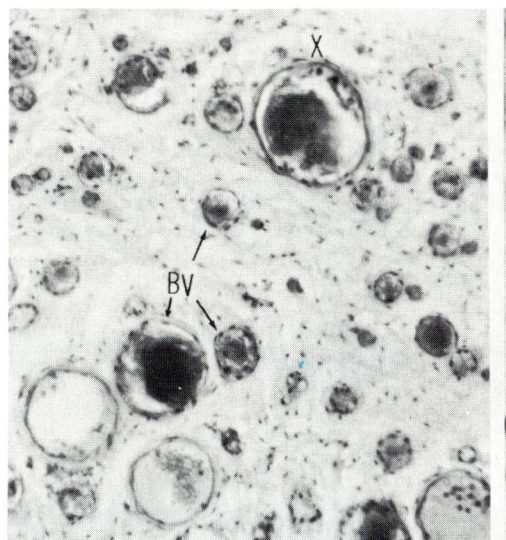
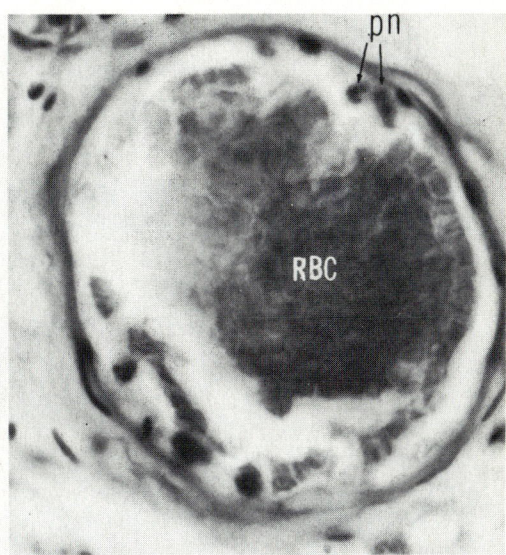

FIG. 7-1 Stasis. *(Left)* Dilated blood vessels (BV), packed with red blood cells. ×240. *(Right)* Higher magnification of blood vessel X in micrograph at left, showing clumping of red blood cells (RBC). Polymorphonuclear leukocytes (pn) are marginating. ×240.

Cell Mediators

The cellular substances include histamine, serotonin (5-hydroxytryptamine; 5-HT), prostaglandins, leukotrienes, various lysosomal components, and some lymphocyte products called lymphokines.

Histamine is normally stored in the granules of mast cells, basophils, and platelets and in the parietal region of the stomach. Physical injury, certain chemical agents, and antigenic challenges of immunoglobulin E (IgE)–sensitized cells cause the release of histamine into the tissues (Fig. 7-2). The histamine acts directly on the local blood vessels, causing an increase in permeability.

5-HT is normally found in the mucosa of the gut, in the brain, and in platelets. When released in tissue as a result of inflammation, 5-HT, like histamine, causes contraction of smooth muscle and increased vascular permeability. Neither histamine nor 5-HT has a chemotactic effect on leukocytes.

Two important groups of potent biologic mediators are synthesized in several kinds of leukocytes: prostaglandins and leukotrienes.

Prostaglandins (PGs) and related biologically active substances are potent chemical transmitters of inter- and intracellular signals that mediate numerous processes in the human body (Pike, 1971). They are derived from arachidonic acid, a 20-carbon polyunsaturated fatty acid in the cell membrane. The enzyme phospholipase breaks down the phospholipid molecules of the disrupted cell membrane to form arachidonic acid. The enzyme cyclooxygenase converts arachidonic acid into two cyclic endoperoxides, G_2 and H_2. These, in turn, are enzymatically modified to make a number of metabolites, including PG E_2, PG $F_2 \alpha$, PG D_2, thromboxane (TX A_2), and prostacyclin (PG I_2). The metabolites each have a role in the function of the cell (Oates, 1982). In inflammation, PGs are found in exudates. They increase vascular permeability, promote chemotaxis, induce fever, and sensitize pain receptors to stimulation by other chemical mediators, such as histamine and bradykinin.

Thromboxane A_2 (TX A_2) is formed when platelets are activated. It enhances platelet aggregation and causes vasoconstriction. On the other hand, prostacyclin (PG I_2), produced by endothelial cells, is a powerful inhibitor of platelet aggregation and is a vasodilator. PG D_2 is produced by basophils and mast cells. It is the principal metabolite of arachidonic acid in mast cells. When these cells are activated by IgE, PG D_2 participates in allergic responses. It is also a potent inhibitor of platelet aggregation. Platelet-activating factor (PAF) is also derived from ba-

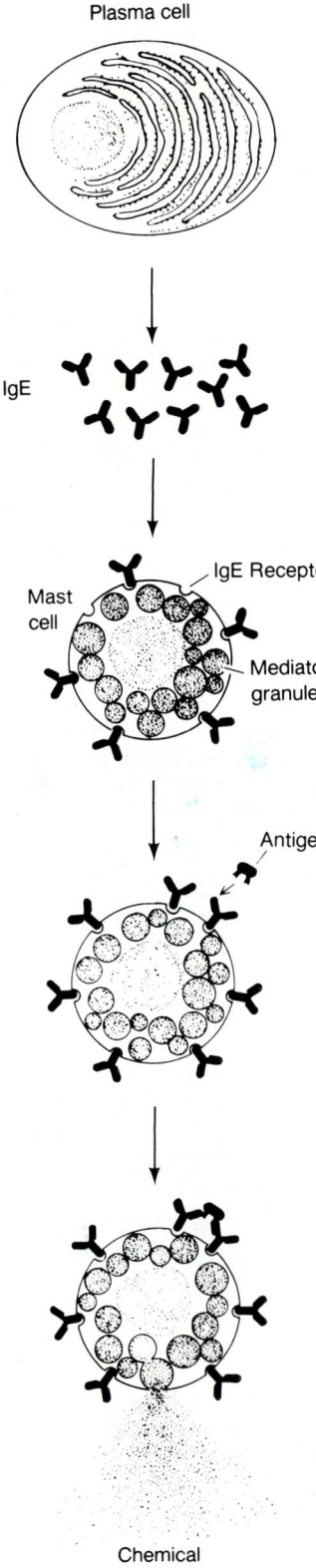

FIG. 7-2 Summary of mast cell's role in immediate hypersensitivity. IgE is secreted by a plasma cell in response to the first appearance of an antigen. The IgE becomes fixed to receptors on the surface of a mast cell. When the antigen is again encountered, epitopes on an antigen molecule are bound by two adjacent IgE molecules. The bridging of the IgE molecules initiates a process whereby mast cell is degranulated and its chemical mediators of the allergic reaction are liberated. (Buisseret PD: Allergy. Sci Am 247:86, August 1982)

sophils, neutrophils, alveolar macrophages, and monocytes. PAF promotes platelet aggregation, chemotaxis, increased vascular permeability (Sanchez-Crespo et al, 1981), serotonin secretion, thromboxane A_2, and some leukotriene production (Voelkel et al, 1982).

In polymorphonuclear leukocytes and reticulocytes, the arachidonic acid is metabolized largely by a 5-lipooxygenase to a series of products called leukotrienes (LTs; Buisseret, 1982). One of these, LT A_4, is converted by the addition of water into LT B_4, which has been found to be a potent chemotactic and enzyme-releasing agent for leukocytes. The addition of glutathione converts LT B_4 into LT C_4. Loss of glutamic acid converts LT C_4 into LT D_4, which in turn forms LT E_4 by the loss of glycine. This last group of leukotrienes (LT C_4, LT D_4, and LT E_4) has been found to be similar to a potent bronchoconstrictor called slow-reacting substance of anaphylaxis (SRS-A; Samuelsson and Hammarström, 1980). In addition to causing smooth-muscle contraction, the leukotrienes are powerful factors in the production of vascular leakage, especially in the terminal arterioles. LT D_4 is also a potent coronary artery vasoconstrictor (Michelassi et al, 1982).

The anti-inflammatory activity of corticosteroids is based partly on their ability to inhibit the liberation of free arachidonic acid from the phospholipids of the cell membrane by phospholipases. On the other hand, aspirin and other nonsteroidal anti-inflammatory drugs block the enzymatic conversion of arachidonic acid to the PGs by inhibiting the cyclooxygenase responsible for oxygenation (Vane, 1971). The formation of leukotrienes is apparently unaffected by the nonsteroidal anti-inflammatory agents.

Plasma Mediators

The plasma-derived factors are usually present in the circulation as inactive precursors. One of these, Hageman factor (Factor XII), is activated by contact with numerous substances, including glass, kaolin, collagen, basement membrane, cartilage, trypsin, kallikrein, plasmin, and bacterial lipopolysaccharides. Once activated, Hageman factor has three important effects: (1) It has prekallikrein activator (PKA) activity; (2) it triggers the clotting cascade; and (3) it triggers the fibrinolytic system.

A fragment of the Hageman factor, prekallikrein activator, activates circulatory prekallikrein to form kallikrein, which then cleaves kininogen to form a kinin, specifically a nonapeptide called bradykinin. Included among bradykinin's effects in inflammation are smooth muscle contraction, dilation of blood vessels, increased vascular permeability, and pain induction (Colman, 1974).

Mediators derived from the clotting system are fibrinopeptides and fibrin degradation products. These may induce vascular leakage and promote leukocyte chemotaxis.

The fibrinolytic system involves plasmin, an enzyme generated from plasminogen. Plasmin digests fibrinogen and fibrin. It plays an important role in activating the Hageman factor and in triggering kinin production. Plasmin is also involved in activating certain portions of the complement cascade, a system of nine factors activated in a particular sequence (Mayer, 1973).

Edema. The leakiness of the endothelium permits blood proteins to seep into the tissue. This results in a change in the osmotic pressure outside the vessel walls, and, hence, more fluid is attracted to the area of injury. This condition is known as edema, the accumulation of fluid within the tissue spaces outside the vessel wall. The edema distends the tissues, causing swelling. The exudate has a high specific gravity and includes albumin proteins, globulins, and fibrinogen, the precursor of fibrin. When fibrinogen leaks into the injured tissue, some clotting occurs in the tissue spaces.

Two pathways have thus far been elucidated for initiating coagulation: (1) the intrinsic system, initiated by surface contact with activation of Hageman factor and Factor XI, and (2) the extrinsic system, initiated by tissue thromboplastin, which requires Factor VII as an intermediary substance. Convergence of these two systems activates Factor X (Stuart-Prower Factor), with which certain precursors react to form fibrinogen (McKay, 1972). Activation of the complement system accelerates blood coagulation by release of a clotting factor from platelets.

The clotting serves a useful purpose, in that it occludes the lymphatics through the formation of thrombi, thereby tending to confine the inflammatory process to the immediate area. The body defenses can then deal with the irritant more effectively. In addition, the fibrin acts as a framework for repair.

Leakage of a small amount of serum proteins into the tissues is called a serous exudate. When a large quantity of plasma proteins leak out, a change in the osmotic pressure occurs. This increased osmotic pressure attracts more fluid into the area and (if the area is dermal) a blister is raised.

Margination of Leukocytes and Chemotaxis. The polymorphonuclear leukocytes (polys) in the bloodstream begin to line the walls of the blood vessels and stick to the endothelial lining (Fig. 7–3)—a process called margination.

There is a marked increase in the number of polys, which marginate or stick to the endothelial wall before migration. Such adherence is the initial step toward leaving the blood vessel (Brubaker, 1974). Shortly, the polys begin to emerge from the vessel walls. They are attracted to the site of injury by chemotaxis.

Chemotaxis has also been demonstrated to occur from activation of the complement system by immune reactions or by the cleavage of complement by proteolytic enzymes released from cells by viruses (Snyderman et al, 1971). Also, collagenases may be modified after injury, leading to the formation of modified tissue proteins that can activate the complement system (Gross et al, 1963). Such activation leads to the release of vasoactive and phlogistic substances, such as anaphylatoxin, which cause the release of a chemotactic histamine product C5a (Bokisch et al, 1968; Mayer, 1973; Snyderman, 1973). Enzymes derived from cells may also act as mediators of the inflammatory response. Those enzymes are usually contained in cell organelles called lysosomes (Fig. 7–4). Among the lysosomal enzymes involved in inflammation are acid proteases, called cathepsins. Release of such lysosomal enzymes following phagocytosis may result in damage to the surrounding cells and tissues.

LIQUEFACTION NECROSIS. The polys contain antibacterial and enzymatic basic proteins (Zeya and Spitznagel, 1963) that digest the irritant. Digestion is mediated by a tripartite system, consisting of an oxidizing enzyme called myeloperoxidase, hydrogen peroxide, and halide ions

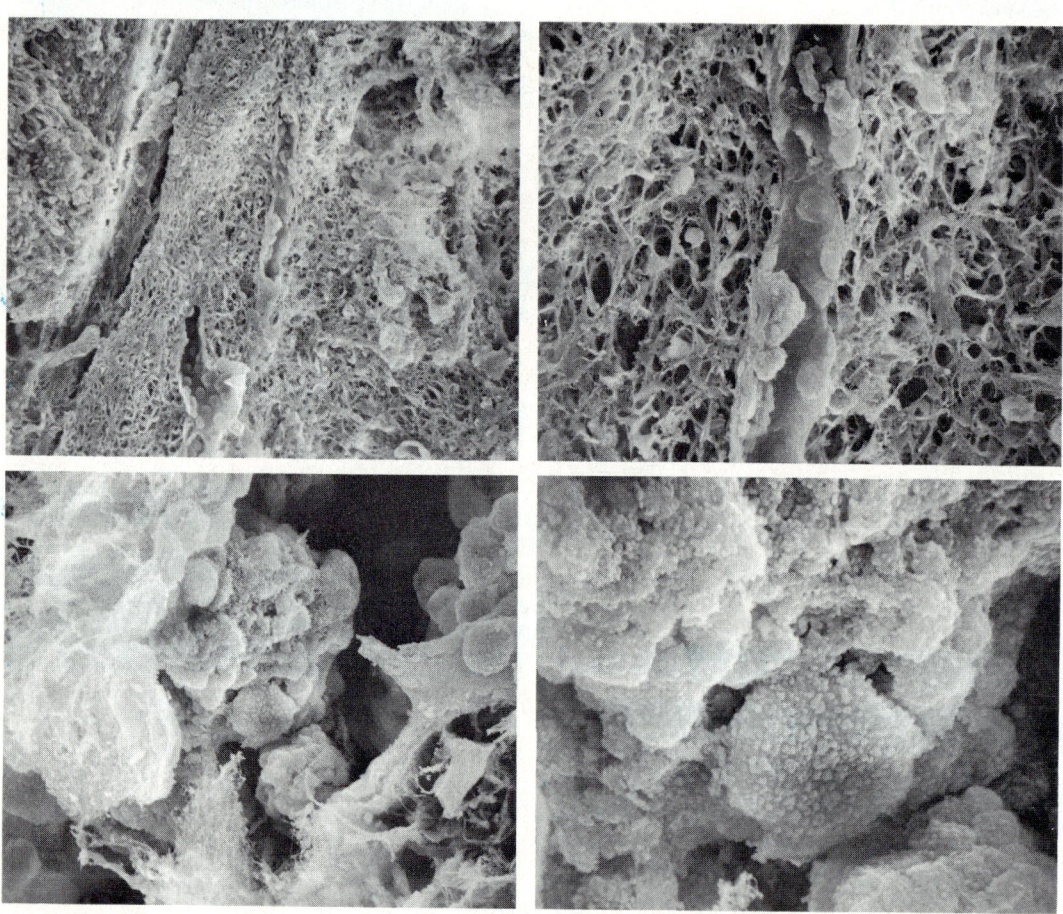

FIG. 7-3 Margination of leukocytes. *(Top, left)* Scanning electron micrograph of coronal pulp. ×100. *(Top, right)* Higher magnification of top left micrograph showing margination of polys in blood vessels. ×500. *(Bottom, left)* and *(bottom, right)* Higher magnifications of marginating polys. Bottom left ×1000; bottom right ×3000.

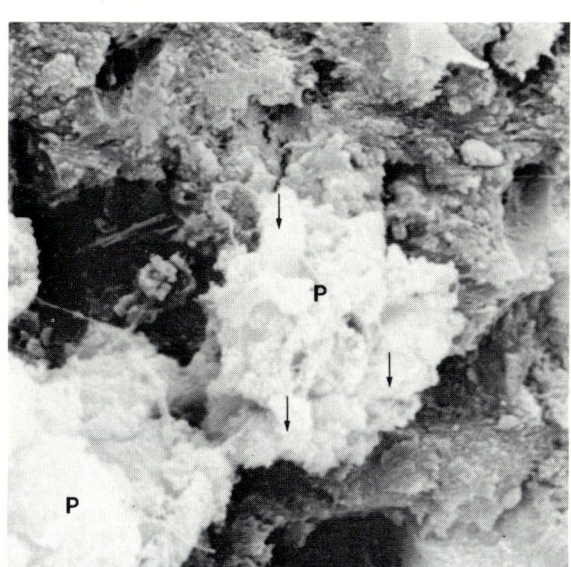
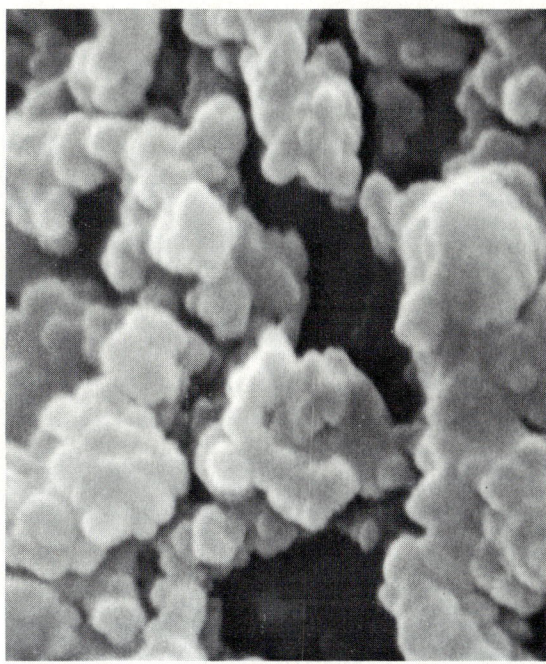

FIG. 7-4 *(Left)* Scanning electron micrograph of polymorphonuclear leukocytes (P), composed of individual packets of lysosomes (arrows). ×5000. *(Right)* Higher magnification of lysosomes composed of spherical subpackets. ×30,000.

(Klebanoff, 1967). Within a short period of time, they themselves degranulate. They then liberate digestive enzymes and other substances from their lysosomes (Fig. 7-5). Greater tissue damage may be caused by the lysosomal enzymes than by microorganisms. Proteolytic (digestive) enzyme activity increases with increased severity and extent of the inflammatory process. Among the proteases that have been identified in inflammatory lesions are chymotrypsin, trypsin, pronase, and collagenase (Bertelli, 1969).

When a large amount of proteolytic enzymes are liberated, the tissue is digested. The resultant digested material, called pus, contains necrotic debris, microorganisms and digestates. When pus is produced, the condition is called an acute suppurative or purulent inflammation (Fig. 7-6). The proteolytic enzymes are liberated mainly after the polys die. Tissues are not digested under normal circumstances because certain antienzymes are present that prevent their digestion. When a tremendous number of polys are attracted to the site of injury, the proteases elaborated overcome the antienzyme effect, and suppuration results.

The polys are also attracted to the site of injury because the pH is on the alkaline side. With the passage of time, there is a drop in pH caused by a disturbance in the intermediate carbohydrate metabolism, resulting in glycolysis and accumulation of lactic acid. As the hydrogen-ion concentration of the exudate increases, the polys are incapable of surviving, and they are replaced by mononuclear phagocytes (macrophages). When the pH falls below 6.5, the leukocytes are killed and liquefaction necrosis (pus) develops.

A leukocytosis-promoting factor liberated from the injured cells at the site of inflammation frequently induces an increase in circulating leukocytes.

CYCLIC NUCLEOTIDES

Cyclic AMP

Cyclic adenosine monophosphate (cyclic AMP) is a second messenger for many hormones. It transmits information to the interior of the cell. Under the control of a cyclic AMP–dependent protein kinase, phosphorylation of various

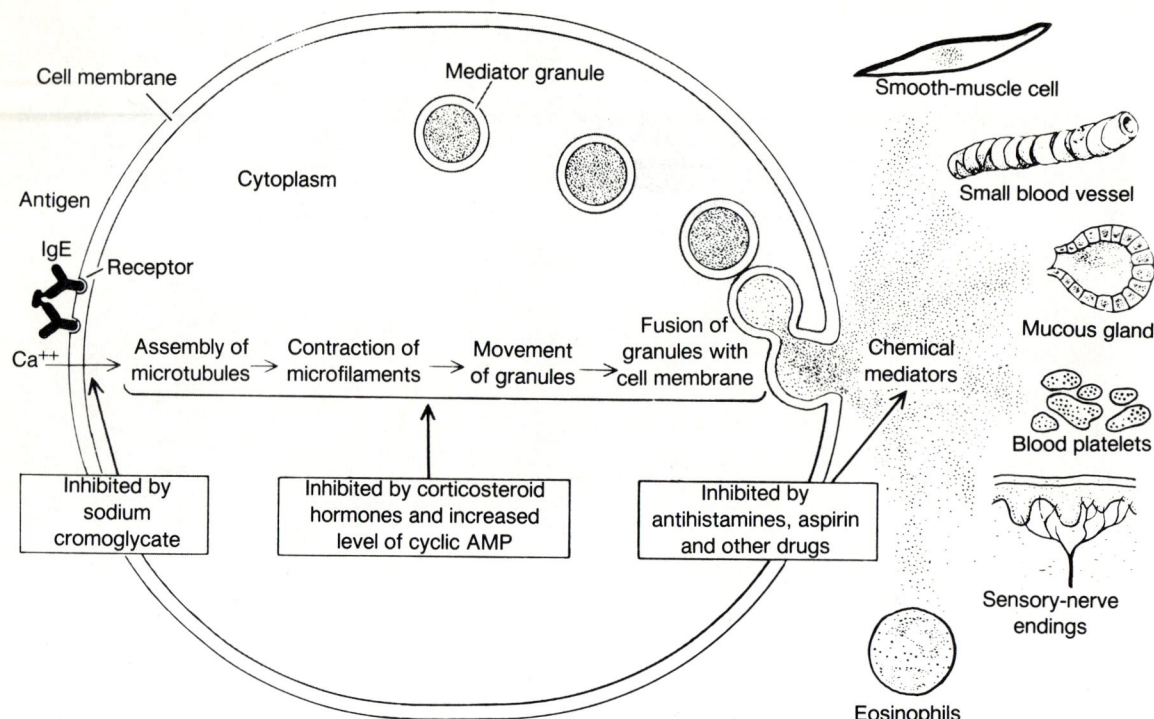

FIG. 7-5 Summary of degranulation and its effects. Calcium ions entering the cytoplasm regulate enzymes controlling microfilaments whose activity makes the granules move to the cell membrane, fuse with the membrane, and discharge their contents: chemical mediators of the allergic reaction. The mediators act on target tissues and cells. For example, they contract smooth-muscle cells, dilate small blood vessels and make them leaky, stimulate secretion by mucous glands, activate blood platelets, irritate nerve endings in the skin, and attract the white blood cells called *eosinophils*. The process is susceptible to drugs at various stages. The entry of calcium ions can be blocked by sodium cromoglycate. The movement of granules can be inhibited by corticosteroid hormones or by agents that increase the cytoplasmic concentration of cyclic adenosine monophosphate (cyclic AMP). Once released, the mediators can sometimes be neutralized by various drugs, including antihistamines and aspirin, or their activity can be counteracted by drugs such as epinephrine. (Buisseret PD: Allergy. Sci Am 247:86, August 1982)

regulatory enzymes directs biosynthetic and biodegradative pathways. The prostaglandins stimulate the enzyme adenylate cyclase in the cell membrane to synthesize cyclic AMP, which in turn retards hydrolytic enzyme release from the lysosomes.

According to the hypothesis of Bourne et al (1974), the character and intensity of inflammatory and immune responses is regulated by certain hormones and mediators. This regulation is mediated by a general inhibitory action of cyclic AMP on the release of mediators from mast cells, basophils, monocytes, and polys. Lymphocyte activation and lymphocyte-mediated cytolysis are also under the influence of cyclic AMP. In addition, the release of PAF, a phospholipid mediator, from monocytes and polys (Lotner et al, 1980), is regulated by cyclic AMP (Alonzo et al, 1982).

Cyclic GMP

Effects opposite to those of cyclic AMP are induced by cyclic guanosine monophosphate (cyclic GMP). Its action is to enhance mediator release, possibly through stimulation of microtubule assembly (Goldstein et al, 1973). Several investigations have indicated that, in pulpitis, there is a relative increase of cyclic GMP over cyclic AMP concentrations (Sproles et al, 1979; Bolanos and Seltzer, 1981).

Acute inflammation occurs soon after the original injury and persists for a short period,

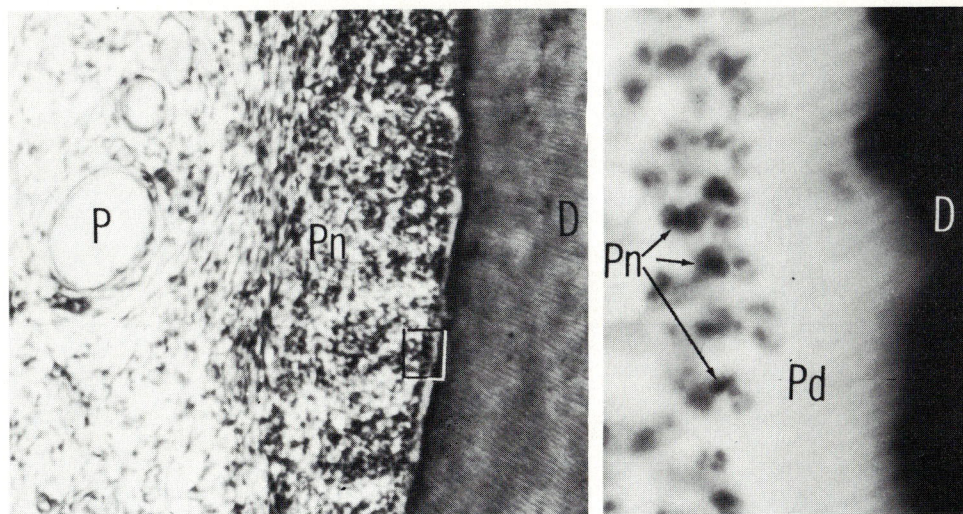

FIG. 7-6 *(Left)* Acute inflammation. The region of pulp injury (P) under the dentin (D) is heavily infiltrated with polymorphonuclear leukocytes (Pn). ×96. *(Right)* Higher magnification of region outlined by rectangle in photomicrograph at *left*. The predominant cell type is the polymorphonuclear leukocyte (Pn). Pd, predentin. D, dentin. ×960.

such as 4 or 5 days to a week. Inflammation that persists beyond this period begins to go into a chronic stage.

CHRONIC INFLAMMATION

The inflammation must be resolved within a short time or it becomes chronic. Inflammation is eliminated because, concurrently with the elaboration of tissue breakdown products, other products are liberated that stimulate the surrounding tissue. Proliferation of other tissue elements occurs and repair of the injured area is begun. Thus, repair commences and continues simultaneously with inflammation.

If the irritant is not eliminated completely, a state of equilibrium develops between the tissue defenses and the irritant. This state of chronic inflammation is characterized by cells of a kind different from those present in acute inflammation.

DEFENSE CELLS (SMALL ROUND CELLS)

Small round cells migrate into the inflamed area and begin to predominate. Prostaglandins are closely associated with this migration. It has been suggested by Giroud and Willoughby (1970) that these mediators are formed partly by the action of complement, and their liberation seems to depend on an intact complement system.

The term small round cells applies to lymphocytes, plasma cells and macrophages (Fig. 7-7). They are called small round cells because there are transitional forms between these cells in many instances. Sometimes it is not clear from their histologic appearance when viewed under the light microscope whether the cells are lymphocytes, macrophages, or plasma cells. The presence of these cells is a response to a change in the pH of the tissue, which now begins to move toward the acid side.

Special Functions. Macrophages are derived from a small pool of rapidly dividing precursor cells in the bone marrow (monocytes). The monocytes are transported to the wound by the bloodstream and there differentiate into macrophages (Fig. 7-8). The function of macrophages includes ingestion of foreign material (Fig. 7-9), antigen-antibody complexes, and initiation of coagulation. Macrophages also adhere to the body's own thymocytes and T cells. This interaction is necessary for a class of immune reactions called T-cell-dependent or cell-mediated immunity (see p 162). Material is digested by enzymes in macrophage lyso-

160 | THE DENTAL PULP

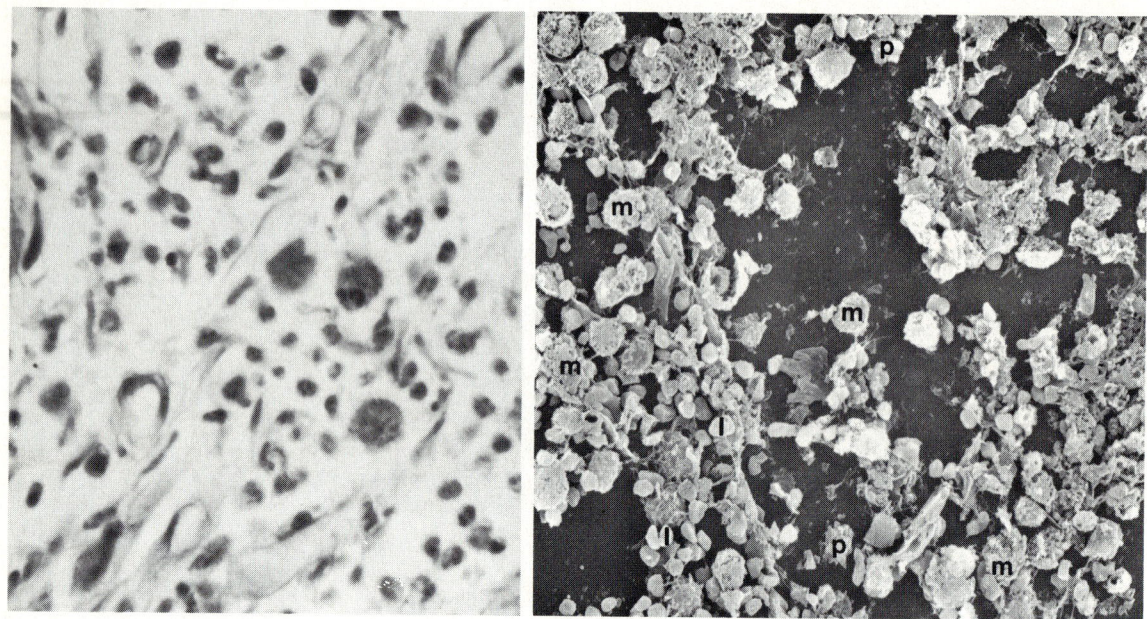

FIG. 7-7 *(Left)* Granulation tissue. ×960. *(Right)* Scanning electron micrograph of tissue section showing chronic inflammatory cells. m, macrophage; l, lymphocyte; p, poly. ×500.

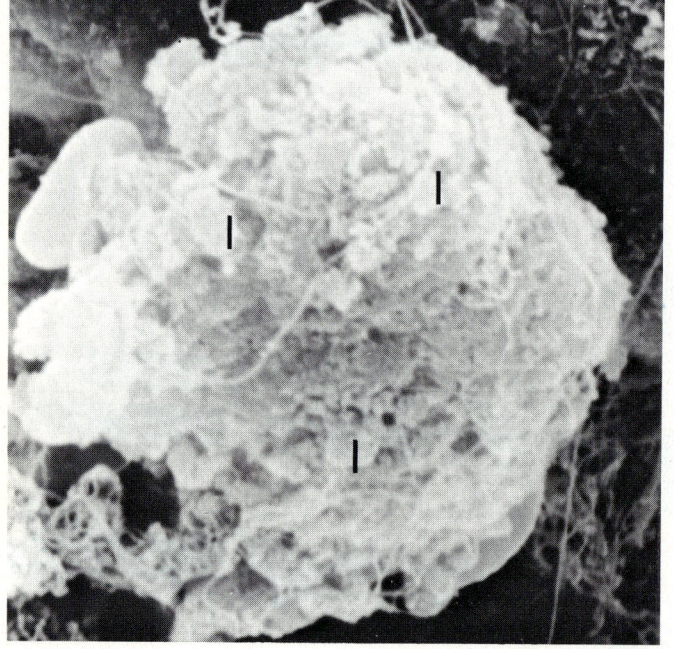

FIG. 7-8 Scanning electron micrograph of macrophage. l, lysosome. ×5000.

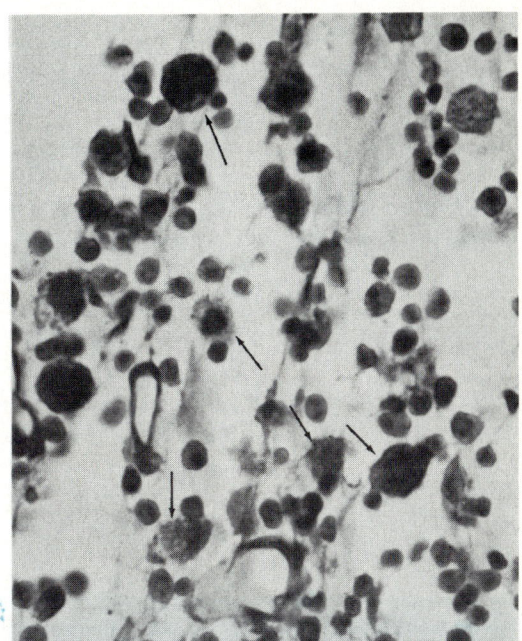

FIG. 7-9 *(Top)* Macrophages (arrows) engorged with carbon particles. ×960. *(Bottom left)* Scanning electron micrograph of tissue section of chronically inflamed pulp showing predominance of macrophages (m). ×500; *(Bottom right)* Higher magnification of dissected macrophage revealing lysosomes (—). ×5000.

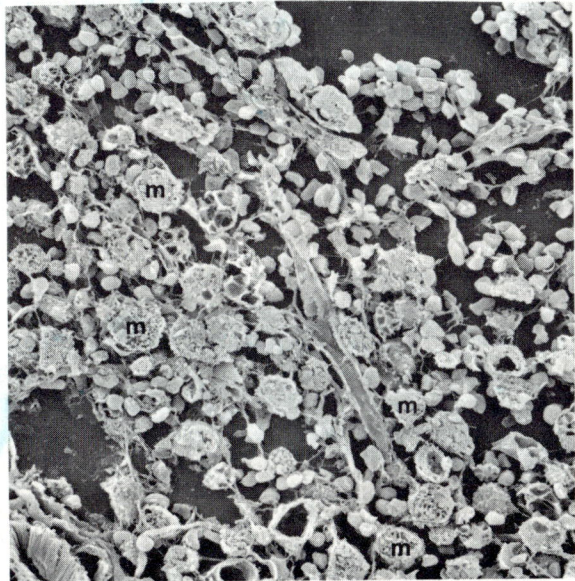
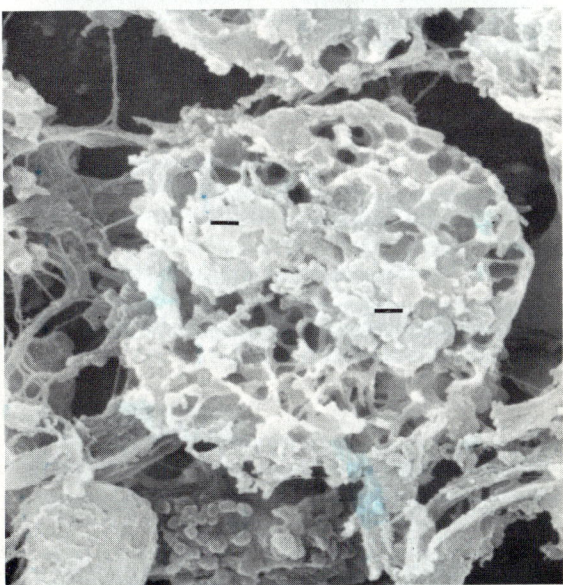

some such as acid phosphatases, nonspecific esterases, proteases, cathepsins, lipases, peroxidases, and collagenases (Pearsall and Weiser, 1970; Salthouse and Matlaga, 1972).

The function of the small lymphocyte is synthesis, storage, and transport of nucleoproteins for use by other cells. The function of the plasma cell (plasmacyte) is synthesis and storage of ribonucleic acid (RNA) and gamma globulins. Thus, infiltrations of small lymphocytes and plasma cells in areas of chronic inflammation and wound healing concentrate proteins for use by other cells to aid in regeneration or replacement.

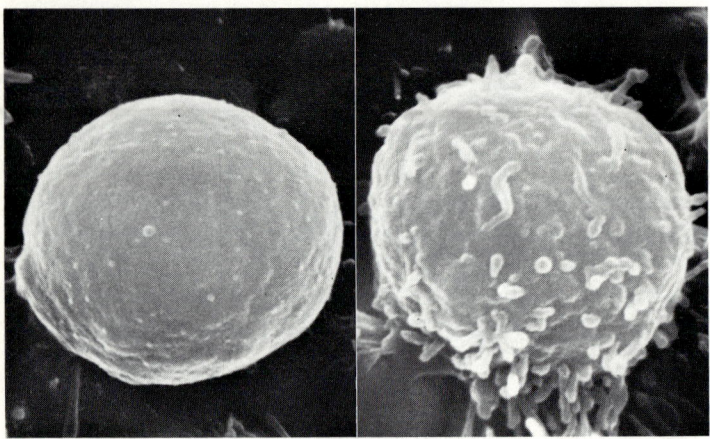

FIG. 7-10 Normal T lymphocyte surface morphology ranges from smooth but slightly irregular, to relatively smooth with small stublike projections, to relatively smooth with a moderate number of surface digitations *(left)*, to intermediate surface morphology with a relatively large number of surface microvilli *(right)*. ×14,000. (Polliack A et al: Identification of human B and T lymphocytes by scanning electron microscopy. J Exp Med 138:607, 1973)

ANTIBODIES

The major mechanism of survival in man is the immune system, designed primarily to recognize, attack, and destroy any foreign matter that may enter the body. The human immune system can specifically respond to and react with an enormous number of different antigens, running the gamut from proteins, through polypeptides and microorganisms, to foreign tissues (Edelman, 1973). The main agents for this function are the lymphocytes (Fig. 7-10). There are two types of lymphocytes, B and T. Both types are derived from the bone marrow (Fig. 7-11). T lymphocytes pass through the thymus gland, where they differentiate and mature into competent lymphocytes. Such maturation is enhanced by prostaglandin release (Garaci et al, 1983). Subsequently, the T cells become seeded in the blood. T cells are activated by antigens; they participate in immune reactions by direct interaction with the antigenic target and by release of lymphokines (mediators of inflammation). The main function of T lymphocytes is the rejection of foreign matter, including fungi, acid-fast bacilli and viruses, and transplanted tissues and organs (cell-mediated immunity). These events occur without the intervention of antibodies. One variety of T cells are known as suppressor T cells. These cells inhibit the immune response of other white cells, preventing inappropriate antibody production. Still others are known as helper T cells. They stimulate B cells to transform when challenged by antigen, resulting in enhanced antibody synthesis. When the regulatory system of suppressor T cells fails, an allergic response may occur through the overproduction of antibody, such as IgE (see Figs. 7-2 and 7-5).

The B lymphocytes are the agents concerned with humoral immunity and are responsible for synthesizing and secreting immunoglobulins and the antibodies they produce into the circulation. At least five major classes of immunoglobulins—IgG, IgM, IgA, IgD, and IgE—have been identified (Roitt, 1971). Subclasses of these may exist. The B cell system appears to be designed to handle a variety of infectious microorganisms. Both B and T cells reside primarily in the lymphoid tissues. From these tissues, the B cells recirculate through the body and continually monitor for the presence of potential attackers.

When a foreign substance or a strange cell enters the body, the lymphocyte starts to work like an internal antiballistic-missile system. The lymphocyte determines whether the macromolecule belongs or does not belong in the body. When the lymphocytes recognize the macromolecules as foreign, an immunologic alarm is triggered.

When the alarm is sounded, the immune system swings into dual action of the B and the T cells. According to Lerner and Dixon (1973), the initial step in the immune response is the contact of an antigen—a foreign substance—with receptor antibodies on the surface of B lymphocytes. Such contact can be changed by interaction of the antigen with macrophages or with T lymphocytes. The antigen-receptor contact changes the expression of the B lymphocyte's genes, thereby setting in motion division and differentiation of the lymphocytes. The daughter lymphocytes become plasma cells

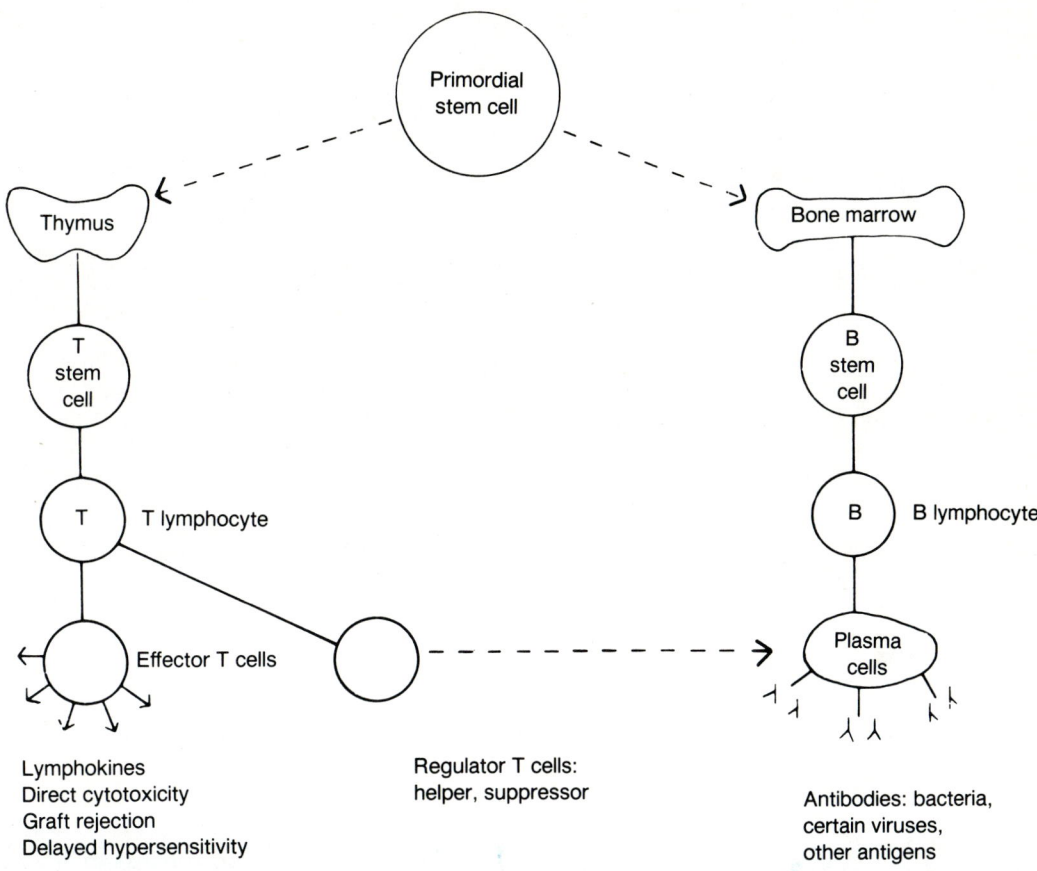

FIG. 7-11 Diagrammatic representation of specific immune pathways. (Legler DW, Arnold RR, Lynch DP, McGhee JR: Immunodeficiency disease and implications for dental treatment. JADA 105:803, 1982. Copyright by the American Dental Association. Reproduced by permission)

(Fig. 7-12) and memory cells. Plasma cells secrete circulating antibodies that attack the antigen. Memory cells are held in reserve and respond to the reappearance of the antigen (Fig. 7-13).

The situation is not so clear with regard to T cells. Although T cells may have specific immunoglobulins on their surfaces, they do not secrete antibodies; only the B cells and their progeny secrete antibody molecules (Jerne, 1973). However, B cells do not respond to antibody formation in the absence of T cells. Thus, the dualistic function of the immune complex acts as a surveillance system of the body.

An in vitro correlate of cellular immunity is a phenomenon called lymphocyte transformation. This is a proliferative response of lymphocytes when leukocytes from an individual with cellular immune hypersensitivity are cultured with a specific antigen (Oppenheim, 1969). The proliferating lymphocytes release soluble mediators of inflammation, including a monocyte chemotactic factor (LDCF), a macrophage inhibitory factor (MIF), and a cytotoxic factor (lymphotoxin). Collectively, these mediators are called lymphokines (Snyderman, 1973).

Thus, antibodies are substances manufactured by the body that combine with and neutralize foreign proteins known as antigens (Fig. 7-14). The combination of antibodies with antigens neutralizes the latter and renders them innocuous. In granulomas, which commonly occur in both the pulp and the periapical tissues, the granulation tissue is rich in lymphocytes and plasma cells; hence, this tissue is a tissue of defense.

Complement System. The components of complement are a complex group of enzymes that, working together with antibodies or other

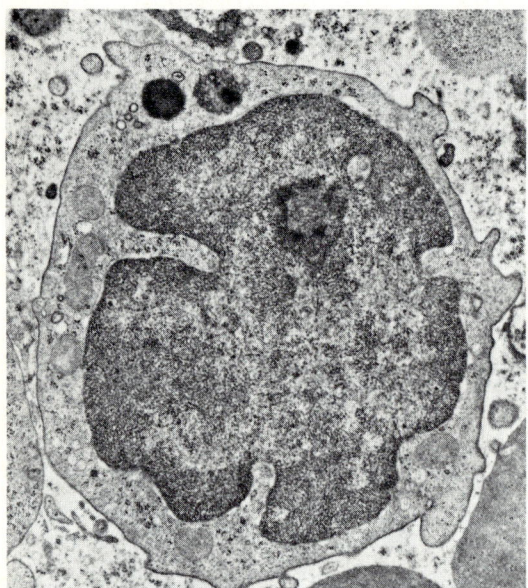 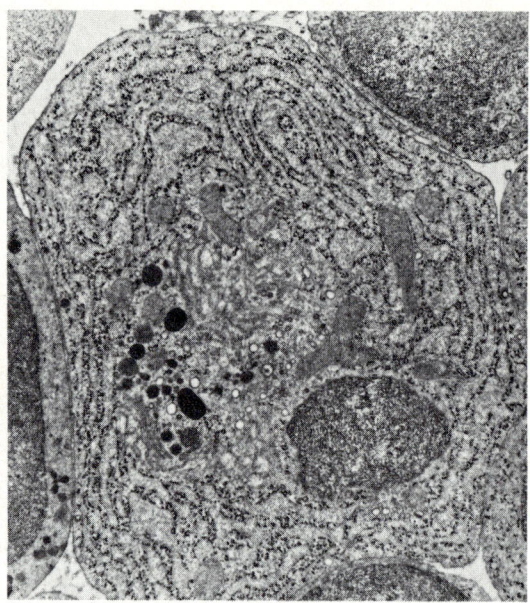

FIG. 7-12 Differentiation in the course of the immune response changes a lymphocyte *(left)* into a plasma cell *(right)*. Noticeable changes include an increase in cell size, a relative decrease in the size of the nucleus, and the formation of organelles involved in synthesis and secretion of antibody, including ribosomes (small black dots) arrayed along the membranous endoplasmic reticulum. Electron micrographs by Joseph Feldman. (Lerner RA, Dixon FJ: The human lymphocyte as an experimental animal. Sci Am 228:82, June 1973)

factors, play a significant role in both immune and allergic reactions. The reactions in which complement participates are humoral, i.e., they take place in the blood serum or other bodily fluids. Cells invading the body are attacked by complement. The invaders are identified as foreign by antibodies, which activate the complement attack. Thus, complement is activated by plasmin and trypsin and by most antigen-antibody complexes. According to Mayer (1973), the relationship between antibody and complement resembles the relationship between the ignition key of an automobile and the engine. Sites on the antibody molecule can combine with a part of the surface of a foreign cell or with another molecule, an antigen. The fit between the ignition key and the ignition lock has the same effect as the fit between the antigen and antibody molecules. The antibody molecule starts the complement system, which, like the automobile engine, actually does the work. Complement, when activated by antibody, threatens not only the invaders, but the host's own cells. Fortunately, this self-destructing activity is reduced by the fixation of complement on the surface of the invading cell by antibody.

There are nine steps in the complement cascade. The complement proteins are designated by the letter C and a subscript number: C_1, C_2, C_3, etc.

When cells are attacked by complement, they swell until the cell ruptures. The cell contents then spill out.

Complement system by-products have several important effects in inflammation. C_{3a} and C_{5a} fragments cause increased vascular permeability by effecting the release of histamine from leukocytes, mast cells, and platelets. C_3 fragments can also induce leukocytosis and help to promote phagocytosis. C_5 fragments are the major complement-derived chemotactic factor. They also help to induce the release of lysosomal enzymes from neutrophils.

Fluorescence Microscopy

Immunoglobulin (receptor) molecules on the surface of the lymphocyte can be visualized by the technique of fluorescence microscopy. First, antibody is prepared against the immunoglobulin molecules of the species supplying the lymphocytes. The antibody is then coupled to a fluorescent dye such as fluorescein. The anti-

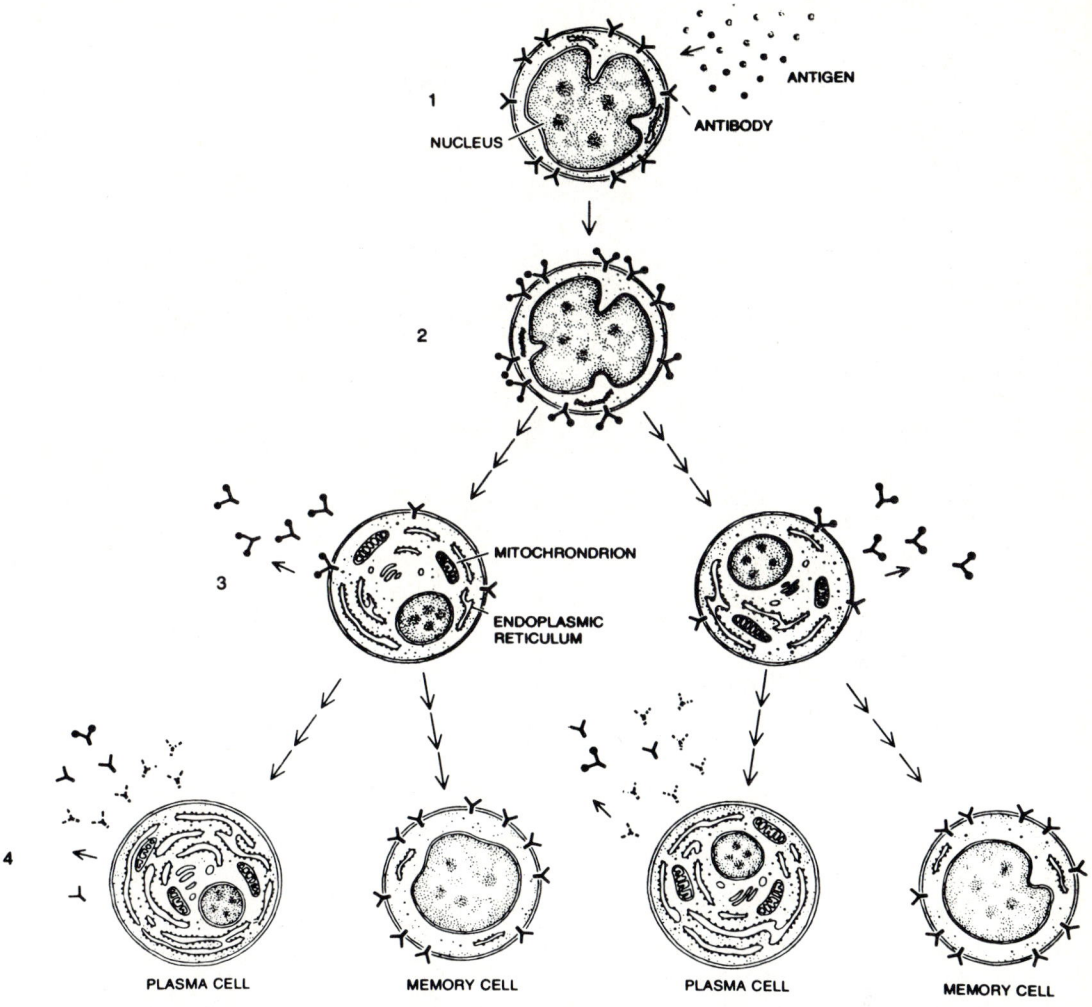

FIG. 7-13 Immune response may begin when a small lymphocyte with antibodies (solid Ys) on its surface encounters antigen molecules (circles) against which its antibody is specific. (1). The antigen is bound to the antibody (2); this event, together with a second signal involving another kind of lymphocyte, induces the small lymphocyte to divide and differentiate (3); surface receptor antibodies are lost and replaced by new ones. The lymphocytes differentiate to become plasma cells and memory cells (4). Plasma cells synthesize and secrete circulating antibody (notched Ys); memory cells, held in reserve, respond sensitively to reappearance of the antigen. (Lerner RA, Dixon FJ: The human lymphocyte as an experimental animal. Sci Am 228:82, June 1973)

body-dye complex reacts with cells and binds to the immunoglobulin molecules on the cell surface. When the cells are exposed to ultraviolet radiation, the fluorescein gives off a characteristic green glow that thus reveals the location of the immunoglobulin molecules on the cell surface.

Fluorescence antibody techniques have been used by Honjo et al (1968, 1970) to study the localization of albumin, gamma globulin, and fibrinogen of inflamed pulps. Gamma globulin was found in most of the plasma cells and sometimes, although rarely, in the cytoplasm of macrophages and polys.

REPAIR

The chemical stimuli that initiate repair are elaborated from the injured cells. Repair is characterized by the proliferation of a large number

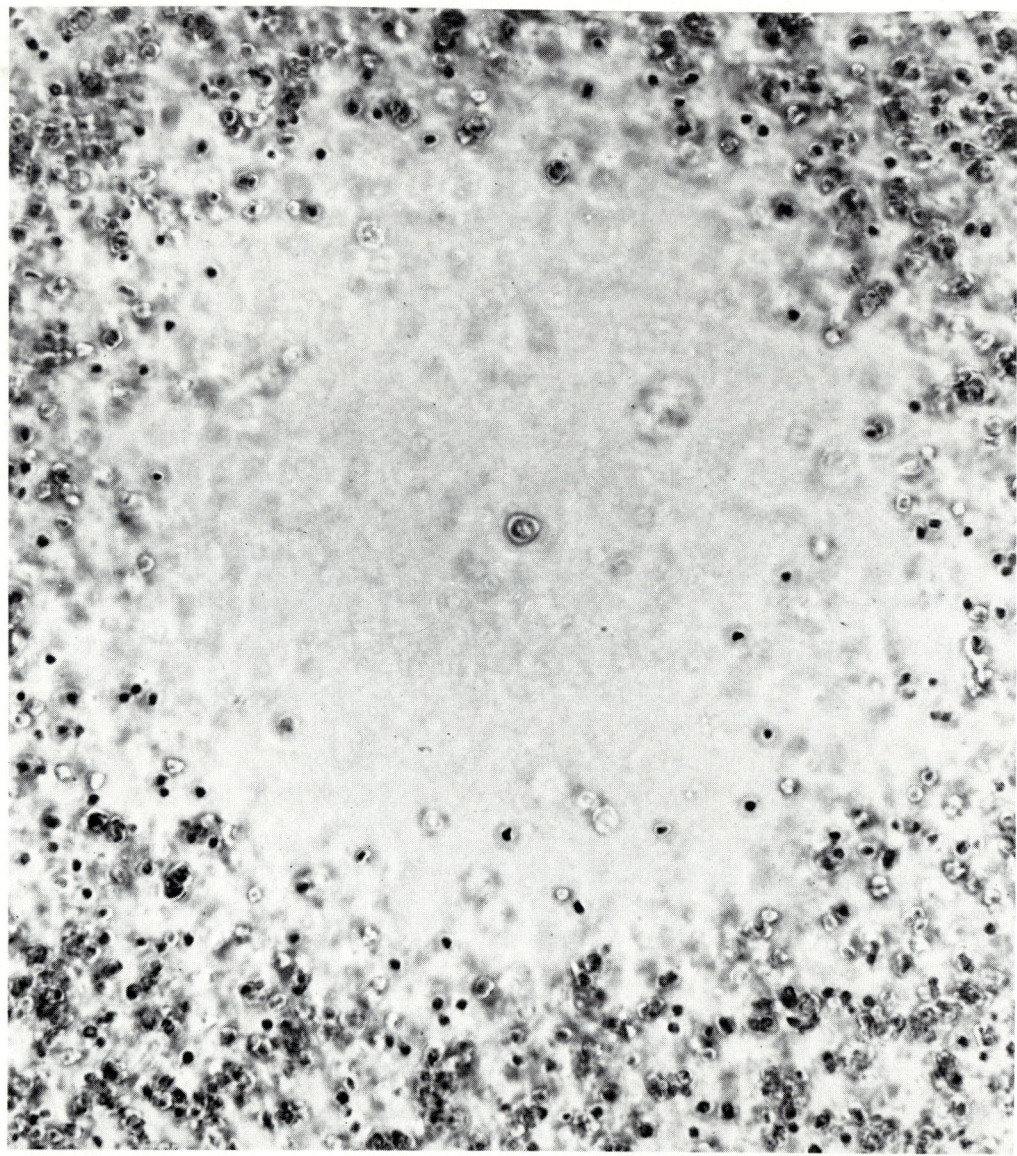

FIG. 7-14 Photomicrograph dramatically illustrating the effect of antibody on an antigen. The cell in the center is a plasma cell, an antibody-secreting lymphocyte of the immune system. It was embedded in a layer of culture medium along with millions of sheep red blood cells. The plasma cell is one that makes antibody against the sheep cells, specifically against epitopes, or small surface patches, on molecules in the surface membrane of the cells. Antibodies secreted by the plasma cell have destroyed the red blood cells in the area into which the antibodies have diffused; the radius of the area of destruction is about ⅕ mm. The technique illustrated here has become a standard one for measuring the immune response to an antigen. (Jerne NK: The immune system. Sci Am 229:52, 1973)

of new fibroblasts from the cells of the adjacent connective tissue (Ross, 1971). According to Ross (1966), the infiltrating fibroblasts are characterized by large nuclei and a prominent nucleolus or nucleoli. Initially, a relatively large amount of poorly developed rough endoplasmic reticulum (rER) is present. Gradually, the endoplasmic reticulum increases, and there is an increase in aggregates of attached ribosomes. A large Golgi apparatus and mitochondria become visible. Aggregates of intracytoplasmic filaments increase. New collagen fibrils are elaborated. In addition, many new blood vessels are formed by the budding of the old vessels. The capillaries send out branches known as capillary loops, and these eventually join other capillaries, resulting in a rich blood supply. This tissue is called granulation tissue (see Fig. 7–7). Thus, granulation tissue consists of new fibroblasts and collagen fibers, new blood vessels and the cells of the chronic inflammatory series. A granuloma is a tumorlike collection of granulation tissue. Actually, the term granuloma is a misnomer, inasmuch as the suffix "-oma" means tumor. However, the term has persisted in the dental literature and is in common usage.

Houck (1963) has demonstrated that, during wound healing, there is a loss of glycoprotein and an increase in the concentration of insoluble collagen, acid polysaccharides, acid-soluble collagen, and insoluble noncollagenous protein in the wound.

In wounds, the amount of proline hydroxylase also is increased (Green and Goldberg, 1968). Such increases represent the presence of hydroxyproline in collagen breakdown products or may reflect decreased cross-linking of the collagen molecules (Martin, 1971).

ENZYMES IN INFLAMMATION

Irritants may be classified as living or nonliving. Living injurious agents are microorganisms: bacteria, fungi, and protozoa. The nonliving injurious agents may be classified as chemical, thermal, mechanical, electrical, and radiant. Viruses also are tissue irritants.

Living irritants elaborate enzymes or injurious agents that can affect cells, fibers, or ground substance. An enzyme is an agent that destroys, inactivates, or catalyzes a highly active substance in the body. All known enzymes are proteins. A specific cell contains perhaps a thousand different kinds of enzymes, and all chemical reactions that take place in cells are catalyzed by enzymes. An enzyme functions by bringing about a specific chemical reaction that it catalyzes by combining reversibly with its particular substrate. For many of the enzymes, this specific substrate is one of the essential metabolites such as a vitamin, a purine, or an amino acid. The unstable enzyme-substrate complex that is thus formed undergoes some sort of molecular rearrangement or fission that yields the intact enzyme plus the products derived from the substrate. The cycle is then repeated because the enzyme has not been consumed in the process. The specificity of the enzyme is determined by its ability to combine with a given substrate but not with unrelated substances. In addition to its substrate, an enzyme usually combines reversibly with a few structural relatives of the substrate. The relative is known as the analogue (the antimetabolite).

Injurious agents are not the only producers of proteolytic enzymes. It is a biologic condition that there must be an enzyme present for every potential substrate in the body. This is because there is a constant buildup and breakdown of tissue within the body. The tissues themselves elaborate the enzymes. Within various cells, multivesicular bodies, called lysosomes, are present that contain digestive enzymes (Goldfischer et al, 1964). The lysosomal enzymes have been implicated in intracellular digestion, autolysis, tissue resorption, and reactions to tissue injury (Weissmann, 1972). The interaction of substrate and enzyme is graphically depicted in the process of inflammation. If an inhibitor were not present in the bloodstream, the proteolytic enzymes released during inflammation would digest all the tissues in the body. It is only when these enzymes are liberated in large quantities at the site of inflammation that they overcome the inhibitor, thereby causing tissue digestion.

ACTION OF ENZYMES ON CELLS

Many enzymes elaborated by injured cells or microorganisms act on the cells and change them during inflammation; a few of these are discussed in the following section.

Ribonucleases and Deoxyribonucleases. Certain enzymes, elaborated by microorganisms, affect the nucleic acids of the cells. These are ribonucleases. There are also deoxyribonucleases, which affect the nucleus of the cell.

Enzymes which are liberated by microorganisms can depolymerize the ribonucleic acid (RNA) and deoxyribonucleic acid (DNA).

Streptodornase is an enzyme that attacks and breaks down the DNA within the nucleus of the cell. Streptokinase, an enzyme that is elaborated by some streptococci, dissolves fibrin. It is therefore also known as a fibrinolysin.

The theory behind the use of streptokinase is that repair occurs more quickly if the fibrin framework is dissolved. Streptokinase also antagonizes bradykinin, a natural polypeptide formed by action of enzymes on a substrate in plasma and present at sites of tissue injury.

Inasmuch as the lymphatic blockade is a natural defense mechanism, it seems reasonable not to interfere with it.

Some microorganisms also elaborate a fibrinolysin that dissolves the fibrin and allows them to invade. For instance, the streptococci, which are the microorganisms most frequently involved in subacute bacterial endocarditis, are invasive because they elaborate fibrinolysins. The penetration of the microorganisms may also be due to the presence of hyaluronidase or a histaminelike substance.

ACTION OF ENZYMES ON GROUND SUBSTANCE

The enzymes that affect the ground substance do so by acting on its components, the glycosaminoglycans, such as hyaluronic acid and chondroitin sulfuric acid.

When hyaluronic acid is depolymerized, microorganisms may penetrate deeper into the tissue. Thus, the hyaluronidase elaborated by the microorganisms contributes to their invasiveness. However, it is possible that the microorganisms may be killed when they do not penetrate. Among the streptococci involved in pulpitis are some that are hyaluronidase elaborators, such as *Streptococcus mitis*.

Another enzyme that acts on a component of ground substance is chondroitin sulfatase. This hydrolyzes chondroitin sulfuric acid, which is a basic component of all hard tissues—dentin, bone, and cementum. The presence of microorganisms that elaborate chondroitin sulfatase in an inflamed pulp may cause depolymerization of the ground substance, resulting in pulp disease. Quintarelli (1960b) has discussed the possibility that cellular as well as bacterial proteolytic enzymes (proteinases and peptidases) play a role in the depolymerization of the ground substance. The release of the protein component of the mucopolysaccharides during inflammation increases the metachromasia of the tissue.

ACTION OF ENZYMES ON FIBERS

Different proteases are liberated from the tissues at different times, depending on the type of inflammation. Proteolytic enzymes can be released from plasma or from the lysosomes of monocytes, fibroblasts, lymphocytes, platelets, and mast cells (Bertelli, 1972).

Some enzymes act on the fibers of connective tissue. Among these are reticulinases and collagenases. The latter depolymerize the collagenous proteins whose basic ingredients are the amino acids proline, hydroxyproline, and glycine. Cathepsins have also been identified as active in the degradation of collagen (Bazin and Delauney, 1972).

Other enzymes, manufactured either by microorganisms or by the body tissues themselves, are involved in inflammation. Many have not yet been identified.

ACTION OF HORMONES

Another group of substances involved in inflammation are hormones. These, too, affect ground substance, fibers, and cells. Inflammation is controlled by hormones. For example, repair is affected in a woman undergoing menopausal changes. The hormones elaborated during this period affect growth and repair. When an excess of estrogen or progesterone is elaborated, the microcirculation is affected. Endothelial swelling, leukocyte adhesion to the vessel walls and aggregation of platelets are induced. Vascular permeability is increased (Lindhe et al, 1969). However, changes occur in the ground substance, rendering it less permeable through hydration. Lurie (1950) has shown that animals are less likely to be infected with tubercle bacilli when they are given extra amounts of estrogen. Conversely, if there is an excess of gonadotrophic hormone, the ground substance binds less water and becomes more permeable, and the microorganisms are able to penetrate more readily, resulting in an increase in infectibility of the tissue.

Steroids. Cortisol and ACTH inhibit the increase in capillary permeability which occurs in the early stages of inflammation. However, when an acid pH develops, neither cortisol nor ACTH can suppress the permeability of the capillaries. Both cortisol and ACTH have been discovered in inflammatory exudates following intravenous injection in rabbits and dogs. Chemotaxis and diapedesis of leukocytes are consequently suppressed.

Cortisone stabilizes the lysosomal membrane, thereby decreasing the capacity of these organelles to release their enzymes (Weissmann and Thomas, 1963). If microorganisms are present, a harmful spread of infection may result (David et al, 1970), inasmuch as the intercellular destruction of microorganisms by neutrophils is reduced. Also, although glucocorticoids do not interfere with phagocytosis of polys, they apparently impair the bactericidal and fungicidal activity of monocytes and interfere with macrophage activity (Claman, 1975).

Wound healing is impaired during cortisone therapy. An excess of cortisone affects both the fibroblasts and the quantity and the quality of the collagen being elaborated by them.

The catabolic actions of glucocorticoids result not only in decreased synthesis but also in increased degradation of protein and RNA. Together with inhibition of glucose and amino acid uptake, the inhibitory actions of glucocorticoids suppress immunologic and inflammatory responses and wound healing (Baxter and Forsham, 1972). The inhibition of antibody production by glucocorticoids results from functional inhibition of both B and T lymphocytes (Gabrielson and Good, 1967; Segal et al, 1972; Beardsley and Cohen, 1978).

Diabetes and Inflammation. Inflammatory reactions are greater in diabetic states, and, conversely, local inflammations cause an intensification of the diabetes. In the diabetic state, the lack of insulin interferes with the transport mechanism of glucose from the blood into the cells, producing an increase in the blood sugar. Cellular dehydration, with a loss of alkali reserve, also occurs (Russel, 1966). Even in the early stages of diabetes, many of the blood vessels, particularly the capillaries, exhibit an increased thickening in their basement membranes (Campbell, 1967). In many instances, vessel lumens become obliterated. Because of the circulatory disorder, the metabolic exchange of the cells adjacent to the injured site is impaired; a more rapid aging process takes place. The pathosis is irreversible even after insulin therapy. The thickened capillaries may play a significant role in infections by acting as a barrier to leukocyte emigration into the sites of acute inflammation (Brayton et al, 1970). Furthermore, gluconeogenesis is augmented at the site of acute inflammation because of increased proteolysis. Hence, the diabetic state is intensified during inflammation.

As a result of atherosclerosis, with occlusion of the blood vessels, microangiopathies and the barrier to leukocytic emigration, infection can spread more readily. Furthermore, the circulatory complications and the complication of infections in this disease can impair healing.

Clinical Correlations. The long-term local use of an anti-inflammatory agent such as cortisone is contraindicated in some disease processes, because the repair mechanism is delayed. Cortisone inhibits the formation of granulation tissue (Boulas, 1959). Since granulation tissue is necessary for repair, its inhibition in certain inflammatory conditions is not desirable.

The systemic use of hormones in the treatment of some inflammatory states is unjustified. The hormonal system is a part of a complete cycle. The elaboration of one hormone affects others. The presence of excessive amounts of some hormones interferes with the proper functioning of other endocrine glands. Normal bodily functions are interfered with. In addition, other endocrine glands are involved in the process of inflammation.

Removal of a local irritant usually stimulates repair. Occasionally, however, persistence of inflammation may be unrelated to poor local treatment. Instead, systemic factors such as hormonal disturbances may be responsible.

On the other hand, sometimes recovery occurs even though local treatment is poor. For example, occasionally, in spite of improper debridement of a root canal, poor mechanical preparation, broken instruments, etc., repair still occurs. This may be due to a favorable systemic and hormonal background.

ROLE OF VITAMINS

Vitamins, especially vitamin C, are significant factors in repair of injured tissue. Vitamin C has an effect on the fibroblasts (cells that elaborate collagen). Good repair depends on properly functioning fibroblasts. A deficiency of vitamin C adversely affects wound repair in experimental animals by altering collagen synthesis. Ross

(1966) has found that the cisternae of the endoplasmic reticulum of the fibroblasts of wounded guinea pigs deficient in ascorbic acid were dilated. The endoplasmic reticulum was also vacuolar and contained ribosomes that had lost their aggregate configuration and were oriented randomly. Large numbers of lipid droplets appeared in the cytoplasm. The extracellular spaces displayed large numbers of fine filaments, fibrin, and extravasated erythrocytes.

When scorbutic animals were treated with vitamin C, collagen synthesis resumed. After 4 hours, the ribosomal aggregates reappeared and collagen fibrils were found extracellularly after 12 hours. Severe injury, produced by burns or surgical procedures in guinea pigs, produces a "biochemical scurvy." In such injured animals, healing is dramatically impaired despite a dietary intake of ascorbic acid normally adequate for growth and repair in unburned guinea pigs (Levenson et al, 1957). Healing was enhanced by the administration of large doses of ascorbic acid during the postburn period. Inasmuch as man, like the guinea pig, requires exogenous vitamin C, it seems logical that the repair of injured pulp or periapical tissues may also be affected by deficiency of dietary vitamin C. Thus, patients should receive an adequate dietary intake of vitamin C during tissue repair (Ringsdorf and Cheraskin, 1982). It is possible that pulp lesions may heal more readily if patients are premedicated with vitamin C and continue to receive it for a while after treatment.

ROLE OF PROTEINS

Protein depletion effectively retards repair of injuries to connective tissue. There is a reduction in fibroblasts and capillaries and a delay in fiber formation (Perez-Tamayo and Ihnen, 1953). When there has been protein deprivation before injury, healing is delayed. In children with advanced protein-calorie malnutrition, cell division fails and chromosomes become structurally abnormal in response to radiation, chemical agents, or viral infections (Armendares et al, 1971). There is evidence that, when proteins become deficient even after healing has occurred, breakdown of the healed area is possible (Levenson et al, 1945; Stahl, 1962). This may be related to lowered resistance to infection (Cannon et al, 1944) or local irritants (Stahl).

INFECTION

The rapidity and the thoroughness with which microorganisms are contained within the immediate region of injury by the lymphatic blockade determine their invasiveness to a large extent. Microorganisms vary in their ability to induce lymphatic occlusion. Thus, some streptococci, by virtue of their elaboration of spreading factors, penetrate readily into the deeper tissues, whereas staphylococci tend to remain localized.

Classically, it has been thought that the inflammatory response is aimed solely at destroying and eliminating microorganisms and other injurious substances, thereby protecting the host from lethal invasion. However, more recent observations show that the cells involved in the immediate reaction to injury, such as polys, contain hydrolytic enzymes in cell organelles, called lysosomes. Such enzymes, when released in the surrounding tissues, produce inflammatory responses. The inflammation sometimes has a component (a cell-mediated immune response) that in itself causes tissue damage. Delayed hypersensitivity increases tissue destruction and reduces the animal's resources for defense against subsequent staphylococcal infections (Goshi et al, 1961). Methods aimed at depressing the hypersensitivity reactions may be useful in the treatment of certain microbial infections (Burke, 1971).

Thus, to think only in terms of infection of an injured pulp is a narrow, limited view. Instead, the kind of infection, the enzymes involved, and other factors, including hypersensitivity and cell-mediated immunity, should be considered. Perhaps a broader view is the host-parasite relationship. Certain microorganisms that are benign under ordinary conditions become damaging to the host when systemic factors are altered. For example, pseudotuberculosis of rats is caused by *Corynebacterium pseudotuberculosis*, which cannot be isolated from the animals in a normal state but multiply extensively when the animals are stressed or are treated with large doses of cortisone. The same microorganisms, when transferred to other healthy animals, do not produce disease. There is also the question, "Do all microorganisms cause damage, or are some of them beneficial?" Some microorganisms are necessary for life. For example, there are microorganisms in the intestinal tract that manufacture enzymes and vitamins. If the bowel is sterilized with antibiotics, many people develop fungal infections and symptoms of avitaminosis. The role of microorganisms in life is dramatized in animals reared under germ-free conditions. They fare poorly under ether or chloroform anesthesia because the liver is unable to detoxify these agents effectively.

BIBLIOGRAPHY

Alonzo F, Sánchez-Crespo M, Mato JM: Modulatory role of cyclic AMP in the release of platelet-activating factor from human polymorphonuclear leukocytes. Immunology 45:493, 1982

Armendares S, Salamanca F, Frenk S: Chromosome abnormalities in severe protein calorie malnutrition. Nature 232:271, 1971

Baserga R, Kisieleski WE: Autobiographies of cells. Sci Am 209:103, 1963

Baxter JD, Forsham PH: Tissue effects of glucocorticoids. Am J Med 53:573, 1972

Bazin S, Delauney A: Role of cathepsins in granulation tissue. J Dent Res (Suppl No 2) 51:244, 1972

Beardsley GP, Cohen HJ: Corticosteroid induced lymphocytopenia in man. Am J Hematol 4:255, 1978

Bertelli A: Proteases in inflammatory reactions. In Proceedings of the International Symposium on Inflammation Biochemistry and Drug Interaction. Amsterdam, Excerpta Medica, 1969

Bertelli A: Enzymes and antienzymes in inflammatory reactions. J Dent Res (Suppl No 2) 51:235, 1972

Bokisch VA, Budzko DB, Müller-Eberhard HJ, Cochrane CG: Cleavage of human C^3 by trypsin into three antigenically distinct fragments including anaphylotoxin. Fed Proc 27:314, 1968

Bolanos OR, Seltzer S: Cyclic AMP and cyclic GMP quantitation in pulp and periapical lesions and their correlation with pain. J Endodont 7:268, 1981

Boulas SH: Dissociation of granulation and epithelization in wounds of rabbits by means of topically applied hydrocortisone. J Invest Derm 32:75, 1959

Bourne HR, Lichtenstein LM, Melmon KL, Henney CS, Weinstein Y, Shearer GM: Modulation of inflammation and immunity by cyclic AMP. Science 184:19, 1974

Brayton RG, Stokes PE, Schwartz MS, Louria DB: Effect of alcohol and various diseases on leukocyte mobilization, phagocytosis and intracellular bacterial killing. New Engl J Med 282:123, 1970

Brubaker LH: Unsticky neutrophils. New Engl J Med 291:674, 1974

Buisseret PD: Allergy. Sci Am 247:86, 1982

Burke JF: Effects of inflammation on wound repair. J Dent Res (Suppl No 2) 50:296, 1971

Campbell MJA: Periodontal disease in the diabetic patient and its treatment. Austral Dent J 12:117, 1967

Cannon PR, Wissler RW, Woolridge RL, Benditt EP: The relationship of protein deficiency to surgical infection. Ann Surg 120:514, 1944

Claman HN: How corticosteroids work. J Allergy Clin Immunol 55:145, 1975

Colman RW: Formation of human plasma kinin. New Engl J Med 291:509, 1974

David DS, Grieko MH, Cushman PJ: Adrenal corticoids after twenty years: a review of their clinically relevant consequences. J Chron Dis 22:637, 1970

Dubos RJ: Bacterial and Mycotic Infections of Man. 4th ed, p 27. Philadelphia, JB Lippincott, 1965

Edelman GM: Antibody structure and molecular immunology. Science 180:830, 1973

Ferguson HW, Lawton FE: Tissue responses in the rat incisor pulp following traumatic injury. Arch Oral Biol 7:407, 1962

Gabrielson AE, Good RA: Chemical suppression of adaptive immunity. Adv Immunol 6:91, 1967

Garaci CR, Favalli C, Gobbo VD, Garachi E: Is thymosin action mediated by prostaglandin release? Science 220:1163, 1983

Giroud JP, Willoughby DA: The interrelationship of complement and prostaglandin-like substance in acute inflammation. J Path 101:241, 1970

Goldfischer S, Essner E, Novikoff AB: The localization of phosphatase activities at the level of ultrastructure. J Histochem Cytochem 12:72, 1964

Goldstein RM, Hoffstein S, Gallin J, Weissmann G: Mechanisms of lysosomal enzyme release from human leukocytes: Microtubule assembly and membrane fusion induced by a component of complement. Proc Natl Acad Sci USA 70:2916, 1973

Goshi K, Cluff LE, Johnson JE: Studies on the pathogenesis of staphylococcal infection. III. The effect of tissue necrosis and antitoxic immunity. J Exp Med 113:259, 1961

Green H, Goldberg B: Differentiation for collagen synthesis in cultured cells. Symposium Int Soc Cell Biol 7:123, 1968

Gross J, Lapiere CM, Tanzer ML: Organization and disorganization of extracellular substances: The collagen system. In Locke M (ed): Cytodifferentiation and Macromolecular Synthesis, pp 175–202. New York, Academic Press, 1963

Honjo H, Tsubakimoto K, Utsumi N, Tsutsui M: Localization of plasma proteins in the human dental pulp. J Dent Res 49:888, 1970

Honjo H, Tsubakimoto K, Sumitani M: Homologous plasma proteins in the human dental pulp. J Osaka Dent Univ 2:147, 1968

Houck JC: Chemistry of inflammation. Ann NY Acad Sci 105:765, 1963

Jerne NK: The immune system. Sci Am 229:52, 1973

Klebanoff SJ: Iodination of bacteria: A bactericidal mechanism. J Exp Med 126:1063, 1967

Le Bell YL, Larmas M: Adenosine-5-triphosphate levels of the human tooth pulp during health and disease. Arch Oral Biol 24:313, 1979

Lerner RA, Dixon FJ: The human lymphocyte as an experimental animal. Sci Am 228:82, 1973

Levenson SM, Davidson CS, Lund CC, Taylor FHL: The nutrition of patients with thermal burns. Surg Gynec Obstet 80:449, 1945

Levenson SM, Upjohn HL, Preston JA, Steer A: Effect of thermal burns on wound healing. Ann Surg 146:357, 1957

Lichtenstein LM: The role of cyclic AMP in inhibiting the

IgE-mediated release of histamine. In Robison GA, Nahas GG, Triner L (eds): Cyclic AMP and cell function. NY Acad Sci 185:403, 1971

Lindhe J, Lundgren D, Stallard R, Östren A: Connective tissue alterations occurring during pregnancy as seen by vital dyes. J Periodont 40:22, 1969

Lotner GL, Lynch JM, Betz SJ, Henson PM: A platelet activating factor derived from human neutrophils. J Immunol 124:676, 1980

Lurie MB: Mechanisms affecting spread in tuberculosis. In The ground substance of the mesenchyme and hyaluronidase. Ann NY Acad Sci 52:1074, 1950

McKay DG: Participation of components of the blood coagulation system in the inflammatory response. Am J Path 67:181, 1972

Martin GR: Recent progress in collagen research. J Dent Res (Suppl No 2) 50:268, 1971

Mayer MM: The complement system. Sci Am 229:54, 1973

Mayer RL: Hyaluronidase and inflammation of the skin. In The ground substance of the mesenchyme and hyaluronidase. Ann NY Acad Sci 52:943, 1950

Meyer KL: The mucopolysaccharides of the interfibrillar substance of the mesenchyme. In The ground substance of the mesenchyme and hyaluronidase. Ann NY Acad Sci 52:943, 1950

Michelassi F, Landa L, Hill RD, Lowenstein E, Watkins WD, Petkau AJ, Zapel WM: Leukotriene D_4: A potent coronary artery vasoconstrictor associated with impaired ventricular contraction. Science 217:841, 1982

Oates JA: The 1982 Nobel prize in physiology or medicine. Science 218:765, 1982

Oppenheim JJ: Immunologic relevance of antigen and antigen antibody complex induced lymphocyte transformation. Ann Allergy 27:305, 1969

Pearsall NN, Weiser RS: The Macrophage. Philadelphia, Lea and Febiger, 1970

Perez-Tamayo R, Ihnen M: The effect of methionine in experimental wound healing. Am J Path 29:233, 1953

Polliack A, Lampen N, Clarkson BD, De Harven E, Bentwich Z, Siegel FP, Kunkel HG: Identification of human B and T lymphocytes by scanning electron microscopy. J Exp Med 138:607, 1973

Quintarelli G: Histochemistry of the gingiva. III. The distribution of amino-peptidase in normal and inflammatory conditions. Arch Oral Biol 2:271, 1960

Quintarelli G: Histochemistry of the gingiva. IV. Preliminary investigations of the mucopolysaccharides of connective tissue. Arch Oral Biol 2:277, 1960a

Quintarelli G: Istochemica Della Gingiva. V. Ulteriori studi sul comportamento della sostanza fondamentale del connettivo. Arch Ital Biol Orale 1:1, 1960b

Ringsdorf WM, Jr, Cheraskin E: Vitamin C and human wound healing. Oral Surg 53:231, 1982

Roitt JM: Essential Immunology. London, Blackwell, 1971

Ross R: The ultrastructure of fibrogenesis. J Dent Res 45:449, 1966

Ross R: Wound healing: Recent progress—future directions. J Dent Res (Suppl No 2) 50:312, 1971

Russel BG: Gingival changes in diabetes mellitus. I. Vascular changes. Acta Path Microbiol Scand 86:161, 1966

Salthouse TN, Matlaga BF: Collagenase associated with macrophage and giant cell activity. Experientia 28:326, 1972

Samuelsson B, Hammarström S: Nomenclature for leukotrienes. Prostaglandins 19:645, 1980

Sánchez-Crespo M, Alonzo F, Inarrea P, Egido J: Nonplatelet mediated vascular action of PAF. Agents Actions 11:30, 1981

Schultz-Haudt S, Bibby BG, Bruce MA: Tissue destructive products of gingival bacteria from nonspecific gingivitis. J Dent Res 33:624, 1954

Segal S, Cohen IR, Feldman M: Thymus-derived lymphocytes: humoral and cellular reactions distinguished by hydrocortisone. Science 175:1126, 1972

Snyderman R: Immunological mechanisms of periodontal tissue destruction. JADA 87:1020, 1973

Snyderman R, Tempel TR, Mergenhagen SE: Chemotaxis of inflammatory cells. J Dent Res (Suppl No 2) 50:304, 1971

Sproles AC, Schilder H, Schaffer LD: Cyclic AMP and cyclic GMP concentrations in normal and pulpitic human dental pulps. J Dent Res 58:2369, 1979

Stahl SS: The effect of a protein-free diet on the healing of gingival wounds in rats. Arch Oral Biol 7:551, 1962

Stahl SS, Sandler HC, Cahn LR: The effects of protein deprivation upon the oral tissues of the rat and particularly upon the periodontal structures under irritation. Oral Surg 8:760, 1955

Voelkel NF, Worthen S, Reeves JT, Henson PM, Murphy RC: Nonimmunological production of leukotrienes induced by platelet-activating factor. Science 218:286, 1982

Weissmann G: Lysosomal mechanisms of tissue injury in arthritis. New Engl J Med 286:141, 1972

Weissmann G, Thomas L: Studies on lysosomes. II. The effect of cortisone on the release of acid hydrolases from a large granule fraction of rabbit liver induced by an excess of vitamin A. J Clin Invest 42:661, 1963

Zeya HI, Spitznagel JK: Antibacterial and enzymatic basic proteins from leukocyte lysosomes: separation and identification. Science 142:1085, 1963

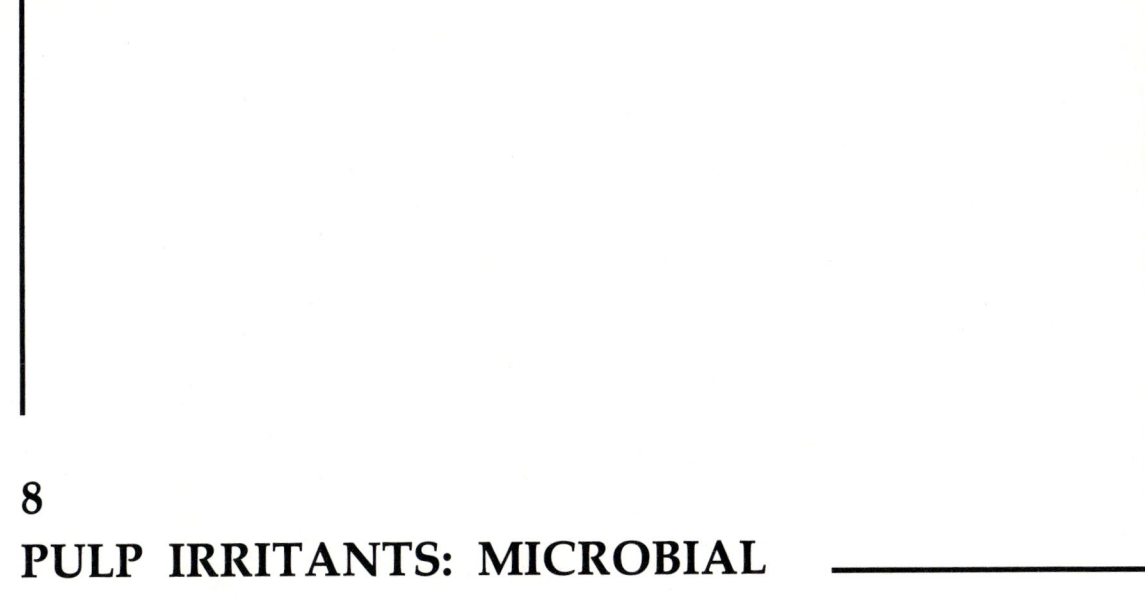

8
PULP IRRITANTS: MICROBIAL

Pulp irritants may be living or nonliving. The living irritants are usually bacterial, but fungi may also be involved, as well as viruses. There are no reports of pulps infected with protozoa. The nonliving irritants may be mechanical, thermal, chemical, or radiant.

One of the local factors, such as dental caries, that affect the odontoblasts and the underlying pulp cells may be classified as microbial.

DENTAL CARIES

Dental caries is a localized, progressive decay of the teeth. The disease is initiated by demineralization of the surface of the tooth by organic acids such as lactic acid (Kuboki et al, 1983), produced by microorganisms localized in plaque. The acid is produced by several different microorganisms, most notably *Streptococcus mutans*. Fermentable carbohydrates, especially sucrose, are the nutrient source (Leverett, 1982; Newbrun, 1982).

Thus, caries of the enamel results from contact of acids and enzymes that accumulate in plaques of microorganisms. The disintegrating substances remain in contact with the tooth surface for an extended period of time. This contact causes demineralization and partial remineralization of the enamel. As the dentin is invaded, proteolysis of the organic matrix occurs.

All of the current theories in regard to the etiology of dental caries (acidogenic, proteolytic, or proteolysis-chelation) implicate microorganisms in the process. Orland et al: (1959) found that caries did not develop in the teeth of germ-free animals, even when the animals were fed a cariogenic diet. However, caries did develop when enterococci and gram-negative bacilli were introduced into the animals' environment.

In experimental animals, caries has been found to be an infectious, transmissible disease (Fitzgerald and Keyes, 1960). Considerable evidence has accumulated to warrant a similar conclusion for humans (Fitzgerald, 1973).

CARIOUS DENTIN

Carious dentin consists of two layers: (1) the outer layer, in which there is irreversible denaturation and infection. This layer is physiologically unmineralizable, and (2) the inner layer, in which the denaturation is reversible and there

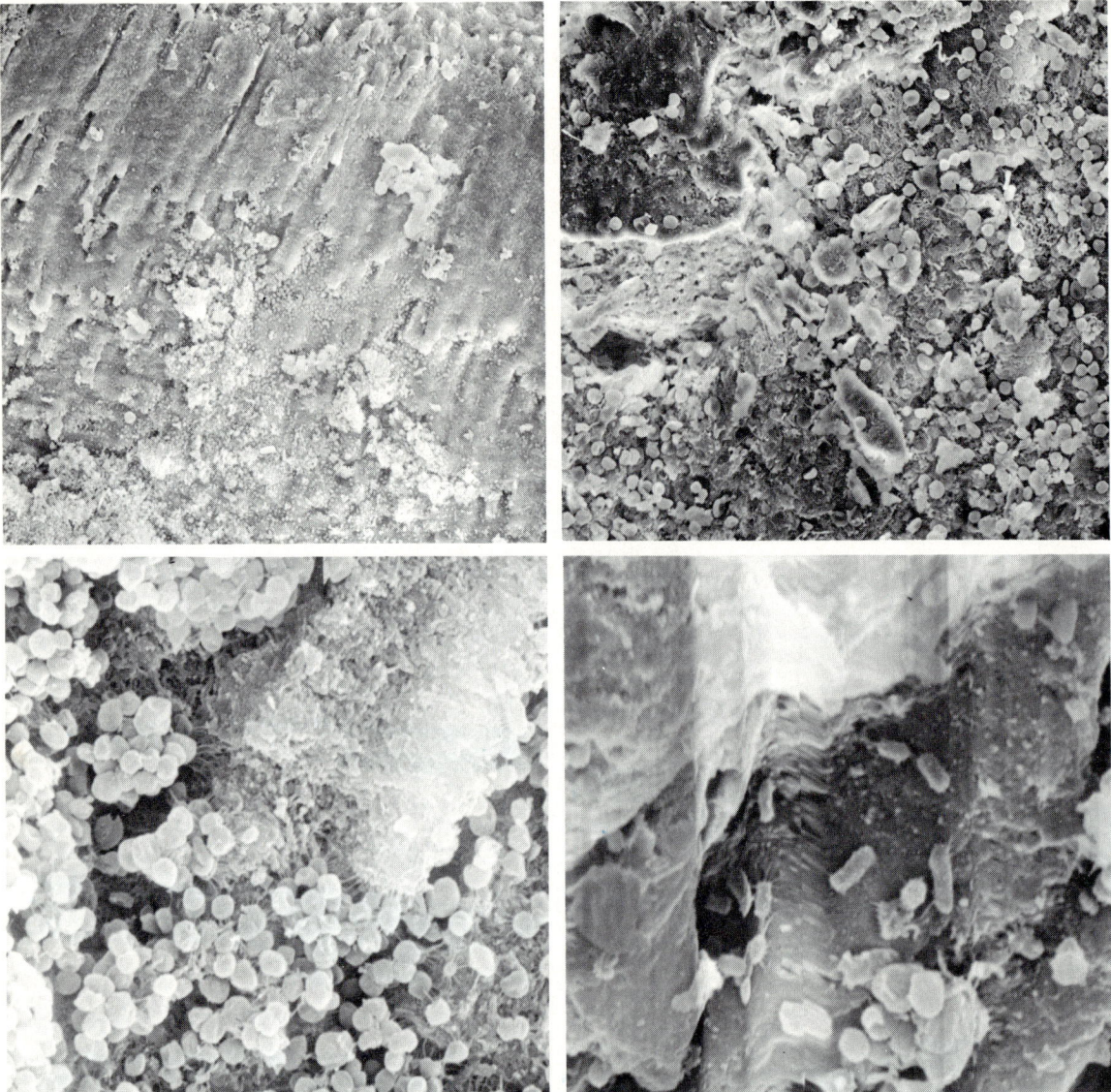

FIG. 8-1 Bacterial invasion of dentin. *(Top, left)* Carious dentin. ×50. *(Top, right)* Higher magnification of top left photomicrograph. Dentinal tubules are disorganized and invaded by microorganisms. ×500. *(Bottom, left)* Bacteria in dentin. ×5000. *(Bottom, right)* Higher magnification of bacteria in dentinal tubules. ×8000.

is no infection. This layer can be remineralized physiologically (Miyauchi et al, 1978).

In the early stages, carious dentin has the morphologic pattern typical of sound dentin. As decalcification progresses, the fibrils of the intertubular matrix are destroyed and the dentinal tubules are distended (Kuboki, 1977). The components of the peritubular matrix appear to consist of fine filaments or granules instead of collagenous fibrils. Although there is a decrease in the density of the crystallite distribution, such decrease is markedly less than in the intertubular areas. The cellular components of many of the tubules become displaced by bacteria (Fig. 8-1). In those tubules, the odontoblastic cell membrane is partially or totally destroyed. Some tubules appear empty, containing neither bacteria nor cellular structure (Symons, 1970).

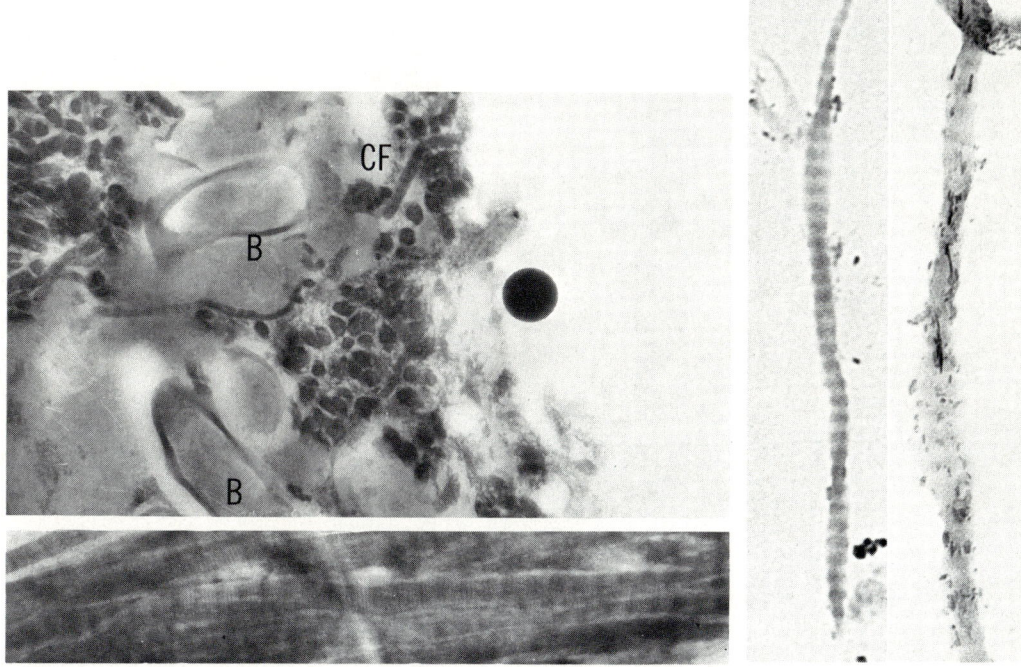

FIG. 8-2 *(Left)* Demineralized, carious permanent human dentin stained with phosphotungstic acid. *(Top, left)* Section of intercanalicular area showing feltwork of collagenous fibrils (CF); bacteria at (B). ×34,600 approx. *(Bottom, left)* Section of intercanalicular matrix; collagenous fibrils exhibit typical banding. ×64,400 approx. *(Middle)* Collagenous fibril isolated from homogenate preparation; note banding and absence of crystallites. ×44,000 approx. *(Right)* Isolated collagenous fibril from homogenate preparation. A few persisting crystallites are associated with the fibril. ×60,000 approx. (Johansen E: Microstructure of enamel and dentin. J Dent Res 43:1007, 1964. Copyright by the American Dental Association. Reproduced by permission)

However, many fibrils, despite the loss of associated crystallites, exhibit typical cross-banding (Llory and Frank, 1969; Fig 8-2). Between the base of the lesion and the dental pulp, the lumens of most of the dentinal tubules become occluded with heavy mineral deposits (Mencis and Darling, 1979). Electron microscope studies indicate that these deposits consist of large crystallites intermingled with the smaller, platelike crystallites usually present (Johansen, 1963; 1964; Fig. 8-3). In addition to the plate-shaped crystals, rhomboid crystals have also been detected in the deep part of the inner carious dentin (Shimizu et al, 1981; Ogawa et al, 1983). Such a mineralization pattern may represent a remineralization process.

Changes in the amino acids of "leathery" carious dentin have been studied by Armstrong (1964). Hydroxyglycine, histidine, lysine, argenine, proline, and hydroxyproline were present in diminished amounts. The largest reduction was in the proline and hydroxyproline contents (30% and 22% respectively). Such reductions might have been produced by the breakdown in peptide bonds of the collagen polypeptide chain by the action of collagenolytic enzymes (collagenases), which are latently bound in dentin (Dayan et al, 1983). After the initial degradation, the collagen is irreversibly denatured (Kuboki et al, 1977). Microorganisms may also be responsible for the elaboration of collagenases, various nonspecific esterases, dehydrogenases, and aminotransferases, all of which play a role in the degradation of dentin lipid, collagen, and ground substance (Larmas, 1972a,b,c).

The uptake of labeled proline under dentin caries was studied autoradiographically by Karjalainen and Söderling (1980). In initial lesions, they found that there was increased labeling of

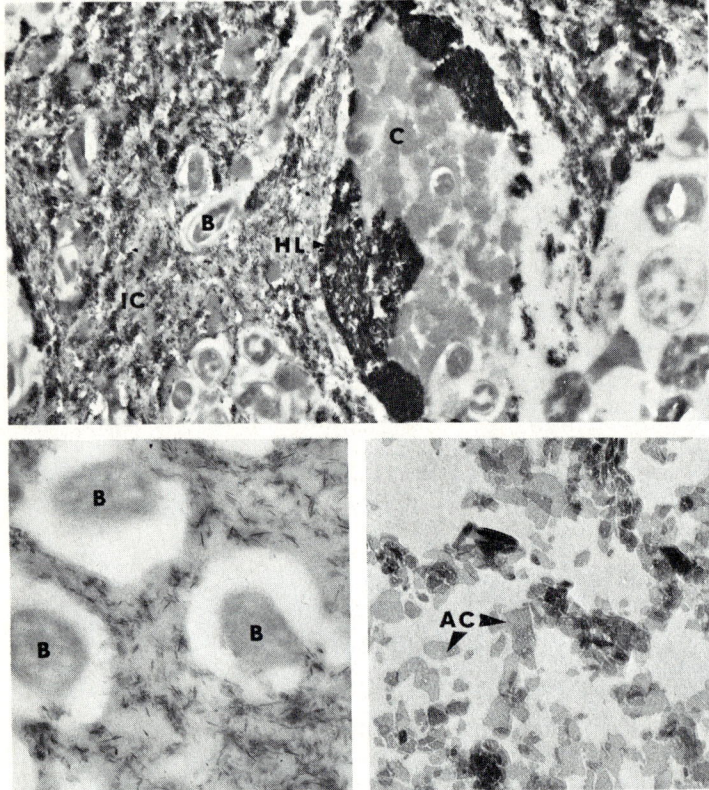

FIG. 8-3 *(Top)* Carious permanent human dentin; inorganic phase. Cross section of dentinal canal. Densely calcified areas (HL) are interposed between the lumen of the canal (C) and the extensively demineralized intercanalicular area (IC); bacteria are seen at B. ×15,000 approx. *(Bottom, left)* Section of intercanalicular area. Bacteria (B) occupy lacunalike spaces; crystallites are seen in edge and broad surface views. ×69,000 approx. *(Bottom, right)* Broad surface view of apatite crystallites (AC) from edge of section. ×105,000 approx. (Johansen E: Microstructure of enamel and dentin. J Dent Res 43:1007, 1964. Copyright by the American Dental Association. Reproduced by permission)

the predentin and decreased labeling of the odontoblastic layer; no alterations were found in the underlying pulp. In advanced lesions, labeling was decreased in the predentin and increased in the odontoblastic layer and the pulp. These findings appear to indicate that initially, caries activates collagen synthesis in a restricted area. However, in the more advanced stages, polypeptide chain formation is increased, but further maturation of collagen is prevented. Alkaline phosphatase, acid phosphatase, and arylsulfatase activities have also been detected in carious dentin (Larmas, 1968). There is also a significant rise in adenosine-triphosphate (ATP) levels in the hard dentin under incipient caries (LeBell and Larmas, 1979). Increased ATP-degrading enzyme activities are also noted in the inflamed pulps of carious teeth (LeBell, 1981).

Formation of a brown pigment in carious dentin was accompanied by an increase of the carbohydrate content from 0.4% to 4.0% of the organic matter. The brown pigment is possibly a reaction product of the newly formed carbohydrate with certain amino acids (Eastoe, 1965), or to degenerative changes in the bacteria (Sarnat and Massler, 1965).

MICROORGANISMS IN CARIOUS DENTIN

Microorganisms or their products most commonly impinge on the dental pulp during the process of dental caries formation. They are always found in caries of the enamel and the dentin and are involved in both demineralization and proteolysis of the enamel and the dentin (see Fig. 8-3). Apparently, tissue fluid from the dental pulp (see Dentinal Pulp Fluid, p. 196) provides a source of nutrition for cariogenic microorganisms (Brown and Wheatcroft, 1966; Brown and Lefkowitz, 1966).

Myriads of microorganisms are found in the superficial layers of carious dentin, while fewer or none are found in the deeper layers, as disclosed by methyl red and ninhydrin staining (Wirthlin, 1970). The microorganisms found in carious dentin are *S. mutans*, lactobacilli, and actinomyces (Loesche and Syed, 1973; McKay, 1976).

According to McKay (1976), bacterial invasion of the dentin occurs in two waves. In the primary invasion, the dentin structure is altered by predominant lactobacilli. A mixed bacterial invasion in the secondary wave is associated with gross dentinal destruction (Edwardsson, 1974).

Controversy has existed as to whether microorganisms precede or follow demineralization of dentin during the process of caries. Older in vitro culture studies (Dorfman et al, 1943; Parikh et al, 1963) have shown that the layer of demineralized but intact dentin under the base of a cavity was almost always sterile. More recently, Al-Marsoomi and Al-Nashi (1980) found that clinically hard dentin was sterile in 50% of extracted carious teeth. In-vivo studies (Crone, 1963; Shovelton, 1968) have indicated that microorganisms may be present in the dentin of a cavity after preparation in at least 36 percent of the cases, even though the dentin floor may clinically appear to be hard. In deep cavities, where a varying amount of softened dentin is permitted to remain, microorganisms are present 68% to 93% of the time (Seltzer, 1940; Shovelton, 1968).

The results of other studies (Whitehead et al, 1960; Fusayama et al, 1966; Shovelton, 1970) emphasize the variability in the detection of microorganisms in dentin.

In electron microscopic studies of carious dentin, some investigators have found that caries of the dentin started in the dentinal tubules and subsequently proceeded into the peritubular and the intertubular matrix. First, demineralization and, then, dissolution of the organic matrix occurred prior to bacterial entrance (Takuma and Kurahashi, 1962).

The electron microscopic studies of Sarnat and Massler (1965) revealed that, in arrested carious lesions, the sclerotic dentinal tubules were free of bacteria. In addition, the deeper layers of active carious lesions were bacteria-free.

FATE OF MICROORGANISMS

What happens to microorganisms in the dentin under a restoration? Schouboe and MacDonald (1962) and Fisher (1966) found that, after considerable periods ranging from 69 to 139 days, the microorganisms in carious dentin sealed in the floor of a cavity by amalgam (a nonantiseptic filling) remained viable and could be cultured. Besic (1943) found that, 1 year after cavities were excavated and filled, the microorganisms tended to die, although, in 30% of the cases, some of them were still viable. It is doubtful that the remaining microorganisms could cause harm (MacGregor, 1962). If a well-fitting restoration is placed so that the microorganisms cannot be reinforced by the saliva, those that remain in the dentin are trapped by the filling material on the outside and, on the pulpal side, by reparative dentin. The microorganisms tend to die. Death of the microorganisms is enhanced by the placement of a calcium hydroxide or zinc oxide-eugenol lining under the restoration (King et al, 1965; Aponte et al, 1966).

The presence of moisture is essential for the growth of microorganisms. However, Dubos (1958) has emphasized that bacteria that survive drying may remain viable for many years. Such dormant bacteria can become active when moisture is reintroduced as a result of marginal percolation of various filling materials, poor marginal seals, or improper condensation of fillings. With the renewal of bacterial activity, the process of caries can begin again.

EFFECTS OF DRUGS

The use of "cavity-sterilizing agents" to kill microorganisms in the dentinal tubules is to be discouraged. It is difficult, if not impossible, to sterilize the base of a cavity with medicaments. Since the medicaments are often more damaging to the dental pulp than are the microorganisms, the use of cavity-sterilizing agents should be avoided. Far greater harm to the pulp results from the use of irritating drugs than from leaving the few microorganisms that may be present within the dentinal tubules. See Dentin Sterilizing Agents, p. 215, in Chapter 10.

DEFENSE AGAINST CARIES

The pulp defends itself against dental caries by producing changes in the primary dentin, by elaborating new dentin, and by inflammatory and immunologic reactions.

DENTINAL CHANGES

In response to the oncoming process of decay, the dentinal tubules of the primary dentin gradually become mineralized, provided the odon-

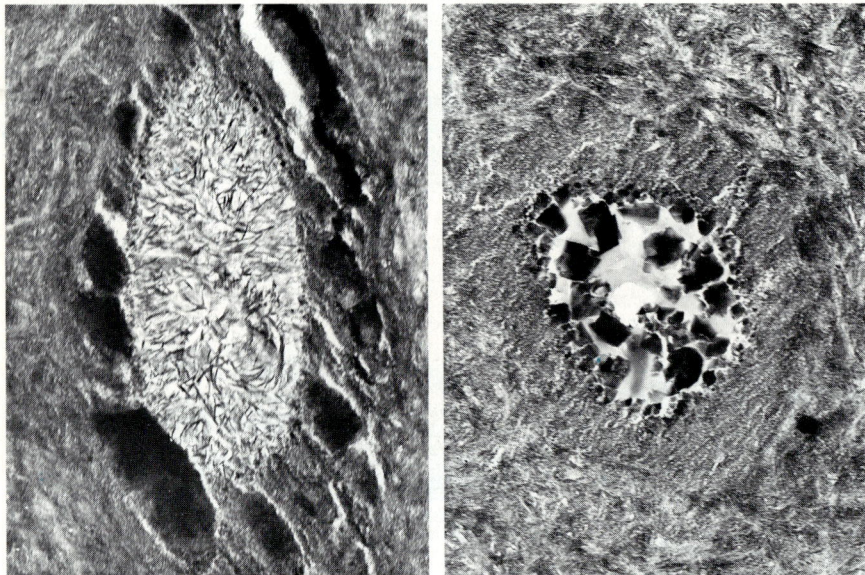

FIG. 8-4 Electron micrographs of dentinal tubule from carious dentin. *(Left)* Note obduration of tubule with needle-shaped crystals. ×38,800. *(Right)* Partial obduration of dentinal tubule with rhombohedral crystals. ×42,500 (Courtesy of Dr. R. M. Frank, Dental Institute, Strasbourg, France)

toblasts remain vital. The distal extension of Tomes' fibers, the protoplasmic processes of the odontoblasts within the dentinal tubules, form peritubular dentin. The peritubular matrix immediately surrounding the odontoblastic process is highly mineralized, in contrast to the remaining intertubular matrix. Sclerosis of the dentin—an increase in peritubular dentin—constitutes the initial defense of the pulp against dental caries, tending to slow down the decay (Trowbridge, 1981). As part of the sclerotic reaction to caries, an increased amount of organic material, collagenous in nature, is elaborated in the dentin, especially in the peritubular and intratubular areas (Levine, 1972). In some cases, large "remineralization (caries) crystals" are deposited in the dentinal tubules beneath the caries (Takuma and Kurahashi, 1962; Frank et al, 1964; Fig. 8-4). Should greater irritation occur, the odontoblasts degenerate and form "dead tracts" (Trowbridge, 1981).

Thus, the opening of the dentinal tubules is followed by a dead tract or sclerotic reaction or both. A band of brown pigment accumulates deep within the lesion (Miller, 1969).

In response to further irritation, as caries progresses, the remaining vital odontoblasts begin to form a less uniform dentin matrix. The dentin thus formed is known as reparative dentin because of its function (Fig. 8-5). The more rapidly the reparative dentin is formed, the less regular is its tubular structure, and this material is often called irregular or amphorous dentin. The reparative dentin is an additional line of defense against further progression of dental caries.

INFLAMMATION UNDER CARIES

Pulp reactions to caries of the enamel have generally been believed to be absent. However, even under white spot lesions of enamel, bacterial products are apparently capable of attracting a few scattered inflammatory cells into the pulp (Brännström and Lind, 1965; Baume, 1970). Nonetheless, both the dentin and the pulp have great resistance to the penetration of microorganisms (Mjör, 1977). After the dentin has become involved by the carious process and reparative dentin has been formed, the pulp may remain relatively normal or the numbers of chronic inflammatory cells may increase slightly (Langeland and Langeland, 1968).

The pulp underlying reparative dentin remains relatively normal until the carious process comes close to it. Just prior to actual exposure by caries, inflammatory changes become manifest (Reeves and Stanley, 1966). The pulp under deep caries, with a thin remaining layer of dentin, is often inflamed and painful but contains no demonstrable bacteria. The degree of inflammation is directly proportional to the depth of dentinal lesion. Bacteria are seldom seen in the unexposed pulp. Scanning and transmission electron microscopic examinations of vital pulps rarely reveal the presence of microorganisms, even under deep carious lesions (Seltzer et al, 1977; Torneck, 1981). When the pulp is exposed, or becomes necrotic, bacteria easily penetrate the infected dentinal tubules (Fig. 8–6). In tissue sections, blood vessels appear dilated and a few scattered inflammatory cells are found extravascularly (Fig. 8–7). This condition, the beginning of inflammation of the pulp, is resolved quickly by placing a sedative dressing such as zinc oxide-eugenol in the cavity. Thus, before exposure, the pulp demonstrates adequate defense capacity against caries. The pulp does not become inflamed until reparative dentin is invaded and wide areas of dentinal tubules are demineralized. This demineralization produces an avenue for ingress of microorganisms or their breakdown products into the pulp.

Experimental Caries-Induced Pulpitis

Pulpitis can be induced in monkey teeth when prepared cavities are sealed with human soft carious dentin (Mjör and Tronstad, 1972; Lervik and Mjör, 1977). When such teeth were examined by transmission electron microscopy, Furseth et al (1980) found that the odontoblastic layers were partly or completely replaced by polymorphonuclear leukocytes (polys). These inflammatory cells also were seen in the dentinal tubules of the predentin and dentin. In some cases, extensive tissue destruction was accompanied by numerous bacteria. Remnants of cells and pulp fibers were seen. The width of the predentin was reduced and the mineralization front was uneven. Similar findings had previously been reported for autogenous caries-induced pulpitis by Torneck (1978).

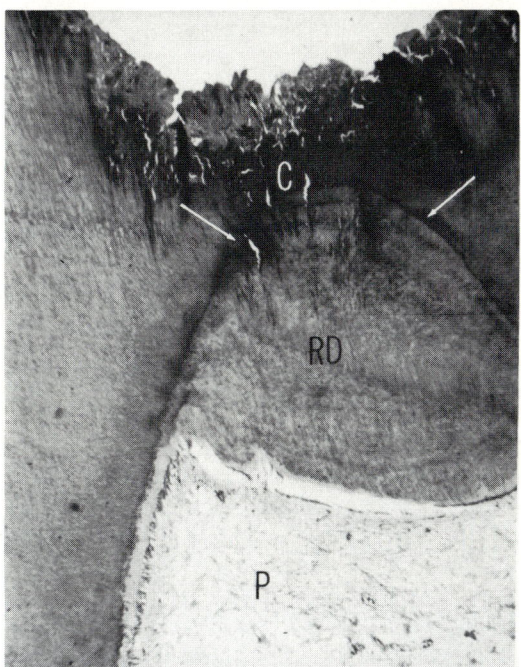

FIG. 8–5 Deep cavity in tooth. The carious process (C) has invaded the original pulp space (arrows). Reparative dentin (RD) has been elaborated as a defense mechanism. The pulp (P) is relatively uninflamed. ×54. (Seltzer S, Bender IB: Modification of operative procedures to avoid postoperative pulp inflammation. JADA 66:503, 1963)

IMMUNOLOGIC REACTIONS TO CARIES

In addition to the dentinal changes, the pulp apparently manufactures antibodies against the antigenic components of dental caries (Torneck, 1981). These immunoglobulins are capable of migrating into the dentin, where they have been detected by Thomas and Leaver (1975) and Okamura et al (1970). Immunoglobulins IgG, IgM (Fig. 8–8), IgA, complement components C_3 and C_4, and secretory component (Fig. 8–9) have been detected by light and electron microscopy and by immunohistochemistry in the cytoplasm of the odontoblasts, in adjacent pulp cells, and in the dentin (Okamura et al, 1980; Ackermans et al, 1981a,b). These components are capable of reacting against the invading caries microorganisms. The presence of bacterial antigens and immunoglobulins in the dentin (and pulp) emphasizes the involve-

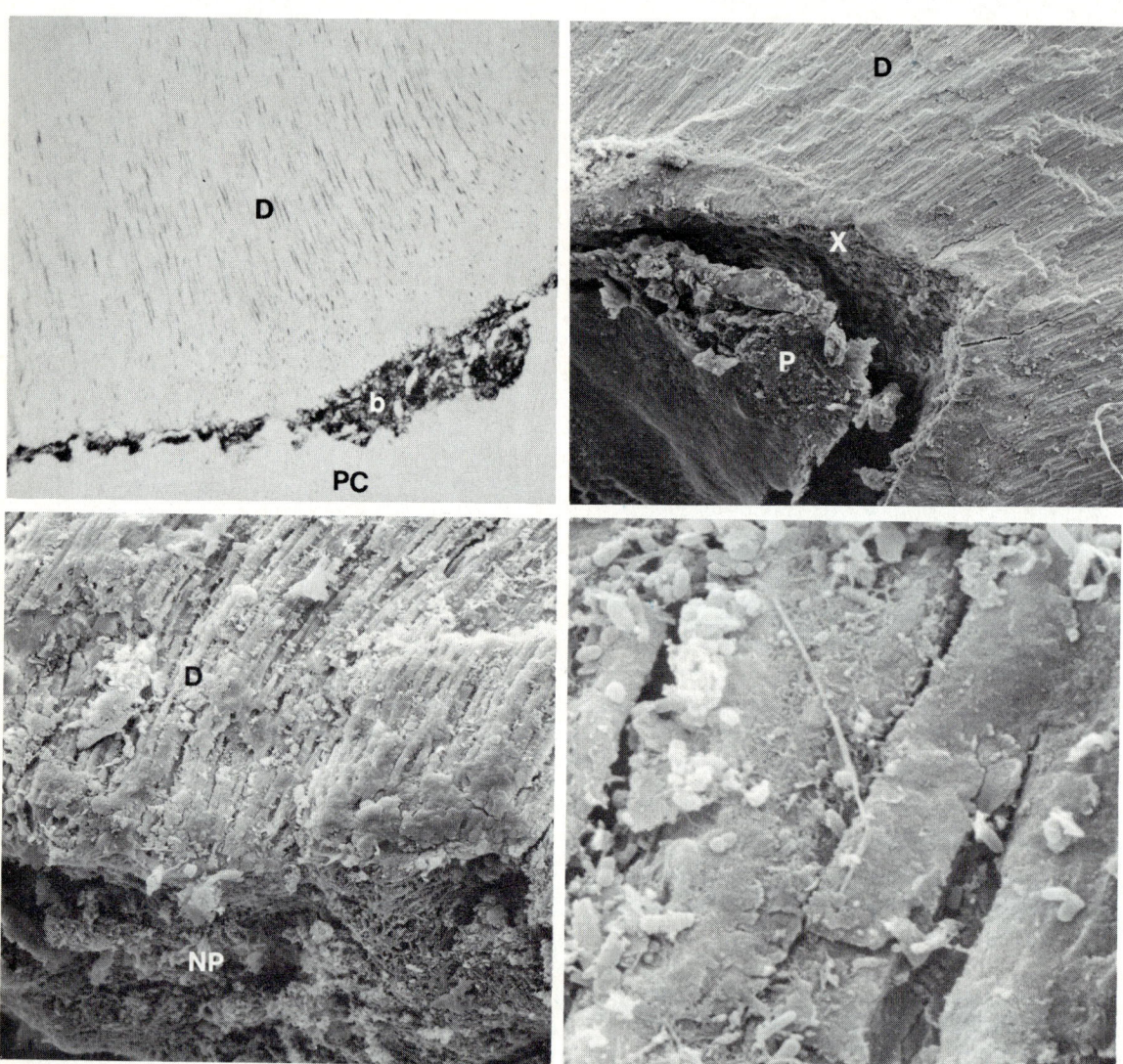

FIG. 8-6 *(Top, left)* Light micrograph showing bacteria (b) in pulp chamber (PC) and dentinal tubules (D) above necrotic pulp. Brown and Brenn stain. ×175. *(Top, right)* Scanning electron micrograph of necrotic pulp (P). D, dentin. ×50. *(Bottom, left)* Higher magnification of area depicted by X in top right. NP, necrotic pulp; D, dentin. ×500. *(Bottom, right)* Bacteria invading dentinal tubules. ×5000.

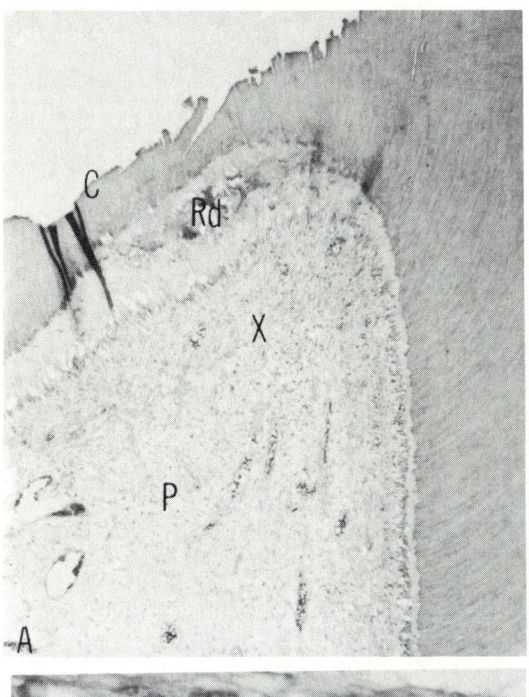

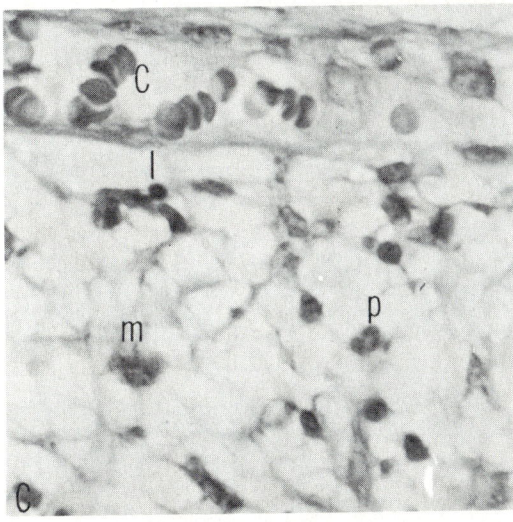

FIG. 8-7 Beginning of inflammation of the pulp under dental caries. *(Top)* Deep carious lesion (C), under which reparative dentin (Rd) has formed. The pulp (P) has a few scattered inflammatory cells within it at region X. ×54. *(Bottom)* Higher magnification of region under pulp horn. Polys (p), lymphocytes (l), and macrophages (m) are present. C, capillary. ×960.

ment of specific immunologic reactions during the carious process.

THE DYNAMICS OF THE DEVELOPMENT OF PULPITIS FROM DENTAL CARIES

The persistence of dental caries for weeks, months, or years provides a continuous stimulus for an inflammatory response within the dental pulp. The pulp protects itself adequately in several ways, depending on the type of caries (active or arrested), and its penetration, the structure of the tooth, the reaction of the underlying dentinal tubules, and the age of the patient (Massler, 1967; Baume, 1970).

The pulp reacts to the process of dental caries by forming sclerotic dentin in the primary dentinal tubules and, also, by the elaboration of reparative dentin under the region of the involved tubules (see Fig. 8-5). In effect, the pulp volume is reduced with the elaboration of reparative dentin, and the aging process of the pulp is accelerated. The formation of reparative dentin increases the collagenous portion of the pulp and decreases its cellular content, thereby reducing pulp defense against further irritants. The amount of reparative dentin elaborated tends to keep pace with the amount of dentin destroyed by the advancing dental caries. In poorly mineralized teeth, the dentinal tubules are massively infected at great depth.

When the caries progresses more rapidly than the elaboration of reparative dentin, the blood vessels of the pulp dilate, and scattered cells of the chronic inflammatory series (macrophages, plasma cells, and lymphocytes, predominantly) become evident in the pulp tissue (Torneck, 1974; see Fig. 8-7). They appear in small numbers initially, but, gradually, as the decay involves the reparative dentin, the number of inflammatory cells increases. At first, in terms of the numbers of inflammatory cells present, the response is mild, inasmuch as the pulp is being only mildly irritated by the products of the carious process. As the decay comes closer to the pulp, more and more macrophages, plasma cells, and lymphocytes are found scattered through the pulp, especially subjacent to the region of the involved dentinal tubules. Finally, a frank exposure occurs (Torneck, 1981; Lin and Langeland, 1981). The pulp reacts at the site of exposure with an infiltration of acute

(Text continues on p. 184)

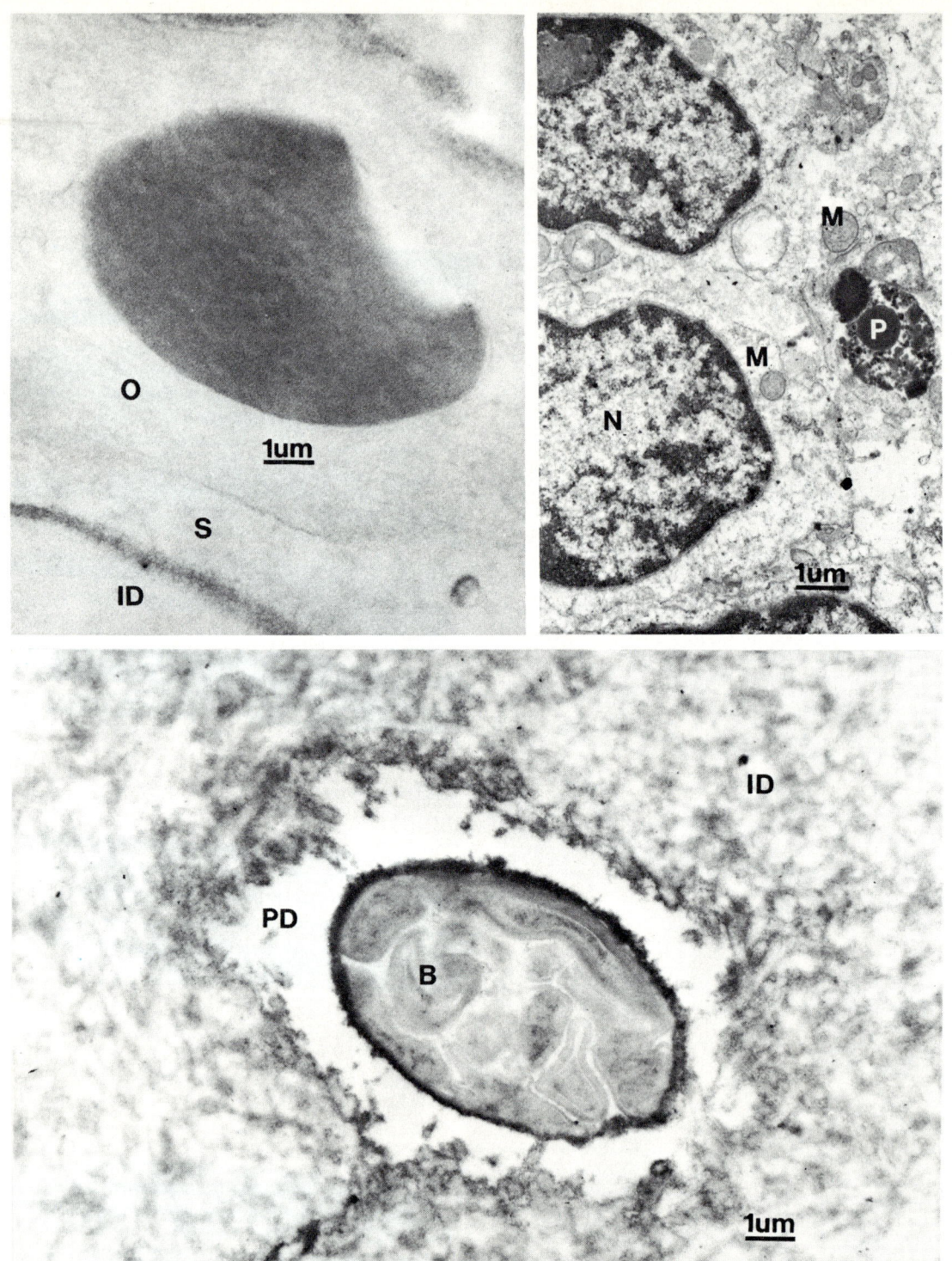

FIG. 8-8 *(Top, left)* Positive reaction for IgM can be seen in a dense vacuole of the odontoblast process (O) of apparently intact inner dentin underlying the carious cone. A dense precipitate is also visible on the wall of the dentinal tubule limited by intertubular dentin (ID). S, organic periodontoblast space. × 60,350. *(Top, right)* An odontoblast underlying the carious cone; positive reactions for SC are present in several dense vacuoles of different sizes. Their heterogeneous aspect and grouping suggests a phagolysosome (P). M, mitochondria.

(Continued)

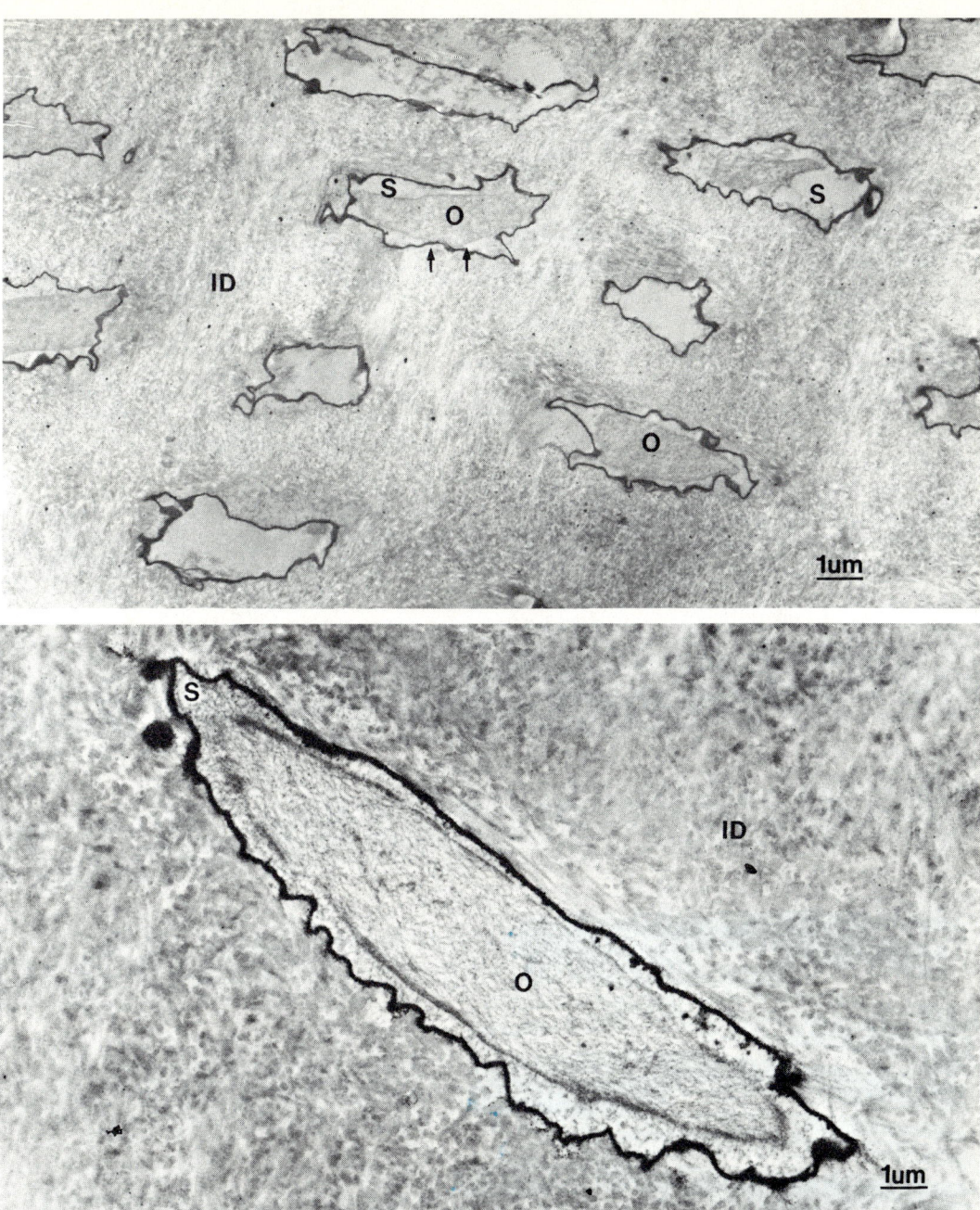

FIG. 8-9 *(Top)* In the inner layer of the carious cone, a strong positive reaction (arrows) for SC is noted along the wall of the dentinal tubule. Note the absence of reaction in the odontoblast process (O). ID, intertubular dentin; S, organic peri-odontoblast space. ×7650. *(Bottom)* Transverse section of a dentinal tubule located in the inner face of the carious cone. A thin and dense positive reaction for IgG is visible on the wall of the dentinal tubule. ID, intertubular dentin; O, odontoblast process; S, organic peri-odontoblast space. ×11,900. (Ackermans F, Klein JP, Frank RM: Ultrastructural localization of immunoglobulins in carious human dentine. Arch Oral Biol 26:879, 1981)

×17,017. *(Bottom)* Cross section of a carious dentinal tubule invaded by several microorganisms (B). A positive reaction for IgG is present on the wall of the dentinal tubule with a less marked precipitate at the border between peritubular dentin (PD) and intertubular dentin (ID). ×26,350. (Ackermans F, Klein JP, Frank RM: Ultrastructural localization of immunoglobulins in carious human dentine. Arch Oral Biol 26:879, 1981)

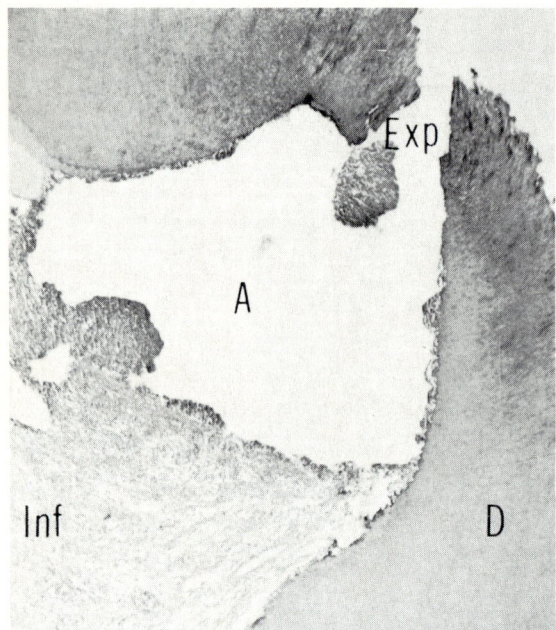

FIG. 8-10 Composite photomicrograph of pulp abscess (A) under carious pulp exposure (Exp). Chronically inflamed pulp tissue (Inf) is present beneath the abscess. D, dentin. ×54.

neck (1978). Protein-carbohydrate complexes become markedly degraded. Concurrently, tissue synthesis occurs in the chronically inflamed areas. Reaggregation and rearrangement of argyrophilic fibrils and metachromatic ground substance predominate. The fibroblasts are probably responsible for the synthesis of the matrix, since they demonstrate a high content

FIG. 8-11 Chronic partial pulpitis. Composite photomicrograph, showing carious exposure (EXP) in the upper portion. The coronal portion of the pulp is inflamed (INF). In the lower portion, the pulp (P) has widely dilated blood vessels (BV), but no inflammatory cells are present. ×54.

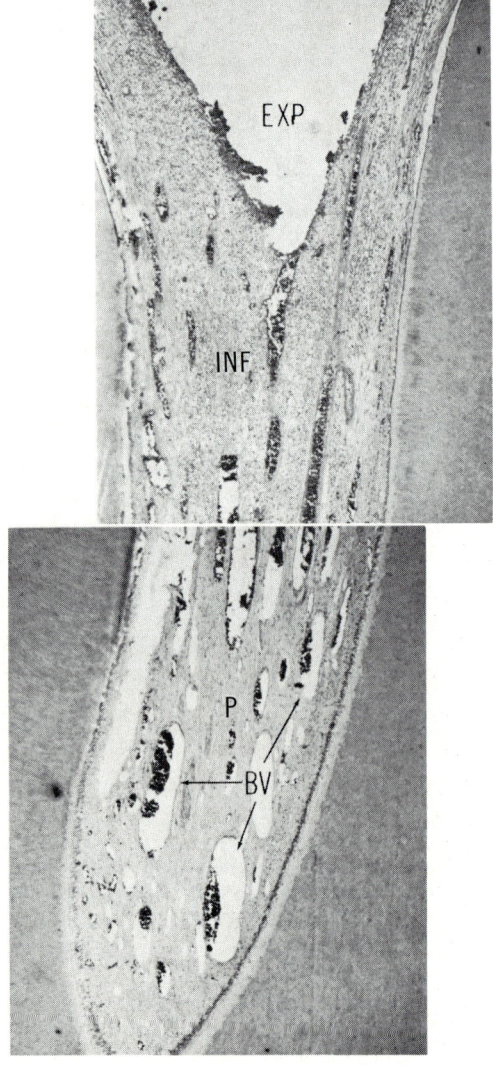

inflammatory cells (i.e., polys), and the chronic pulpitis then becomes acute.

Clinically, a small abscess develops within the coronal portion of the pulp under the region of the exposure (Fig. 8-10). Here, dead or dying polys, together with other dead cells, are present. Many polys are evident surrounding the area of pus, and the cells of the chronic inflammatory series are found farther away from the central area of irritation. The remainder of the pulp may be uninflamed (Fig. 8-11), or, if the exposure has been present for a long time, the pulp may have been converted to granulation tissue (Fig. 8-12). Dystrophic mineralizations may be formed in long-standing granulation tissue (Fig. 8-12). The inflammatory cells themselves mineralize and are eventually incorporated in the mineralized mass (Fig. 8-13). Histochemical studies (Zerlotti, 1969) have indicated that, during the acute phases of caries-induced pulpitis, tissue components break down. Argyrophilic and collagen fibers become fragmented and disrupted. Intracellular digestion of these fibers by fibroblasts has been reported by Ten Cate et al (1976) and by Tor-

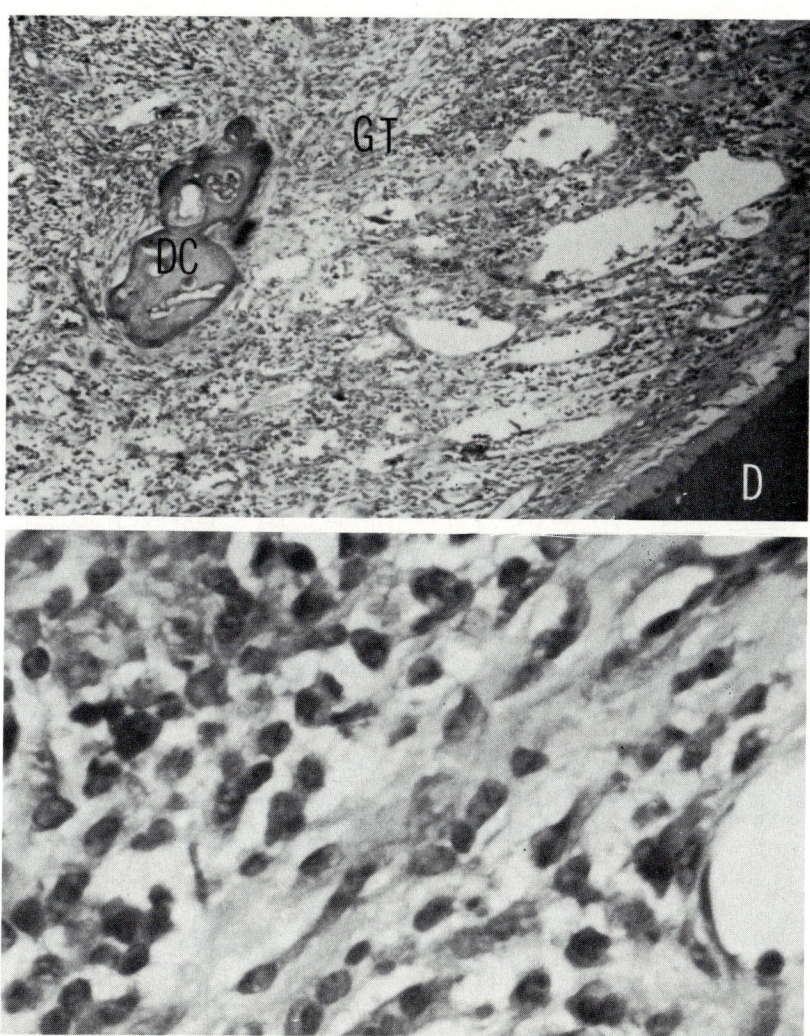

FIG. 8-12 Chronic total pulpitis. *(Top)* The pulp has been converted to granulation tissue (GT). A small region of dystrophic calcification (DC) has formed. D, dentin. ×96. *(Bottom)* Higher magnification of the cells of the granulation tissue. The cells are macrophages, lymphocytes, and plasma cells. ×960.

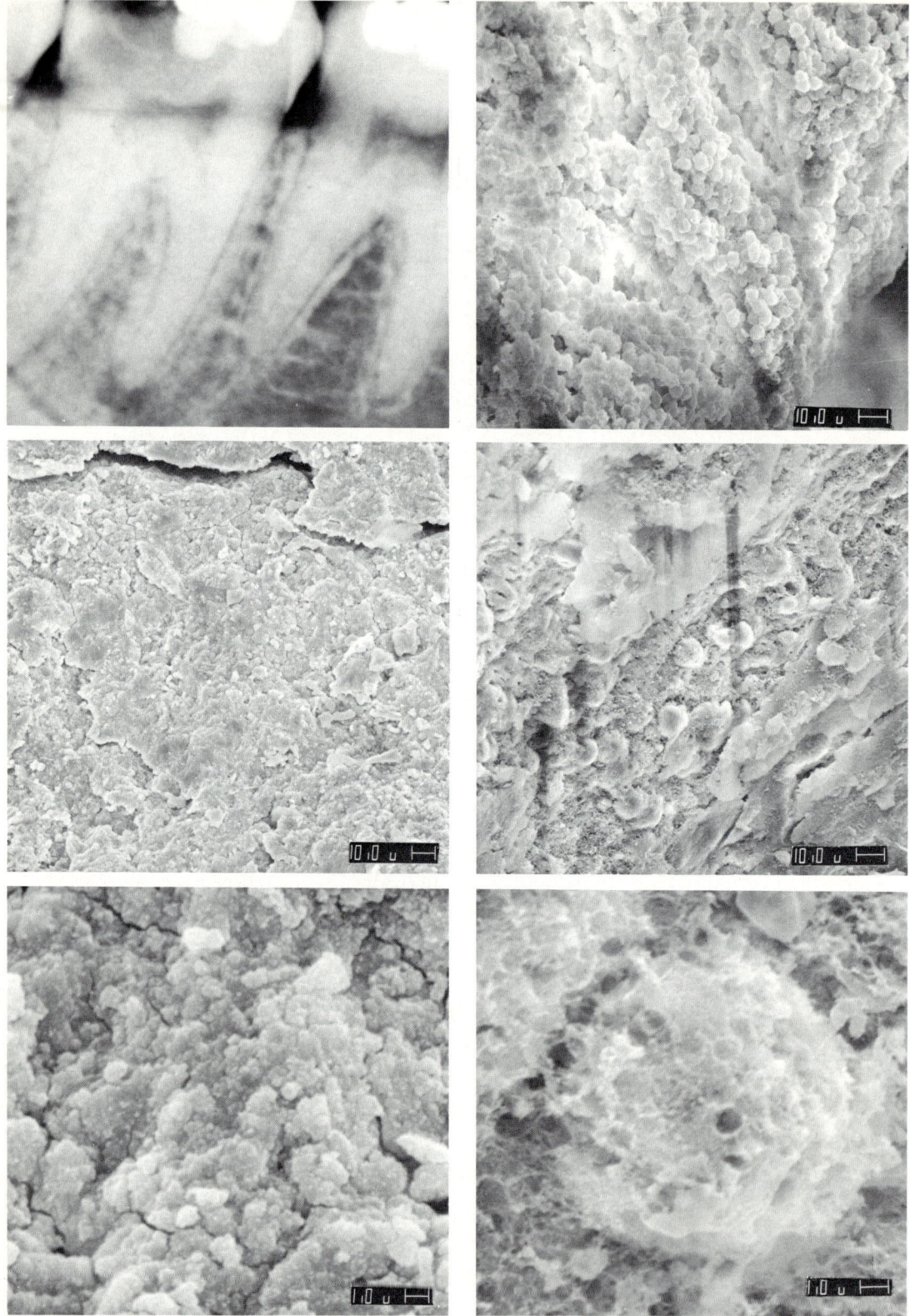

of ribonucleic acid (RNA), as well as granule-containing glycoproteins, acid mucopolysaccharides, sialic acid, and proteins bearing free ε-amino groups of lysine-hydroxylysine.

When a pulp has been exposed by dental caries, the lesion may be called ulcerative pulpitis or pulpitis, open-form, inasmuch as the surface covering of the pulp (the dentin) has been removed, leaving the pulp exposed to the oral fluids. Chronic pulpitis, open-form, usually requires endodontic treatment, since, generally, the prognosis for capping an exposed, chronically inflamed pulp is poor. Recovery is possible but unlikely. Instead, the entire pulp may become acutely inflamed, or total necrosis may ensue. If left untreated, the pulpitis may become painful as a result of food packing or pressure, or chronic pulpitis may gradually involve the entire pulp and, consequently, the periapical tissues as well.

The pulp that remains chronically inflamed for a long time exhibits many new capillary buds, an abundance of fibroblasts, and collagen fibers. Scattered throughout are many macrophages, lymphocytes, and plasma cells. When the inflammation persists for long periods, fibroblasts or undifferentiated mesenchymal cells elaborate dentinal matrix, which, with subsequent mineralization, narrows the root canal.

Thus, following exposure by dental caries, chronic inflammation develops in the pulp, but this is not due to the perpetuation of an acute reaction; rather, it begins insidiously, as a low-grade smoldering response that never has the classic features of the acute form. This process usually continues for longer periods, perhaps years.

Thus, breakdown of the pulp from caries results in the formation of an abscess directly beneath the region of the invading microorganisms, perhaps mediated by the release of lysosomal hydrolases from the polys (Taichman, 1970). In the remainder of the coronal pulp tissue, the chronic inflammatory infiltrate with its rich content of macrophages, lymphocytes, and plasma cells may indicate the presence of an antibody-mediated hypersensitivity reaction. Excessive antigens available in high concentrations from the microorganisms involved in the carious process may cause synthesis of immunoglobulins. The immune antigen-antibody precipitates thus formed may, in the presence of complement, become chemotactic for polymorphonuclear leukocytes (Ward et al, 1965, 1966). Phagocytosis of these immune precipitates (Uriuhara and Movat, 1964) may then result in cell degradation, with release of lysosomes into the pulp tissue. The liberation of proteases (Movat et al, 1964) would then result in the formation of a pulp abscess. Immune complexes have been detected in experimentally induced pulpal Arthus reactions in rabbits (Adamkiewicz and Pekovic, 1980) and in monkeys (Bergenholtz et al, 1977). The rich granulation tissue barrier below the abscess prevents further spread of inflammation into the radicular pulp tissue. Gradually, with repeated episodes of poly-mediated Arthus-type reactions, the immune response reaches into the radicular tissue, and eventually into the periapical tissues, where a typical granulomatous lesion develops.

The chronic inflammation may be partial or total, depending on the extent and amount of pulp tissue involved. The pulp tissue in the radicular portion of the tooth is usually uninflamed, except for the presence of dilated blood vessels. As the exposure progresses, the partial necrosis of the pulp may be followed, in some instances, by total pulp necrosis. In other instances, the apical pulp tissue may remain chronically inflamed for long periods. Necrosis may be of the coagulation type, or it may be liquefactive or gangrenous, in which case there is a combination of coagulation and liquefactive necrosis. Drainage appears to be a factor determining whether or not partial or total necrosis occurs. If the pulp is open to the oral fluids, drainage occurs, and the apical pulp tissue may remain uninflamed or chronically inflamed. If the opening becomes closed as a result of food packing or restoration, the entire pulp may become necrotic more rapidly. Figure 8–14 depicts the reaction of the pulp to dental caries.

◀ **FIG. 8–13** *(Top, left)* Radiograph of lower left second molar with deep carious exposure. *(Middle, left)* Carious dentin. ×400. *(Bottom, left)* Microorganisms in carious dentin. ×4000. *(Top, right)* Inflammatory cells (lymphocytes and macrophages) in mid-root area. ×500. *(Middle, right)* Inflammatory cells surrounded by mineralized material. ×500. *(Bottom, right)* Lymphocyte. ×5000. (Seltzer S, Rainey E, Gluskin AH: Correlation of scanning electron microscope and light microscope findings in uninflamed and pathologically involved human pulps. Oral Surg 43:910, 1977)

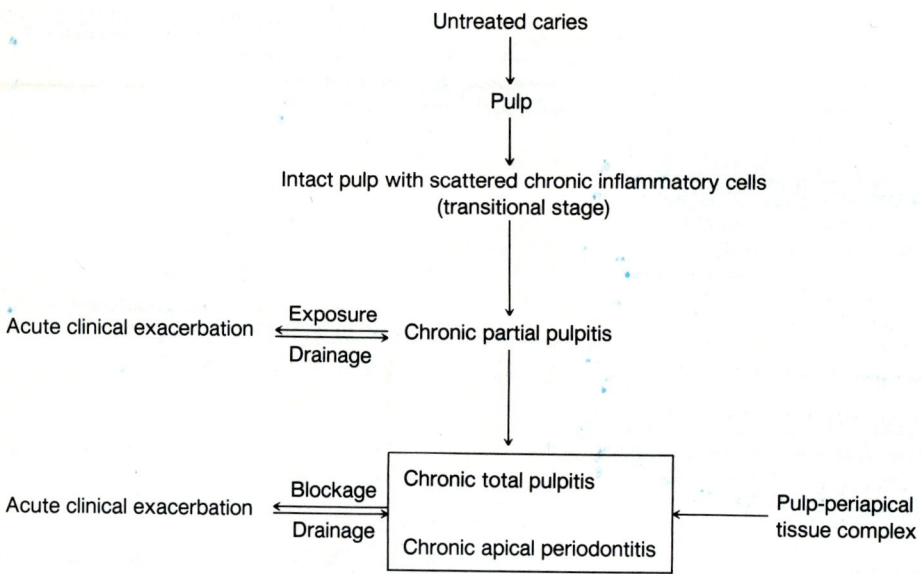

FIG. 8-14 Pulp reactions to dental caries.

INDIRECT PULP CAPPING

What procedure should be employed in deep-seated caries where there is danger of exposing the pulp if all of the decay is excavated? Should all of the decay be excavated, resulting in exposure, or should some decay be left, in order to avoid exposure of the pulp? The latter procedure is referred to as indirect pulp capping. In our view, pulps that are uninflamed, in a transitional stage, or in a stage of chronic partial pulpitis without liquefaction necrosis (See Chap. 18, Differential Diagnosis) are amenable to indirect pulp capping procedures. If, in the operator's judgment, removal of the "last spoonful" of decay would result in a pulp exposure, the leaving of some decay in the tooth is justified in all cases not involving partial or total necrosis of the pulp. Cotton's experiments (1974) have led him to a similar conclusion. Soft, mushy or leathery decay always should be removed. Only when the dentin is intact, yet demineralized, can this procedure be expected to yield successful results.

If the pulp is exposed, a hazard to recovery even greater than the decay results. In the act of exposing the pulp, tissue is crushed and blood vessels are opened, thereby creating hemorrhage within the pulp. When bleeding occurs inside the pulp chamber (where it is not visible), the pressure of the hemorrhage kills other pulp cells. The pulp-capping material that must then be placed directly on the pulp is irritating (see Chap. 14, Pulp Capping and Pulpotomy). Therefore, it is better *not* to subject the pulp to these hazards, if they are avoidable. It is preferable to leave some of the decay and place a calcium hydroxide or zinc oxide-eugenol dressing. Should the operator wish, he may remove the remaining carious dentin a month or 6 weeks later with greater assurance that a pulp exposure will not occur. Reentry to the cavity for the complete removal of carious dentin has been recommended by Leung et al (1980). Whether this is necessary has not yet been definitely determined.

Indirect pulp capping is clinically successful. Numerous investigators have used calcium hydroxide (Law and Lewis, 1961; Sawusch, 1982; Fairbourn et al, 1980; Leung et al, 1980); others have used zinc oxide-eugenol (Jordan and Suzuki, 1971; Hutchins and Parker, 1972; Fairbourn et al, 1980). In all of these investigations, the results were decidedly favorable in terms of a clinically successful outcome.

The number of microorganisms remaining in the dentin is reduced by the use of indirect pulp capping agents, such as zinc oxide-eugenol or calcium hydroxide (Fisher, 1972; Fairbourn et al, 1980; Leung et al, 1980). When used for

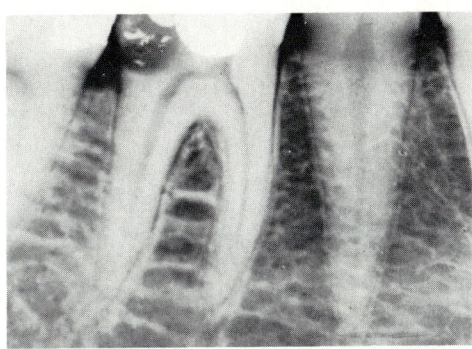 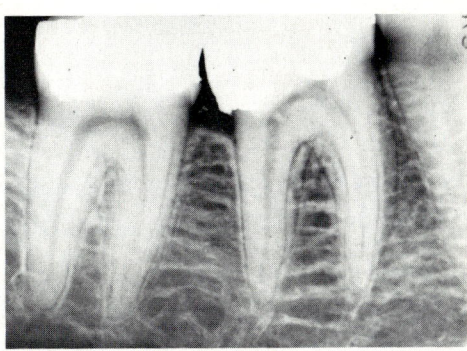

FIG. 8-15 Indirect pulp capping. *(Left)* Deep carious lesion of lower left first molar. Patient was symptom-free. Complete removal of decay would have resulted in pulp exposure. Instead, gross caries was removed and a zinc oxide-eugenol dressing was placed. *(Right)* Eight years later: the tooth is still asymptomatic, and the pulp is vital.

indirect pulp capping, calcium hydroxide has also been shown to stimulate remineralization of demineralized dentinal tubules, as determined by their increased phosphorus content (Eidelman et al, 1965).

A number of studies have demonstrated that demineralized dentin is capable of undergoing remineralization (Solomons and Neuman, 1960; Bang and Urist, 1967; Levine, 1972; Alacam and Yilmaz, 1983). It is possible that dentin demineralized from caries contains sufficient organic matrix and nuclei of calcium and phosphate ions to initiate remineralization once the cavity is sealed from the saliva. The dentin under calcium hydroxide and zinc oxide-eugenol has been demonstrated to become denser, probably as a result of additional mineralization in the walls of the dentinal tubules (Mjör, 1960; Eidelman et al, 1965; Ehrenreich, 1968).

There does not appear to be a significant advantage for any specific type of calcium hydroxide preparation. Okada et al (1979) compared the effects of various commercial preparations with aqueous suspensions of calcium hydroxide as indirect pulp-capping agents on 100 vital human teeth. They found no correlation between clinical and histopathologic results. Clinically, the treatment of all of the cases was deemed successful, involving insignificant pain. In all of the cases, histopathologic changes varied from none to a slight to moderate hyperemia; a slight to moderate degree of hemorrhage, and an absence of, or a mild degree of, round cell infiltration. There were minimal dentin changes. Histologically, the aqueous suspension of calcium hydroxide caused fewer changes, whereas use of the commercial preparations produced the best clinical results. No increased calcific deposits in the pulp or narrowing of the root canals was observed in the absence of pulp exposures.

In deeply carious teeth, it may be advisable to use hand instruments to remove undermined enamel walls. The decay then may be excavated and zinc oxide-eugenol placed into the cavity, provided the operator is sure that a pulp exposure is not present. When doubt exists, calcium hydroxide should be used. All demineralized dentin need not be removed. Leathery, mushy, disorganized dentin should be removed, but intact demineralized dentin need not be. Transitional inflammatory pulpal states may thus be resolved (Fig. 8-15).

Only when a massive invasion of microorganisms occurs, as in a pulp exposure, does an infection ensue (Fig. 8-16). Removal of most of the decay results automatically in removal of large numbers of microorganisms and their toxic products. Thus, the number of irritants is reduced and the possibility of repair enhanced. Zinc oxide-eugenol not only has mild antibacterial action but also is hygroscopic, thereby removing some of the moisture in the leathery decay and thus creating an environment less favorable to the growth of microorganisms.

ANACHORESIS

Microorganisms can reach the dental pulp by anachoresis, a process in which microorganisms carried by the bloodstream from another source

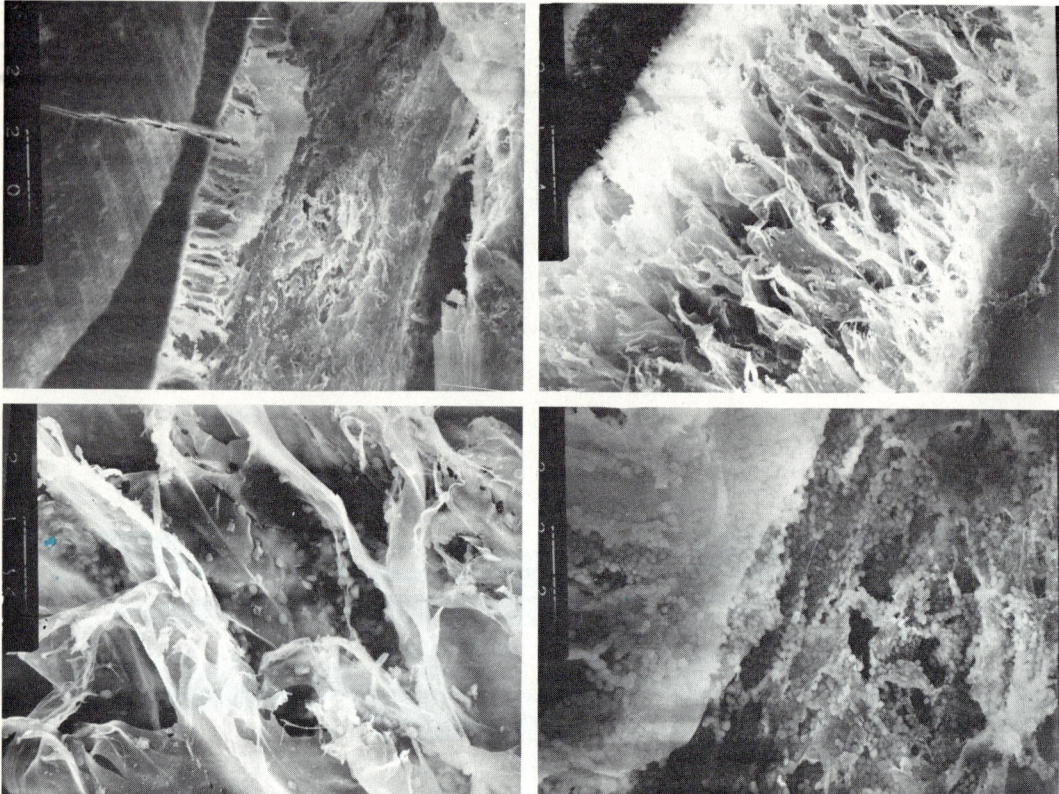

FIG. 8-16 *(Top, left)* Scanning electron micrograph of cariously exposed pulp. ×250. *(Top, right)* Higher magnification of odontoblastic layer. ×300. *(Bottom, left)* Higher magnification of disrupted odontoblasts shown in top right frame, revealing bacteria in tissue. ×1000. *(Bottom, right)* Deeper pulp tissue invaded by masses of bacteria. ×1000.

localize on inflamed tissue. Robinson and Boling (1941) prepared cavities in cats' teeth and placed croton oil (a severe irritant) and milder irritants on the dentin of the prepared cavities. Then they injected a culture of known microorganisms into the bloodstream. They found that the test microorganism localized in the inflamed pulps of 72% of the teeth as compared with only 8.5% in the controls. During the process of inflammation in the pulp caused by the croton oil, blood vessels became leaky, and the microorganisms escaped into the inflamed area.

In other experiments on rats, Burke and Knighton (1960) and Smith and Tappe (1962), in separate studies, extended Robinson and Boling's experimental design to include histopathologic and statistical data covering longer periods of observation. Localization of injected microorganisms in pulps occurred with greater frequency in the increasingly severe pulp inflammations resulting from blows, heat injury and pulp exposure. When the interval between injury and bacterial injection was increased, the incidence of bacterial localization was reduced.

BACTERIAL INVASION AS A RESULT OF PRESSURE

Bacterial invasion of the pulp through the dentinal tubules may be caused by pressure. In vitro experiments by Michelich et al (1980) have demonstrated that a hydrostatic pressure of 240 cm Hg was sufficient to filter bacteria across 1 mm of acid-etched dentin in less than 20 minutes. Hydrostatic pressures exceeding 240 cm Hg may develop on exposed dentin during mastication.

Bacteria can be introduced into the pulp when a modeling compound or a wax impression is taken of dentin that is moist with saliva. The penetration of bacteria depends on the depth of the cavity preparation, inasmuch as pressure can force the bacteria through the dentinal tubules more readily in deep preparations. If the pulp is already chronically inflamed, the introduction of bacteria through pressure on the tubules may result in infection of the pulp. This is similar to the anachoretic phenomenon of Robinson and Boling.

BACTEREMIA ASSOCIATED WITH OPERATIVE MANIPULATION

Wagoner and Kruger (1963) reported that detectable bacteremia can occur following Class 1 and Class 2 cavity preparations. In a series of 50 cases, preoperative bacteremia was demonstrated in four patients.

Eight blood cultures were positive following cavity preparations, and five were positive after the application of the matrix band. The researchers claimed that four cases developed bacteremia following Class 1 preparations in the absence of periodontal disease. They found no relationship between tooth mobility and the incidence of bacteremia. However, it is unlikely that a detectable bacteremia actually occurs after operative procedures. In our studies, bacteremia could not be detected when teeth were subjected to vital pulp extirpation, even when the root canals were exposed to oral fluids and filed vigorously for 10 minutes. Bacteremia was not produced when the instrumentation was confined in the root canal. Beechen et al (1956) also could not demonstrate detectable bacteremia after pulpotomy procedures.

Microorganisms can be detected in the pulps of all teeth that have been extracted with forceps. Microorganisms that are present in the gingival crevice or pocket of the tooth are pumped into the bloodstream and thence into the pulp vessels through the rocking action of the forceps. Therefore, detection of the presence of microorganisms in the pulp of an extracted tooth has little significance.

In clinical practice, the few microorganisms that get into the pulp usually are engulfed by the defense cells and are quickly phagocytized. However, if the pulp should be injured severely as a result of cumulative traumata, such as may be caused by repeated crown preparations, leaky temporary restorations and application of drugs together with pressure, a severe inflammatory response would occur in the pulp. If an impression of such a tooth bathed in saliva is taken with modeling compound, the pressure could force microorganisms through the dentin, and they may localize in the pulp.

Since development of infection depends on the virulence and concentration of the microorganisms, as well as other factors, it does not necessarily follow that, every time bacteria are introduced into the pulp because of pressure, an infection will develop locally or a bacteremia will ensue. Conversely, pulp injury is not necessarily related to the presence of microorganisms. For example, as a result of a blow to the tooth; hemorrhage of ruptured blood vessels occurs within the pulp; the circulation is impaired, and the pulp may die. An area of rarefaction may develop, yet there is no positive culture. On the other hand, a root canal infection sometimes may be detected when a patient has received a blow on an intact anterior tooth and the pulp has become necrotic (Brown and Rudolph, 1957; MacDonald et al, 1957; Chirnside, 1957). Inasmuch as there is no apparent direct connection between the pulp chamber or pulp canal and the external environment, a positive culture might result from anachoresis, in the following manner. In patients with periodontal disease, a transient bacteremia is caused occasionally by chewing. The microorganisms, temporarily in the bloodstream, could then localize and grow on the inflamed pulp tissue.

PERIODONTAL INVOLVEMENT

Pulps may become infected by microorganisms through accessory canals in all teeth and, especially, through lateral canals in the furcation regions of molars in periodontally involved teeth. In teeth with deep pockets in which the attachment apparatus has receded, accessory or lateral canals act as avenues through which microorganisms enter the pulp and cause pulp inflammation.

Pulpitis can be induced in monkey teeth by sealing lyophilized material, from oral bacteria isolated from human dental plaque, for 32 hours into deep cavities (Bergenholtz and Lindhe, 1975).

SYSTEMIC INFECTIONS

Although the dental pulp may become infected by almost any microorganism that is capable of infecting connective tissue, reports of such systemic infections invading the pulp are rather sparse. Stanley (1973) has reported that the microorganisms of tuberculosis, leprosy, actinomycosis, and aspergillosis have been recovered from the pulps of patients with those diseases.

BIBLIOGRAPHY

Ackermans F, Klein JP, Frank RM: Ultrastructural localization of immunoglobulins in carious human dentine. Arch Oral Biol 26:879, 1981a

Ackermans F, Klein JP, Frank RM: Ultrastructural location of streptococcus mutans and streptococcus sanguis antigens in carious human dentine. J Biol Buccale 9:203, 1981b

Adamkiewicz VW, Pekovic DD: Experimental pulpal arthus allergy. Oral Surg 50:450, 1980

Akpata ES, Blechman H: Bacterial invasion of pulpal dentin wall in vitro. J Dent Res 61:435, 1982

Alacan T, Yilmaz T: In vivo remineralization of carious dentin treated with 10% solution of stannous fluoride. J Endodont 9:313, 1983

Armstrong WG: Chemistry of carious enamel and dentin. J Dent Res 43:1002, 1964

Bang G, Urist MR: Recalcification of decalcified dentin in the living animal. J Dent Res 46:722, 1967

Baume LJ: Dental pulp conditions in relation to carious lesions. Int Dent J 20:309, 1970

Beechen II, Lasten DJ, Garbarino VE: Transitory bacteremia as related to the operation of vital pulpotomy. Oral Surg 9:902, 1956

Bergenholtz G, Ahlstedt S, Lindhe J: Experimental pulpitis in immunized monkeys. Scand J Dent Res 85:396, 1977

Bergenholtz G, Lindhe J: Effect of soluble plaque factors on inflammatory reactions in the dental pulp. Scand J Dent Res 83:153, 1975

Besic FC: The fate of bacteria sealed in dental cavities. J Dent Res 22:349, 1943

Brännström M, Lind PO: Pulpal response to early dental caries. J Dent Res 44:1045, 1965

Brown LR, Lefkowitz W: Influences of dentinal fluids on experimental caries. J Dent Res 45:1493, 1966

Brown LR, Rudolph EE: Isolation and identification of microorganisms from unexposed canals of pulp-involved teeth. Oral Surg 10:1094, 1957

Brown LR, Wheatcroft MG: Effect of the diffusion of microbial growth factors through tooth substance on production of carious lesions in vitro. J Dent Res 45:830, 1966

Burke GW, Jr, Knighton HT: The incidence of microorganisms in inflamed dental pulps of rats following bacteremia. J Dent Res 39:205, 1960

Chirnside IM: A Bacteriological and histological study of traumatized teeth. N Zeal Dent J 53:176, 1957.

Chirnside IM: Bacterial invasion of non-vital dentin. J Dent Res 40:134, 1961

Cotton WR: Bacterial contamination as a factor in healing of pulp exposures. Oral Surg 38:441, 1974

Dayan D, Binderman I, Mechanic GL: A preliminary study of activation of collagenase in carious human dentine matrix. Arch Oral Biol 28:185, 1983

Dorfman A, Stephan RM, Muntz JA: In vitro studies on sterilization of carious dentin. II. Extent of infection in carious lesions. JADA 30:1901, 1943

Eastoe JE: The chemical composition of bone and tooth. Adv Fluor Res Dent Car Prev 3:5, 1965

Edwardsson S: Bacteriological studies on deep areas of carious dentine. Odont Revy 25 (Suppl 32) 1974

Ehrenreich DW: A comparison of the effects of zinc oxide-eugenol and calcium hydroxide on carious dentin in human primary molars. J Dent Child 35:451, 1968

Eidelman E, Finn SB, Koulourides T: Remineralization of carious dentin treated with calcium hydroxide. J Dent Child 32:218, 1965

Fairbourn DR, Charbeneau GT, Loesche WJ: Effect of improved Dycal and IRM on bacteria in deep carious lesions. JADA 100:547, 1980

Fisher FJ: The viability of micro-organisms in carious dentine beneath amalgam restorations. Brit Dent J 121:413, 1966

Fisher FJ: The effect of a calcium hydroxide/water paste on micro-organisms in carious dentine. Brit Dent J 133:19, 1972

Fitzgerald RJ: The potential of antibiotics as caries-control agents. JADA 87:1006, 1973

Fitzgerald RJ, Keyes PH: Demonstration of the etiologic role of streptococci in experimental caries in the hamster. JADA 61:9, 1960

Fitzgerald RJ: Ecologic factors in dental caries. The fate of antibiotic-resistant cariogenic streptococci in hamsters. Am J Path 42:759, 1963

Frank RM, Wolff F, Gutmann B: Microscopie électronique de la carie au niveau de la dentin humaine. Arch Oral Biol 9:163, 1964

Furseth R, Mjör IA, Skogedal O: The fine structure of induced pulpitis in a monkey (cercopithecus aethiops). Arch Oral Biol 24:883, 1980

Fusayama T, Okuse K, Hosoda H: Relationship between hardness, discoloration, and microbial invasion in carious dentin. J Dent Res 45:1033, 1966

Hutchins DW, Parker WA: Indirect pulp capping: clinical evaluation using polymethyl methacrylate reinforced zinc oxide-eugenol cement. J Dent Child 39:55, 1972

Johansen E: Ultrastructural and chemical observations on dental caries. In Sognnaes R (ed): Mechanisms of Hard Tissue Destruction, pp 187–211. Washington, DC, Pub No 75, Am Ass Adv Sci 1963

Johansen E: Microstructure of enamel and dentin. J Dent Res 43:1007, 1964

Jordan RE, Suzuki M: Conservative treatment of deep carious lesions. J Canad Dent Ass 37:337, 1971

Karjalainen S, Söderling E: The autoradiographic pattern of the in vitro uptake of proline by the coronal areas of intact and carious human teeth. Arch Oral Biol 24:909, 1980

Keyes PH, Jordan HV: Factors influencing the initiation, transmission, and inhibition of dental caries. In Mechanisms of Hard Tissue Destruction, pp 261–283. Washington, Pub No 75, Am Ass Adv Sci 1963

Kuboki Y, Liu C-F, Fusayama T: Mechanism of differential staining in carious dentin. J Dent Res 52:713, 1983

Kuboki Y, Ohgushi K, Fusayama T: Collagen biochemistry of the two layers of carious dentin. J Dent Res 56:1233, 1977
Langeland K: Management of the inflamed pulp associated with deep carious lesion. J Endodont 7:169, 1981
Langeland K, Langeland LK: Indirect capping and the treatment of deep carious lesions. Int Dent J 18:326, 1968
Larmas M: Histochemical studies on phosphatase and arylsulfatase activity in human carious dentin. Acta Odont Scand 26:357, 1968
Larmas M: A chromatographic and histochemical study of nonspecific esterases in human carious dentine. Arch Oral Biol 17:1121, 1972a
Larmas M: Alanine and aspartate aminotransferases in sound and carious human dentine. Arch Oral Biol 17:1133, 1972b
Larmas M: Histochemical demonstration of various dehydrogenases in human carious dentine. Arch Oral Biol 17:1143, 1972c
Law DB, Lewis TM: The effect of calcium hydroxide on deep carious lesions. Oral Surg 14:1130, 1961
Le Bell Y: Ca^{2+}- and Mg^{2+}-activated ATP hydrolysis in human tooth pulp. J Dent Res 60:128, 1981
Le Bell Y, Larmas M: Adenosine-5′-triphosphate levels of the human tooth pulp during health and disease. Arch Oral Biol 24:313, 1979
Lervik T, Mjör IA: Evaluation of techniques for the induction of pulpitis. J Biol Buccale 5:137, 1977
Leung RL, Loesche WJ, Charbeneau GT: Effect of Dycal on bacteria in deep carious lesions. JADA, 100:193, 1980
Leverett DH: Fluorides and the changing prevalence of dental caries. Science 217:26, 1982
Levine RS: The distribution of hydroxyproline in the dentine of carious human teeth. Arch Oral Biol 17:127, 1972
Levine RS: Remineralization of human carious dentine in vitro. Arch Oral Biol 17:1005, 1972
Lin LB, Langeland K: Light and electron microscopic study of teeth with carious pulp exposures. Oral Surg 51:292, 1981
Llory H, Frank RM: Ultrastructure de la dentine cariée. Actualités Odontostomat 88:507, 1969
Loesche WJ, Syed SA: The predominant cultivable flora of carious plaque and carious dentine. Caries Res 7:201, 1973
McKay GS: The histology and microbiology of acute occlusal dentine lesions in human permanent premolar teeth. Arch Oral Biol 21:51, 1976
MacDonald JB, Hare GO, Wood AWS: The bacteriologic status of the pulp chambers in intact teeth found to be nonvital following trauma. Oral Surg 10:318, 1957
Al-Marsoomi A, Al-Nashi Y: Bacteriology of deep-seated carious lesions. Oral Surg 49:89, 1980
Massler M: Pulpal reactions to dental caries. Int Dent J 17:443, 1967
Massler M, Pawlak J: The affected and infected pulp. Oral Surg 43:929, 1977
Mendis BRRN, Darling AI: A scanning electron microscope and microradiographic study of closure of human coronal dentinal tubules related to occlusal attrition and caries. Arch Oral Biol 24:725, 1979
Michelich VJ, Schuster GS, Pashley DH: Bacterial penetration of human dentin in vitro. J Dent Res 59:1398, 1980
Miller WA: Spread of carious lesions in dentin. JADA 78:1327, 1969
Miller WA: Fat staining in carious dentin. J Dent Res 48:109, 1969
Miyauchi H, Iwaku M, Fusayama T: Physiological recalcification of the carious dentin. Bull Tokyo Med Dent Univ 25:169, 1978
Mjör IA: Bacteria in experimentally infected cavity preparations. Scand J Dent Res 85:599, 1977
Mjör IA: Microscopic changes in dentin. Alabama Dent Rev 8:1, 1960
Mjör IA: Histologic studies of human coronal dentine following cavity preparations and exposure of ground facets in vivo. Arch Oral Biol 12:247, 1967
Mjör IA, Kvam E: Dental pulp reactions following the exposure of coronal dentine in vivo. Acta Odont Scand 27:145, 1969
Mjör IA, Tronstad L: Experimentally induced pulpitis. Oral Surg 34:102, 1972
Movat HZ, Uriuhara T, Macmorine DL, Burke JS: A permeability factor released from leukocytes after phagocytosis of immune complexes and its possible role in the Arthus reaction. Life Sciences 3:1025, 1964
Newbrun D: Sugar and dental caries: A review of human studies. Science 217:418, 1982
Ogawa K, Yamashita Y, Ichijo T, Fusayama T: The ultrastructure and hardness of the transparent layer of human carious dentin. J Dent Res 62:7, 1983
Okada T, Ito A, Asai Y: Clinico-pathological studies of the effects of various kinds of calcium hydroxide compounds as indirect pulp capping agents on human vital pulp tissues. Bull Tokyo Dent Coll 20:61, 1979
Okamura K, Maeda M, Nishikawa T, Tsutsui M: Dentinal response against carious invasion: Localization of antibodies in odontoblastic body and process. J Dent Res 59:1368, 1980
Okamura K, Tanaka A, Kakehi A, Maeda M, Tsutsui M: Plasma components in deep carious lesions of human carious dentin. J Dent Res 58:2010, 1979
Orland FJ, Blayney JR, Harrison RW, Reyniers JA, Trexler PC, Erwin RF, Gordon HA, Wagner M: Experimental caries in germ free rats inoculated with enterococci. JADA 50:259, 1959
Parikh SR, Massler M, Bahn A: Microorganisms in active and arrested carious lesions of dentin. NY Dent J 29:347, 1963
Paterson RC, Pountney SK: Pulp response to dental caries induced by *streptococcus mutans*. Oral Surg 53:88, 1982
Reeves R, Stanley HR: The relationship of bacterial penetration and pulpal pathosis in carious teeth. Oral Surg 22:59, 1966
Robinson HBG, Boling LR: Anachoretic effect in pulpitis. JADA 28:268, 1941
Sarnat H, Massler M: Microstructure of active and arrested dentinal caries. J Dent Res 44:1389, 1965
Schouboe T, MacDonald JB: Prolonged viability of organisms sealed in dentinal caries. Arch Oral Biol 7:525, 1962
Seltzer S: The bacteriologic status of the dentin after cavity preparation. JADA 27:1799, 1940
Seltzer S, Bender IB, Kaufman IJ: Histologic changes in dental pulps of dogs and monkeys following application

of pressure, drugs, and microorganisms on prepared cavities, Part I. Part II, Changes observable more than one month after application of traumatic agents. Oral Surg 14:327, 856, 1961

Seltzer S, Rainey E, Gluskin AH: Correlation of scanning electron microscope and light microscope findings in uninflamed and pathologically involved human pulps. Oral Surg 43:910, 1977

Shimizu C et al: Carious change of dentin observed on longspun ultrathin sections. J Dent Res 60:1826, 1981

Shovelton, DS: A study of deep carious dentine. Int Dent J 18:392, 1968

Shovelton, DS: Studies of dentine and pulp in deep caries. Int Dent J 20:283, 1970

Skogedal O, Tronstad L: An attempt to correlate dentin and pulp changes in human carious teeth. Oral Surg 43:135, 1977

Smith LS, Tappe GD: Experimental pulpitis in rats. J Dent Res 41:17, 1962

Solomons CC, Neuman WF: On the mechanisms of calcification: the remineralization of dentin. J Biol Chem 235:2502, 1960

Stanley HR: The effect of systemic diseases on the human pulp. In Siskin M (ed): The Biology of the Human Dental Pulp, p 606. St. Louis, CV Mosby, 1973

Symons NBB: Electron microscopic study of the tubules in human carious dentine. Arch Oral Biol 15:239, 1970

Taichman NS: Mediation of inflammation by the polymorphonuclear leukocyte as a sequela of immune reactions. J Periodont 41:228, 1970

Takuma S, Kurahashi Y: Electron microscopy of various zones in a carious lesion in human dentine. Arch Oral Biol 7:439, 1962

Ten Cate AR, Deporter DA, Freeman E: The role of fibroblasts in the remodeling of periodontal ligament during physiologic tooth movement. Am J Orthodont 69:155, 1976

Thomas M, Leaver AG: Identification and estimation of plasma proteins in human dentine. Arch Oral Biol 20:217, 1975

Torneck CD: Changes in the fine structure of the dental pulp in human caries pulpitis. Inflammatory infiltration. J Oral Path 3:83, 1974

Torneck CD: Intracellular destruction of collagen in the human dental pulp. Arch Oral Biol 23:745, 1978

Torneck CD: 1. A report of studies into changes in the fine structure of the dental pulp in human caries pulpitis. J Endodont 7:8, 1981

Trowbridge HO: 2. Pathogenesis of pulpitis resulting from dental caries. J Endodont 7:52, 1981

Uriuhara T, Movat HZ: Allergic inflammation. IV. The vascular changes during the development and progression of the direct, active and passive Arthus reaction. Lab Invest 13:1057, 1964

Wagoner RP, Kruger GO: Bacteriological investigation of bacteremias following restorative dental procedures utilizing blood sampling techniques. J Dent Res Abs 135, 1963

Ward PA, Cochrane CG, Müller-Eberhard HJ: The role of serum complement in chemotaxis of leukocytes in vitro. J Exp Med 122:327, 1965

Ward PA: Further studies on the chemotactic factor of complement and its formation in vivo. Immunol 11:141, 1966

Whitehead FIH, MacGregor AB, Marsland EA: Experimental studies of dental caries. II. The relationship of bacterial invasion to softening of the dentine in permanent and deciduous teeth. Brit Dent J 108:261, 1960

Wirthlin MR, Jr: Acid-reacting stains, softening, and bacterial invasion in human carious dentin. J Dent Res 49:42, 1970

Zerlotti E: Histochemical changes in the connective tissue of the dental pulp during inflammation. Oral Surg 27:664, 1969

9
MECHANICAL AND THERMAL IRRITANTS

When the dentist drills a tooth, sterilizes a cavity, applies a cavity liner or base, or performs other common operative procedures, he almost always causes some damage to the pulp. Sometimes, the ensuing inflammation of the pulp is slight; for example Mjör (1967) and Mjör and Kvam (1969) have shown that the pulp can protect itself well from exposure of the coronal dentin to the oral environment through shallow grinding; the surface layer of the dentin becomes hypermineralized. Not infrequently, however, pulp reactions are intense.

Severe pulp damage may develop in a tooth with an originally normal pulp after full crown preparation. The chemicals used to sterilize the dentin or in dental cements cause injury to the pulp tissues. Extremes of heat and cold are damaging to pulp tissue. The mechanical irritants, pressures used in dentistry, such as those used for impression taking, foil malleting, and so forth, are capable of producing pulp damage. Trauma occurring to a tooth as a result of a fall causes injury. X-irradiation causes damage to pulp tissue. If an individual receives large doses of radiation in the region of the head or the neck for carcinoma, the pulps of the teeth may be injured.

In this and the following chapters, the various pulp irritants and some of the conditions favorable and unfavorable to the health of the pulp are discussed in detail.

"DENTISTOGENIC" (IATROGENIC) PULPITIS

Some commonly used operative procedures endanger the health of the tooth more than do the disease processes they are intended to correct. Decay, in many instances, is much less harmful than the operative procedure used to treat it — a state of affairs that should cause sober reflection on the part of the practicing dentist. Pulp inflammation for which the dentists' own procedures are responsible may well be designated "dentistogenic pulpitis" (i.e., "dentist-induced" pulpitis — similar to the term iatrogenic, "physician-induced").

REASONS FOR PREVENTING PULPITIS

The effect of postoperative inflammation may be to shorten the period during which the pulp remains vital and to impair resistance of the pulp to subsequent irritation. If the dentist, by modifying his operative techniques, can reduce damage to the pulp, he will minimize the possibility that the tooth eventually will require endo-

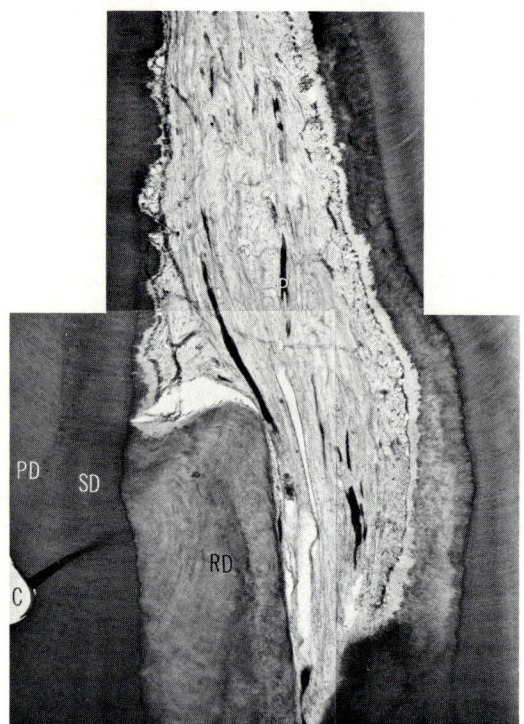

FIG. 9-1 Composite photomicrograph, showing reparative dentin formation, in response to dental caries. C, a portion of the cavity. Below the primary (PD) and the secondary dentin (SD), the pulp (P) has elaborated reparative dentin (RD). ×54.

dontic treatment or extraction. Such modification is possible when the causes of pulp irritation are understood. The operative procedures least likely to cause significant postoperative inflammation are presented.

When a tooth becomes carious, the pulp tissue responds to the irritation by laying down reparative dentin subjacent to the involved dentinal tubules (Fig. 9-1). This process mitigates further effects of irritation on the underlying pulp tissue, thereby tending to preserve the vitality of the pulp. However, when previously uninvolved dentin is operated on, as in extension for prevention or full crown preparation, tubules are cut that are not protected by reparative dentin. A cavity preparation one square millimeter in area would uncover 12,000 to 50,000 dentinal tubules, according to the observations of Melková (1966) and Brännström and Åström (1972). According to Garberoglio and Brännström (1976), the number of dentinal tubules varies according to location. By scanning electron microscopy, they examined the coronal dentin of human teeth in various age groups. Near the pulp, they found about 45,000 tubules per mm^2. In the middle dentin, there were 29,500 tubules per mm^2. At the periphery, the number of tubules decreased to 20,000/mm^2. There were no differences in the numbers of tubules based upon age.

The cutting of primary dentin renders the involved odontoblasts more vulnerable to damage than those that were previously exposed to the process of decay. Thus, the process of reaction to decay seems to afford some protection to the pulp from ensuing operative trauma.

Dentinal Pulp Fluid

Fluid flow from the dental pulp through the dentin and enamel has been demonstrated in vivo (Bergman et al, 1966; Steinman and Leonora, 1975; Pashley et al, 1981a,b). Larger protein molecules in the fluid are apparently unable to penetrate the dentinoenamel junction.

Cutting of the dentinal tubules or odontoblastic processes causes changes in the injured protoplasm that result in leakage of fluid. Brännström's experiments (1963) demonstrated that this outward flow of fluids causes displacement of the odontoblastic nuclei into the dentinal tubules through capillary action. Haldi and Wynn (1963) and Stüben and Kreudenstein (1957) suggested that the fluid is a capillary transudate from the pulp, because they found electrophoretic evidence that the pulp fluid from a dog's tooth contains the same protein fractions as the blood plasma. Numerous serum and plasma proteins have also been found, by immunofluorescent techniques, to be adsorbed on dentin and the odontoblasts (Okamura et al, 1979 a,b).

In addition, glucose, potassium, sodium, chlorine, magnesium, urea, and alkaline phosphatase concentrations are similar in the dentinal fluid and the blood plasma, as determined by chemical and electron microprobe analysis (Haldi et al, 1965; Coffey et al, 1970). However, the dentinal fluid may also contain a component elaborated by the odontoblastic processes (Haljamäe and Röckert, 1970) and soluble ground substance of dentin (Paunio, 1966). Systemically administered chemotherapeutic agents, such as sulfonamides and penicillin, also have been detected in the dental pulp fluid in the same concentration as in the blood plasma (Haldi and John, 1965).

When the pulp of a tooth is examined histolog-

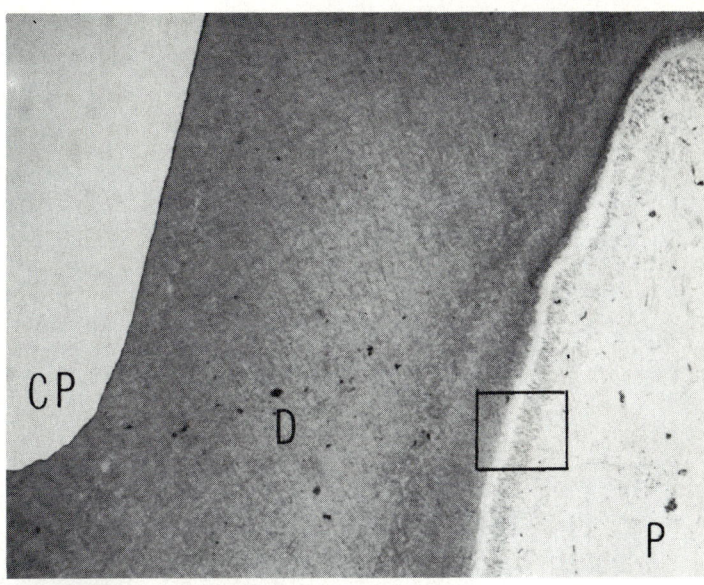
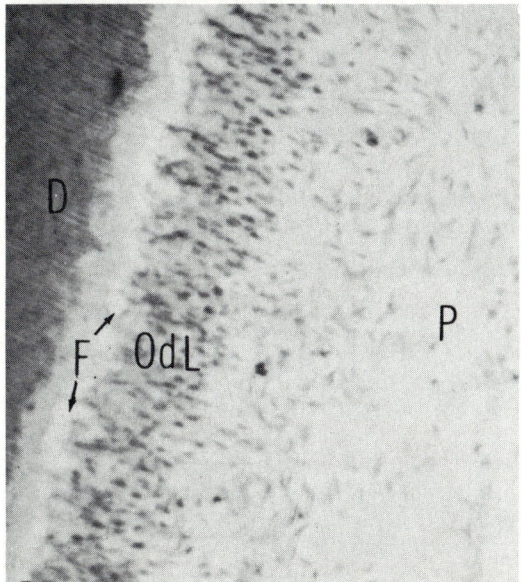

FIG. 9-2 Mild reaction to moderately deep cavity preparation. *(Top)* Cavity preparation (CP) with several millimeters of dentin (D) remaining causes little visible reaction within the dental pulp (P). ×54. *(Bottom)* Higher magnification of region outlined by rectangle in top picture. The odontoblastic layer (OdL) is only mildly disturbed by slight accumulation of fluid (F). P, pulp. ×240.

ically after an operative procedure such as cutting of the dentin, the odontoblastic layer subjacent to the cavity preparation typically exhibits changes attributable to the fluid exudate; these include displacement of odontoblastic nuclei, disturbance of the pulpodentinal membrane and various degrees of inflammation of the pulp. The amount of odontoblastic disturbance, the degree of inflammation, and the subsequent repair are influenced by a number of factors that are discussed in the following sections.

DEPTH OF CAVITY PREPARATIONS

Cavity preparation causes an increased rate of dentin collagen turnover (Hoppenbrouwers et al, 1982) and some odontoblastic cell damage (Kawahara and Yamagami, 1970). Protein synthesis by the odontoblasts directly under, and adjacent to, the cavity preparation is curtailed (Searles, 1975).

The deeper a cavity is cut and, therefore, the

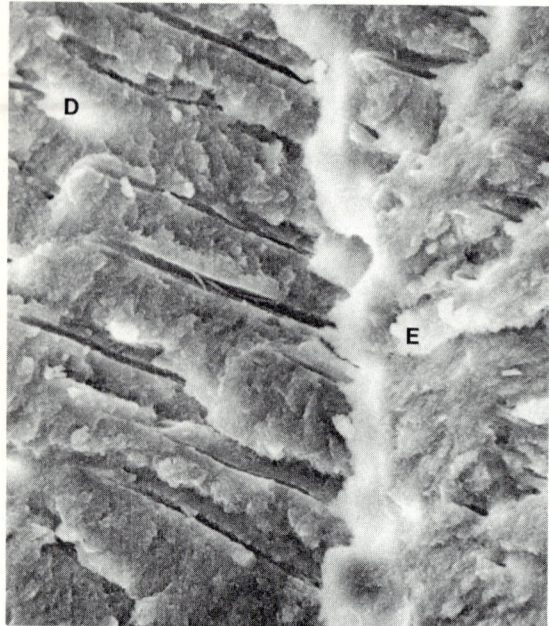

FIG. 9-3 Scanning electron micrograph of dentinoenamel junctional area of human incisor. Odontoblastic processes are absent. D, dentin; E, enamel. ×1800.

Pashley's experiments (1979, 1981) have shown that a reduction in dentin thickness markedly increases its permeability to ^{125}I. The closer the dentin preparation is to the pulp, the greater the number of dentinal tubules per unit surface area. Closer to the pulp, there is also an increase in the diameter of each tubule. Both of

FIG. 9-4 *(Top)* Moderately deep cavity preparation (C) in the dentin (D) causes increase quantitatively in the production of reparative dentin (Rd) by the pulp (P). ×54. *(Bottom)* Higher magnification of region outlined by rectangle in top picture. The odontoblastic layer (OdL) of the pulp (P) is thinned under the reparative dentin (Rd). D, dentin. ×960.

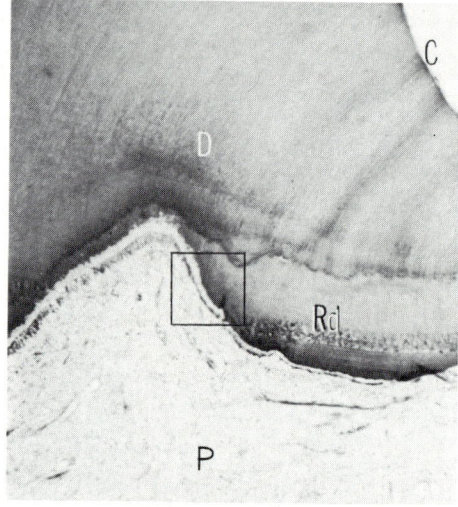

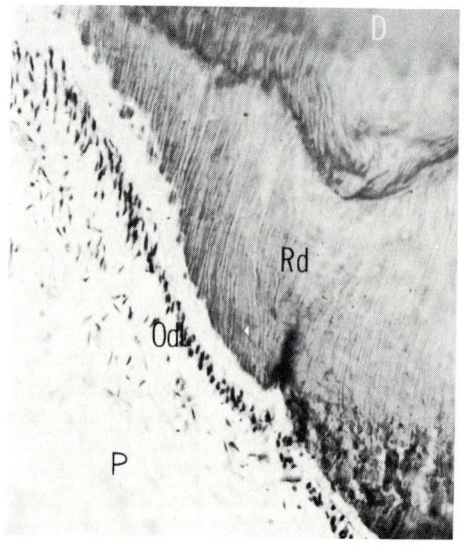

closer the odontoblastic nucleus is approached, the more severe is the injury to the odontoblast. A superficial cavity preparation that cuts the odontoblastic processes close to the dentinoenamel junction usually produces only mild irritation (Fig. 9-2). Whether such a shallow preparation actually results in cutting of the odontoblastic processes is yet to be settled. Light and electron miscroscope studies by Brännström and Garberoglio (1972), Holland (1976), Garberoglio and Brännström (1976), and Thomas (1979, 1983) indicate that, in cats and man, the odontoblastic processes do not extend to the dentinoenamel junction (DEJ; Fig. 9-3). Other investigators (Kelley et al, 1981; Grossman and Austin, 1983) have found the processes at or near the DEJ in the dentinal tubules of monkey tooth samples examined by scanning electron microscopy. Regardless, the underlying odontoblasts are stimulated to produce regular reparative dentin. As the cavity depth is increased, and with the cutting of the odontoblastic processes, there is an increase in irritation, with a consequent increase in the rate of production of reparative dentin (Fig. 9-4).

these factors contribute to an increase in diffusional surface area in dentin.

The degree of inflammatory reaction of the pulp also is increased proportionately, in direct relation to the depth of the cavity preparation. When not more than 0.5 mm of dentin remain between the base of a cavity and the pulp, each decrease of 0.1 mm produces progressively more severe pulp inflammation in low-speed preparations without coolant.

When low-speed preparations are made with proper cooling devices, the floor of the preparation can be brought much closer to the pulp (0.3 mm) with less danger of severe inflammatory response. With high-speed preparations also (200,000 rpm and more), the damage is less severe, provided adequate cooling is delivered at the interface between the bur and the dentin.

The effects of further operative procedures on the pulp are influenced by the depth of the cavity preparation. For example, if a cavity of medium size is prepared, the use of zinc phosphate cement is acceptable. However, when the cavity is deep, zinc phosphate cement is irritating, and a sedative dressing such as zinc oxide-eugenol should be used instead, to allay the inflammation induced in the pulp, prior to filling. The degree of inflammatory response is in no way related or proportional to the pain produced. The absence of postoperative pain is not an indicator of the absence of pulp inflammation.

RELATIONSHIP OF DEPTH OF PREPARATION TO REPARATIVE DENTIN FORMATION

The relationship between increased rate of reparative dentin formation and increased depth of cavity preparations holds only if the dentin remaining between the pulp and the dentinoenamel junction is at least half the original thickness. At that level, the maximal threshold of stimulation is reached. Further cutting of the dentin causes greater injury to the odontoblasts. The rate of formation of reparative dentin begins to decrease and the structure becomes irregular. The reparative dentin lacks its usual tubular structure and is poorly mineralized. At greater depths, with less thickness of remaining dentin, formation of reparative dentin becomes inhibited temporarily, and the odontoblastic cells show signs of atrophy.

The speed of reparative dentin formation after cavity preparation depends on variation in cavity depths. On microscopic examination the formation of reparative dentin was found to begin earlier in shallow cavities and later in deep cavities. In deep cavity preparations, the odontoblasts require a longer period for recovery. However, once reparative dentin formation begins in deep cavities, its rate is more rapid but the quality is poorer than that of the dentin formed under shallow cavity preparations.

SPEED OF ROTATION

When dentin is cut by rotary instruments at various speeds, an odontoblastic reaction will occur; the injury varies in degree only. The greatest amount of odontoblastic damage occurs at speeds up to 50,000 rpm with both belt-driven and turbine-driven instruments. The least amount of damage occurs at speeds of 150,000 to 250,000 rpm, provided that a coolant is used properly. Marsland and Shovelton (1957) and Langeland (1961) reported that very low speeds (300–500 rpm) produced an absence of, or a reduction in, odontoblastic reactions.

According to Marsland and Shovelton (1957), speeds from 5000 to 15,000 rpm are more destructive to the human odontoblast than speeds under 3000 rpm without coolants. Swerdlow and Stanley (1958) showed that, at 20,000 rpm, odontoblastic damage occurs whether or not a coolant is used. However, the reactions in the "nonspray" specimens were much more severe. From 50,000 to about 250,000 rpm, if the coolant is delivered properly, reactions are minimal.

Without the use of a coolant, there is no safe speed. However, with sharp burs at 3000 to 5000 rpm, without coolant, there is less damage than at ultra-high speeds without coolant (Riethe, 1969).

High-speed cutting is disadvantageous when burs are countersunk into the dentin, since water is excluded in a confined region. Burns of the dentin following the use of high-speed instruments have been demonstrated histologically (Fig. 9–5). The integrity of the pulp is threatened and the charred dentinal tubules are more susceptible to subsequent decay.

Numerous investigators have suggested that ultra-high speeds be used for the removal of enamel and superficial dentin and the finishing of the preparations be made with very low speeds. It may be concluded from the evidence thus far at hand that speeds of 3000 rpm or less and 200,000 rpm and above are the safest, pro-

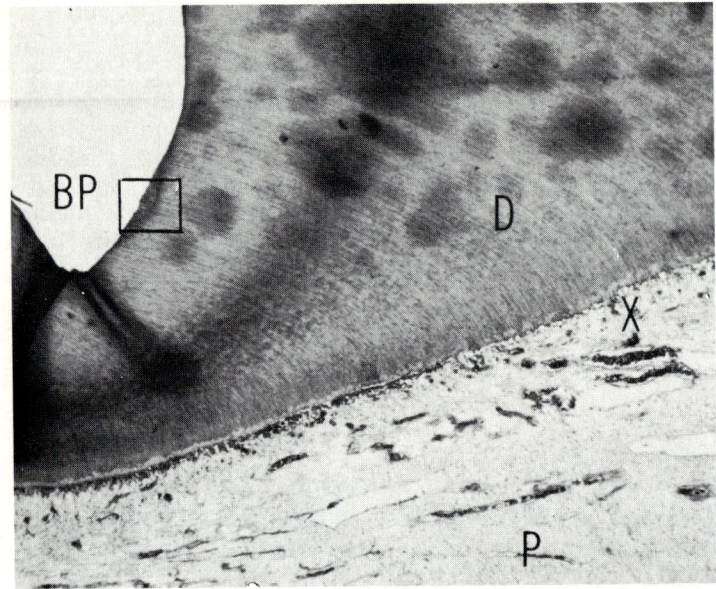

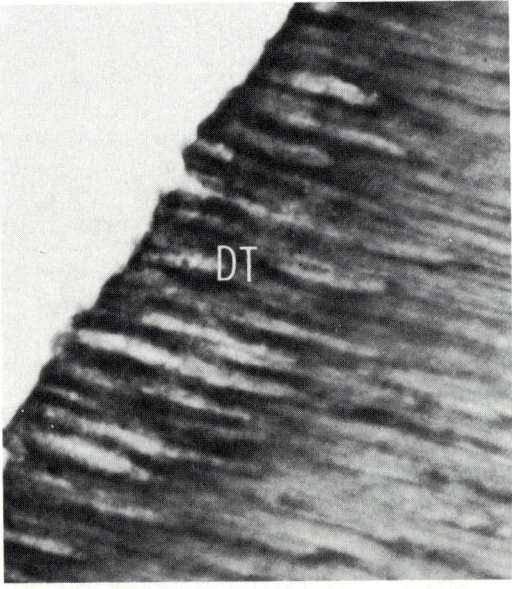

FIG. 9-5 Burn of the dentin, caused by high-speed preparation. *(Top)* Region of bur preparation (BP) of dentin (D). The odontoblastic layer of the pulp (P) is damaged at region X. ×54. *(Bottom)* Higher magnification of region outlined by rectangle. The charred dentinal tubules (DT) are more vulnerable to subsequent decay. ×960.

vided that a proper coolant is employed. Speeds between 3000 and 30,000 rpm, even with coolant, are most deleterious to the pulp.

HEAT AND PRESSURE

The factors of heat and pressure are discussed together because the two irritants frequently impinge on the pulp simultaneously. Usually, heat is generated in the tooth in operative procedures by cutting instruments and impression materials. Heat may also be delivered to the tooth through bleaching techniques on the enamel, and by electrosurgical procedures for gingivoplasty. The effects of these procedures on the pulp are discussed at the end of this section.

Factors in the production of heat within the dental pulp as a result of cavity preparation are: the depth of the preparation; the speed of rotation of the bur or stone; the size, the shape and composition of the bur or stone; the amount and direction of pressure on the cutting instrument; the amount of moisture in the field of operation; the direction and kind of coolants employed; the tissue being cut (i.e., whether it is enamel or dentin) and the length of time the instrument is in continuous contact with the tissue.

DRY CAVITY PREPARATION

Suchard (1979) found that several dry preparations on the same tooth did not cause significantly more damage to the pulp than wet cooling procedures. However, as in many other clinical studies, his findings were not equated with depth of cavity preparations.

Numerous other investigators have found that dry cavity preparation causes greater trauma to the pulp than preparation under water spray (Cotton et al, 1965; Hamilton and Kramer, 1967). Prolonged dehydration with air causes odontoblastic displacement and pulpal edema, a condition that cannot be reversed by moistening the dentin after cavity preparation (Morrant, 1977).

Grinding and drilling of tooth structure without a coolant produces both reversible and irreversible pulp changes. The circulation of the dental pulp is affected by elevation of temperature. The heat produced by cavity preparations on cats' teeth inhibited sympathetic nerve activation, resulting in vasodilatation of the pulpal vessels (Forssell-Ahlberg and Edwall, 1977). A 5°C to 7°C temperature elevation in rat pulps increased capillary permeability (Pohto and Scheinin, 1958). Pulp temperatures above 46°C caused irreversible changes, such as stasis and thrombosis in the pulp blood vessels (Pohto and Scheinin, 1958; Laurichesse and Santoro, 1972).

The intrapulpal pressure is also affected by excessive heat generation (Beveridge and Brown, 1965). Initially, there is a drop of intrapulpal pressure. Normal values gradually return, followed by a rise in intrapulpal pressure (Van Hassell and Brown, 1969), possibly as a result of release of chemical mediators such as various amines, leading to persistent vasodilatation. The consequent escape of plasma proteins into the interstitial fluid of the pulp would lead to a lowering of the osmotic pressure and an accumulation of fluid in the pulp chamber.

Kramer (1963) demonstrated that even the enamel temperature increases substantially when teeth are cut with turbines employed without adequate water coolant. He pointed out (1967) that this increased enamel temperature may not necessarily cause pulp damage, since dentin is a good insulator. However, Brown et al (1978) showed that thermal stress, especially produced by dry cutting, may cause enamel to fracture. The induced high temperatures ultimately affect the dentin, and the pulp may be adversely affected as well. Furthermore, dentinal damage may contribute to the breakdown of tooth structure at the margins, resulting in marginal leakage and recurrent caries.

NATURE OF CUTTING INSTRUMENT

Marsland and Shovelton (1957) and Weiss et al (1963) demonstrated that thermal damage was greater with steel burs than with carbide burs. This probably is related to the greater heat produced by steel burs, as shown by Peyton (1958). With proper cooling, carbide burs produce negligible pulp damage. However, uncooled carbide burs and diamond instruments produce severe damage to the dental pulp which is uncompensated for by intermittent grinding or variations in preparation time. Even with the use of a coolant, diamond instruments are capable of producing damage to the pulp (Shovelton and Marsland, 1958), but this may be related to the additional pressure (Stanley and Swerdlow, 1960). At any rate, the damage is not severe, since the use of the coolant reduces the reactions to a minimum. From a practical standpoint, cavities prepared with rough diamond instruments reportedly provide better retention for resin fillings than do cavities prepared with steel burs (Aker et al, 1979).

Simultaneous increases of rotational speeds and pressure by various types of rotary cutting instruments (carbide burs, steel burs, and diamond stones) cause tooth temperature increases (Peyton, 1955). Such temperature elevations increase inflammatory responses in the pulp. Stanley and Swerdlow (1959) found that even the use of coolants did not minimize inflammatory responses when the operative technique required an applied force above 8 oz. Apparently, increased bur pressure also may cause displacement of odontoblastic nuclei into the dentinal tubules (Brännström, 1962).

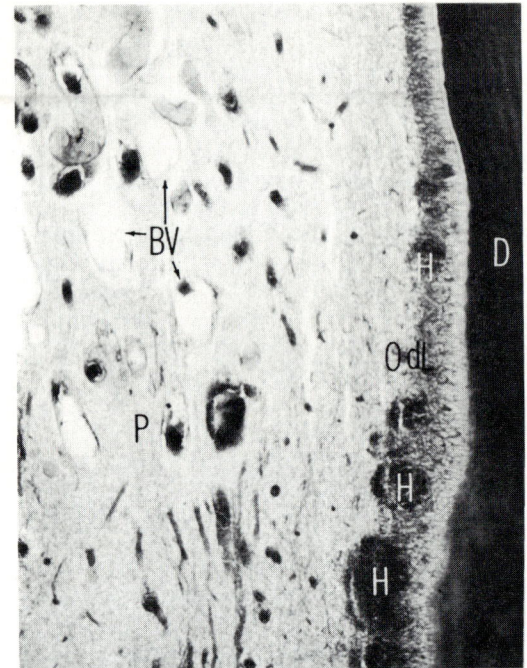

FIG. 9-6 Pulp damage, from the use of large wheels. A crown preparation has been made. The odontoblastic layer (OdL) is damaged and a number of hemorrhages (H) have occurred. The blood vessels (BV) of the deeper pulp tissue (P) are dilated. D, dentin. ×54.

Effects of Heat from Tooth Bleaching

A rise in pulp temperature that occurs in some tooth bleaching procedures did not produce deleterious pulp changes in dogs' teeth (Seale et al, 1981). Cohen (1979) and Robertson and Melfi (1980) used 35% hydrogen peroxide solution and a heating device on the dentin of vital human teeth stained by tetracyclines. They found a lack of, or mild, inflammatory responses in the pulps 1 hour to 30 days later.

Effects of Heat from Electrosurgery

Heat may be delivered to the pulp by electrosurgical gingivoplasty. Whether such heat is damaging to the pulp has been investigated by Robertson et al (1978) and by Krejci et al (1982). Robertson et al found that when the electrode tip contacted Class 5 amalgam restorations in monkey teeth, and the electrosurgical current was delivered for not more than 1 second with a fully rectified unit, the pulps became severely damaged. No corresponding damage to the pulps resulted from the application of the current to unrestored teeth. In the study of Krejci et al on dogs, care was taken to limit the contact of the activated electrode with the gingival restorations to no more than 0.2 to 0.4 seconds, which they claimed would be more compatible with clinical usage. Under those circumstances, there were no adverse pulpal effects. However, longer periods of exposure to the electrosurgical currents produced severe pulpal damage.

Spangberg et al (1982) found that even the placement of a calcium hydroxide base, covered by copal varnish, under the metallic restorations did not prevent pulpal damage.

SIZE OF WHEELS AND BURS

The size of the wheels and the burs that are used is significant. The larger sizes produce greater pulp damage, owing to increased heat generation. The peripheral speed of large disks is significantly higher than that of a small disk at the same rpm. In addition, when a large instrument is used, a greater area at a time is cut. The coolant cannot get to the tooth as readily, resulting in more severe reactions (Fig. 9-6). The manufacturers have attempted to avoid this by placing holes in the wheels, but, even with them, the coolant cannot get to the region of contact of tooth and wheel as readily as it would with a smaller instrument. Stanley and Swerdlow (1960) have shown that less severe reactions develop when smaller instruments are employed, compared with those resulting from the use of larger instruments.

HAND INSTRUMENTS

The effects on the pulp of the use of hand instruments are not definitely known. Direct experimental evidence that deals with this question is unavailable, although Massler (1959) has noted that damage to the pulp seemed to be more severe when hand instruments were used for cavity preparation, as compared with burs. With the use of hand instruments, heat is not generated, but pressure is introduced which can cause pulp damage.

SMEAR LAYER

When cavities are prepared, an amorphous layer of dentinal debris remains attached to the dentin. The nature of the cutting instrument is unrelated to the development of this layer. Thus, cutting of the dentin with a high-speed tungsten carbide bur or with diamond points, or preparing cavities with hand chisels all produce a "smear layer" (Brännström et al, 1979). Neither water spray nor hydrogen peroxide-ethanol solution can successfully restore the dentin surface to normal. However, polishing with pumice (Dahl, 1978), treatment with a microbicidal fluoride solution (Brännström and Johnson, 1974), acid etching (Brännström and Nordenvall, 1977), or application of a combination of 0.2% EDTA and surface-active antibacterial solutions can effectively remove the smear layer (Brännström et al, 1980).

COOLANTS

As has been shown, heating of dentin has a deleterious effect on the human pulp, and recovery may not be complete.

In order to reduce or eliminate the heat generated by the cutting procedures, coolants must be employed. The coolants in use are an air spray; a combination of water and air, as a water spray; water applied through a hollow bur; and water, as a jet stream.

Air Spray

Schuchard and Watkins (1960) inserted thermocouples in vital teeth. Various types of cavity and crown preparations were made with instruments rotating at varying speeds with or without air or air-water spray coolants. The average of observed temperature rise on all cuts was $-10°C$ ($14°F$) without coolant. When an air coolant was employed, the average rise in temperature was reduced to $-17°C$ ($1°F$). Subsequently, Schuchard (1967) concluded that there is no significant heat rise and pulp damage with air cooling. Similar conclusions were reached by Bhaskar and Lilly (1965). In addition, Carson et al (1979) found, through the use of thermography, that there were no significant differences in the cooling effectiveness between air-water spray and air alone.

Biologic reactions cannot be measured with a thermocouple or with thermography. For example, if a thermocouple should be placed on one side of the hand and a hot instrument applied to the other side, the small increase in temperature registered by the thermocouple would have no significance as a measure of the severe damage to the cells caused by the application of the hot instrument. Similarly, dentin is vital tissue which contains protoplasmic extensions of cells. These can be damaged even though the thermocouple records no signficant rise in temperature. However, the experiments do indicate that dentin is a good insulating material and a poor conductor of heat.

DRYING OF DENTIN

Air blasts are damaging to the pulp. It has been shown by Langeland (1972) that a blast of air on the dentin, with either an ordinary chip syringe or compressed air, for 10 seconds is enough to produce displacement of odontoblastic nuclei. Thus, the use of air spray or air coolant, especially during deep cavity preparation, presents a potential hazard to the pulp, and, therefore, cavity cutting should not be performed with air cooling alone. During cavity toilet, the cavity should not be dried with air blasts; cotton pellets should be used instead.

The use of the rubber dam leads to desiccation of the dentin and consequent odontoblastic injury and displacement. Operating on the tooth under dry conditions is detrimental. Cavities can be prepared safely under the rubber dam with a water spray if suction equipment is used to evacuate the accumulated water. The use of desiccating drugs, such as alcohol or chloroform, on dentin is contraindicated. (See Chap. 10, Chemical Irritants.)

From a clinical standpoint, it appears that, although greater cellular damage occurs initially from the use of air coolant, repair may ensue in the absence of other irritating factors (Cotton, 1967; Dachi and Stigers, 1968). Recovery depends on factors such as the state of health of the pulp at the time of cavity preparation, the depth and the extent of the preparation, the extent of the tissue damage and the presence of a sufficient number of cells capable of differentiation (Stanley, 1961).

Water Spray

Most investigators have shown that there is less likelihood of pulp damage when water is used as the coolant (Stanley and Swerdlow, 1960; Zach and Cohen, 1962). Zach and Cohen (1962; 1965) and Marsland and Shovelton (1970) found that the immediate damage to the dental pulp was greater in air-cooled than in water-cooled teeth, up to 15 days postoperatively. Furthermore, up to 7 weeks, repair processes were more advanced in the pulp of the water-cooled specimens. After longer periods, the pulps of both groups did not differ significantly.

Even for short periods of time, water cooling has an advantage over the other methods. The temperature elevations are significantly reduced. Furthermore, with water cooling, the rate of removal of debris is improved (Lloyd et al, 1978).

Kim et al (1983) found that the pulpal microvasculature was altered in dogs' teeth that were subjected to full crown preparations both with and without water spray. The pulpal blood flow was reduced by 12% in the tooth prepared with water spray. After 1 hour, the blood flow returned to within 7% of the control. Without water spray, there was a 44% reduction of blood flow. After 1 hour, the pulpal blood flow was even further decreased.

These findings indicate that the coolant plays a significant role in controlling the inflammatory reaction in the pulp. To ignore cooling the tooth with water while operating at higher speeds is an invitation to disaster. As Bodecker (1939) pointed out so graphically, it is comparable with "cooking the pulp in its own juice."

However, teeth that are inundated with water are not necessarily protected. When speeds of 50,000 rpm and over are used, water in the form of a jet stream must be employed because the speed at which the bur revolves creates an area of turbulence, tending to deflect the water from the dentin being prepared (Langeland, 1972). The water must have sufficient pressure to penetrate the area of turbulence. To be effective, the water should be delivered directly at the point of contact between the bur and the tooth. Frequently, instruments containing only one aperture for water are unable to fulfill this requirement. If the instrument is moved to the side opposite the one from which the stream of water is coming, the water will be obstructed by the tooth, especially in the deeper parts of the cavity. To prevent such obstruction, the water should be delivered from both sides. When crosscut fissure burs are used, for efficient cooling, the water should strike the bur at several different levels, thereby keeping wet the entire contacting area of bur and tooth. If such instruments were made available, a shower-head type of aperture would be preferable. Actually, owing to the centrifugal force of the bur and the shunting away of the water, the tooth still can be burned —and, incongruously, an odor of burning tooth tissue is frequently evident. Intermittent grinding does not necessarily reduce the severity of the injury. In the absence of properly directed coolant, intermittent grinding is of no benefit; the tooth is burnt a little at a time. During cavity cutting, if an odor of burning dentin becomes obvious (an odor similar to the odor of burned chicken feathers), sufficient cooling at the point of cutting is not present. The quantity of coolant alone is not significant. The contact of water with bur and the dentin simultaneously is of paramount importance. For example, in the preparation of pinledge inlays with high-speed turbines, the coolant cannot be delivered to the contact area, and pulp damage can occur.

High-speed cutting should be done with a brush stroke similar to that employed by a painter using water colors. In this way, the bur and the tooth can be covered simultaneously by the coolant.

TEMPERATURE OF COOLANTS

The temperature of the water cooling used during cavity preparation apparently has little significant effect on the pulp. Croft and Stanley (1966) found no significant histopathologic differences between three groups of teeth in which cavity preparations were made with different coolant temperatures ranging from 12.5°C (54.5°F) to 18°C (64.4°F). Frank et al (1972) found that even subfreezing temperatures produced only a transient fall in intrapulpal blood pressure, a condition that was quickly reversible.

The lowering of pulp temperatures in rats' and monkeys' teeth below $-10°C$, through the use of a cryosurgical unit, was found to produce damage to the odontoblasts and the microvasculature (Shepard, 1976; Dowden et al, 1983). When a cryosurgical instrument with circulating liquid nitrogen at $-196°C$ was applied to mandibular osseous defects in dogs for 3 minutes, no severe damage to the pulps of neighboring teeth was noted after 6 weeks (Pollan et al, 1974). Thus, it appears that the temperature of coolants used clinically would have no significant effects on the dental pulp.

With the increase of speeds of rotation of cutting instruments, not only is greater heat generated but there is also an increase in vibrations, which affects the pulp.

Searles (1967) has pointed out that mechanical vibration during high speed drilling may be responsible for protein denaturation of the odontoblasts. The denaturation causes morphologic changes leading to destruction of the odontoblasts.

EXTENSIVENESS OF PREPARATION

The extensiveness of the preparation has an influence on the amount of heat generated. Zach and Cohen (1958) demonstrated that, in cavities prepared on the teeth of Rhesus monkeys with high-speed instruments, the pulp damage was roughly proportional to the amount of tooth structure removed. Schuchard and Watkins (1961) had similar results in their experiments. Class 1 and Class 5 cavity preparations produced a much lower heat reaction than did mesioocclusodistal (MOD) or full crown preparations.

In Class 1 preparations with high speeds, it is not desirable to sink a bur directly into a tooth fissure, because the coolant will not be able to reach the cutting area and extensive injury to the pulp will result (Fig. 9–7). It is best to increase the width and the depth of the fissure gradually by shallow, angular cuts.

In three-quarter crown preparations, it is desirable to use intruments rotating at high speed for gross cutting and finish the grooving part of the preparation with burs revolving at low speed. With high-speed instruments, the coolant cannot reach the depth of the preparation, and vision is obstructed. The cavity preparation with high-speed instruments should be widened and deepened gradually so that proper cooling will result. Pulp damage thus will be prevented or minimized.

Full crown shoulder preparations are more harmful to the pulp than are shoulderless ones, because, in the former, the preparations are much deeper into the dentin and closer to the pulp. A full crown shoulder preparation in a young tooth is especially hazardous because there is not as much thickness of dentin.

In crown and bridge procedures, the paralleling of walls to facilitate a path of insertion for the finished bridge is frequently hazardous. During full crown preparation, occasionally a pinkish to brownish discoloration becomes obvious in the dentin (Fig. 9–8). This is caused by pulp hemorrhage. Pulp recovery in such circumstances is questionable. If the pulp is actually exposed, the prognosis is even more doubtful. The treatment of choice is endodontics. The operator should not wait for painful symptoms to develop, because successful outcome of endodontic treatment is more likely before an area of rarefaction develops.

In order to avoid the danger of pulp damage or exposure from excessive cutting, a double cast-

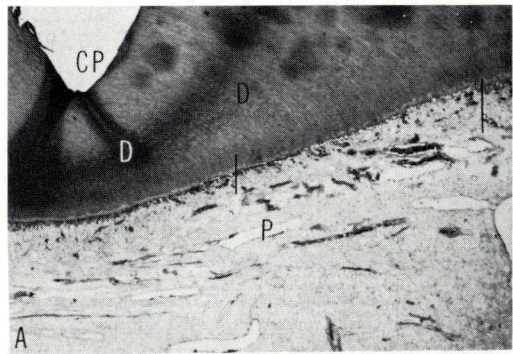
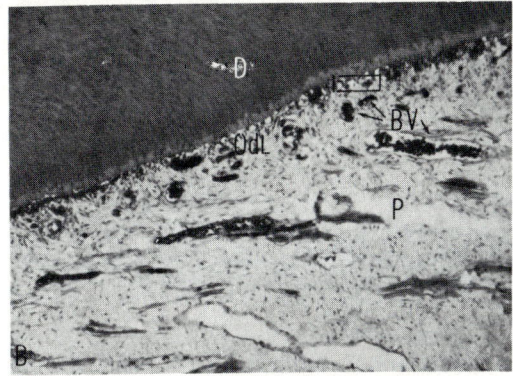
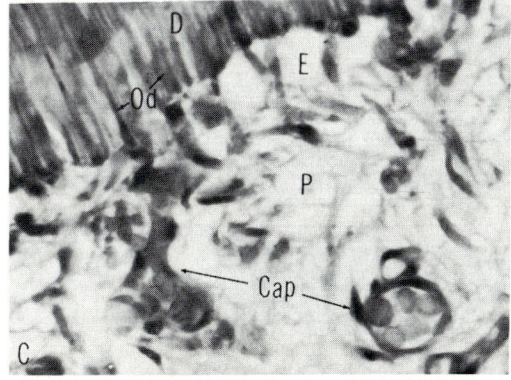

FIG. 9–7 Burn of the pulp, caused by sinking a bur that was revolving at high speed directly into the dentin. *(Top)* Region of preparation (CP) of dentin (D). Pulp (P) in region between black lines is affected. ×54. *(Center)* Higher magnification of region between black lines in top picture. The odontoblastic layer (OdL) of the pulp (P) is damaged. Blood vessels (BV) are dilated. D, dentin. ×135. *(Bottom)* Higher magnification of region outlined by rectangle in center picture. Odontoblasts (Od) are displaced into the dentin (D). Edema (E) has occurred in the pulp (P). Capillaries (Cap) are dilated. ×960.

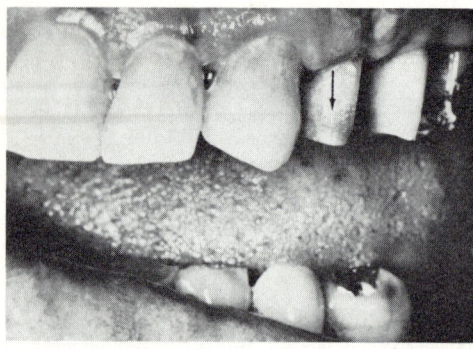 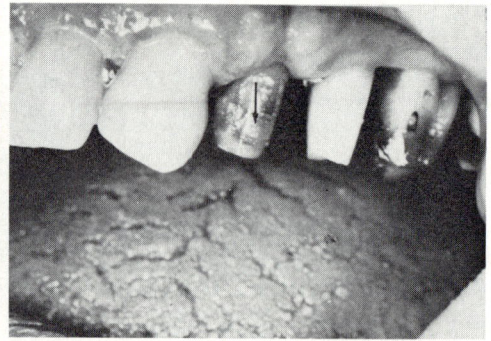

FIG. 9-8 Hemorrhage of tooth, due to crown preparation. *(Left)* An upper first premolar has been prepared for a full crown. A pinkish discoloration due to pulp hemorrhage has occurred (arrow). *(Right)* One week later, the tooth is stained more intensely (arrow) by decomposition of the erythrocytes.

ing technique may be employed. The telescoping of one crown over another crown helps to avoid excessive cutting.

USE OF PINS

In pinledge or pitledge preparations, the use of high-speed instruments should be avoided because the coolant is prevented from reaching the depth of the preparation.

Friction grip or cement type pin techniques to increase retention of large amalgam fillings should be used with caution. Often, carious destruction or fracture of a tooth leaves little remaining dentinal tissue. The insertion of pins introduces the hazard of dentinal fractures or unnoticed pulp exposures. Moreover, the deep insertion of the pin can increase pulpal irritation of an already chronically inflamed pulp. As has been mentioned (see Chap. 8, Pulp Irritants: Microbial), all carious lesions produce chronic inflammation in the pulp and the degree of inflammation is directly proportional to the depth and extensiveness of the decay.

The cementation of pins with zinc phosphate cement adds another hazard of irritation to the pulp (see Chap. 10, Chemical Irritants). The use of fast-setting zinc oxide-eugenol or carboxylate cements could reduce or prevent the inflammation in a normal pulp. However, under clinical conditions, with the persistent presence of inflammation in the pulps of decayed teeth, the hazards of pin insertion demand caution regardless of technique used.

To mitigate the extra irritation from the pins, the application of calcium hydroxide in the prepared holes has been advocated (Suzuki et al, 1973). Their experiments on dogs' teeth have shown that, with the use of this drug, the insertion of pins reduced the inflammatory reaction in the experimental teeth, as compared with controls. Furthermore, if pulp exposure occurred, the pulps of noncarious teeth treated with calcium hydroxide did not become necrotic. Conversely, when pins were inserted into pulp exposures without the prior application of calcium hydroxide, pulpal necrosis did occur. The response to pin insertion was minimal if some remaining dentin was present. However, dentinal cracks and slight inflammatory changes persisted for the duration of the experiment (28 days).

REBOUND RESPONSE

Bernier and Knapp (1958) described pulp injury (which they called the rebound response) attributable to the high energy which is released by ultrasonic cutting or by ultra-high speeds. They held that, when a cavity is prepared on one side of a tooth, reactions occur on the opposite side.

Shovelton and Marsland (1958), Zach and Cohen (1958), and Holden (1962) also referred to odontoblastic displacement or degeneration in the tubules on the side opposite to that of the cut dentinal tubules. However, as discussed by Stanley (1961) and Langeland (1961), some controversy exists about the actuality of the occurrence of the rebound phenomenon. In tissue cultures, Kawahara and Yamagami (1970) found no significant cellular damage due to vibration with high-speed dental drills used with a water coolant, casting doubt on the existence of

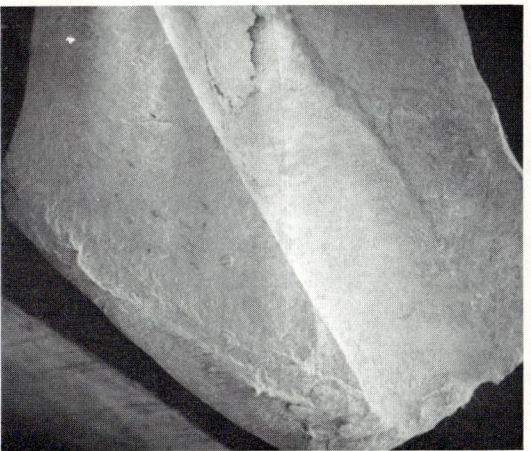 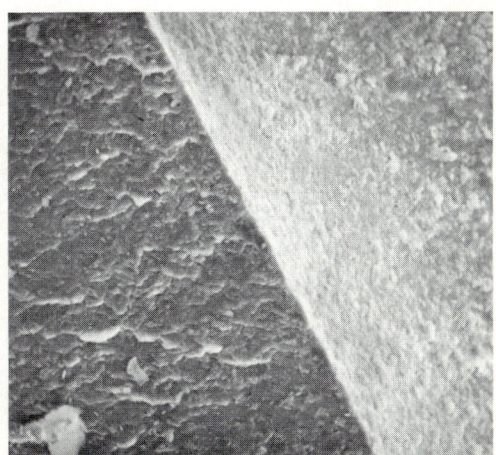

FIG. 9-9 *(Left)* Scanning electron micrograph of apical portion of pulp canal obliterated by hard tissue formation. ×40. *(Right)* Higher magnification of calcified canal. Normal dentin is on left. ×180.

a rebound phenomenon. Nonetheless, Searles (1975) found that the odontoblasts opposite the site of cavity preparation showed a decrease in cellular activity when labeled isotopes (tritiated proline) were administered to rats. The exact cause remains conjectural.

OTHER PHYSICAL TRAUMATA

BLOWS

Physical trauma such as a blow, with or without fracture, may cause hemorrhage in the pulp, resulting in nutritional disturbances to the cells, hyalinization of the pulp tissue, excessive mineralization and tooth discoloration (Arwill et al, 1967; Stanley et al, 1978). In such a traumatic injury to a tooth, it is impossible to predict the extent of damage to the pulp. Generally, the greater the trauma to the tooth, the higher the incidence of pulp necrosis. The pulp may recover completely or it may become necrotic, depending on the severity of the hemorrhage, on whether or not the apex is completed and on the establishment of infection. In teeth with incomplete root formation, the chances for pulp regeneration are enhanced. The incidence of pulp necrosis is usually low (Andreasen, 1970), and long-term prognosis for most cases has been reported to be favorable (Jacobsen and Zachrisson, 1975; Jacobsen and Kerekes, 1977; Zadik et al, 1979).

In favorable cases, the color of the tooth may return to normal. In many instances, the odontoblasts or other pulp cells react by elaborating huge quantities of reparative dentin, mostly atubular, which tend to obliterate almost the entire pulp space (Fig. 9-9).

In some teeth, the hard tissue formed is similar to bone or cementum. In time, such teeth may develop periapical areas of rarefaction, rendering treatment exceedingly difficult. In others, repair is favorable.

FRACTURES

Crown Fractures

Clinical observations (Ellis, 1970) suggest that when the pulp is not exposed, the chances for pulp survival increase when the crown is fractured, compared to traumatized teeth without crown fractures. Should the crown fracture expose the pulp, pulp capping or pulpotomy is usually highly successful. Cvek (1978) studied the status of the pulps of patients with crown-fractured incisors whose ages ranged from 7 to 16 years. Their pulps exhibited a high frequency of healing following a partial pulpectomy and pulp covering with calcium hydroxide.

Root Fractures

After impact accidents, intra-alveolar root fractures (IARFs) occur most often in the upper anterior teeth of juveniles. Blackwood (1959)

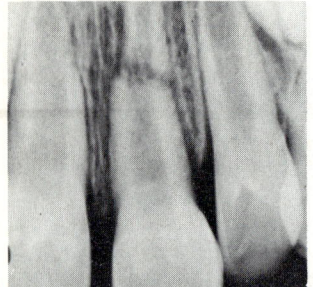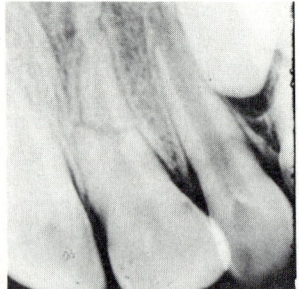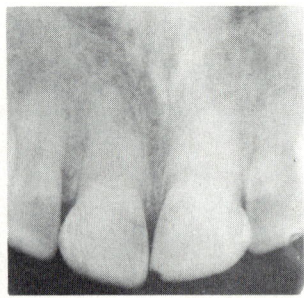

FIG. 9-10 *(Left)* Root fracture in 1956. *(Middle)* Four years later. *(Right)* Twenty years later. Both centrals respond to electric pulp testing, are clinically functional, and are normal in color. Both teeth show the same degree of pulp obliteration.

and Andreasen and Hjørting-Hansen (1967) have described four possible reactions to IARFs: (1) healing with calcification of the pulp; (2) healing with interposition of connective tissue between the fragments; (3) healing with interposition of bone and connective tissue; and (4) persistence of granulation tissue between the fragments. Most of the fractured teeth fall into the last category. In favorable cases, the fragments are repaired by the deposition of cementum, uniting the fractured segments (Michanowicz et al, 1971).

Higher recovery or survival rates of pulps occur in permanent teeth with transverse IARFs than in traumatized teeth with no root fractures (Bender and Freedland, 1983). Pulp vitality is affected by the extent of apical maturation, the location of the fracture site, and the skill of the operator in treating traumatic injuries, with early stabilization. The more apical the fracture, the more favorable the pulp prognosis (Zachrisson and Jacobsen, 1975). When the entire fracture is within the alveolus above the epithelial attachment, the chances for pulp recovery are enhanced. However, when the fracture site is close to the gingival crevice, the prognosis is poorer.

Clinical observations reveal that root fractures in young permanent teeth have a high potential for healing (75%-80%), and pulp vitality may be maintained without additional therapy (Fig. 9-10). Long-term histologic studies show that hard tissue forms between the fragments. Healing is enhanced when there is no fragment dislocation and there is early fracture fixation (Boulger, 1928; Michanowicz et al, 1971; Andreasen, 1981).

The incidence of pulp necrosis in permanent teeth with transverse IARFs varies from 20% to 40% (Austin, 1930; Andreasen, 1981); in traumatized, luxated, or subluxated teeth with no IARFs, the incidence of pulp necrosis increases from 38% to 59% (Rock, 1974; Weiskopf, 1961).

TRAUMATIC OCCLUSION

Clinical observations have led to the postulation that excessive occlusal forces may cause pulp changes such as increased pulp stones, pulpitis, and necrosis (Natkin and Ingle, 1963; Ramfjord and Ash, 1966). However, Landay et al (1970) found that light occlusal forces produced by the placement of high amalgam restorations in rats' teeth had not caused significant pulpal changes over short periods (up to 6 months). Subsequently, stainless steel pins were placed in the upper molars to produce heavier sustained occlusal forces on the opposing teeth (Cooper et al, 1971). No pulp changes were observed up to 7 months. Thereafter, concentrations of macrophages and lymphocytes became evident in the pulps of the traumatized teeth. In addition, there were disruptions of the odontoblastic layer and deposition of reparative dentin on the floor of the pulp chamber and in the root canals.

POLISHING OF RESTORATIONS

Polishing of restorations without taking precautions for dissipation of heat is dangerous to the pulp (Aplin et al, 1967). A significant elevation in temperature occurs as a result of friction. Sandpaper discs or rubber cups, run dry at high speeds, can generate sufficient heat to damage the pulp. The generated heat can also cause enamel to fracture (Brown et al, 1978). Therefore, polishing instruments should be run intermittently at low speeds, or in conjunction with coolants in order to reduce heat generation (Christensen and Dilts, 1968).

IMPRESSIONS

The taking of impressions for inlay and crown fabrication also exposes the pulp to serious hazards. Modeling compound must be heated to render it sufficiently soft to accomplish its purpose. When the compound is applied to cavity or full crown preparations, a great deal of pressure is exerted on the pulp. Both heat and pressure impinge on the dentin simultaneously.

Temperatures inside the pulp chamber can be significantly elevated when impressions are taken with modeling compound that has been heated in an open flame. Intrapulpal temperatures remain high for more than 3 minutes, rising to an average of 52°C (120°F) which is an increase of 15°C (59°F), unless the modeling compound is rapidly chilled (Grajower et al,

FIG. 9-11 Cross section of tooth following crown preparation and impression with plasticine. Hemorrhages (H) have occurred into the odontoblastic layer (OdL) of the pulp (P). ×96.

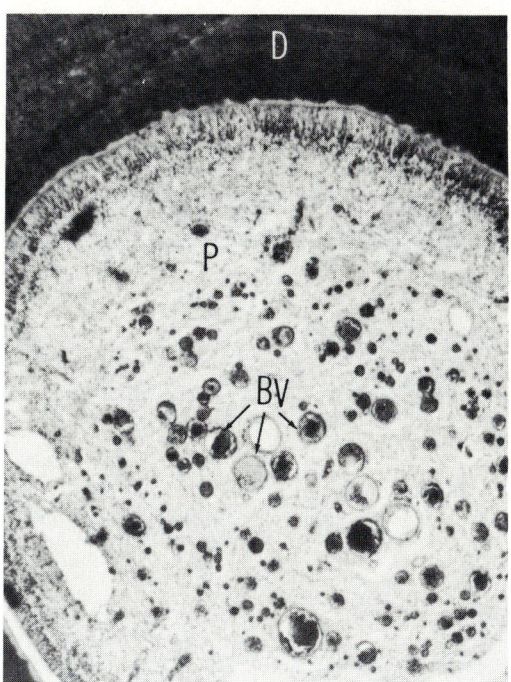

FIG. 9-12 Cross section of a tooth, following crown preparation and impression with modeling compound. The blood vessels (BV) are distended and filled with polymorphonuclear leukocytes. Edema of the odontoblastic layer of the pulp (P) has occurred. ×54.

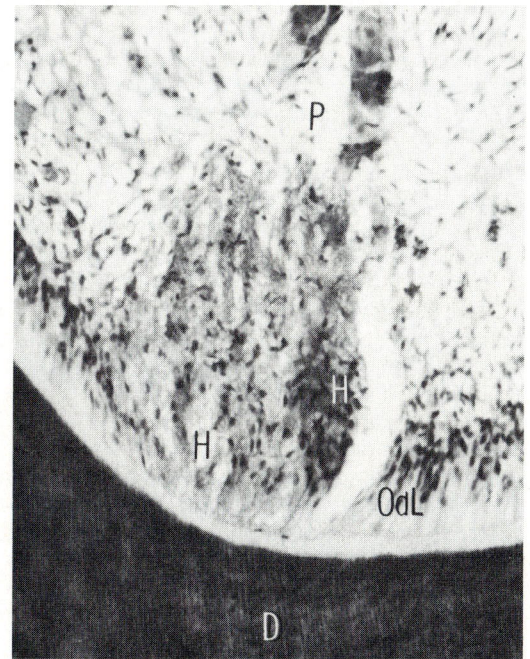

1975). Such a heat rise may cause pulpitis. Histologically, Lindholm (1975) found that crown preparation plus modeling compound impressions caused a significant widening of pulp arterioles, and irregularities in the odontoblastic layer. We investigated the effects of pressure alone on the dental pulp by using plasticine in a copper band for taking an impression of a full crown preparation. Examination of histologic sections revealed edema, hemorrhage and displacement of odontoblastic nuclei (Fig. 9-11). In further experiments, modeling compound was employed for the impressions, thereby subjecting the pulp to both heat and pressure. The tissue sections revealed a greater inflammatory reaction in the pulp. Increased hemorrhages and edema were evident in both the odontoblastic layer and the deeper pulp tissue (Fig. 9-12).

To avoid some of these deleterious effects, the use of rubber base impression materials may be recommended. These materials generate no

THE EFFECT OF TOOTH MOVEMENT ON THE DENTAL PULP

Pulp injury may occur following rapid tooth movement. When a tooth is moved quickly by separating instruments, hemorrhages are produced in the periodontal ligament. The ensuing pulp inflammation is associated with edema, and the tooth may become extremely sensitive. Also, the pulp of the tooth may become inflamed because of interference with the blood supply.

ORTHODONTICS

The forces involved in orthodontic tooth movement create disturbances in the circulation of the pulp that are similar in many ways to those found in periodontally involved teeth (see Chap. 15, The Interrelationship of Pulp and Periodontal Disease). In young, experimentally intruded teeth, circulatory disturbances result in degeneration of the odontoblasts. The alterations are more severe in teeth with completed apices. In teeth with incomplete root end formation, malformations of the root are induced (Stenvik and Mjör, 1970).

The changes are proportionately more severe with increasingly greater forces. Interference with the blood supply of the pulp takes place, resulting in reduction of the supply of nutrients to the odontoblasts. Some of the odontoblasts degenerate and the other cells of the pulp may undergo atrophy (Tschamer, 1974). There is increased deposition of reparative dentin in both the coronal and the radicular portions of the pulp and a concurrent increase in dystrophic mineralization (Fig. 9–13). In time, the root canals are extremely narrowed. In some instances, they appear to have been completely obliterated by the dentin and calcific deposition. The pulp cells may undergo atrophy, with eventual necrosis (Delivanis and Sauer, 1982; Fig. 9–13). In most cases, the damage to the pulp is reversible. Following orthodontics, a significant alteration of nerve axons has not been detected in studies by Bunner and Johnson (1982). All of these changes generally produce no symptoms, but the symptoms may be masked by the pain produced when changes in force are made by the orthodontist.

Pulp changes are also attributable to the introduction of orthodontic forces beyond the limits of physiologic tolerance of the periodontal liga-

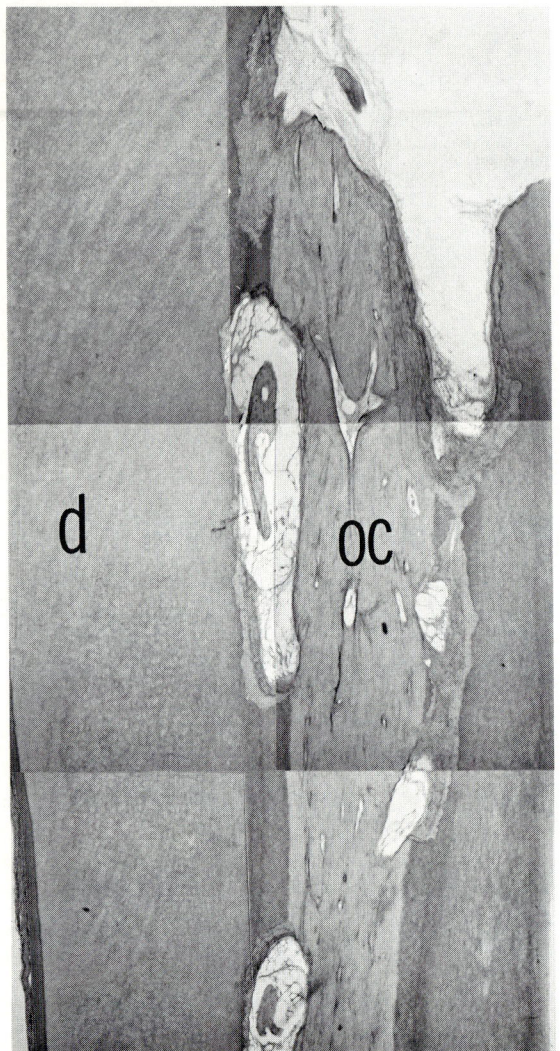

FIG. 9-13 Composite photomicrograph, showing obliteration of the pulp by excessive orthodontic tooth movement. The pulp has been replaced by hard tissue—osteocementum (oc)—resembling bone. d, Dentin. ×54.

heat and little pressure. Langeland and Langeland (1965) investigated the effects of rubber base impression materials on the pulp and found no irritation.

The hydrocolloid impression material also is used for impressions for inlay and crown and bridge preparations. With this material, pressure is not employed and the heat is not as damaging as that of modeling compound.

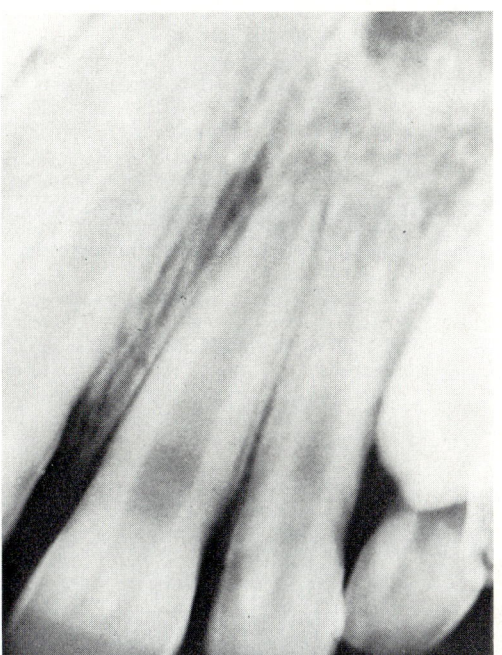 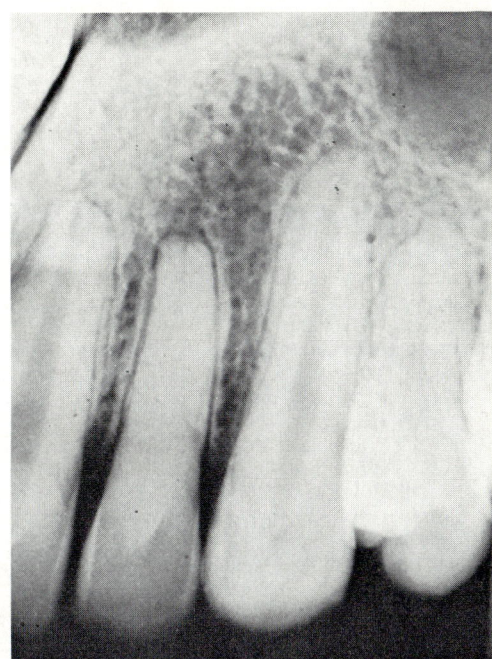

FIG. 9-14 Effect of orthodontic tooth movement on the dental pulp. *(Left)* Upper right first and second incisors before orthodontic treatment. *(Right)* The same teeth, 5 years later, after completion of orthodontic treatment. The pulp of the second incisor is practically obliterated. There also has been shortening of the roots of the incisors by resorption. (Courtesy of Dr. Richard Snyder, Philadelphia)

ment. As a consequence, blood vessels in the periodontal ligament may rupture, with resultant hemorrhage. When this occurs along the lateral aspects of the roots, there is loss of the nutritional supply to some pulp cells. These cells will atrophy and die. However, if the hemorrhage occurs from one of the larger vessels supplying the pulp, the entire pulp may become necrotic. At first, the color of the tooth becomes pinkish or reddish because erythrocytes enter the dentinal tubules. As time goes by, the red blood cells decompose, liberating hemoglobin which breaks down to hemosiderin (a dark yellow, iron-containing pigment) and other blood pigments. The tooth color gradually changes to yellowish, then to various hues ranging from slate-grey to bluish-black. Usually, a pericementitis is present initially, but this gradually subsides. Eventually, a periapical area of rarefaction may become visible in the radiograph. Another radiographic finding which affords a clue to pulp necrosis is the width of the pulp chamber and the root canal. When the pulp becomes necrotic, it ceases to elaborate dentin. As a result, in time, the width of the root canal and the pulp chamber appears greater in this tooth than its neighbor.

Orthodontic tooth movement may also be responsible for excessive resorption of the apical cementum and dentin of the tooth. The root ends become shortened and blunted, although pulp vitality is not necessarily affected (Fig. 9-14).

Care must be exercised in performing operative procedures on teeth that are undergoing, or those that have undergone, orthodontic tooth movement. The pulps are not able to withstand as readily the irritating effects of some manipulations, and pulp inflammation and necrosis may readily ensue. More frequent inspection of the teeth for detection of incipient caries is indicated. Cavity preparations should be made as soon as the beginnings of carious lesions are detected, in order to keep the preparations shallow. Frequent removal of bands for inspection purposes is to be recommended.

BIBLIOGRAPHY

Aker DA, Aker JR, Sorenson S: Effect of methods of tooth enamel preparation on retentive strength of acid-etch composite resins. JADA 99:185, 1979

Andreasen JO: Luxation of permanent teeth due to trauma. Scand J Dent Res 78:273, 1970

Andreasen JO: Traumatic injuries of the teeth, 2nd ed, Chaps 5 and 6, Munksgaard, Copenhagen, 1981

Andreasen JO, Hjørting-Hansen E: Intra-alveolar root fractures: radiographic and histological study of 50 cases. J Oral Surg 25:414, 1967

Aplin AW, Sorenson FM, Cantwell KR: Temperature change in dental polishing. J Dent Res 46:325, 1967

Arwill T, Henschen B, Sundwall-Hagland I: The pulpal reaction in traumatized permanent incisors in children aged 9–18. Odont Tids 75:130, 1967

Austin LT: Review of forty cases of retained fractured roots of anterior teeth. JADA 17:1930, 1930

Bender IB, Freedland JB: Clinical considerations in the diagnosis and treatment of intra-alveolar root fractures. JADA 107:595, 1983

Bergman G, Lindén LÅ, Röckert H: An attempt to analyse the enamel fluid. ORCA Proc 4:163, 1966

Bernier JL, Knapp MJ: Methods used in evaluation of high-speed dental instruments and some results. Oral Surg 12:234, 1957

Bernier JL, Knapp MJ: A new pulpal response to high-speed dental instruments. Oral Surg 11:167, 1958

Beveridge EE, Brown AC: The measurement of human dental intrapulpal pressure and its response to clinical variables. Oral Surg 19:655, 1965

Bhaskar SN, Lilly GE: Intrapulpal temperature during cavity preparation. J Dent Res 44:644, 1965

Blackwood HJJ: Tissue repair in intra-alveolar root fractures. Oral Surg 12:360, 1959

Bodecker CF: Demonstration of possible ill effects of heat on the pulp caused by rapid operative technic. JADA 26:527, 1939

Boulger EP: Histologic studies of a specimen of fractured roots. JADA 15:1778, 1928

Brännström M: Dentinal and pulpal response. VI. Some experiments with heat and pressure illustrating the movement of odontoblasts into the dentinal tubules. Oral Surg 15:203, 1962

Brännström M: Dentin sensitivity and aspiration of odontoblasts. JADA 66:366, 1963

Brännström M, Åström A: The hydrodynamics of the dentine; its possible relationship to dentinal pain. Int Dent J 22:219, 1972

Brännström M, Garberoglio R: The dentinal tubules and the odontoblast process. A scanning electron microscope study. Acta Odont Scand 30:291, 1972

Brännström M, Glantz P-O, Nordenvall K-J: The effect of some cleaning solutions on the morphology of dentin prepared in different ways. An in vitro study. J Dent Child 46:19, 1979

Brännström M, Johnson G: Effects of various conditioners and cleaning agents on prepared dentin surfaces: A scanning electron microscopic investigation. J Prosth Dent 31:422, 1974

Brännström M, Nordenvall K-J: The effect of acid etching on enamel, dentin, and the inner surface of the resin restoration. J Dent Res 56:917, 1977

Brännström M, Nordenvall K-J, Glantz P-O: The effect of EDTA-containing surface-active solutions on the morphology of prepared dentin: An in vivo study. J Dent Res 59:1127, 1980

Brown WS, Christenson DO, Lloyd BA: Numerical and experimental evaluation of energy inputs, temperature gradients and thermal stresses during restorative procedures. JADA 96:451, 1978

Bunner M, Johnson D: Quantitative assessment of intrapulpal axon response to orthodontic movement. Am J Orthodont 82:244, 1982

Carson J, Rider T, Nash D: A thermographic study of heat distribution during ultra-speed cavity preparation. J Dent Res 58:1684, 1979

Christensen G, Dilts WE: Thermal change during dental polishing. J Dent Res 47:690, 1968

Coffey CI, Ingram MJ, Bjorndal AM: Analysis of human dentinal fluid. Oral Surg 30:835, 1970

Cohen SC: Human pulpal response to bleaching procedures on vital teeth. J Endodont 5:134, 1979

Cooper MB, Landay MA, Seltzer S: The effects of occlusal force on the pulp. II. Heavier and longer term forces. J Periodontol 42:353, 1971

Cotton WR: Pulp response to an airstream directed into human cavity preparations. Oral Surg 24:78, 1967

Cotton WR, Gorman WJ, Lamb JR: Pulp response to cavity drying in rat teeth. J Dent Res 44:801, 1965

Croft L, Stanley HR: The effect of a chilled coolant on the human pulp during cavity preparation. Oral Surg 22:66, 1966

Cvek MA: A clinical report on partial pulpotomy and capping with calcium hydroxide in permanent incisors with complicated crown fracture. J Endodont 4:232, 1978

Dachi SF, Stigers RW: Pulpal effects of water and air coolants used in high-speed cavity preparations. JADA 76:95, 1968

Dahl BL: Effect of cleansing procedures on the retentive ability of two luting cements to ground dentin in vitro. Act Odont Scand 36:137, 1978

Delivanis HP, Sauer GJR: Incidence of canal calcification in the orthodontic patient. Am J Orthodont 82:58, 1982

Dowden WE, Emmings F, Langeland K: The pulpal effects of freezing temperatures applied to monkey teeth. Oral Surg 55:408, 1983

Ellis RG: The Classification and Treatment of Injuries to the Teeth of Children, 5th ed. Chicago, Year Book Medical Publishers, 1970

Forssell-Ahlberg K, Edwall L: Influence of local insults on sympathetic vaso-constrictor control in feline dental pulp. Acta Odont Scand 35:103, 1977

Frank U, Freundlich J, Tansy MF, Chaffee RB, Jr, Weiss RC, Kendall FM: Vascular and cellular responses of teeth after localized controlled cooling. Cryobiology 9:526, 1972

Garberoglio R, Brännström M: Scanning electron microscopic investigation of human dentinal tubules. Arch Oral Biol 21:355, 1976

Grajower R, Kaufman E, Stern N: Temperature of the pulp chamber during impression taking of full crown preparations with modelling compound. J Dent Res 54:212, 1975

Crossman ES, Austin JC: Scanning electron microscope observations on the tubule content of freeze-fractured peripheral vervet monkey dentine (cercopipthecus pygerythrus). Arch Oral Biol 28:279, 1983

Haldi J, John K: Sulfanilamide and penicillin in the pulp fluid of the dog following administration of these compounds. J Dent Res 44:1386, 1965

Haldi J, Law ML, John K: Comparative concentrations of various constituents of blood plasma and dental-pulp fluid. J Dent Res 44:427, 1965

Haldi J, Wynn W: Protein fractions of the blood plasma and dental-pulp fluid of the dog. J Dent Res 42:1217, 1963

Haljamäe H, Röckert H: Potassium and sodium content in dentinal fluid. Odont Revy 21:369, 1970

Hamilton AI, Kramer IRH: Cavity preparation with and without waterspray. Brit Dent J 123:281, 1967

Holden GGP: Some observations on the vibratory phenomenon associated with high speed air turbines and their transmission to living tissue. Brit Dent J 113:265, 1962

Holland GR: The extent of odontoblast process in the cat. J Anat 121:133, 1976

Hoppenbrouwers PMM, Borggreven JMPM, Thé GST, Maltha JC: The effect of cavity preparation on the metabolism of protein in dentin. J Dent Res 61:1035, 1982

Jacobs HR, Thompson RE, Brown WS: Heat transfer in teeth. J Dent Res 52:248, 1973

Jacobsen I, Kerekes K: Long-term prognosis of traumatized permanent anterior teeth showing calcifying processes in the pulp cavity. Scand J Dent Res 85:588, 1977

Jacobsen I, Zachrisson BU: Repair characteristics of root fractures in permanent anterior teeth. Scand J Dent Res 83:355, 1975

Kawahara H, Yamagami A: In vitro studies of cellular responses to heat and vibration in cavity preparation. J Dent Res 49:829, 1970

Kelley KW, Bergenholtz G, Cox CF: The extent of the odontoblast process in rhesus monkeys (macaca mulatta) as observed by scanning electron microscopy. Arch Oral Biol 26:893, 1981

Kim S, Grayson A, Kim B, Schacter W: Effects of tooth preparation on pulpal blood flow in dogs. AADR Abstr 286, J Dent Res 62:199, 1983

Kramer IRH: The effects on the dental tissues of restorative techniques and materials. Brit Dent J 115:26, 1963

Kramer IRH: The effects of cavity preparation on the dental pulp. Austral Dent J 12:565, 1967

Krejci RF, Reinhardt RA, Wentz FM, Hardt AB, Shaw DH: Effects of electrosurgery on dog pulps under cervical metallic restorations. Oral Surg 54:575, 1982

Landay MA, Nazimov H, Seltzer S: The effects of excessive occlusal force on the pulp. J Periodont 41:3, 1970

Langeland K: Management of the inflamed pulp associated with deep carious lesion. J Endodont 7:169, 1961

Langeland K: Tissue Changes in the Dental Pulp. Oslo, Oslo Univ. Press, 1957

Langeland K, Langeland LK: Pulp reactions to crown preparation, impression, temporary crown fixation, and permanent cementation. J Pros Dent 15:129, 1965

Laurichesse JM, Santoro JP: The microcirculation of the dental pulp. I. Techniques of intravital microscopy. Rev Odontostomat 19:297, 1972

Lindholm K: The effect of crown preparation and compound impressions on the diameter of the pulp arteriole. Proc Finn Dent Soc 71:10, 1975

Lloyd BA, Rich JA, Brown WS: Effect of cooling techniques on temperature control and cutting rate for high-speed dental drills. J Dent Res 51:675, 1983

Marsland EA, Shovelton DS: Effect of cavity preparation on the human dental pulp. Brit Dent J 102:213, 1957

Marsland EA, Shovelton DS: Repair in the human dental pulp following cavity preparation. Arch Oral Biol 15:411, 1970

Massler M: Discussion in histologic evaluation of pulp reactions to operative procedures. Oral Surg 12:1370, 1959

Melková V: The ultrastructure of the surface of predentine. Scripta Medica 39:101, 1966

Michanowicz AE, Michanowicz JP, Abou-Rass M: Cementogenic repair of root fractures. JADA 82:569, 1971

Mjör IA: Histologic studies of human coronal dentine following cavity preparations and exposure of ground facets in vivo. Arch Oral Biol 12:247, 1967

Mjör IA, Kvam E: Dental pulp reactions following the exposure of coronal dentine in vivo. Acta Odont Scand 27:145, 1969

Morrant GA: Dental instrumentation and pulpal injury. J Brit Endo Soc 10:55, 1977

Natkin E, Ingle JI: A further report on alveolar osteoporosis and pulpal death associated with compulsive bruxism. J Am Soc Periodont 1:260, 1963

Okamura K, Tsubakimoto K, Uobe K, Nishida K, Tsutsui M: Serum proteins and secretory components in human carious dentin. J Dent Res 58:1127, 1979a

Okamura K, Tanaka A, Kahehi A, Maeda M, Tsutsui M: Plasma components in deep lesions of human carious dentin. J Dent Res 58:2010, 1979b

Pashley DH: 2. The influence of dentin permeability and pulpal blood flow on pulpal solute concentrations. J Endodont 5:355, 1979

Pashley DH, Kehl T, Pashley E, Palmer P: Comparison of in vitro and in vivo dog dentin permeability. J Dent Res 60:763, 1981

Pashley DH, Nelson R, Williams EC, Kepler EE: Use of dentine-fluid protein concentrations to measure pulp capillary reflection coefficients in dogs. Arch Oral Path 26:703, 1981a

Pashley DH, Nelson R, Pashley EL: In-vivo fluid movement across dentine in the dog. Arch Oral Biol 26:707, 1981b

Paunio K: Chemical studies on interstitial fluid in the hard tissues. J Dent Res 45:630, 1966

Peyton FA: Temperature rise in teeth developed by rotating instruments. JADA 50:629, 1955

Peyton FA: Effectiveness of water coolant with rotary cutting instruments. JADA 56:664, 1958

Peyton FA: Response to shaping cavities with modern high speed instruments. New York J D 28:262, 1958

Pohto M, Scheinin A: Microscopic observations in living dental pulp. II. Effect of thermal irritants on circulation of the pulp in the lower rat incisor. Acta Odont Scand 16:315, 1958

Pollan LD, Kruger GO, Reynolds DC, Mopsik ER: Osseous cryosurgery and its effect on adjacent pulpal tissues. Oral Surg 38:668, 1974

Ramfjord SP, Ash MM: Occlusion, pp 151, 238. Philadelphia, WB Saunders, 1966

Riethe P: Preparation and pulp. Deutsch Zahnaerztl Z 24:695, 1969

Robertson PB, Lüscher B, Spangberg LS, Levy BM: Pulpal and periodontal effects of electrosurgery involving cervical metallic restorations. Oral Surg 46:702, 1978

Robertson WD, Melfi RC: Pulpal response to vital bleaching procedures. J Endodont 6:645, 1980

Rock WP, Gordon PH, Friend LA, Grundy MC: The relationship between trauma and pulp death in incisor teeth. Brit Dent J 136:236, 1974

Schuchard A: Surface temperature response by use of air coolant in restorative procedures. JADA 75:1188, 1967

Schuchard A, Watkins C: Temperature response to increased rotational speeds. J Dent Res 39:738, 1960

Schuchard A, Watkins C: Temperature response to increased rotational speeds. J Pros Den 11:313, 1961

Seale NS, McIntosh JE, Taylor AN: Pulpal reaction to bleaching of teeth in dogs. J Dent Res 60:948, 1981

Searles JC: Light and electron microscope evaluation of changes induced in odontoblasts of the rat incisor by the high-speed drill. J Dent Res 46:1344, 1967

Searles JC: Radioautographic evaluation of changes induced in the rat incisor by high-speed cavity preparation. J Dent Res 54:174, 1975

Shepard JP: Effects of lowered temperatures on rat pulp and gingivae. Oral Surg 42:386, 1976

Shovelton DS, Marsland EA: A further investigation of the effect of cavity preparation on the human dental pulp. Brit Dent J 105:16, 1958

Sicher M: The odontoblast. The Bur 54:2, 1953

Spangberg LS, Helldén L, Robertson PB, Levy BM: Pulpal effects of electrosurgery involving based and unbased cervical amalgam restorations. Oral Surg 54:678, 1982

Stanley HR: Traumatic capacity of high-speed and ultrasonic dental instrumentation. JADA 63:749, 1961

Stanley HR, Jr, Swerdlow H: Reaction of the human pulp to cavity preparation: Results produced by eight different operative grinding technics. JADA 58:49, 1959

Stanley HR, Jr, Swerdlow H: Biological effects of various cutting methods in cavity preparation: The part pressure plays in pulpal response. JADA 61:450, 1960

Stanley HR, Weisman MI, Mechanowicz AE, Bellizzi R: Ischemic infarction of the pulp: Sequential degenerative changes of the pulp after traumatic injury. J Endodont 4:325, 1978

Steinman RR, Leonora J: Effect of infusing selected chemical compounds on dentinal fluid movement in the rat. J Dent Res 54:567, 1975

Stenvik A, Mjör IA: Pulp and dentine reactions to experimental tooth intrusion. Am J Orthodont 57:370, 1970

Stüben VJ, von Kreudenstein TS: Dentinstoffwechselstudien. VI. Papierelektrophoretische Untersuchungen über die Zusammensetzung der Dentinliquorproteine. Deutsch Zahnärztl Z 12:500, 1957

Suchard A: Pulpal response to cooling armamentaria at ultra high speeds. J Pros Dent 41:58, 1979

Suzuki M, Goto G, Jordan RE: Pulpal response to pin placement. JADA 87:636, 1973

Thomas HF: The extent of the odontoblast process in human dentin. J Dent Res 58 (Spec Iss D):2207, 1979

Thomas HF: The effect of various fixatives on the extent of the odontoblast process in human dentine. Arch Oral Biol 28:465, 1983

Tschamer H: The histology of pulpal tissue after orthodontic treatment with activators during late adolescence. Zahnärztl Prax 25:530, 1974

Van Hassel HJ, Brown AC: Effect of temperature changes on intrapulpal pressure and hydraulic permeability in dogs. Arch Oral Biol 14:301, 1969

Von Kreudenstein TS: The biochemistry of dental lymph. NY Dent J 24:343, 1958

Weiskopf J, Gehre G, Graichen K-H: Ein Beitrag zur Behandlung von Luxationen und Wurzelfracturen um Frontzahngebeit. Stoma (Heidelberg) 14:100, 1961

Weiss MB, Massler M, Spence JM: Operative effects on adult dental pulp. Dent Prog 4:6, 1963

Zach L, Cohen G: Biology of high speed rotary operative dental procedures. I. Correlation of tooth volume removed and pulpal pathology (abstr). J Dent Res 37:67, 1958

Zach L, Cohen G: Thermogenesis in operative techniques. J Pros Dent 12:977, 1962

Zach L, Cohen G: Pulp response to externally applied heat. Oral Surg 19:515, 1965

Zachrisson BU, Jacobsen I: Long-term prognosis of 66 permanent anterior teeth with root fracture. Scand J Dent Res 83:345, 1975

Zadik D, Chosack A, Eidelman E: The prognosis of traumatized permanent anterior teeth with fracture of the enamel and dentin. Oral Surg 47:173, 1979

10
CHEMICAL IRRITANTS

The pulp is subjected frequently to chemical irritation from materials in general use in dentistry. Various filling materials produce some irritation (ranging from mild to severe), as do various medicaments used for desensitization or dehydration of the dentin. Also irritating to the pulp are medicaments that are used, albeit rarely, for sterilization of the dentin after removal of decay.

DENTIN STERILIZING AGENTS

Bacteria have been found in the dentinal tubules in deep carious lesions and are involved in the process of tooth decay (see Chap. 8). Thus, the use of antibacterial agents to destroy the microorganisms may seem to be justified, provided the antibacterial agent is not in itself injurious to the pulp. However, since many antibacterial substances are, the need to remove the bacteria by treatment with an antibacterial agent has not been completely justified (Mjör, 1977). Despite evidence that the pulp may be damaged (Langeland, 1981), many compounds (each with its advocates) have been used for sterilization of dentin: phenols and phenolic derivatives such as thymol, eugenol, and beechwood creosote; silver nitrate; and combinations of drugs, such as parachlorophenol and penicillin. A brief discussion of some of the sterilizing agents that are still employed follows.

PHENOL

Phenol, which has been used extensively in the past, is both cytotoxic and a poor sterilizing agent.

It has been stated that phenol combines with organic matter in the dentinal tubules and forms a coagulum that blocks the tubules and limits the action of the phenol. This concept has been disproved by radioactive tracer studies, which have demonstrated that the phenol actually increased, rather than decreased, the permeability of the dentinal tubules (Amler and Bevelander, 1951; Martin, 1951). Therefore, greater pulp damage can occur with its use (Fig. 10–1).

The poor disinfectant and the highly irritating qualities of phenol make its use as a dentin sterilizing agent undesirable and detrimental.

SILVER NITRATE

Silver nitrate has been employed for dentin sterilization by many clinicians.

Both histologic and isotope studies confirm that, when silver nitrate is used on dentin,

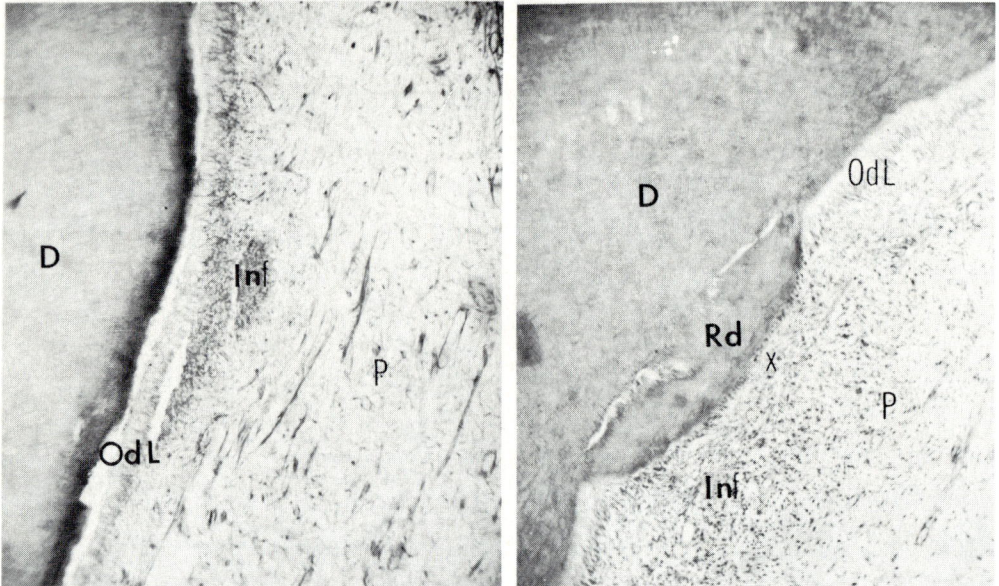

FIG. 10-1 Effect of phenol on the dental pulp. *(Left)* Buccolingual section of the upper left second molar of a dog. Phenol had been applied to the base of a shallow cavity in the dentin (D) 3 months previously. The pulp (P) is inflamed. There is a small collection of inflammatory cells (Inf) within and below the odontoblastic layer (OdL). ×100. *(Right)* Buccolingual section of the lower left first molar of a dog. Three months after the application of phenol to a deep cavity in the dentin (D), the pulp (P) is still inflamed (Inf). Reparative dentin (Rd) has been elaborated subjacent to the cavity preparation. The odontoblastic layer (OdL) is thinned at region X. ×100. (Seltzer S, Bender IB, Kaufman IJ: Oral Surg 14:856, 1961)

blockage of the dentinal tubules does not occur. In fact, increased uptake of the isotope of silver nitrate-impregnated dentin takes place. Silver salts diffuse rapidly through the dentinal tubules and, regardless of the depth of the cavity, eventually reach the pulp tissue (Fig. 10-2). The depth of penetration of the silver increases with time, and the silver nitrate can penetrate into dead tracts, irregular dentin, sclerosed dentin, and calcific barriers (Langeland, 1981).

Numerous studies have demonstrated the irritating potential of silver nitrate to the pulp. In spite of precipitation with formalin or eugenol, irritation continues for long periods, since precipitation is not limited primarily to the surface of the dentin. A resultant inflammatory reaction occurs in the pulp (Fig. 10-3).

CAMPHORATED PARACHLOROPHENOL AND PENICILLIN

A combination of parachlorophenol and penicillin was found by Burkman et al (1954) to be an effective sterilizing agent for deep cavities. However, histologic studies by Langeland (1981) have shown that camphorated phenol and penicillin cause pulpal inflammation.

The local use of penicillin is contraindicated because of its potential for sensitization of the patient and the serious sequelae of such occurrences. Besides, it is doubtful that dentin of pulp infections can be "sterilized" by individual antibiotics (Langeland, 1981).

EUGENOL

Eugenol, mixed with zinc oxide in a paste form, is often applied to deep cavities to allay pain associated with inflammation of the pulp. Eugenol is the active ingredient in many over-the-counter "toothache" drops; it has always been thought to have anodyne properties. When loosely mixed with zinc oxide, eugenol can inhibit the action potential in the nerve fibers of the dental pulp of the cat (Trowbridge et al, 1982). Other studies on crayfish (Ozeki, 1975) and on bullfrogs (Kozam, 1977) have demon-

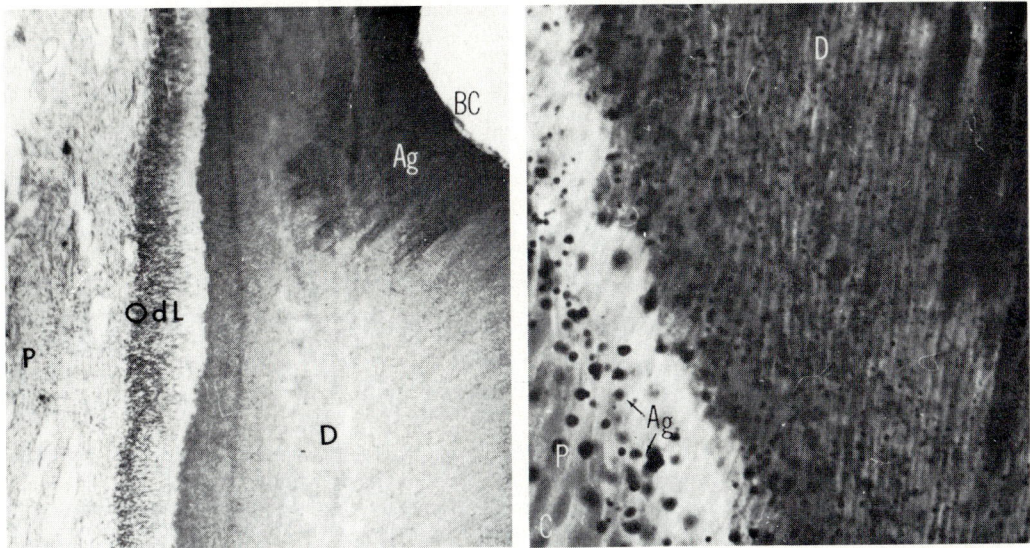

FIG. 10-2 Penetration of silver nitrate. *(Left)* Silver nitrate was applied to the base of a medium-depth cavity (BC) and the animal was sacrificed immediately afterward. Silver particles (Ag) have penetrated the dentin (D). OdL, odontoblastic layer, P, pulp. ×35. *(Right)* Silver nitrate was applied to a deeper cavity. The silver particles (Ag) have penetrated the dentin (D) and are present more profusely within the pulp (P). ×450.

FIG. 10-3 Pulp irritation with silver nitrate. *(Top)* Silver nitrate has penetrated the dentinal tubules (D) of a monkey molar and silver particles have been deposited within the pulp (P), which is severely inflamed. The blood vessels (BV) are stained black by the silver particles. ×54. *(Bottom)* Higher magnification of a capillary in the pulp (P). The endothelial lining is stained black by the silver nitrate. ×960.

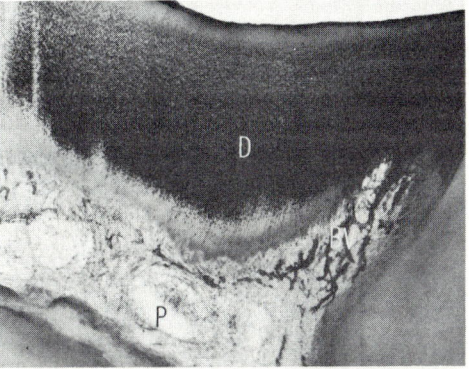

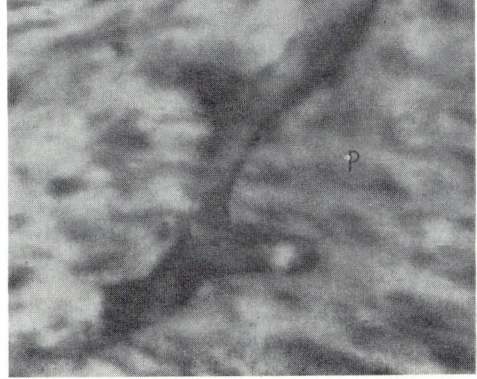

strated that 100 to 200 ppm eugenol can block nerve impulse transmission.

Zinc oxide-eugenol, when applied to dentin, may be considered inhibitory rather than destructive of microbial growth (McKnight, 1967; Cox et al, 1978). The inhibition of growth of the microorganisms may be due to the hygroscopic property of the zinc oxide-eugenol. Removal of the moisture from the substrate may inhibit the growth of the microorganisms.

The use of a zinc oxide-eugenol paste has been found beneficial in the treatment of deep-seated caries when the caries is near the pulp.

All investiagors agree that zinc oxide-eugenol is not irritating to the pulp if applied to dentin. In contrast however, when zinc oxide-eugenol is placed on an exposed pulp, a marked inflammatory reaction occurs. The presence of an inter-

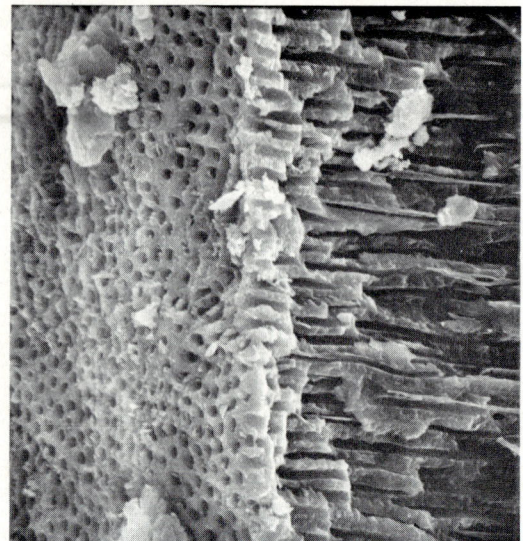

FIG. 10-4 Scanning electron microscope photomicrograph of dentin treated with ethylenediaminetetraacetic acid (EDTA). Note the widened dentinal tubules. ×1000.

vening layer of dentin appears to be necessary to prevent an inflammatory response.

CLEANSING AND DRYING MEDICAMENTS

A tooth cavity preparation creates a "smeared" surface layer of debris that is not removed by ordinary washing and drying (Boyde and Knight, 1970; Dahl, 1977; Øilo, 1978). Removal of this layer enhances bonding of resin fillings to enamel and dentin (Retief, 1972; Gwinnett and Buonocore, 1972; Lee and Swartz, 1972). The smear layer may be removed by polishing with pumice (Dahl, 1978), acid etching (Brännström and Johnson, 1974; Brännström and Nordenvall, 1977; Pashley et al, 1978), or treatment with surface-active cleansing solutions combined with ethylenediaminetetra-acetic acid (Brännström et al, 1980).

Hydrogen peroxide, alcohol, and combinations of alcohol and chloroform have been used for cleansing and drying the dentin prior to the application of cements or filling materials. These drugs, when applied to dentin, usually produce pain. Alcohol injures the odontoblasts becasue it denatures the protein of the protoplasmic processes. Isotope studies have indicated that, when applied to the dentin of dogs' teeth, alcohol permitted increased penetration of ^{32}P from the cavity surface. Acid from zinc phosphate cements penetrates the dentin to a greater extent after the dentin has been treated with alcohol.

Hydrogen peroxide solutions are potentially damaging. Pohto and Scheinin (1959) found that hydrogen peroxide, applied to deep dentin of rat incisors, can penetrate the dentin and cause the formation of emboli in the pulp. Rupture of blood vessels results. The pressure of the liberated oxygen interferes with and disrupts the circulation. Even when applied to the enamel of dogs' teeth, a 35% solution of hydrogen peroxide produced severe but reversible pulp inflammation (Seale et al, 1981).

Blasting of the dentin with compressed air or an air syringe for a period of 10 seconds produces odontoblastic displacement (Langeland, 1963).

Thus, it appears that drying of the cavity by rinsing with warm water and rubbing with cotton pellets produces the least damage.

Other cavity cleansing agents may have a demineralizing effect on the dentinal tubules, possibly resulting in enhanced bacterial invasion (Fig. 10-4). Brännström and Nyborg (1973) have recommended a cavity cleanser consisting of chlorhexidine and dodecyldiaminoethyl glycine in a 3% sodium fluoride solution. Their studies indicated that such a solution eliminated all residual bacteria from a cavity preparation without any irritating effect on the pulp.

ACID ETCHANTS

Acids, such as citric and phosphoric, or experimental chemical cleanser solutions have been used to remove the smeared layer (Bowen, 1978; Mjör et al, 1982).

Scanning electron microscope studies by Lee et al (1973) have demonstrated that the surface of the dentin was demineralized by exposure to a 50% solution of phosphoric or citric acid for from 1 to 5 minutes; the dentinal tubules beneath the surface were apparently unaffected.

In vitro, acid etching of dentin discs markedly increased dentin permeability (Pashley, 1979), a condition that was reversed by treatment with 3% solution of potassium-hydrogen oxalate (Pashley et al, 1978). Such dentin changes permitted penetration of colonies of *Streptococcus mutans* into the dentinal tubules; similar unetched dentin was not penetrated by the bacteria (Michelic et al, 1980).

Pulp reactions to acid etchants have generally

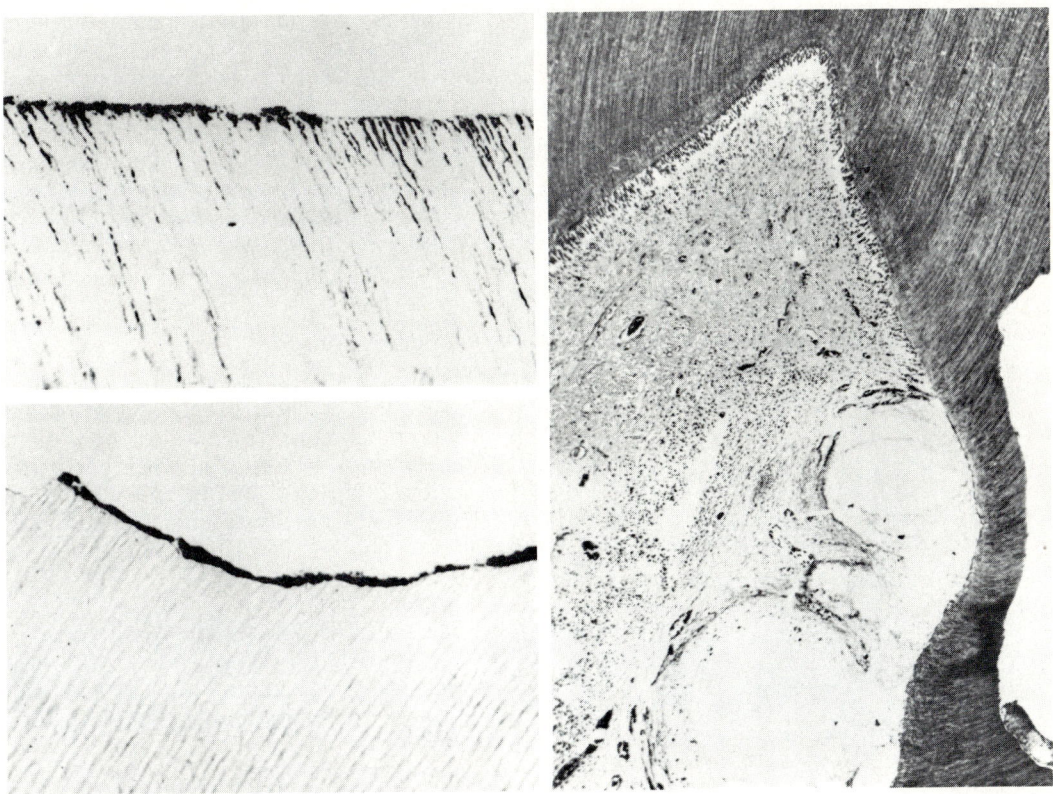

FIG. 10-5 *(Top, left)* Acid-treated cavity. Dentinal tubules are filled with bacteria. Brown-Brenn stain. ×250. *(Bottom, left)* Untreated cavity in tooth contralateral to that shown at top, left. Bacterial layer on bottom of cavity is thick, but only one tubule was penetrated by bacteria. Brown-Brenn stain. ×440. *(Right)* Acid-treated cavity shown at top, left. Distance to pulp is 0.16 mm. Pulp beneath cavity is necrotic. Hematoxylin and Eosin. ×35. (Vojinović O, Nyborg H, Brännström M: Acid treatment of cavities under resin fillings: bacterial growth in dentinal tubules and pulpal reactions. J Dent Res 52:1189, 1973. Copyright by the American Dental Association. Reproduced by permission)

been rated as mild to moderate (Macko et al, 1978). However, Vojinović et al (1973), Eriksen (1973), Stanley et al (1975), and Cotton and Siegel (1978) found that citric acid treatment of cavity walls prior to filling with composite resins resulted in severe inflammatory reactions in the pulp. Furthermore, bacteria were found in almost all acid-treated dentinal tubules, in contrast with the tubules of nontreated resin-filled control teeth (Fig. 10-5; Brännström and Vojinović, 1976). Etching apparently increases pulp inflammation because it removes the debris that accumulates over the dentinal tubules when they are cut, thereby facilitating the penetration of irritants into the dentinal tubules.

Whether removal of the smeared layer is desirable has not yet been determined. The use of calcium hydroxide bases or liners before acid pretreatment of enamel is highly recommended.

DESENSITIZING AND REMINERALIZING AGENTS

Sensitivity of dentin occurs following cervical erosions, coronal fractures, gingival recessions, and gingivectomies and after dentin is cut during cavity or crown preparation. Clinicians are sometimes under the erroneous impression that the application of drugs such as phenol, silver nitrate, zinc chloride, formalin, and other protein coagulants desensitize the dentin by coagulating the protoplasm within the dentinal tubules, thereby blocking the tubules. Anderson (1963) has demonstrated that, contrary to the

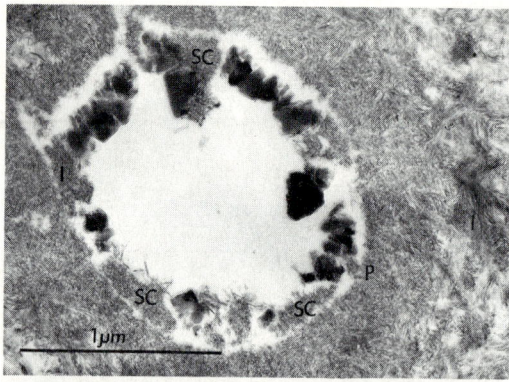

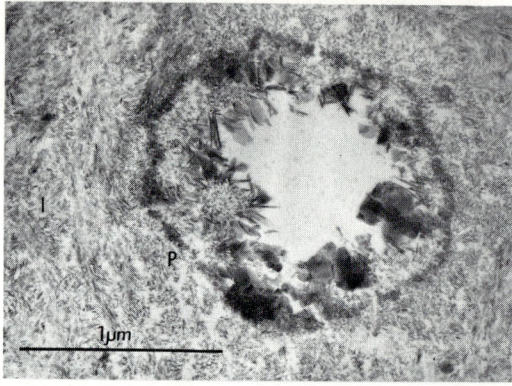

FIG. 10-6 *(Top)* Tubule near the experimental surface in a decalcification lesion produced in sclerosed dentin. The fluoride treatment has protected the peritubular zone and, to a lesser extent, the intratubular minerals from being decalcified by the acid buffer. Remains of the dense, preexisting, obturating mineral are seen as patches (SC) along the periphery of the lumen. These areas consist of minute crystals, similar in size to those found in the peritubular zone (P). The large, irregular crystals forming a single layer along the edge of the tubule are considered to represent precipitates induced by the decalcification procedure. I, intertubular dentin. ×50,000. *(Bottom)* Tubule near the surface of the lesion in a specimen of sclerosed dentin. Large crystals precipitated during the decalcification procedure form a single layer along the border of the lumen. The needlelike crystals presumably represent platelike crystals in edge view. P, peritubular zone; I, intertubular dentin. ×50,000. (Selvig KA: Effect of fluoride on the acid solubility of human dentine. Arch Oral Biol 13:1297, 1968)

belief of many clincians, silver nitrate does not reduce the sensitivity of dentin after cavity preparation. Such drugs, purposely applied to reduce sensitivity and prevent the penetration of acids from cements and silicates, are harmful. There appears to be no valid argument for desensitization of the dentin prior to filling. More appropriately, an insulator, such as calcium hydroxide, should be used.

Numerous surface agents, described below, have been used to control hypersensitive dentin. Despite many claims of efficacy, about 20% to 30% of patients who received no treatment or sham treatment have reported abatement of symptoms (Hernandez et al, 1972; Uchida et al, 1980).

Calcium Fluoride

Martin (1951) reduced the sensitivity and permeability of dentin by applying a 2% sodium fluoride solution followed by a solution of calcium chloride, thereby precipitating insoluble calcium fluoride within the dentinal tubules. The blocked dentinal tubules were rendered impermeable to radioactive phosphorus.

Sodium Fluoride

The use of sodium fluoride for desensitization of the teeth (Lukomsky, 1941; Lefkowitz, 1962) was based on its ability to stimulate the formation of reparative dentin, which is less permeable than primary dentin and, theoretically, should protect the pulp better against further irritation.

Amler and Bevelander (1951) found that sodium fluoride application increased permeability to ^{32}P.

Selvig et al (1968) found by microradiography that topical application of 2% sodium fluoride solution to acid-demineralized human dentin resulted in the production of a radiopaque zone, 5 μ to 20 μ in width, at the surface of the lesion. The fluoride-treated dentin was more acid resistant than nontreated dentin, as demonstrated by reduced depth and severity of subsequent acid decalcification (Fig. 10-6). Neutral fluoride-treated dentin contains high concentrations of fluorine, although only a small fraction of the fluoride, probably calcium fluoride, is retained in the insoluble formed apatite structure. Such precipitations may present mechanical barriers to stimuli, preventing their transmission to the odontoblastic processes (Tal et al, 1976).

Although 2% sodium fluoride solution has been found effective for reducing cervical sensitivity (Gedalia et al, 1978), reports on the human pulpal effects following its application on dentin are controversial. Severe pulp inflammations, which persisted for months, have been reported by some investigators (Lefkowitz and Bodecker, 1945; Rovelstad and St. John, 1949).

One of us found a high incidence of pulpal inflammation in 24 young human premolars following the application of 2% sodium fluoride solution in moderately deep cavities (Seltzer; Fig. 10-7). Others (Weiss and Massler, 1969; Furseth and Mjör, 1973) have reported that the pulps were relatively unaffected when cavities were treated with a 2% sodium fluoride solution for 2 minutes, covered with zinc oxide-eugenol or calcium hydroxide and restored with amalgam. Thus, the contradictory results may be related to the prevention of subsequent leakage of restorations. An alternative possibility is that Furseth and Mjör's results could be attributable to the reaction of calcium hydroxide and sodium fluoride, resulting in the precipitation of calcium fluoride within the dentinal tubules, similar to Martin's observations.

Desensitization may be due to the fact that fluorine is an enzyme inhibitor or poison. Many odontoblasts may be killed or injured and cease to function. Therefore, sodium fluoride solutions, especially high concentrations, should not be used on freshly cut dentin.

Ionization

Electrical currents have been used to facilitate the penetration of substances through dentin. Pashley et al (1978) found that the penetration of labeled iodine or lidocaine through dentin discs prepared from human third molars, was increased by iontophoretic currents. These findings indicate that iontophoresis may be useful for increasing the permeation of therapeutic agents through dentin for the treatment of hypersensitive dentin.

Ionization of a sodium fluoride solution on the exposed dentin has been recommended for desensitization of hypersensitive dentin. Murthy et al (1973) found that iontophoresis with a 1% solution of sodium fluoride produced the best results for desensitization when compared with topical application of a 33.3% sodium fluoride paste or with iontophoresis of the patient's own saliva. Scott (1962) reported minor pulp damage caused by the ionization of a 1% solution of sodium fluoride for 1 milliampere minute on the freshly cut dentin of bicuspids and deciduous cuspids. Additional investigations by Gangarosa and Park (1978), Gangarosa et al (1981), and Carlo et al (1982) have confirmed that cervical hypersensitivity can be treated effectively by iontophoretic applications of a 2% sodium fluoride solution. A high percentage of patients obtained significant relief from sensitivity induced by a blast of air and application of an explorer to

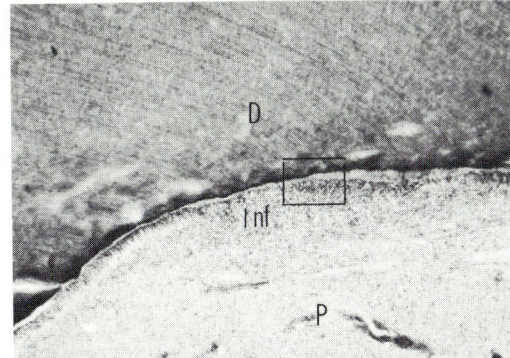
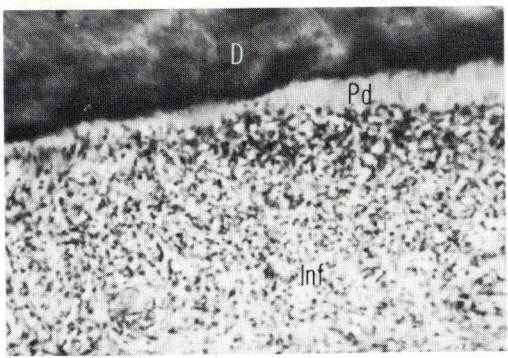

FIG. 10-7 Effect of a 2% solution of sodium fluoride on the pulp. *(Top)* Inf, chronic inflammation of the pulp (P), 6 weeks after application of sodium fluoride in a moderately deep cavity in the dentin (D). ×54. *(Bottom)* Higher magnification of region outlined by rectangle in picture at top. Inf, chronic inflammatory cells in the pulp. The predentin (Pd) is widened. D, dentin. ×240.

the sensitive surface. The desensitizing effect was long-lasting and caused no harm to the pulp in dogs' teeth (Walton et al, 1979). Jensen (1964) and Johnson et al (1982) found that an iontophoretic toothbrush,* used with a fluoride dentifrice, markedly reduced tooth hypersensitivity.

The mechanism by which iontophoresis produced desensitization is not clear. Zadok et al (1976) suggested that the action causes an increased uptake of fluoride into dentin, as compared to topical application of fluoride only. Lefkowitz et al (1963) found that the ionizing current, not the fluoride, was responsible for the desensitization and the production of reparative dentin. In our view, however, the deliberate in-

---

* A negatively charged applicator with which sodium fluoride was applied to the positively charged tooth with a current flow.

duction of reparative dentin is not biologically acceptable.

Stannous Fluoride

Stannous fluoride has been applied, by a variety of techniques, for the arrest of caries. It has also been shown to reduce the solubility of enamel (Abramovich and Sabelli, 1974), of dentin (Sandoval and Shannon, 1969), and of root surfaces (Gordon, 1969). Its effect on the pulp when applied to freshly cut dentin of the teeth of experimental animals and humans has been investigated by Myers et al (1971) and Brännström and Nyborg (1971). Effects of solutions ranging from 4% to 30% were studied. Histologic examinations after 3 to 62 days indicated minimal pulpal responses to the lower concentrations, except when the solutions were placed on undetected pulp exposures.

Radiographic (Fig. 10–8) and microradiographic studies (Wei et al, 1968) have also indicated that a 10% stannous fluoride solution is capable of rapidly remineralizing carious dentin in vitro (Fig. 10–9). Electron micrographs demonstrated a deposit of electron-dense material in the dentin matrix following treatment with this stanous fluoride solution (Fig. 10–10). X-ray diffraction indicated that the material was probably a tin phosphate (Wei and Forbes, 1968).

Shanon (1971), measuring the reduction of dentin solubility after application of aqueous solutions of stanous fluoride ranging from 30% to 1%, found that a 1% solution was as effective as the higher concentrations. Use of a 1% solution would thus constitute a biologically sounder approach in clinical practice.

A 0.4% stanous fluoride gel has been reported effective for reducing the hypersensitivity of root surfaces exposed by periodontal disease (Miller et al, 1968).

Other Sodium Fluoride Solutions

Topical applications of different forms of sodium fluoride solutions have been recommended for dentin desensitization and caries reduction. A 0.9% solution of sodium silicofluoride (Massler, 1955), and a 6% solution of sodium monofluorophosphate have been reported beneficial in relieving hypersensitivity of exposed dentin and cementum (Ericsson, 1961; Bolden et al, 1968; Hazen et al, 1968; Kanouse and Ash, 1969). Furthermore, there was a significant reduction in the incidence of caries (Peterson, 1979).

Acidulated sodium fluoride solutions have also been used for dentin desensitization. The fluoride combines with the apatite structure to form calcium fluoride, which interferes with the transmission of pain stimuli to the pulp. According to Laufer et al (1981), the fluoride concentration of dentin treated with acidulated fluoride is significantly higher than that treated with neutral fluoride.

Glucocorticoids

Topical applications of glucocorticoids to freshly prepared cavities have been used for reducing sensitivity of teeth. The topical application is therapeutically effective for the amelioration of pain, possibly owing to the control of the edema that develops after acute inflammation. The therapeutic benefits have been attributed primarily to the suppression of the inflammatory response that follows cell injury.

Glucocorticoids alter the vascular response to injury by reducing dilatation and decreasing the permeability of the capillary endothelium. Glucocorticoids also inhibit granulocyte adherence, like all anti-inflammatory drugs. The reduction of cell stickiness or margination causes fewer polymorphonuclear leukocytes to aggregate at the site of injury. Thus, the inflammation is suppressed by confining fluids and the inflammatory cells inside the venules.

The suppression of the inflammatory response occurs regardless of whether the inciting agent is mechanical, chemical, bacterial, or immunologic. The administration of the drug is primarily palliative. The underlying cause of the disease remains; the inflammatory manifestations are merely suppressed. According to Stanley (1968), immediately after corticosteroid application to cavity preparations, the intensity of the inflammatory reactions in the pulps was reduced. Dachi and Stigers (1967) found that application of prednisone to cavities reduced thermal sensitivity in teeth restored with amalgam. On the other hand, Langeland et al (1971) found that the application of corticosteroids to dentin did not prevent or reduce acute or chronic pulp inflammation or resorption or apposition of dentin. A possible basis for such reduced sensitivity is the finding of Mjör and Furseth (1968) that corticosteroids applied topically to dentin caused many of the dentinal tubules to become obliterated by a highly electron dense, mineralized material.

Probably no harm results to the pulp from a single topical application of steroids to dentin.

CHEMICAL IRRITANTS | 223

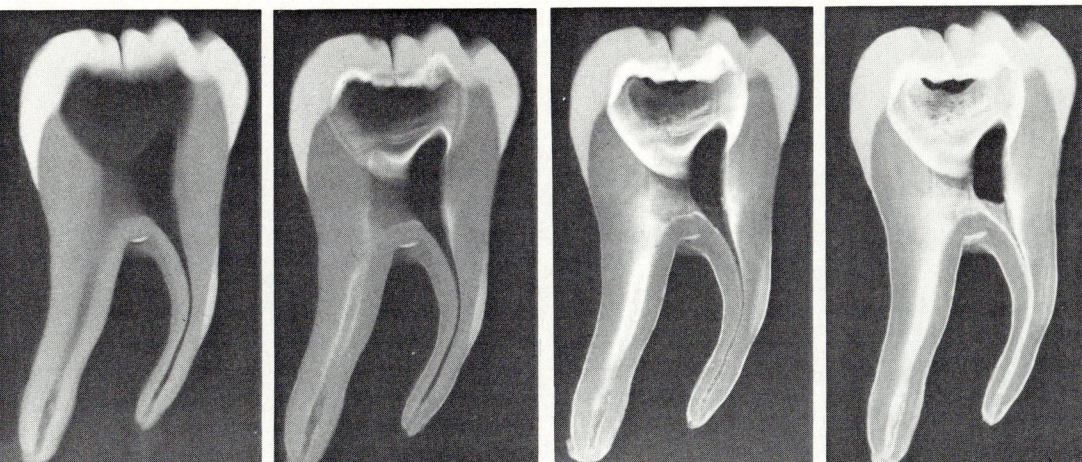

FIG. 10-8 Radiographic appearance of a longitudinal section, 1 mm thick, of a tooth with an active carious lesion, prior to treatment *(left)*, and after immersion in a 10% solution of stannous fluoride, for 30 minutes *(center, left)*, for 24 hours *(center, right)* and for 48 hours *(right)*. Notice the gradual increase in radiodensity with time, in the carious dentin, demineralized enamel, and circumpulpal dentin. (Wei SHY, Kaqueler JC, Massler M: Remineralization of carious dentin. J Dent Res 47:381, 1968. Copyright by the American Dental Association. Reproduced by permission)

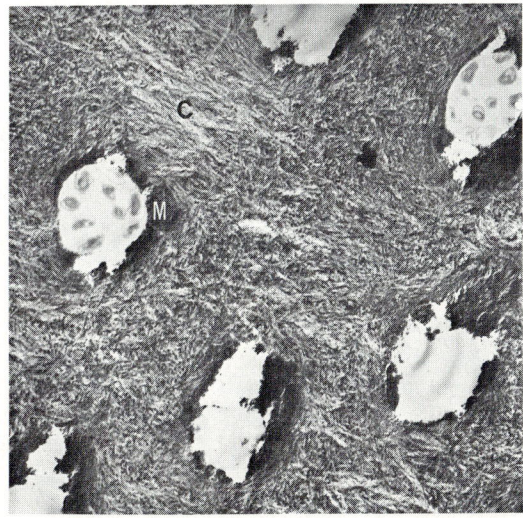

FIG. 10-9 Transmission electron photomicrograph of typical carious dentin, showing the presence of bacteria within the tubules and the dense peritubular distribution of mineral (M). The collagenous matrix (C) can be clearly seen and appears relatively intact despite advanced caries and demineralization. ×7860. (Wei SHY, Kaqueler JC, Massler M: Remineralization of carious dentin. J Dent Res 47:381, 1968. Copyright by the American Dental Association. Reproduced by permission)

FIG. 10-10 Electron photomicrograph of a cross section through an active carious lesion of dentin after immersion in sodium fluoride solution (1%) for 24 hours. Notice the needle-shaped apatite crystallites (A), the peritubular deposition of dense mineral (M), and bacterial inclusion bodies (B). ×17,500. (Wei SHY, Kaqueler JC, Massler M: Remineralization of carious dentin. J Dent Res 47:381, 1968. Copyright by the American Dental Association. Reproduced by permission)

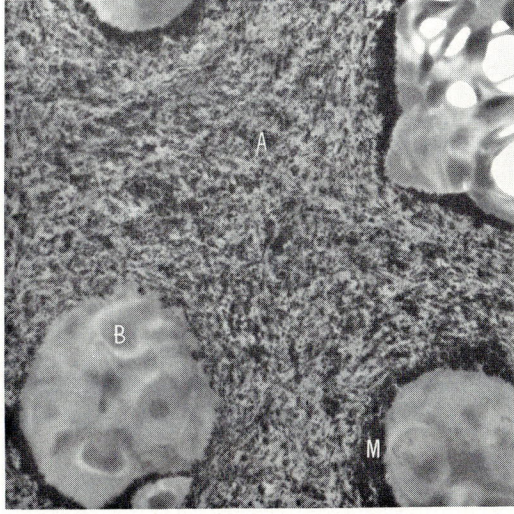

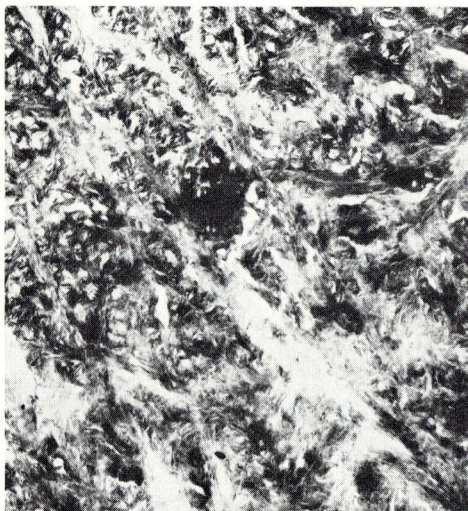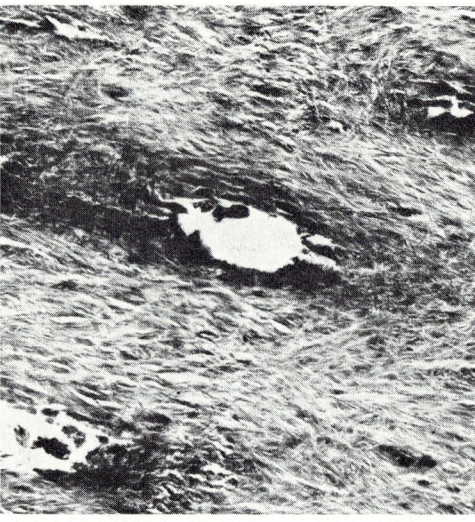

FIG. 10-11 *(Left)* Electron micrograph from the subsurface region. The lumen of a dentinal tubule is obliterated by mineral deposits, and the deposits appear continuous with the surrounding matrix. *(Right)* In the deeper portions of dentin, the tubules were patent and apparently empty, with no evidence of bacteria or other organic material. (Hiatt HH, Johansen E: Root preparation. I. Obturation of dentinal tubules in treatment of root hypersensitivity. J Periodontol 43:373, 1972)

Strontium Chloride

Shapiro et al (1970) noted that patients using a dentifrice containing 10% strontium chloride had significantly less root hypersensitivity after 4 weeks than a group of control patients. After 8 weeks, no significant differences were observed between the two groups.

It has been claimed that strontium chloride in a concentration of 0.048 mol/liter can cause blockage of neural transmission of stimuli. However, Anderson and Matthews (1966) found that application of a saturated solution of strontium chloride to freshly cut cavities for 30 seconds did not reduce pain sensation when the cavities were stimulated osmotically.

The effects on the pulp of a solution containing strontium chloride and sodium fluoride in an oxicellulose gel have been studied by Auvenshine and Eames (1972). After 45 days, they found some pulp changes, such as displacement of odontoblastic nuclei and areas of hemorrhage, which they attributed to the trauma of extraction. Further and more controlled investigations are indicated.

Calcium Hydroxide

A paste made of calcium hydroxide and sterile distilled water was tested by Levin et al (1973) on the necks of 118 teeth in 50 patients. Both they and Green et al (1977) confirmed the effectiveness of calcium hydroxide in reducing or eliminating hypersensitivity. Relief was immediate in the majority of the teeth; poorer results were obtained in teeth treated with magnesium hydroxide and distilled water. However, after 6 months, 40% of the control teeth also were free of hypersensitivity, indicating that hypersensitivity tends to resolve itself spontaneously with the passage of time.

Calcium Acid Phosphate

Hiatt and Johansen (1972) have found that rubbing exposed tooth roots with a fine-ground paste of calcium acid phosphate reduced sensitivity to touch, foods, and temperature changes. Electron microscopic examinations revealed that, in such teeth, most of the dentinal tubules were blocked with a crystaline material that resembled calcium acid phosphate (Fig. 10-11).

Potassium Nitrate

Solutions and toothpastes containing potassium nitrate have also been advocated for control of dentin hypersensitivity. Prolonged effective desensitization occurred when various concentrations were applied to exposed dentin or cementum (Hodosh, 1974). Treatment with solutions ranging from 1% to 15% were effective, but the results were better with more concentrated solutions. Saturated solutions by weight yielded the most favorable results. Green et al (1977) and Tarbet et al (1980) confirmed Hodosh's observations through the use of other pain-inducing modalities, such as thermal, electrical, and mechanical stimuli. In contrast to controls and to the application of calcium hydroxide, cessation of hypersensitivity occurred almost immediately following application of potassium nitrate and the relief lasted for 3 months. Subsequently, Tarbet et al (1982) compared the efficacy of four different toothpastes, including those containing strontium chloride, dibasic sodium citrate, and formaldehyde, on dentinal sensitivity. They found that the potassium nitrate was significantly superior to the other toothpastes. However, as a group, the other toothpastes also provided significant reductions in sensitivity.

Potassium nitrate appears to be a safe chemical that does not cause adverse effects on the pulps of the teeth (Tarbet et al, 1981). In fact, Hodosh et al (1983) have advocated its use as a pulp capping agent. The desensitizing mechanism is not understood. It is unlikely that the rapidity of desensitization is due to a process of crystallization within the dentinal tubules that would prevent dentinal nerve excitation.

AN ALTERNATIVE METHOD

Rubbing the sensitive area of dentin with an orangewood stick eliminates the sensation of pain. Whether the friction and the small amount of heat generated, or the packing of dentin filings, or the cellulose products from the stick have a stimulating effect on the odontoblasts is not known. Quite frequently, these painful sensations disappear spontaneously with no treatment whatsoever.

CAVITY LINERS AND TEMPORARY AND PERMANENT FILLING MATERIALS (AND RELATED PROCEDURES)

Chemical irritation of the pulp is induced by the ingredients of cavity liners and temporary and permanent filling materials. Cavity liners produce only minor pulp reactions and are included for discussion in this chapter because they are used primarily for the prevention of pulp inflammation.

CAVITY LINERS

Cavity liners have been employed to reduce the sensitivity of freshly cut dentin and to protect the pulp from the injurious effects of filling materials, particularly composite acrylic resins, silicates, and zinc phosphate cements (Eames et al, 1979).

In vitro tests indicate that most acrylic resins exhibit antibacterial activity when freshly prepared. This activity is lost with further polymerization on aging (Updegraff et al, 1971). Silicates also exhibit antibacterial activity. Nonetheless, unlined cavities restored with silicates or composite resins have been shown to contain dense accumulations of bacteria, presumably from contraction of the restorations (Qvist et al, 1977). Toxic products from such bacteria may be instrumental in causing inflammation of the pulp (Brännström et al, 1979).

Varnishes

Most cavity liners are varnishes. Rosin or other resins are dissolved in a volatile organic solvent, such as chloroform or acetone. Such liners may also contain calcium hydroxide, zinc oxide, or other additives.

Cavity liners of the varnish type have limited value for protection of pulp against silicates or cements. They reduce, but do not completely inhibit, the irritation. Zander (1946) and Swartz et al (1968) have shown that a resin varnish, when applied to experimental cavities, did not protect the pulp from the deleterious effects of silicates. There is evidence that some liners reduce the degree of dentin dehydration by various filling materials (Johnson and Brännström, 1971) and aid in the prevention of recurrent caries around amalgam restorations (Ellis and Brown, 1967). In clinical practice, it has been observed that teeth with cavities that were lined only with varnish and filled with silicates remained sensitive for varying periods of time. In many, the pulps became necrotic, and periapical areas of rarefaction developed. These complications may be attributed to bacterial penetration that could not be prevented even with a double application of copalite (Brännström and Nordenvall, 1978). Even following three subsequent varnish applications, the permeability of the smear layer of dentin was not reduced (Dippel et al, 1979).

In clinical practice, deep cavities should receive a base of calcium hydroxide or zinc oxide and eugenol. The varnish should then be applied over the sub-base. Going (1964) has pointed out that the varnish should be applied with a cotton pellet, in a thin coat and uniformly. Ether evaporates from older varnishes. Use of the resultant thicker, more viscous liquid leaves a thick, irregular coating on the tooth. Therefore, the bottle containing the varnish should be kept tightly stoppered. If the varnish hardens, it should be thinned before use with the appropriate ether solvent. In shallow cavities, under composites and amalgams, a benzalconium hydrochloride shellac primer in an alcohol solution, with ethyl acetate as a solvent, offers good protection against bacterial growth and thermal changes. This liner is approximately 5 μm to 6 μm thick (Brännström, 1981).

Polystyrene and Methylcellulose Liners

Cavity liners composed of polystyrene, zinc oxide-eugenol, and calcium hydroxide preparations have a potential for pulp protection. The polystyrene is a thin film that acts as a barrier. Zinc oxide-eugenol and calcium hydroxide also prevent irritating materials from penetrating the dentinal tubules. Zinc oxide-eugenol is the treatment of choice for deep-seated carious lesions. Zinc phosphate cement may be placed over this liner for greater tensile strength.

Cavity liners made up of mixtures of calcium hydroxide and zinc oxide suspended in a chloroform solution of polystyrene* as suggested by Zander et al (1950), and those that contain calcium hydroxide in a methylcellulose base,† as suggested by Berk (1950), have proved effective in protecting the pulp against irritation by silicates. Also, they reduce the sensitivity of the pulp to thermal stimuli.

Fluoride Liners. Cavity liners incorporating fluorides, such as calcium monofluorophosphate ($CaFPO_4$) and potassium fluorozirconate (K_2ZrF_6), have been found effective in reducing thermal conduction into the pulp by metal restorations and in decreasing acid solubility of dentin (Söremark et al, 1969; Brännström and Nyborg, 1969). An absence of irritating effects on the pulp has been reported (Brännström, 1969).

A modification of the formula of Zander et al, in which diiodide dithymol and calcium fluorophosphate have been added,‡ has been shown to provide equally good pulp protection against sili-

---

* Chambar (L.D. Caulk Company, Milford, Delaware)
† Pulpdent (Pulpdent Corp. of America, Boston, Massachusetts)
‡ Tubulitec, AB Forsergs Dentaldepot, Stockholm, Sweden

cates and amalgams (Brännström and Nyborg, 1969; 1971). Used as a cavity cleaner, this solution has also been found by Brännström and Nyborg (1974) to eliminate debris and bacteria on cavity walls. Eriksen (1973) has also found that this liner reduces, but does not eliminate, pulpal irritation caused by some composite resins.

Calcium Hydroxide

Calcium hydroxide is relatively insoluble and acts as a mechanical barrier when applied to dentin. It may cause sclerosis of the primary tubules, and it does not stimulate the elaboration of reparative dentin.

The presence of the Ca^{2+} ion may activate adenosine triphosphatase (ATPase), which may then enhance dentin mineralization (Abiko, 1977; Guo and Messer, 1976), a finding not confirmed by Brännström et al (1976). In low concentrations, calcium hydroxide, when applied to dentin, may also stimulate mitosis of pulp fibroblasts (Torneck and Wagner, 1980; Torneck et al, 1983). When applied to pulp exposures, $Ca(OH)_2$ does stimulate reparative dentin formation.

Calcium hydroxide acts as a chemical neutralizer for the acidity of silicate and zinc phosphate cements and prevents penetration of the acid into the pulp (Fig. 10–12). Calcium hydroxide placed on the dentin acts as a physical barrier also, because of its relative insolubility.

Calcium hydroxide is an insoluble base that dissociates, to a limited degree, into Ca^+ and OH^- ions. The hydroxyl ions are available for neutralizing the H^+ ions from the acids of the cements. There is a significant elevation of pH in the dentin subjacent to calcium hydroxide application after 1 to 3 days (Hasselgren et al, 1982). However, in the larger silicate restorations, the amount of hydroxyl ions liberated by the calcium hydroxide may not be sufficient to neutralize the acidity of silicates. Some free acid may remain unneutralized. Langeland (1959) has shown that deleterious pulp changes may occur under silicates lined with calcium hydroxide. The liberation of acidic ions from a silicate continues for prolonged periods because the silicate remains in a gel state. Therefore, according to Swartz et al (1968), in deep cavities in which large silicate restorations are employed, it is advisable to apply zinc phosphate cement over the calcium hydroxide for additional protection of the pulp.

Radiographic density of the dentin of teeth has been used as a tool for measuring the sclerosis of dentinal tubules. This is accomplished by magnifying the radiograph and then measuring the density of the shadow of the dentin with an instrument called a densitometer and comparing the results with those of controls.

The densitometric studies of Klein (1961) and Mjör et al (1961) have shown that dentin becomes denser under calcium hydroxide because of sclerotic changes. In electron microscopic studies, Mjör and Furseth (1968) found that the dentinal tubules were obturated, partially or completely, by an electron-dense, crystalline material. Increase in density has been observed clinically under cortisone and zinc oxide-eugenol and after the application of parachlorophenol and penicillin.

In extremely deep cavities, in which there may be microscopic exposures, it is recommended that calcium hydroxide be applied, followed by zinc oxide-eugenol or zinc phosphate cement under the completed restoration. Where pulp exposures do not exist, zinc oxide-eugenol is the least irritating and the most palliative cement, possibly because of its hygroscopic and anodyne properties. It removes moisture from the dentinal tubules, thus relieving pressure on an inflamed pulp. On the other hand, calcium hydroxide does not significantly alter or depress nerve impulse activity (Trowbridge et al, 1982) and therefore should not be used to treat painful pulpitis.

Dropsin

Dropsin,* according to the manufacturer, is a cavity liner made by mixing a liquid with a powder. The liquid consists of 25% phosphoric acid, 8% aluminum hydroxide, and 67% distilled water. The powder contains zinc oxide, calcium hydroxide, magnesium oxide, and aluminum hydroxide. Studies conducted by Plant and Tyas (1970) on monkey and human teeth indicated that the material was well tolerated by the pulp. However, Eriksen (1971) found that Dropsin was permeable and did not protect the pulps of monkey teeth when it was used as a liner under composite resins.

PIT AND FISSURE SEALANTS

A number of materials have been advocated for sealing pits and fissures in the enamel surfaces of teeth in an effort to prevent the development of caries. Among these materials are cyanoacrylates, polyurethanes, polycarboxylates and a

* Svedia, Enköping, Sweden

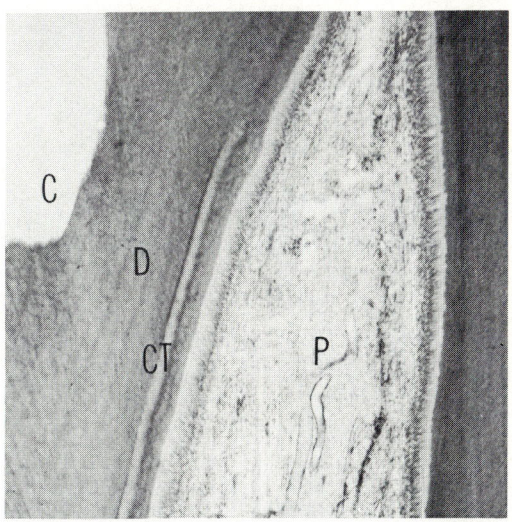

FIG. 10-12 Calcium hydroxide under cement base. When placed on the dentin (D) of a prepared cavity (C) of a dog tooth, calcium hydroxide reduces or prevents the deleterious effects of the acid from zinc phosphate cement. The pulp (P) is uninflamed 6 weeks after therapy. A calcio-traumatic response (CT) is evident in the dentin. ×54. (Seltzer S, Bender IB: JADA 66:503, 1963)

reaction product of bisphenol A and glycidyl methacrylate (Buonocore, 1973). With the last-mentioned material, the enamel is usually prepared for bonding by the application of a 50% solution of phosphoric acid for 1 minute. The adhesive, containing the reaction product of 3 parts bisphenol A and glycidyl methacrylate and 1 part methacrylate monomer to which is added an ultraviolet-light-sensitive catalyst (benzoin methyl ether), is then applied by brush to the involved surfaces. The adhesive is then hardened by exposure to long-wave ultraviolet light. Studies have indicated that the number of microorganisms from the dentin of the sealed teeth were substantially lower than that from the dentin of control teeth (Handelman et al, 1973). However, although acid treatment of dentin may cause pulpal reactions (Vojinović et al, 1973), the effects of acid etching of enamel on the dental pulp probably are not harmful.

TEMPORARY FILLING MATERIALS AND BASES

Various bases and cements are used to insulate the pulp from thermal diffusion through metallic restorations and from the irritating action of

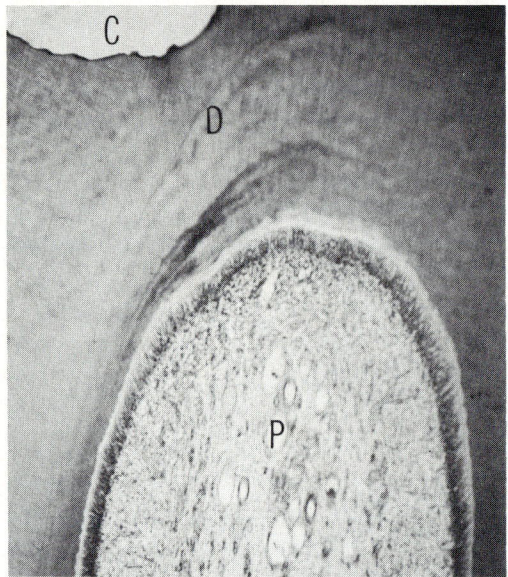

FIG. 10-13 The effect of zinc oxide-eugenol, used as a temporary filling material. Zinc oxide-eugenol which was placed on the dentin (D) of a prepared cavity (C) in a dog's tooth has a palliative effect on the pulp (P), as evidenced by the mildness of the inflammatory response. ×54. (Seltzer S, Bender IB: JADA 66:503, 1963)

chemical constituents of various restorative materials, and to provide resistance to occlusal forces. In general, the thickness of the base is probably the most significant factor for thermal insulation (Braden, 1964; Voth et al, 1966). However, other factors, such as pH, setting characteristics, bond strength, compressive strength, adhesiveness, solubility, permeability, irritational, or sedative qualities, must be evaluated (ADA, 1972; Qvist and Stoltze, 1982). Our discussion of the commonly used cements and bases concerns primarily the biologic aspects of these materials and their effects on dentin and pulp.

Zinc Oxide-Eugenol

Zinc oxide-eugenol is a temporary filling material that is also used frequently as a liner under other restorative materials. Under both in vitro and in vivo conditions, Tibbetts et al (1976) have shown that a zinc oxide-eugenol base under amalgam restorations is a better thermal insulator than calcium hydroxide or zinc phosphate cements. Of all the filling materials, it has always been considered the safest from a biologic standpoint. Most investigators have agreed that there was little pulp irritation following the application of zinc oxide-eugenol to a cavity (Fig. 10-13).

However, tissue culture studies have shown that zinc oxide-eugenol is toxic to pulp cells (Das, 1981), and some reports have suggested that zinc oxide-eugenol may be more irritating to the pulp than zinc phosphate cement (Brännström and Nyborg, 1976; Brännström et al, 1981). Furthermore, Brännström's group has claimed that zinc oxide-eugenol should not be applied to deep cavities without an intervening liner. The type of eugenol used in the mixture may be responsible for some of the irritating effects. Webb and Bussell (1981) found that commercial eugenol contains a number of impurities. When tested on the connective tissue of rats, purified eugenol produced less of an inflammatory response than the commercial variety. The greater the amount of free eugenol in the mixture, the greater the chance of pulpal irritation. In our view, there is little likelihood that a thick mixture of zinc oxide-eugenol will irritate the pulp.

Traditionally, zinc oxide-eugenol has been used as an anodyne for pulpal pain. The sedative effects are apparently due to eugenol's ability to block or reduce nerve impulse activity (Trowbridge et al, 1982).

Radioactive tracer studies and our scanning electron microscope and microprobe analysis studies (Fig. 10-14) have shown that it provides a better marginal seal than the zinc phosphate cements, although leakage increases with time (Norman et al, 1963). It is an effective insulating material and prevents galvanic action of the amalgam, thus inhibiting corrosion. Another advantage is that there is no heat rise during setting (Plant and Jones, 1976). Its disadvantages as a temporary filling material are its softness, its slowness in setting, and the ease with which it may be displaced by biting stress before setting. However, some of these disadvantages can be overcome by adding cotton or asbestos fibers to the mixture. The addition of zinc acetate accelerates setting, producing a hard cement. When it is anticipated that the zinc oxide-eugenol will be removed, it should be applied to a moistened cavity surface. Unless the cavity is so moistened, the dentin becomes sensitive on removal of the zinc oxide-eugenol, because the latter is hygroscopic (Johnson and Brännström, 1971). According to Scott (1979), the frequency of nerve impulse firings is increased in freshly dehydrated dentin. Such frequency is reduced when water is applied to the opened dentinal tubules. Zinc oxide-eugenol also has a slight demineralizing action on dentin, chelating calcium (Rotberg and deShazer, 1966).

The use of zinc oxide-eugenol under silicates is contraindicated because it may discolor the silicate material. Its use is also contraindicated under composites because it prevents complete polymerization. Also, greater penetration of isotopes results. In extremely deep cavities in anterior teeth, a sub-base of calcium hydroxide followed by a base of zinc phosphate cement may be used under the silicate in preference to zinc oxide-eugenol.

Modified Zinc Oxide-Eugenol Cements. To compensate for its low strength, a major disadvantage of zinc oxide-eugenol, products incorporating polymethyl methacrylate in the powder have been developed as intermediate restorative materials (IRM; Jendresen and Phillips, 1969). The cements are formed from mixing a powder containing zinc oxide, aluminum oxide, polymethyl methacrylate, and resin with a liquid containing o-ethoxybenzoic acid and eugenol. Such materials can be inserted without elaborate cavity preparation and remain in the cavity for a long period until a more permanent type of restoration can be placed. When inserted in cavities prepared in swine and human teeth, the pulps showed mild, reversible damage (Coleman and Kirk, 1965; Bhaskar et al, 1969). On the other hand, studies by Brännström et al (1981) showed that, despite preventing bacterial ingrowth from the tooth surface, IRM may cause inflammation in human pulps when inserted in deep cavities with a remaining dentin thickness of less than 0.5 mm. Until further studies are made, no definitive conclusions can be drawn regarding the pulpal effect of IRM.

FLUORIDE-MODIFIED ZINC OXIDE-EUGENOL. Wolf et al (1973) have modified zinc oxide-eugenol by adding to it a 14% concentration of $CaFPO_4$; the final product contained approximately 2% fluoride. In vitro and in vivo studies of the dentin of human tooth cavities in which the base was placed were made after several weeks. Both the microhardness and the fluoride content of the dentin covered by the $CaFPO_4$-supplemented liner were increased. In contrast, there was no effect on the microhardness in the dentin of control cavities lined solely with zinc oxide-eugenol.

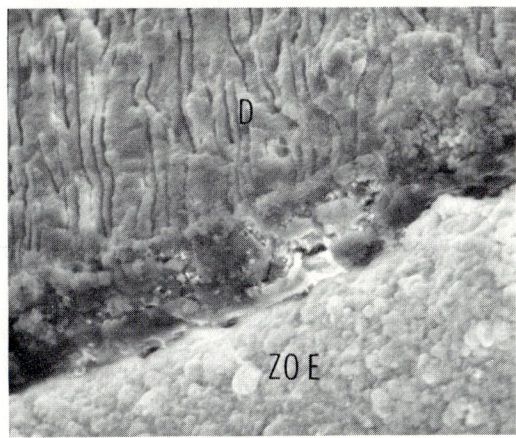

FIG. 10-14 Scanning electron micrograph of zinc oxide-eugenol (ZOE) and dentin (D) interface, showing close adaptation. ×600.

Zinc Phosphate Cement

Zinc phosphate cement can cause severe pulpal damage because of its inherent irritating properties (Brännström and Nyborg, 1960). Kim has found that phosphoric acid, when applied to the capillaries of the hamster cheek pouch, causes stasis of red blood cells (RBCs), eventually resulting in autolysis. Toxicity is more pronounced when the cement is placed in deep cavity preparations. In shallow or medium-depth cavities, damage is proportionately less severe (Fig. 10-15). Zinc phosphate cement is not as irritating as silicate cement because it crystallizes and sets much faster than the latter. Thus, the hydrogen ions are not liberated for as long a period. In deep cavities in anterior teeth, zinc phosphate cement should not be used without an intervening liner of zinc oxide-eugenol or calcium hydroxide. Thick mixes should be used to minimize pulp irritation and marginal leakage. When thinner mixes are employed, pH values of 1.5 to 1.6 have been recorded. There is a delay in crystallization, which prolongs the irritating effects, and greater heat is generated. Nixon (1962) has demonstrated that pH values of 4.8 are maintained and neutralization of the cement is never achieved, even after crystallization.

The pulp may be affected by the components of the material, the heat that is liberated in setting, and the marginal leakage that permits the ingress of irritants from saliva. Brännström and Nyborg (1974, 1977) and Watts (1979) attributed pulpal injury from the cement to the

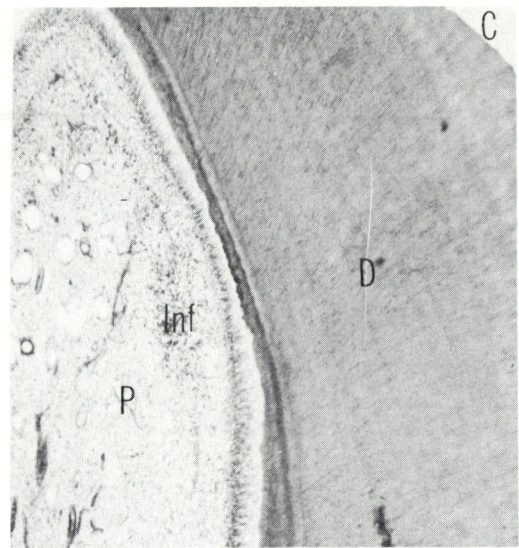

FIG. 10-15 Zinc phosphate cement placed on the dentin (D) of a prepared cavity of moderate depth (C) in a dog's tooth caused inflammation (Inf) of the pulp (P), which still persists 6 weeks after treatment. ×54. (Seltzer S, Bender IB: JADA 66:503, 1963)

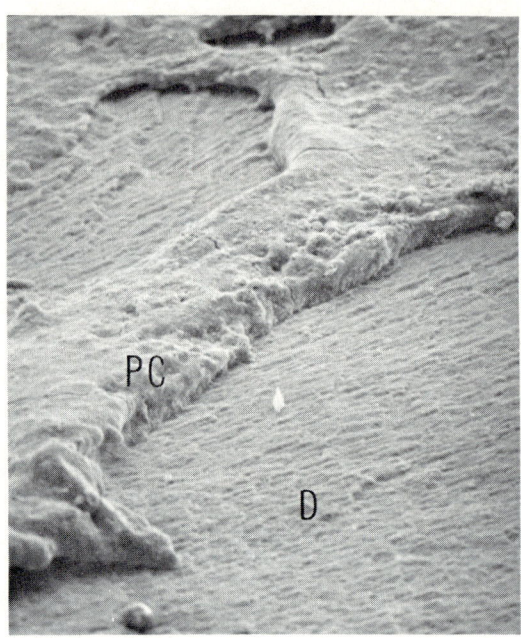

FIG. 10-16 Scanning electron micrograph of zinc polycarboxylate cement and dentin interface, showing close adaptation of cement (PC) to dentin (D). ×180.

marginal leakage, rather than to its toxic chemical properties. Isotope studies have shown that, when labeled phosphoric acid was mixed with the powder and the cement placed on dentin of prepared cavities, the isotope penetrated into the underlying dentin along the dentinal tubules. Also, marginal penetration of the isotopes was increased. The addition of amalgam alloy materially reduces disintegration, marginal and bulk fracture of the zinc phosphate cement (Wolcott et al, 1962; Mahler and Armen, 1962).

Polyacrylic (Polycarboxylate) Cements

Efforts have been made to formulate an improved cement that would have the manipulative qualities and strength of zinc phosphate cement with a reduced irritancy and toxicity. Furthermore, adhesion to tooth structure would reduce marginal leakage.

Such a cement, formulated by Smith (1968), is composed of a modified zinc oxide powder and an aqueous solution of a polyacrylic acid. The cement bonds to both dentin and enamel by chelation (Fig. 10-16). However, the bonding to enamel is stronger than the bonding to dentin (Beech, 1973; Kawahara et al, 1979). Concentrated acids and fluoride solutions greatly reduce the bond strength (Beech, 1978).

The cement demonstrates strong antibacterial properties in vitro (Beagrie, 1979). Cytotoxic tests have been made in tissue culture (Spangberg et al, 1974; Kawahara et al, 1979) and on the prepared cavities of dog, monkey, and human teeth. No perceptible difference in pulp reactions from those of control teeth filled with zinc oxide and eugenol have been noted by Truelove et al (1971), Barnes and Turner (1971), Safer et al (1972), and El-Kafrawy et al (1974). However, Plant (1971) did find that the zinc polycarboxylate cements produced inflammatory reactions that were absent in zinc oxide-eugenol filled cavities under similar test conditions.

Cyanoacrylate Cements

Cyanoacrylate cements are composite-type polymers that can be polymerized to hard products by the use of basic, inorganic materials that also serve as fillers. These cements are adhesive (Beech, 1972) and bacteriostatic (Jandinski and Sonis, 1971). A number of homologues of alkyl 2-cyanoacrylates in the form of methyl, ethyl, n-butyl, and isobutyl have been formulated into dental cements and pit and fissure sealants. According to Bhaskar et al (1966), histotoxicity is decreased as the chain length is increased. Pulpal effects of an isobutyl cyanoacrylate cement have been investigated by Bhaskar et al (1969). They found that mild to moderate inflammatory responses were induced in the pulps of miniature pigs after 3 weeks. There was also an increased deposition of reparative dentin, as compared to that under zinc oxide-eugenol. They concluded that these cements were biologically acceptable, particularly as indirect pulp capping agents.

When n-butyl cyanoacrylate was used as a liner under amalgam restorations, in vitro experiments demonstrated leakage patterns similar to those of copal resins (Stark et al, 1969).

According to Fukushi and Fusayama (1980), the use of ethylcyanoacrylate is preferable to methylcyanoacrylate because of its greater adhesion, lesser leakage, and lesser pulp irritation. They believe that methylcyanoacrylate has an adverse effect on the pulp, probably because it is hydrolyzed more readily to formaldehyde, which is irritating. Pulp irritation may also be due to the fact that cyanoacrylate on polymerization removes water from the dentinal tubules (Matsui et al 1967).

Calcium Hydroxide Cements

To eliminate the necessity of placing a sub-base of calcium hydroxide followed by a base of zinc phosphate cement or zinc oxide-eugenol, cements containing calcium hydroxide have been developed. They are formulated, in general, of two pastes that are mixed together. According to Accepted Dental Therapeutics (1982), one formula consists of a base containing calcium phosphate (tribasic) 31.4%; calcium tungstate 17.6%; zinc oxide 8.7%; in a glycol salicylate base. The catalyst consists of calcium hydroxide, 51.0%; zinc oxide, 9.23%; zinc stearate, 0.29% in ethylene toluene sulfonamide.* Another formula contains calcium hydroxide, a resin, barium sulfate, and titanium dioxide.† These cements are antibacterial (Fisher and McCabe, 1978; Fairbourn et al, 1980; Leung et al, 1980). However, the antibacterial effect is not long-lasting (Fitzgerald et al, 1983). When set, they provide a hard base over which a permanent restoration can be placed. Favorable results when used in primary and permanent teeth have been reported by Delaney and Seylor (1966) and Tronstad and Mjör (1972).

Calcium hydroxide cements are hydrolytically unstable, releasing calcium and hydroxide ions and salicylates when in contact with water. The rate of erosion is controlled by plasticizers (Prosser et al, 1982). Thus, in time, these cements tend to decompose and disappear from the dentin (Akester, 1979). However, such decomposition may be advantageous, since the large amounts of calcium released at high alkalinity promote sterilization and calcification of carious dentin.

GLASS IONOMER CEMENTS

Glass-ionomer cements are reaction products of an ion-leachable glass powder and a poly-anion (alkenoic-acid) in aqueous solution. The combination forms a hard polysalt gel (Crisp and Wilson, 1974). The setting characteristics are improved by the addition of low-molecular-weight chelating agents, such as hydroxycarboxylic acids (D-tartaric acid), which are now employed in all commercial variants of the glass-ionomer cements* (Prosser et al, 1982).

There are a variety of clinical applications for glass-ionomer cements, such as their use as restorative and sealing materials. A more finely ground powder has enabled the glass ionomer cements to be used also as a translucent luting cement, as a cavity liner, as a restoration for erosion lesions, and as a sealer for occlusal pits and fissures (McLean and Wilson, 1977). Glass-ionomer cements adhere tightly to enamel and to dentin (Hotz et al, 1977), but the enamel bond is stronger (Maldonado et al, 1978).

When tested in cell culture, freshly prepared material was found to be toxic to fibroblasts and macrophages, but the toxicity decreased after setting (Dahl and Tronstad, 1976; Kawahara et al, 1979; Meryon et al, 1983). Despite a low pH (Iwaku et al, 1980), these cements have been found by Nordenvall et al (1979), Kawahara et al (1979), and Pameijer et al (1981) to cause insignificant pulp damage. Others (Tobias et al, 1978; Cooper, 1980), however, tested the effects of several different preparations on pre-

---

* Dycal (L.D. Caulk Co., Milford, Delaware)
† Hydrex (Kerr Manufacturing Company, Detroit, Michigan)

* De Trey's ASPA, Chem Bond Cement (AD International Ltd., London); Caulk ASPA (L.D. Caulk Co., Milford, Delaware); Fuji Ionomer (G.C. Dental Industrial Corp., Tokyo)

pared human cavities. They found a greater degree of pulp inflammation than that caused by zinc oxide-eugenol.

Gutta-Percha

Gutta-percha is an organic substance used for temporary fillings. Because of its poor marginal sealing and other irritating properties, gutta-percha has an injurious effect on the pulp. Frequently, the tooth is sensitive after the removal of the temporary filling. This sensitivity is attributable to marginal leakage that permits oral fluids to penetrate the freshly cut dentin. Gutta-percha does not seal the dentinal tubules (Johnson and Brännström, 1971); fluids and bacteria from the mouth are pumped into the dentin, and the odontoblasts are injured.

The heat and pressure associated with the materials' insertion may also contribute to the sensitivity.

Langeland (1961), Johnson and Brännström (1971), and Mjör and Tronstad (1972) have shown that the material itself is irritating to the pulp. Langeland excluded the possibility of heat damage by cooling the gutta-percha to a temperature at which it could be handled comfortably by the fingers. The chances for marginal leakage were reduced by covering the applied gutta-percha with zinc oxide-eugenol, followed by amalgam. In spite of these precautions, pulp inflammation, characterized by displaced odontoblastic nuclei and the presence of polymorphonuclear leukocytes, lymphocytes, plasma cells, macrophages, and circulatory disturbances, was induced. Jarby (1962) found similar changes, related to depth of cavity preparation. If the base of the cavity was less than 0.2 mm from the pulp, inflammatory changes occurred. However, the gutta-percha in shallower cavities (depth of remaining dentin 0.5 mm) produced no pulp changes.

Proprietary Preparations

Cavit* is a proprietary name for a temporary filling material that contains zinc oxide, calcium sulfate, zinc sulfate, glycol acetate, polyvinyl acetate, polyvinyl chloride acetate, triethanolamine, and a red pigment. The material sets when saliva reacts with calcium sulfate and with zinc oxide-zinc sulfate. It has been reported to have excellent sealing qualities (Brännström and Vojinović, 1976), possibly caused by water sorption. It is less antibacterial than zinc oxide-eugenol (Krakow et al, 1977). In tissue culture, it is mildly toxic (Antrim, 1976). The effects of Cavit on the dental pulps of monkey and human teeth have been studied by Widerman et al (1971), Brännström and Vojinović (1976), and Provant and Adrian (1978). They found that it caused no severe pathologic alterations in the pulp.

Cavit can be recommended as a temporary filling material, especially for teeth undergoing root canal therapy (Parris and Kapsimalis, 1960).

---

* Premier Dental Products, Philadelphia

BIBLIOGRAPHY

Abiko Y: Studies on calcium-stimulated adenosine triphosphatase in the albino rabbit dental pulp: its subcellular distribution and properties. J Dent Res 56:1558, 1977

Abramovich A, Sabelli CA: Action of *Streptococcus mutans* on dental enamel pretreated with stannous fluoride. J Dent Res 53:94, 1974

Accepted Dental Therapeutics, 39th ed, p 301. Chicago, American Dental Association, 1982

Akester J: Disappearing dycal. Brit Dent J 146:369, 1979

American Dental Association: Recommended standard practices for biological evaluations of dental materials. JADA 84:382, 1972

Amler MH, Bevelander G: Dentin permeability to radioactive phosphorus after specific time intervals following the application of various drugs. NYJ Dent 21:195, 1951

Anderson DJ: Chemical and osmotic excitants of pain in human dentine. In Anderson DJ (ed): Sensory Mechanisms in Dentine. New York, Macmillan, 1963

Anderson DJ, Matthews B: An investigation into the reputed desensitizing effect of applying silver nitrate and strontium chloride to human dentine. Arch Oral Biol 11:1129, 1966

Andres CJ, Stookey GK, Muhler JC: Studies concerning the effect on the dental pulp in dogs of a stable stannous fluoride solution applied to freshly cut dentine. J Oral Ther Pharm 4:113, 1967

Antrim DD: Evaluation of the cytotoxicity of root canal sealing agents on tissue culture cells in vitro: Grossman's Sealer, N_2 (permanent), Rickert's sealer, and Cavit. J Endodont 2:111, 1976

Armstrong WD, Simon, WJ: Penetration of radiocalcium at the margins of filling materials, a preliminary report. JADA 43:684, 1951

Association Reports, American Dental Association: Status report on the glass ionomer cements. JADA 99:221, 1979

Auvenshine R, Eames WB: The biological effects of a desensitizing solution on the gingival and pulp tissues. J Ala Dent A 56:17, 1972

Barnes DS, Turner EP: Initial response of human pulp to zinc polycarboxylate cement. J Canad Dent A 37:265, 1971

Beagrie GS: Pulp irritation and silicate cement. J Dent 45:67, 1979

Beech D: Adhesion in the oral environment: Biophysical and biochemical considerations. Int Dent J 28:338, 1978

Beech DR: Bonding of alkyl 2-cyanoacrylates to human dentin and enamel. J Dent Res 51:1438, 1972

Beech DR: Adhesion of polycarboxylate cement to human dentin. J Dent Res (Abst No 114) 52:959 1973

Berk H: Effect of calcium hydroxide-methyl cellulose paste on the dental pulp. J Dent Child 17:65, 1950

Bhaskar SN, Cutright DE, Beasley JD, Boyers RC: Pulpal response to four restorative materials. Oral Surg 28:126, 1969

Bhaskar SN, Frisch J, Margetis PM, Leanard F: Application of a new chemical adhesive in periodontal and oral surgery. Oral Surg 22:526, 1966

Bolden TA, Volpe AR, King WJ: The desensitizing effect of a sodium monofluorophosphate dentifrice. Periodontics 6:112, 1968

Boyde A, Knight PJ: Scanning electron microscopic studies of the preparation of the embrasure walls of class II cavities. Brit Dent J 129:557, 1970

Braden M: Heat conduction in teeth and the effect of lining materials. J Dent Res 43:315, 1964

Brännström M: Dentin and Pulp in Restorative Dentistry. p 102. Nacka, Sweden, Dental Therapeutics AB, 1981

Brännström M: New aspects of dentin isolation. Zahnärztl Welt 78:611, 1969

Brännström M, Isacsson G, Johnson G: The effect of calcium hydroxide and fluorides on human dentine. Acta Odont Scand 34:59, 1976

Brännström M, Johnson G: Effects of various conditioners and cleaning agents on prepared dentin surfaces. J Prosth Dent 31:422, 1974

Brännström M, Nordenvall K-J: Bacterial penetration, pulpal reaction and the inner surface of concise enamel bond. Composite fillings in etched and unetched cavities. J Dent Res 57:3, 1978

Brännström M, Nordenvall K-J: The effect of acid etching on enamel, dentin, and the inner surface of the resin restoration. J Dent Res 56:917, 1977

Brännström M, Nordenvall K-J, Glantz P-O: The effect of EDTA-containing surface-active solutions on the morphology of prepared dentin: An in vivo study. J Dent Res 59:1127, 1980

Brännström M, Nordenvall K-J, Torstenson B: Pulpal reaction to IRM cement: An intermediate restorative material containing eugenol. J Dent Child 48:259, 1981

Brännström M, Nyborg H: Bacterial growth and pulpal changes under inlays cemented with zinc phosphate cement and epoxylite CBA 9080. J Prosth Dent 31:556, 1974

Brännström M, Nyborg H: Cavity treatment with a microbicidal fluoride solution. Growth of bacteria and effect on the pulp. J Prosth Dent 30:303, 1973

Brännström M, Nyborg H: Dentinal and pulpal response. IV. Pulp reaction to zinc oxyphosphate cement. A morphologic study on dog and man. Odont Revy 11:37, 1960

Brännström M, Nyborg H: Pulpal protection by a cavity liner applied as a thin film beneath deep silicate restorations. J Dent Res 50:90, 1971

Brännström M, Nyborg H: Pulpal reaction to composite resin restoration. J Prosth Dent 27:181, 1972

Brännström M, Nyborg H: Pulpal reaction to polycarboxylate and zinc phosphate cements used with inlays in deep cavity preparations. JADA 94:308, 1977

Brännström M, Nyborg H: Pulp reactions to a temporary zinc oxide-eugenol cement. J Prosth Dent 35:185, 1976

Brännström M, Nyborg H: Pulp reaction to fluoride solution applied to deep cavities: An experimental histological study. J Dent Res 50:1548, 1971

Brännström M, Soremark R: The penetration of ^{22}Na ions around amalgam restoration with and without cavity varnish. Odont Revy 13:331, 1962

Brännström M, Vojinović O: Response of the dental pulp to invasion of bacteria around three filling materials. J Dent Child 43:83, 1976

Buonocore MG: Adhesives in the prevention of caries. JADA 87:1000, 1973

Burkman NW, Schmidt HS, Crowley MC: A preliminary report of an investigation to study the effectiveness of certain drugs for sterilizing carious dentine. Oral Surg 7:647, 1954

Carlo GT, Ciancio SG, Seyrek SK: An evaluation of iontophoretic application of fluoride for tooth desensitization. JADA 105:452, 1982

Castagnola L, Garberoglio R: Can varnishes influence the formation of fissures between the cavity and the filling material? Schweiz Mschr Zahnheilk 78:766, 1968

Coleman JM, Kirk EEJ: An assessment of a modified zinc oxide-eugenol cement. Brit Dent J 118:482, 1965

Cooper IR: The response of the human dental pulp to glass ionomer cements. Int Endo J 13:76, 1980

Cotton WR, Siegel RL: Human pulp response to citric acid cavity cleanser. JADA 90:639, 1978

Cox ST, Hembree JH, McKnight JP: The bacterial potential of various endodontic materials for primary teeth. Oral Surg 45:947, 1978

Crisp S, Wilson AD: Reactions in glass ionomer cements: III. The precipitation reaction. J Dent Res 53:1420, 1974

Dachi SF, Stigers RW: Reduction of pulpal inflammation and thermal sensitivity in amalgam-restored teeth treated with copal varnish. JADA 74:1281, 1967

Dahl BL: Dentine/pulp reactions to full crown preparation procedures. J Oral Rehabil 4:427, 1977

Dahl BL: Effect of cleansing procedures on the retentive ability of two luting cements to ground dentin in vitro. Acta Odont Scand 36:137, 1978

Dahl BL, Tronstad L: Biological tests of an experimental glass ionomer (Silicopolyacrylate) cement. J Oral Rehabil 3:19, 1976

Das S: Effect of certain dental materials on human pulp tissue in tissue culture. Oral Surg 52:76, 1981

Delaney JM, Seyler AE: Hard set calcium hydroxide as a sole base in pulp protection. J Dent Child 33:13, 1966

Dippel HW, Hoppenbrowers PMM, Borggreven JMPM: Influence of smear layer on the permeability of dentin. J Dent Res (Special Issue D) 58:2249, 1979

Dorfman A, Stephan RM, Muntz JA: In vitro studies on sterilization of carious dentin. II. Extent of infection in carious lesions. JADA 30:1901, 1943

Dorfman A, Stephan RM, Muntz JA: Effect of various procedures on the human dental pulp. Oral Surg 14:210, 1961

Dorfman A, Stephan RM, Muntz JA: Effective duration of

some agents used for dentin sterilization. J Dent Res 21:115, 1942

Dorfman A, Stephan RM, Muntz JA: Effectiveness of antibacterial agents used in cavity sterilization. J Dent Res 21:269, 1942

Eames WB, Hendrix K, Mohler HC: Pulpal response in rhesus monkeys to cementation agents and cleaners. JADA 98:40, 1979

El-Kafrawy AH, Dickey DM, Mitchell DF, Phillips RW: Pulp reaction to a polycarboxylate cement in monkeys. J Dent Res 53:15, 1974

Ellis JM, Brown LR: Application of an in vitro cariogenic technic to study the development of carious lesions around dental restorations. J Dent Res 46:403, 1967

Ericsson Y: Fluorides in dentifrices—investigations using radioactive fluorine. Acta Odont Scand 19:41, 1961

Eriksen HM: Tissue reactions and sealing properties of Tubulitec and Dropsin. J Dent Res 50:1223, 1971 (Abstr No 11)

Eriksen HM: Pulpal responses to composite dental materials lined with Tubulitec or Dropsin. Scand J Dent Res 81:285, 1973

Evans JA, Massler M: Nonreaction of pulp to fluoride application. J Dent Child 35:91, 1968

Fairbourn DR, Charbeneau GT, Loesche WJ: Effect of improved Dycal and IRM on bacteria in deep carious lesions. JADA 100:547, 1980

Fischer FJ, McCabe JF: Calcium hydroxide base materials. Brit Dent J 144:341, 1978

Fitzgerald M, Cox CF, Bergenholtz G, Syed SA, Heys DR, Baker JD: Observations of $Ca(oH)_2$ bases after one year placement in monkeys. AADR Abst #733, J Dent Res 62:250, 1983

Fukushi Y, Fusayama T: Effect of cyanoacrylate treatment of cavity walls. J Dent Res 59:662, 1980

Furseth R, Mjör IA: Pulp studies after 2 per cent sodium fluoride treatment of experimentally prepared cavities. Oral Surg 36:109, 1973

Gangarosa LP: Iontophoretic application of fluoride by tray technique for desensitization of multiple teeth. JADA 102:50, 1981

Gangarosa LP, Park NH: Practical considerations in iontophoresis of fluoride for desensitizing dentin. J Prosth Dent 39:173, 1978

Gedalia I, Brayer L, Kalter N, Richter M, Stabholtz A: The effect of fluoride and strontium application on dentin: in vivo and in vitro studies. J Periodont 49:269, 1978

Going RE: Cavity liners and dentin treatment. JADA 69:415, 1964

Gordon GE: The effect of stannous fluoride on the solubility of the root surfaces of human teeth. M.S. Thesis, University of Texas Dental Branch, 1969

Green BL, Green ML, McFall WT: Calcium hydroxide and potassium nitrate as desensitizing agents for hypersensitive root surfaces. J Periodont 48:667, 1977

Guo MK, Messer HH: Properties of Ca^{2+}, Mg^{2+} activated adenosine triphosphatase from rat incisor pulp. Arch Oral Biol 21:637, 1976

Gwinnett AJ, Buonocore MG: A scanning electron microscope study of pit and fissure surfaces conditioned for adhesive sealing. Arch Oral Biol 17:415, 1972

Handelman SL, Buonocore MG, Schoute PC: Progress report on the effect of a fissure sealant on bacteria in dental caries. JADA 87:1189, 1973

Hardwick JL: Sterilization of carious dentin. Proc Roy Soc Med (Sec Odont), 42:815, 1949

Harrison LM: Cavity varnishes shown ineffective. J Dent Child 33:174, 1966

Hasselgren G, Kerekes K, Nellestam P: pH changes in calcium hydroxide-covered dentin. J Endodont 8:502, 1982

Hazen SP, Volpe AR, King WJ: Comparative desensitizing effect of dentifrices containing sodium monofluorophosphate, stannous fluoride and formalin. Periodontics 6:230, 1968

Hernandez F, Mohammed C, Shannon I, Volpe A, King W: Clinical study evaluating the desensitizing effect and duration of two commercially available dentifrices. J Periodont 43:367, 1972

Hiatt WH, Johansen E: Root preparation. I. Obturation of dentinal tubules in treatment of root hypersensitivity. J Periodont 43:373, 1972

Hiatt WH, Johansen E: Histologic evaluation of pulp reactions to operative procedures. Oral Surg 12:1235, 1357, 1959

Hodosh M: A superior desensitizer—potassium nitrate. JADA 88:831, 1974

Hodosh M, Hodosh SH, Shklar G, Hodosh AJ: Potassium nitrate: An effective treatment for pulpitis. Oral Surg 55: 419, 1983

Hotz P, McLean JW, Sced I, Wilson AD: The bonding of glass ionomer cements to metal and tooth substrates. Brit Dent J 142:41, 1977

Jandinski J, Sonis S: In vitro effects of isobutyl cyanoacrylate on four types of bacteria. J Dent Res 50:1557, 1971

Jarby S: Response of the dental pulp to heated filling materials. Odont Tids 70:1, 1962

Jendresen MD, Phillips RW: A comparative study of four zinc oxide and eugenol formulations as restorative materials. II., J Prosth Dent 21:300, 1969

Jensen AL: Hypersensitivity controlled by iontophoresis: Double blind clinical investigation. JADA 68:216, 1964

Johnson G, Brännström M: Dehydration of dentin by some restorative materials. J Prosth Dent 26:307, 1971

Johnson G, Brännström M: Pain reaction to cold stimulus in teeth with experimental fillings. Acta Odont Scand 29:639, 1971

Johnson RH, Zulguar-Nain BJ, Koval JJ: The effectiveness of an electro-ionizing toothbrush in the control of dentinal hypersensitivity. J Periodontol 53:353, 1982

Kanouse MC, Ash MM, Jr: The effectiveness of a sodium monofluorophosphate dentifrice on dental hypersensitivity. J Periodontol 40:15, 1969

Kawahara H, Imanishi Y, Oshima H: Biological evaluation on glass ionomer cement. J Dent Res 58:1080, 1979

Klein AI: Association between deciduous dentin sclerosis and calcium hydroxide methylcellulose base material. JADA 63:92, 1961

Kozam G: The effect of eugenol on nerve transmission. Oral Surg 44:799, 1977

Krakow AA: Destoppelaar JD, Gron P: In vivo study of temporary filling materials used in endodontics in anterior teeth. Oral Surg 43:615, 1977

Langeland K: Histologic evaluation of pulp reactions to operative procedures. Oral Surg 12:1235, 1357, 1959

Langeland K: Effect of various procedures on the human dental pulp. Oral Surg 14:210, 1961

Langeland K: Management of the inflamed pulp associated with deep carious lesion. J Endodont 7:169, 1981

Langeland K: Pulpal response to caries and operative procedures. JDAS Af 18:101, 1963

Langeland K, Dowden WE, Tronstad L, Langeland LK: Human pulp changes of iatrogenic origin. Oral Surg 32:943, 1971

Laufer B, Mayer I, Gedalia I, Deutsch D, Kaufman HW, Tal M: Fluoride-uptake and fluoride-residual of fluoride-treated human root dentine in vitro determined by chemical, scanning electron microscopy and x-ray diffraction analyses. Arch Oral Biol 26:159, 1981

Lee HL, Swartz ML: Evaluation of a composite resin crown and bridge luting agent. J Dent Res 51:756, 1972

Lefkowitz W: Pulp response to ionization. J Prosth Dent 12:966, 1962

Lefkowitz W, Bodecker CF: Sodium fluoride: Its effect on the dental pulp. Ann Dent 3:141, 1945

Lefkowitz W, Burdick HC, Moore, DL; Desensitization of dentin by bioelectric induction of secondary dentin. J Prosth Dent 13:940, 1963

Leung RL, Loesche WJ, Charbeneau GT: Effect of Dycal on bacteria in deep carious lesions. JADA 100:193, 1980

Levin MP, Yearwood LL, Carpenter WN: The desensitizing effect of calcium hydroxide and magnesium hydroxide on hypersensitive dentin. Oral Surg 35:741, 1973

Lukomsky EH: Fluorine therapy for exposed dentin and alveolar atrophy. J Dent Res 20:649, 1941

McKnight JP: The effect of zinc oxide and eugenol on microorganisms in the dental pulp. J Dent Child 34:166, 1967

McLean JW, Wilson AD: The clinical development of the glass ionomer cements. Formulation and properties. Aust Dent J 22:31, 1977

Macko DJ, Rutberg M, Langeland K: Pulpal response to the application of phosphoric acid to dentin. Oral Surg 45:930, 1978

Mahler, DB, Armen GK, Jr: Addition of amalgam alloy to zinc phosphate cement. J Prosth Dent 12:157, 1962

Maldonado A, Swartz ML, Phillips RW: An in vitro study of certain properties of a glass ionomer cement. JADA 96:785, 1978

Martin ND: The permeability of the dentine to P^{32} using the direct tissue radioautography technique. Oral Surg 4:1461, 1951

Massler M: Desensitization of cervical cementum and dentin by sodium silicofluoride. J Dent Res 34:731, 1955

Matsui A, Buonocore M, Sarda O, Yamaki M: Tissue reactions to methyl- and ethyl-2-cyanoacrylate adhesives. J Dent Res 46:389, 1967

Meryon SD, Stephens PG, Browne RM: A comparison of the in vitro cytotoxicity of two glass-ionomer cements. J Dent Res 62:769, 1983

Michelic VJ, Schuster GS, Pashley DH: Bacterial penetration of human dentin in vitro. J Dent Res 59:1398, 1980

Miller JT, Shannon IL, Kilgore WG, Bookman JE: Use of a water-free stannous fluoride-containing gel in the control of dental hypersensitivity. J Periodont 39:54/490, 1968

Mjör IA: Bacteria in experimentally infected cavity preparations. Scand J Dent Res 85:599, 1977

Mjör IA, Finn SB, Quigley MB: The effect of calcium hydroxide and amalgam on non-carious, vital dentine. Arch Oral Biol 3:283, 1961

Mjör IA, Furseth R: The inorganic phase of calcium hydroxide- and corticosteroid-covered dentine studied by electron microscopy. Arch Oral Biol 13:755, 1968

Mjör IA, Tronstad L: Experimentally induced pulpitis, Oral Surg 34:102, 1972

Mosteller JH: The use of prednisolone in the elimination of postoperative thermal sensitivity: A clinical study. J Prosth Dent 12:1176, 1962

Murthy KS, Talim ST, Singh I: A comparative evaluation of topical application and iontophoresis of sodium fluoride for desensitization of hypersensitive dentin. Oral Surg 36:448, 1973

Myers CL, Stanley HR, Hayde JB: Response of the primate dental pulp to a concentrated stannous fluoride solution. J Dent Res 50:517, 1971

Nixon GS: Zinc phosphate cement. Dent Pract 12:322, 1962

Nordenvall K-J, Brännström M, Torstensson B: Pulp reactions and microorganisms under ASPA and Concise composite fillings. J Dent Child 46:449, 1979

Norman RD, Swartz ML, Phillips RW: Studies on film thickness, solubility, and marginal leakage of dental cements. J Dent Res 4:950, 1963

Øilo G: Adhesive bonding of dental luting cements; influence of surface treatment. Acta Odont Scand 36:265, 1978

Ozeki M: The effects of eugenol on the nerve and muscle in crayfish. Comp Biochem Physiol 50:183, 1975

Pameijer CH, Segal E, Richardson J: Pulpal response to a glass-ionomer cement in primates. J Prosth Dent 46:36, 1981

Parris L, Kapsimalis P: Effect of temperature change on the sealing properties of temporary filling materials. Oral Surg 13:982, 1960

Pashley DH: 2. The influence of dentin permeability and pulpal blood flow on pulpal solute concentrations. J Endodont 5:355, 1979

Pashley DH, Livingston MJ, Outhwaite WC: Dentin permeability: Changes produced by iontophoresis. J Dent Res 57:77, 1978

Pashley DH, Livingston MJ, Reeder OW, Horner J: Effects of the degree of tubule occlusion on the permeability of human dentine. Arch Oral Biol 23:1127, 1978

Peterson JK: A supervised brushing trial of sodium monofluorophosphate dentifrices in a fluoridated area. Caries Res 13:68, 1979

Plant CG: Effect of zinc polycarboxylate cement on the dental pulp. J Dent Res 50:682, 1971 (Abst No 87)

Plant CG, Jones DW: The damaging effects of restorative materials: Part 1. Brit Dent J 140:373, 1976

Plant CG, Tyas MJ: Lining materials with special reference to Dropsin: a comparative study, Brit Dent J 128:486, 1970

Pohto M, Scheinin A: Mikroskopiska undersökninger av levande tandpulpa, Götesborgs tandläkaresällskaps artikelserie. N:0289, 1959

Prosser HJ, Jerome SM, Wilson AD: The effect of additives on the setting properties of a glass-ionomer cement. J Dent Res 61:1195, 1982

Provant DR, Adrian JC: Dental pulp reaction to cavit temporary filling material. Oral Surg 45:305, 1978

Qvist V, Stoltze K: Identification of significant variables for pulpal reactions to dental materials. J Dent Res 61:20, 1982

Retief DH: Effect of conditioning the enamel surface with phosphoric acid. J Dent Res 51:839, 1972

Rotberg SJ, deShazer DO: The completing action of eugenol on sound dentin. J Dent Res 45:307, 1966

Rovelstad GH, St John WE: Condition of the young dental pulp after the application of sodium fluoride to freshly cut dentin. JADA 39:670, 1949

Safer DS, Avery JK, Cox CF: Histopathologic evaluation of the effects of new polycarboxylate cements on monkey pulps. Oral Surg 33:966, 1972

Sandoval E, Shannon IL: Stannous fluoride and dentin solubility. Tex Rep Biol Med 27:111, 1969

Scott D: Mechanism and control of pain. In Grossman L (ed): p 35: Masson Publishing USA, Inc, 1979

Scott HM: Reduction of sensitivity by electrophoresis. J Dent Child 24:225, 1962

Seale NS, McIntosh JE, Taylor AN: Pulpal reaction to bleaching of teeth in dogs. J Dent Res 60:948, 1981

Selvig KA, Sand HF, Mörch T: The effect of topically applied fluorides on the acid resistance of human dentin studied by means of microradiography. Odont T 76:171, 1968

Shannon IL: Treatment of cavity preparations with stannous fluoride. J Oklahoma State Dent A 62:6, 1971

Shapiro WB, Kaslick RS, Chasens AI: The effect of a strontium chloride toothpaste on root hypersensitivity in a controlled clinical study. J Periodont 41:42/702, 1970

Smith DC: A new dental cement. Brit Dent J 124:381, 1968

Smith DC: A review of the zinc polycarboxylate cements. J Canad Dent A 37:22, 1971

Söremark R, Hedin M, Röjmyr R: Studies on incorporation of fluoride in a cavity liner (varnish). Odont Revy 20:189, 1969

Spangberg L, Rodrigues H, Langeland K: Biologic effects of dental materials. 4. Effect of polycarboxylate cements on Hela cells in vitro. Oral Surg 37:113, 1974

Spangberg L, Rodrigues H, Langeland K: Biologic effects of dental materials. 5. Effect of cavity liners on Hela cells in vitro. Oral Surg 37:284, 1974

Stanley HR: (Discussion) The use of corticosteroid-antibiotic preparations in endodontic therapy. In Grossman, LI (ed): Fourth Int Conf Endo, pp 83–86. Philadelphia, University of Pennsylvania, 1968.

Stanley HR, Going RE, Chauncey MH: Human pulp response to acid pretreatment of dentin and to composite restorations. JADA 91:817, 1975

Stark MM, Nicholson RJ, Soelberg KB: Marginal seal afforded by n-butyl and isobutyl cyanoacrylates as cavity liners. J Prosth Dent 21:380, 1969

Swartz ML, Niblack BF, Alter EA, Norman RD, Phillips RW: In vivo studies on the penetration of dentin by constituents of silicate cements. JADA 76:573, 1968

Tal M, Oron M, Gedalia I, Ehrlich J: X-ray diffraction and scanning electron microscope investigation of fluoride-treated dentin in man. Oral Biol 21:285, 1976

Tarbet WJ, Buckner A, Stark MM, Fratarcangelo PA: Clinical evaluation of a new treatment for dentinal hypersensitivity. J Periodont 51:535, 1980

Tarbet WJ, Buckner A, Stark MM, Fratarcangelo PA, Augsburger R: The pulpal effects of brushing with a 5 percent potassium nitrate paste used for desensitization. Oral Surg 51:600, 1981

Tarbet WJ, Silverman G, Fratarcangelo PA, Kanapka JA: Home treatment for dentinal hypersensitivity: a comparative study. JADA 105:227, 1982

Tibbetts VR, Schnell RJ, Swartz ML, Phillips RW: Thermal diffusion through amalgam and cement bases: Comparison of in vitro and in vivo measurements. J Dent Res 55:441, 1976

Tobias RS, Browne RM, Path MRC, Plant CG, Ingram DV: Pulpal response to a glass-ionomer cement. Brit Dent J 144:345, 1978

Torneck CD, Moe H, Howley TP: The effect of calcium hydroxide on porcine pulp fibroblasts in vitro. J Endodont 9:131, 1983

Torneck CD, Wagner D: The effect of calcium hydroxide cavity liner on early cell division in the pulp subsequent to cavity preparation and restoration. J Endodont 6:719, 1980

Tronstad L, Mjör IA: Pulp reactions to calcium hydroxide-containing material. Oral Surg 33:961, 1972

Trowbridge H, Edwall L, Panopoulos P: Effect of zinc oxide-eugenol and calcium hydroxide on intradental nerve activity. J Endodont 8:403, 1982

Truelove EL, Mitchell DF, Phillips RW: Biologic evaluation of a carboxylate cement. J Dent Res 50:166, 1971

Uchida A, Wakano Y, Fukuyama D, Miki T, Iwayama Y, Okada H: Controlled clinical evaluation of a 10% strontium chloride dentifrice in treatment of dentin hypersensitivity following periodontal surgery. J Periodont 51:578, 1980

Vojinović O, Nyborg H, Brännström M: Acid treatment of cavities under resin fillings: Bacterial growth in dentinal tubules and pulpal reactions. J Dent Res 52:1189, 1973

Voth ED, Phillips RW, Swartz ML: Thermal diffusion through amalgam and various liners. J Dent Res 45:1184, 1966

Walton RE, Leonard L, Sharawy M, Gangarosa L: Effects on pulp and dentin of iontophoresis of sodium fluoride on exposed roots in dogs. Oral Surg 48:545, 1979

Watts A: Bacterial contamination and the toxicity of silicate and zinc phosphate cements. Brit Dent J 146:7, 1979

Webb JG, Bussell NE: A comparison of the inflammatory response produced by commercial eugenol and purified eugenol. J Dent Res 60:1724, 1981

Wei SHY, Forbes WC: X-ray diffraction analysis of carious dentine treated with stannous fluoride. Arch Oral Biol 13:407, 1968

Wei SHY, Kaqueller JC, Massler M: Remineralization of carious dentin. J Dent Res 47:381, 1968

Weiss MB, Massler M: Pulp reaction to fluorides. IADR Program and Abstracts, No 663, 1969

Widerman FH, Eames WB, Serene TP: The physical and biologic properties of Cavit. JADA 82:378, 1971

Williams JI, Yates JL, Hembree JH, McKnight JP: The

frozen-aluminum-slab-mixing technique. The effect on zinc phosphate cements. J Dent Child 46:398, 1979

Wilson AD, Paddon JM, Crisp S: The hydration of dental cement. J Dent Res 58:1065, 1979

Wolcott RB, Shiller WR, Kraske LM: Clinical evaluation of temporary restorative materials. J Prosth Dent 12:782, 1962

Wolf D, Gedallia, I, Reisstein I, Goldman J, and Stieglitz H: Effect of addition of $CaFPO_3$ to a zinc oxide-eugenol base liner on the microhardness and fluoride content of dentin. J Dent Res 52:467, 1973

Zadok J, Gedalia I, Weinman J, Daphni L: Fluoride uptake by root dentin after immersion in 2% NaF solution with iontophoresis. J Dent Res 55:310, 1976

Zander HA: The reaction of dental pulps to silicate cements, JADA 33:1233, 1946

Zander HA, Glenn JF, Nelson CA: Pulp protection in restorative dentistry. JADA 41:563, 1950

11
PERMANENT RESTORATIONS

PERMANENT RESTORATIVE MATERIALS

SILICATES

For many years, silicate cement was the most popular anterior esthetic restorative material. However, its popularity has declined because of its high solubility, color instability, and tendency to produce severe damage to the pulp, especially when used without a liner.

When applied to the cut dentin of rat incisors, Pohto and Scheinin (1967) noted that the silicate cement liquid penetrated a dentin layer 30 μ to 40 μ thick in 10 to 30 seconds. The penetration was associated with the liberation of carbon dioxide that entered the pulp and resulted in thrombosis of the entire vascular system of the pulp.

Silicates also cause a centrifugal flow of fluid in the dentinal tubules (Johnson and Brännström, 1971), which may result in displacement of the odontoblasts. Inflammation is thus initiated. In teeth in which a silicate filling has been in place for 1 week, sections show a dense collection of acute inflammatory cells in the pulp under the region of the cut dentinal tubules. Reparative dentin formation is inhibited initially, owing to the death of the underlying odontoblasts and other pulp cells. In cavities of moderate depth (more than 0.5 mm from the pulp), other pulp cells assume the function of elaborating reparative dentin, which they produce in haphazard fashion. The reparative dentin may be elaborated so rapidly that pulp cells are frequently trapped within it, causing the reparative dentin to look like osteodentin (Fig. 11–1).

The effect of silicate on the pulp is influenced by the depth of the cavity preparation: the closer the silicate is placed to the pulp, the more severe the inflammatory reaction. In deep cavities, where less than 0.5 mm of dentin remains between the base of the cavity and the pulp, chronic inflammation may persist for 6 months to a year, often resulting in total pulp necrosis. In teeth with silicate fillings several months old, examination of tissue sections reveals the persistence of the inflammatory response. The blood vessels are very much dilated, and in some regions of the pulp, abscesses have formed. The inflammation extends throughout a large area of the coronal portion of the pulp (Fig. 11–2).

Unlike the effects of other restorative materials, the deleterious effects of silicates on the pulp are progressive (Spangberg et al, 1973). Silicates continuously produce irritation because they do not crystallize but remain in a gel state, constantly liberating toxic products. The

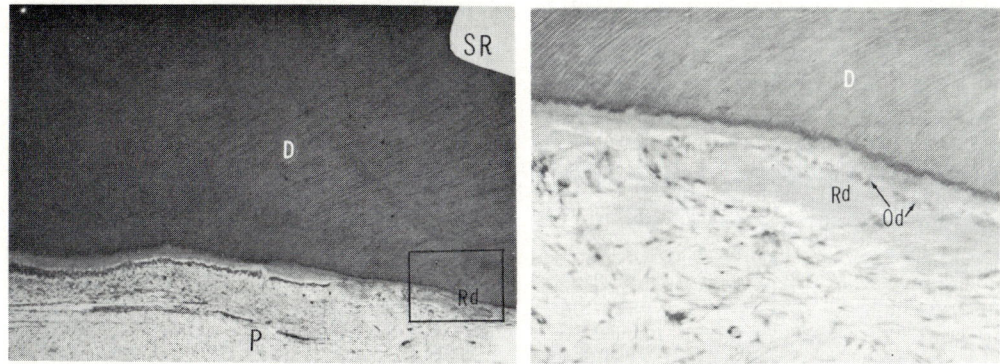

FIG. 11-1 Pulp irritation by silicate. *(Left)* Following the placement of a silicate restoration (SR) on the dentin (D) of a prepared cavity, a reaction has taken place in the pulp (P). Reparative dentin (Rd) has been elaborated. ×54. *(Right)* Higher magnification of region outlined by rectangle in picture at left. The reparative dentin (Rd) has been elaborated so rapidly that odontoblasts (Od) have been trapped in it. D, dentin, ×96. (Seltzer S, Bender IB: JADA 66:503,1963)

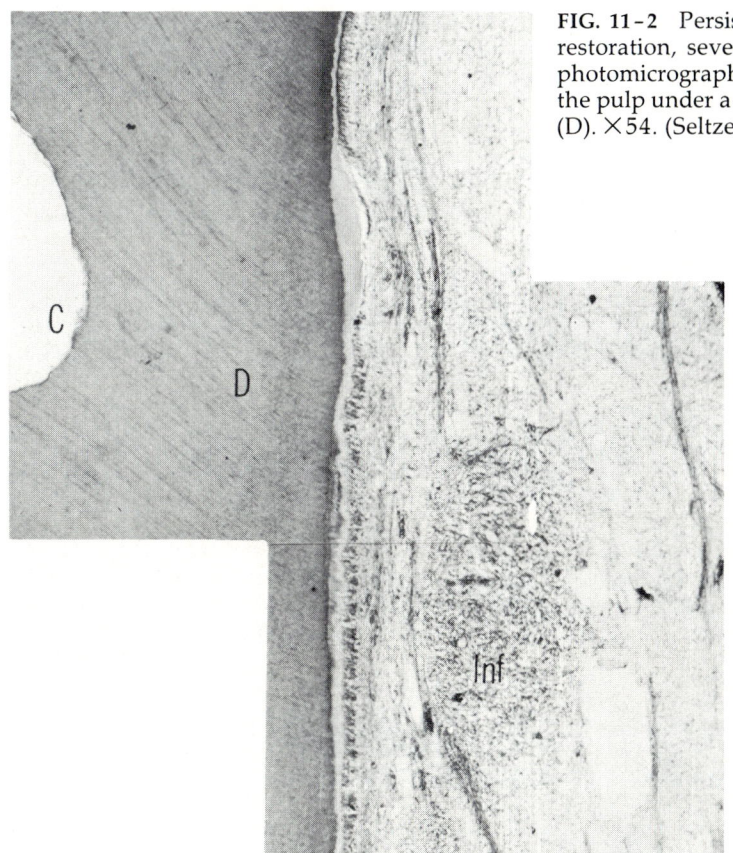

FIG. 11-2 Persistence of inflammation under a silicate restoration, several months after treatment. Composite photomicrograph, showing chronic inflammation (Inf) of the pulp under a silicate-restored cavity (C) in the dentin (D). ×54. (Seltzer S, Bender IB: JADA 66:503, 1963)

acidity of the silicate has been implicated. Radioactively tagged phosphorus of phosphoric acid in silicates has been shown to penetrate the dentin into the pulp (Swartz et al, 1968). However, phosphoric acid solutions have not uniformly induced inflammatory pulp responses in experimental cavities (Johnson et al, 1970). Roydhouse (1961) has postulated that a response of antigen-antibody type to dissolved silica fractions may also be involved.

Often, the patient is unaware that anything is wrong with the pulp. Eventually, the periapical tissues become involved. Areas of rarefaction develop that may be discovered accidentally in a routine full-mouth radiograph. The upper lateral incisors and the lower anteriors are affected most frequently, because these teeth are small and because even shallow preparations are close to the pulp. Young teeth, particularly, are susceptible to the irritating effects of silicates because of the wider dentinal tubules and the greater size of the pulp chamber.

Silicates have been shown by isotope studies and studies of bacterial penetration (Mortensen et al, 1965) to have distinct marginal leakage which does not change appreciably with the passage of time. Bacteria have also been demonstrated to persist in the dentinal tubules under silicate restorations (Brännström and Nyborg, 1971; Hansen and Bruun, 1971), possibly owing to the persistent marginal leakage. Thus, it appears as if pulpal damage under silicates is not due solely to chemical irritation of the filling, but results from irritation caused by bacterial growth in the gap between the filling and cavity walls (Brännström and Vojinović, 1976; Watts, 1979; Tobias et al, 1982). Therefore, it is imperative to use a zinc oxide-eugenol or calcium hydroxide liner to maximize protection of the pulp from both bacterial and chemical irritants.

El Kafrawy and Mitchell (1963) have shown that the reparative dentin formed under caries or as a result of previous operative procedures affords protection against the deleterious effects of silicates. Clinically, silicates confer high resistance to recurrent caries, possibly owing to the fluorides in the material.

RESTORATIVE RESINS

Acrylic (methyl methacrylate) resins, originally unfilled, were extensively used by many clinicians, both as cements and filling materials. They underwent considerable shrinkage during the polymerization process, resulting in marginal leakage with recurrent caries and consequent pulp damage. Moreover, the monomer itself was irritating to the pulp (Langeland, 1966). They are no longer in vogue as restorative materials. Epoxy resins with catalyst systems that are filled with glass or quartz, known as composite or filled resins, have been developed. These resins are a 3-dimensional combination of at least two chemically different materials with a distinct interface separating the components (Bowen et al, 1972).

Most of the composite resins consist principally of a resin binder, a thermosetting methacrylate, which is the reaction product of an epoxy resin and methacrylic acid (BIS-GMA). Various fillers, such as fused silica and glasses have been added to increase strength, durability and radiopacity. The fillers are coated with silanes to enhance their bonding to the resin (Bowen, 1966). Formulations include special coupling agents to improve bonding between composite filler materials and dentin and enamel (Chandler et al, 1970).

Newer composite restorative materials and filler systems, catalysts and methods of curing, such as ultraviolet and visible light, have been developed (Bassiouny and Grant, 1978). In these newer composites, the size of the particles of the filler may range from 0.04 μm to 5 μm, with various size mixtures (Council Report, 1982). These have been called microfilled or smooth surface composite resins.

Tests of tooth-pulp reactions have not been made for all composite resins. However, on the basis of results for many that have been tested, it may generally be concluded that all composite resins, with or without resin liners, irritate the dental pulp (Fig. 11–3). Some have been found to be more irritating than others (Stanley et al, 1975; Nordenvall et al, 1979; Valcke et al, 1980; Inokoshi et al, 1982). The resins exhibit little or no antibacterial activity after polymerization or water leaching (Updegraff et al, 1971).

Many investigators have claimed that pulp damage is generally mild (Heys et al, 1977) and has not resulted from the composite resin itself (Brännström and Nyborg, 1972). Some credence for this hypothesis is found in the studies of Stanley et al (1979), who evaluated pulp responses to eight ingredients of composite materials individually. None were found to cause significant inflammation. Instead, microorganisms introduced through leakage or left on the cavity walls during restoration placement were re-

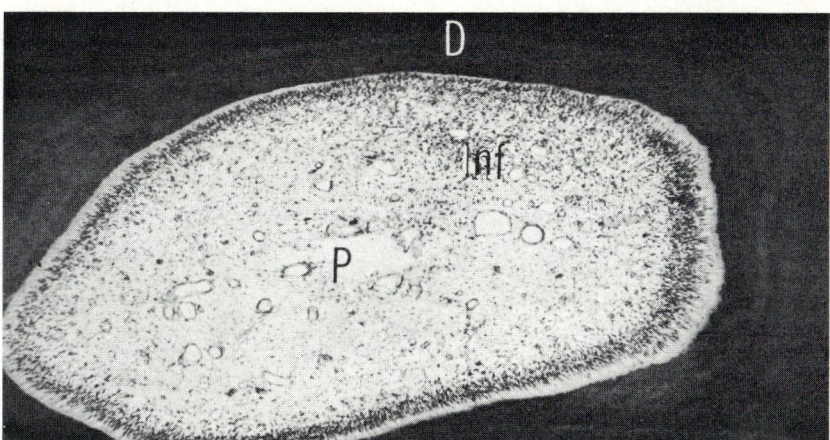

FIG. 11-3 Pulp reaction to acrylic resin. One week after the insertion of an acrylic resin in a cavity of a dog's tooth, the pulp (P) is acutely inflamed (Inf). D, dentin. ×54.

sponsible for the deleterious pulpal effects (Dickey et al, 1974; Skogedal and Eriksen, 1976; Brännström and Nordenvall, 1978; Leidal, 1979). The number of bacteria apparently increases with time (Qvist, 1975; Inokoshi et al, 1982), and the kind of microbial flora under the restorations resembles that of dental plaque (Mejare et al, 1979). According to Bergenholtz (1977), bacterial components from human plaque, when applied to cavities prepared in monkeys' teeth, caused inflammatory pulp reactions.

The resin liners do little to protect the pulp from the toxic effects of the restorative material (Langeland et al, 1966; Suarez et al, 1970). In fact, tissue culture studies indicate that the resin liners have greater cytotoxicity than the composite materials (Spangberg et al, 1974). Contraction of the resin results in a space beneath it that usually contains a dense accumulation of bacteria (Brännström and Nyborg, 1971; Dickey et al, 1974). Thus, cavities in which composite resins are to be placed should be lined with calcium hydroxide and covered with zinc phosphate cement prior to insertion of the filling material (Langeland et al, 1970; Tobias et al, 1973). Such a procedure reduces or eliminates the irritational effects of the composite resin (Meyers et al, 1976; Inokoshi et al, 1982). The polycarboxylate or zinc phosphate cements also have no adverse effect on polymerization of the composite resins (Special Report of the American Academy of Restorative Dentistry, 1980). On the other hand, zinc oxide-eugenol liners should not be used with composite resins inasmuch as they inhibit complete polymerization.

Adhesive Restorative Resins

In addition to conventional restorative resins, several new resins are reported to be adhesive to both enamel and dentin. Etching of the tooth structure with phosphoric or citric acid is supposed to enhance adhesion. However, the ability of acid etchants to enhance long-term adhesion in dentin has been questioned (Special Report, 1980).

Several reports indicate that with the use of these newer adhesive resins, pulpal damage is slight to absent (Fusayama et al, 1979; Heida et al, 1978; Inokoshi et al, 1982). Futhermore, according to Inokoshi et al, covering of the etched dentin with a liner such as calcium hydroxide is both undesirable and contraindicated. However, long-term studies of adhesive resins are needed to determine whether the bond remains firm. As Hoppenbrouwers et al (1982) have noted, the high dentinal collagen turnover after cavity preparation may induce a replacement of the collagen bond to the adhesive by new dentinal matrix. Alternatively, the bond may denature the immediately adjacent collagen to such a degree that it would not be involved in the turnover process. However, the collagen of the next layer would be renewed, possibly resulting in a structure-weakening effect.

GOLD INLAY

Gold inlays are potentially damaging to the pulp, but not because of irritation inherent in the gold itself. Several other factors are involved. The first is the thinner mixture of zinc phosphate cement with which the inlay is inserted, which acts as an irritant due to the acidity and heat resulting from the setting of the cement. The second factor is the large amount of pressure, generated in seating the inlay, brought to bear on the dentinal tubules during cementation. Such pressure on the pulp is one of the most deleterious factors and injures the odontoblastic layer. A third factor is the predisposition of cast gold restorations to marginal leakage due to poorly adapted margins or excessive use of cement. The end result is dissolution of the cement, recurrent caries, and pulp involvement (Going, 1979).

Inflammation is reduced in shallow or moderately deep preparations because the thicker dentin acts as a protective shield and, therefore, the zinc phosphate cement is not able to cause as much irritation. Deep inlay preparations for greater strength and stability may enhance the restoration mechanically. However, biologically, the pulp is placed in greater jeopardy. Brännström and Nyborg (1960) found moderate to severe inflammatory responses in the pulps of both dogs' teeth and human teeth that were restored with gold inlays. Brännström and Nyborg (1977) have concluded that the inflammation was caused by debris-containing bacteria left behind on the dentin after cavity preparation. These findings underline the importance of removing grinding debris and bacteria before inlay cementation.

Poorly fitting inlays result in future pulp diseases because of the ensuing marginal percolation and recurrent decay.

The pressure of cementation of a tight-fitting inlay may cause a pulpitis, and frequently pain results. Preparations for inlay restorations subject the tooth to the superimposition of many irritants, from which the pulp has a poorer chance of recovering. After the preparation of a tooth for an inlay, an impression is taken. The use of modeling compound, particularly, is damaging because of impingement of combined pressure and heat. When many irritants are superimposed in sequence, the pulp may become acutely inflamed, with hemorrhage, edema, and other characteristic inflammatory changes. The use of cavity liners is recommended to allay these injurious effects. However, even when recovery occurs, leakage may ensue with the passage of time as a result of the washing-out of the cementing medium around less than perfect margins. Isotope studies have demonstrated the poor sealing qualities of zinc phosphate cements. Recurrent decay and pulp involvement are likely sequelae. According to Mondelli et al (1978), the application of two layers of cavity varnish to the cavosurface cavity margins affords the best protection against marginal leakage.

GOLD FOIL

Gold foil has always been considered to have excellent marginal sealing qualities, a distinct advantage for a restorative material. However, reports of studies of the marginal sealing properties of gold foil are conflicting. Fisher (1949), using dyes, and Armstrong and Simon (1951), using radioactive tracers, found distinct marginal penetration around gold foil restorations. The penetration was less than that found around the margins of zinc phosphate and silicate cements, but more than that around zinc oxide-eugenol and amalgam. Going et al (1960) found that, among these filling materials, the better marginal seal was provided by gold foil. Apparently, gold foil restorations that are hand condensed result in greater marginal isotope penetration than do those condensed mechanically (Thye, 1967). The insertion of gold foil irritates the pulp (Thomas et al, 1969). The mechanical malleting of the dentin is the offending factor (Fig. 11–4). Once the foil is inserted and the malleting is stopped, the irritant is removed. If the duration of application of the malleting force is short, there is a reasonable chance for pulp recovery. Recovery is more rapid in the pulps of teeth restored with gold foil than in those restored by some other means because the irritation ceases on completion of insertion of the filling material (Fig. 11–5). In silicate-filled teeth, for example, the irritation is continuous.

The effects of the pressure of gold foil insertion on the pulps of the teeth of dogs have been investigated by James and Schour (1955). Histologic studies revealed that a severe, acute reaction occurred immediately after insertion of the filling. This reaction was even more severe than that observed under silicates. The inflammatory reaction in the pulp probably was due to the pressure transmitted to the pulp cells through the dentin. Histologic sections of some human teeth following the insertion of gold foil fillings displayed chronic inflammation with the presence of a granuloma subjacent to the cavity even after 90 days (Fig. 11–5). Should inflammation persist, internal resorption may ensue (Burke

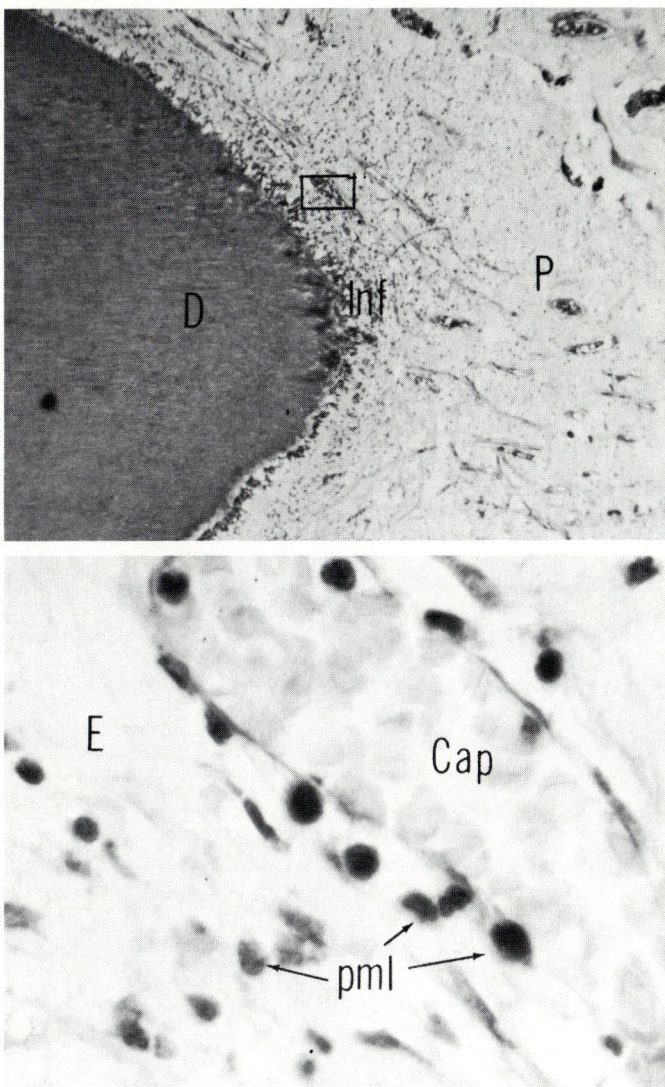

FIG. 11-4 The effects of gold foil insertion. *(Top)* Pulp reaction in a shallow cavity preparation of the dentin (D). A small region of acute inflammation (Inf) is present in the pulp (P) 1 week later. ×54. *(Bottom)* Higher magnification of region outlined by rectangle in picture at top. A dilated capillary (Cap) is shown. Polymorphonuclear leukocytes (pml) are present in the edematous tissue spaces (E). ×960.

and Cermak, 1971). In other teeth, repair was evident without any inflammatory response. In human teeth, cavity depth has an important influence on pulp reactions to gold foil restorations. The thicker the layer of the remaining dentin, the less the inflammatory response.

The use of gold foil should be avoided in the teeth of youngsters because pulps are larger and the dentin is less thick. Also, the dentinal tubules are wider in young persons than in older people. Consequently, the possibility of inducing pulp inflammation is enhanced.

AMALGAM

Amalgam is one of the safest filling materials, even though minor inflammatory pulp responses have been reported to occur after its insertion (Möller and Granath, 1973). Of all of the permanent filling materials, amalgam is the least irritating to the pulp, even when liners are not employed. However, liners are necessary in order to prevent discomfort due to the thermal conductivity of the metal (Dachi and Stigers, 1967) and to help reduce the effects of the pres-

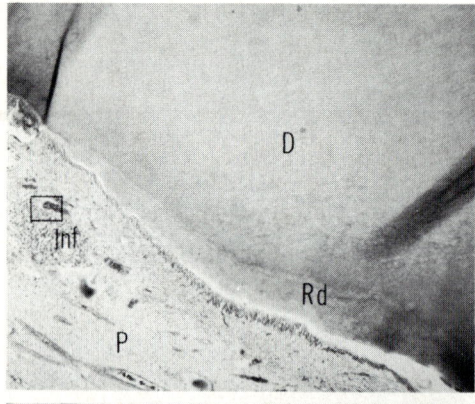
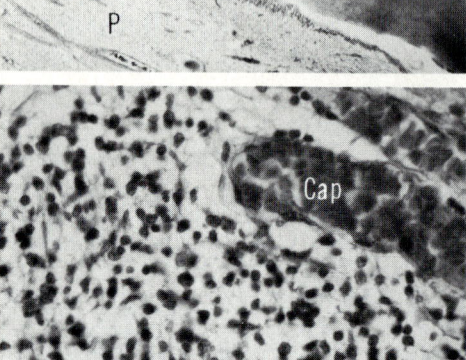
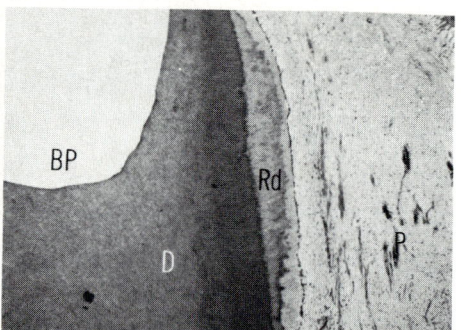

FIG. 11-5 Inflammation, several months after gold foil insertion. *(Top)* Two months after restoration, the pulp (P) still has a small region of inflammation (Inf). Reparative dentin (Rd) has been elaborated. D, dentin. ×54. *(Bottom, left)* Higher magnification of region outlined by rectangle in picture at top, showing chronic inflammatory cells around dilated capillary (Cap). *(Bottom, right)* In another tooth, 8 months after restoration with gold foil, the pulp (P) has recovered. BP, base of cavity preparation in the dentin (D). Reparative dentin (Rd) has been elaborated. ×54.

sure of amalgam condensation. In shallow cavities, pulp reactions under amalgam are lacking or of minimal intensity (Fig. 11-6). In deeper cavities, inflammation that occurs after amalgam insertion is mild to moderate, and the pulp recovers readily. Some investigators have claimed that inflammation was absent even in deep cavities but that there was inhibition of reparative dentin formation, owing to a paralysis of the odontoblasts.

One of the disadvantages of amalgam restorations is their poor aesthetic appearance, which limits their use to posterior teeth. Corrosion also must be considered when amalgam restorations are inserted. The galvanic action of the amalgam produces a corrosion of the outer and inner surfaces of the amalgam. The intensity of amalgam corrosion is directly related to the porosity of the amalgam. Thus, zinc-free amalgams, which have a greater degree of porosity and microleakage (Granath, 1971) than those with zinc, corrode more intensely (Jørgensen, 1972; Jørgensen and Esbensen, 1973). Moreover, the corrosion can be greatly increased by contamination with moisture such as occurs when the amalgam is mulled in the hands. However, old amalgam fillings exhibit less marginal fluid exchange, probably because debris from corrosion products eventually plugs the marginal spaces. Unfortunately, marginal corrosion frequently leads to fracture of the amalgam (Grieve, 1971). If the width of the defect exceeds 50 μm, the risk of the development of secondary caries increases (Jørgensen and Wakumoto, 1968; Hals et al, 1974).

Massler and Barber (1953) and Schoonover and Souder (1951) have shown that dentin discoloration results from galvanic action from the amalgam, causing the transmission of mercury ions through the dentinal tubules, where they are precipitated as sulfides. The quantity of mercury ions reaching the pulp has been found to be insignificant by Frykholm (1957). Kurosaki and Fusayama (1973) and Halse (1975) found, by electron probe microanalysis, that tin and zinc, but no mercury or silver, penetrated decalcified dentin under amalgam restorations. The use of insulating bases completely prevents the penetration, in addition to preventing thermal shock to the pulp.

Copper Amalgam

High copper-content amalgam alloys have been increasingly utilized in dentistry because of their higher compressive strengths and resistance to creep and corrosion. They also exhibit less marginal breakdown (Fan and Leinfelder, 1982). However, copper has been found to be toxic in various cell culture systems (Leirskar, 1974; Takahashi, 1975). In general, the pulpal inflammatory response in unlined monkey teeth cavities was initially greater under high copper content amalgam than in cavities filled with conventional silver amalgams (Mjör et al, 1977; Skogedal and Mjör, 1979). The results were influenced by time and by the thickness of remaining dentin (Skogedal and Mjör, 1979; Heys et al, 1979). With the passage of time, the pulps under high-copper amalgam alloys exhibited slight inflammation and extensive irregular reparative dentin formation; the alloys with a low-copper content produced no reparative dentin in some teeth. In other teeth, reparative dentin formation varied in quantity from small to large, and the structure was distinctly regular (Skogedal and Mjör, 1979). On the other hand, Heys et al (1979) found no differences in the pulp response to high-copper and to conventional amalgam alloys. The disparity in the results of the two studies may be due to the fact that, in the latter study, the cavities were lined.

A zinc oxide-eugenol cavity liner should be used under copper-containing and conventional silver amalgams to protect the pulp and to prevent corrosions (Swerdlow and Stanley, 1962; Skogedal and Mjör, 1979; Heys et al, 1979).

The success of amalgam as a filling material is attributed, in part, to the relatively small volume changes that occur after it is inserted. In our experiments, test bacteria could not penetrate at the margins of amalgam fillings. However, Mortensen et al (1965) did find that temperature cycling increased bacterial penetration of amalgam cavity interfaces. Brännström and Söremark (1962) found that radioactive sodium could penetrate around the margins of fresh amalgam restorations and that such penetration was prevented by insulating with calcium hydroxide varnish.

The use of varnishes under amalgams and at the margins has been recommended (Castagnola and Garberoglio, 1968). Two coats of copal resin varnish should be applied to all surfaces of the cavity, including cavosurface margins. Such procedures eliminate potential irritation of the

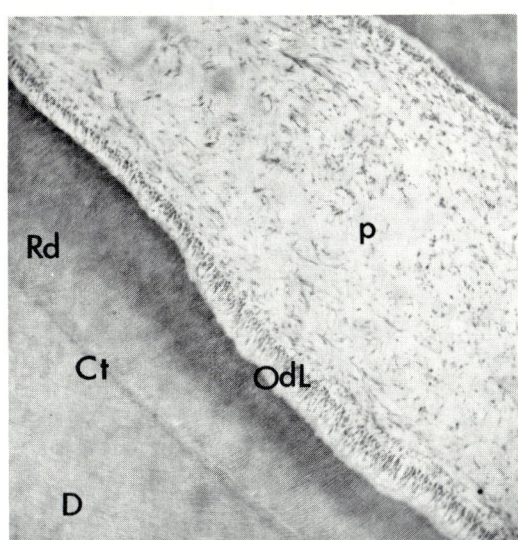

FIG. 11-6 Pulp reaction to amalgam, 3 months after cavity preparation and amalgam restoration. The pulp (p) has recovered from the initial injury. Ct, calcio-traumatic response in the dentin (D). Reparative dentin (Rd) has been elaborated by the odontoblasts (OdL). ×100. (Seltzer S, Bender IB, Kaufman IJ: Oral Surg 14:856, 1961)

pulp and postoperative tooth sensitivity (Going 1979). The varnish has been shown to decrease the penetration of radioisotopes through the margins of amalgam restorations (Swartz and Phillips, 1960; Phillips et al, 1961; Dolven, 1966). However, varnishes help reduce the space but do not eliminate it (Wing and Lyell, 1966), and bacteria may penetrate this space (Harrison, 1966). Furthermore, Mateer and Reitz (1972) have found that the common cavity liners do not block the galvanic current flow through the body-tissue–saliva circuit to the oral amalgam interface. Such a current flow develops as a result of the exposure of amalgam to two electrolytes—saliva and dentinal pulp fluid. The amalgam-dentin interface becomes negative, with migration of tin into the dentin. The oral amalgam interface is positive. The resultant current flow continues to enhance the amalgam corrosion. Amalgams incorporating small amounts of stannous fluoride have been developed. Such amalgams have been found to reduce enamel solubility and increase the fluoride content of the adjacent tooth structure (Jerman, 1970; Souganidis et al, 1981). Unfortunately, addition of stannous fluoride to amalgam has been found to increase the amalgam's corrosive properties when immersed and tested in Ringer's solution (Stoner et al, 1971).

Metal Pins for Amalgam Reinforcement

The insertion of metal pins into dentin may be hazardous to the pulp. Dentinal cracks and fractures may be induced and inadvertent pulp exposure may result (Rud and Omnell, 1970; Arvidson and Wróblewski, 1978). Pulp studies are limited, and the results controversial. Dolph (1970) has found that when the pins were inserted into human dental pulps aseptically, repair and regeneration occurred after 100 days. Even saliva-contaminated pins have been reported to cause reversible pulp damage. Abraham and Baum (1972) placed saliva-contaminated metal pins directly into the pulps. Histologic examinations, made from 4 to 211 days later, revealed slight to severe inflammation in less than half of the teeth. They interpreted their results to mean that the pulps were not severely affected and that repair had ensued. On the other hand, Langeland et al (1971) found that despite the use of a water spray the pulps of the teeth in which pins had been inserted were inflamed. Suzuki et al (1973) also found that when gold-plated stainless steel, threaded pins were placed into the pulps of dogs, severe inflammatory responses leading to necrosis were induced. Such responses were minimized when a calcium hydroxide preparation was placed on the end of the pin prior to insertion.

CROWN AND BRIDGE PROCEDURES

Various procedures involved in crown and bridge fabrication, other than preparation, may affect the pulps.

Impression materials, such as modeling compound, can cause damage through excessive transfer of heat to the tooth. Elastic impression materials apparently cause less damage, although few tests have been made (Langeland and Langeland, 1965).

Acrylic cements and acrylic splints that are fabricated in the mouth over prepared teeth are potentially damaging to the pulp. The odontoblasts are injured by this material. In addition, elevations of pulp temperatures occur after in vivo polymerization of acrylic resins. The exothermic reaction that evolves during the curing process of the resin on the teeth causes a temperature increase exceeding 5.5°C (Zach and Cohen, 1965), a rise that can cause irreversible pulp damage. Grajower et al (1979) performed in vitro experiments with varying flow rates of water through the pulp chamber. Their findings indicate that heat would not be effectively dissipated by the blood circulation in the pulp during the curing of temporary acrylic-resin crowns.

In the cementation of a bridge, the zinc phosphate cement is introduced as a thin mix in order to facilitate the seating of the bridge and to permit the excess cement to escape. A great deal of pressure is needed to seat the bridge. Frequently, when the bridge is tried in the mouth and the occlusion is acceptable, premature contact becomes obvious subsequent to cementation. Extensive grinding for correction of the occlusion may be needed. If the gold is not very thick, perforation of the cast crown may result. In order to prevent such perforation, as well as to facilitate seating of the bridge and reduce the pressure that is generated, "escape hatches" are recommended. A hole is drilled through the crown with a No. 701 fissure bur before cementation. This allows the excess cement to escape before setting has occurred and also prevents the tremendous pressure on the preparation, thereby reducing pulp damage. Subsequently, this small opening can be plugged with gold foil or amalgam. The use of escape hatches is particularly necessary for long crowns in which air may be trapped.

Zinc phosphate cement has certain deficiencies that prevent its classification as an ideal material for permanent crown and bridge cementation. Among these are its tendency to disintegrate in the oral fluids with the passage of time, especially in crowns with inadequate marginal fit, and the initial pulp irritation of phosphoric acid liquid, due to its low pH (Eames et al, 1979). To neutralize the toxic effects of the acid, an aqueous suspension of calcium hydroxide or a loose mix of zinc oxide-eugenol should be placed on the preparation before cementation. Besides neutralizing the acidity, calcium hydroxide can also reduce the permeability of the dentin by increasing sclerosis of the dentinal tubules. Mjör and Pindborg (1973), using a methylene blue dye, found that there was a greater reduction of dentin permeability following the application of calcium hydroxide than after zinc oxide-eugenol. Since the hydroxyl ion may prevent complete setting by interfering with the crystallization of the cement, the calcium hydroxide should be placed only on the

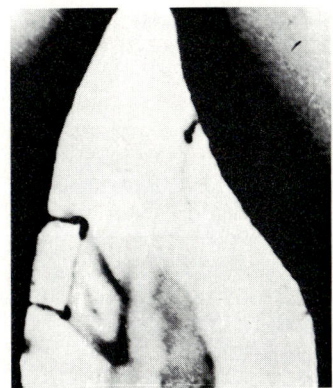 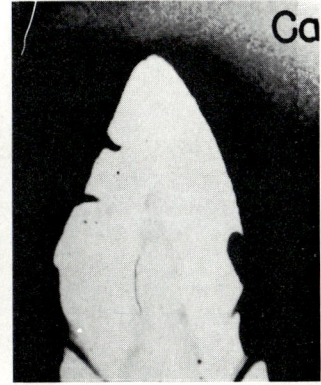 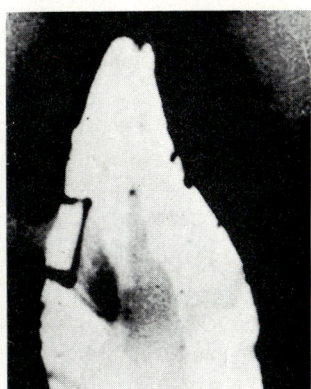

FIG. 11-7 Marginal leakage, demonstrated by autoradiography. Penetration of radiocalcium through the margins of cavities filled with various materials. *(Left)* Amalgam. *(Center)* Silicate. *(Right)* Acrylic resin. ×5. (Going RE, Massler M, Dute HL: Marginal penetration of dental restorations by different radioactive isotopes. J Dent Res 39:273, 1960. Copyright by the American Dental Association. Reproduced by permission.)

prepared dentin of the tooth, avoiding the cavity margins. Another method is to place the calcium hydroxide on the prepared tooth during the period of temporary cementation of the cast crown. During the interval before final cementation with zinc phosphate, sclerosis of the dentinal tubules can occur.

The strength of all cements is directly related to their hydration. The strongest cements are the most hydrated, have the greatest modulus, and deform the least (Special Report, 1980). Phosphoric acid cements are the most hydrated. Their hydration and strength increases with age (Wilson et al, 1979). To improve the physical qualities of zinc phosphate cements, the mixing should be done on a refrigerated aluminum slab. This prolongs the working time, significantly reduces the setting time at oral temperatures, increases the powder to liquid ratios, with a decrease in film thickness and a significant increase in compressive strength (Williams et al, 1979; Windeler, 1979).

In an effort to overcome some of the deficiencies of zinc phosphate cement, other cements such as zinc polycarboxylate, cyanoacrylate, composite resins, and the glass ionomer cements have been formulated. These cements, after being tested for adhesion to dentin, setting time, film thickness, solubility, compressive strength, and pulp reactions, have failed to fulfill their physical and clinical expectations. The polyacrylic acid cements are less hydrated and weaker than phosphoric acid cements. The biologic compatibility of the glass ionomer cements is similar to that of the polycarboxylate cements. They should be used on crowns with large thicknesses of remaining dentin (Association Reports, 1979). In teeth with deep preparations, Tobias et al (1978) recommended that a base of calcium hydroxide or zinc oxide material be used. We concur with this recommendation.

MARGINAL LEAKAGE

Marginal leakage around various filling materials has been implicated as a causative factor in tooth hypersensitivity, tooth discoloration resulting from breakdown of restorative materials, bacterial ingrowth, recurrent caries and pulp pathosis. Unfortunately, none of the filling materials available today exhibits perfect marginal seals against the oral fluids (Fig. 11-7). With temporary filling materials, the greatest leakage occurs around gutta-percha and the least around zinc oxide-eugenol. The permanent filling materials, such as composite resins, silicates, amalgams, and glass ionomer cements, exhibit varying degrees of microleakage. The extent of such leakage has been illustrated by the use of dye solutions, radioactive tracers (Going, 1959, 1972; Jennings and Ranley, 1972; Douglas et al, 1980), and bacteria (Brännström and Nyborg, 1971, 1972; Qvist, 1977). Numerous studies have shown that microleakage is responsible for bacterial penetration. Acrylic resins exhibit considerable leakage. The amount of bacterial penetration depends upon the type of composite resin (whether hydrophilic or hydrophobic) and whether or not etchants and liners have been used. Most composite resins are hydrophilic, readily absorbing water and oral fluids. Without chemical bonding of the resin to tooth structure, the interface becomes filled with water or saliva (Craig, 1979), promoting leakage. Newer hydrophobic fluomethacrylate composite resins may reduce or eliminate marginal leakage (Douglas et al, 1978, 1980).

Inokoshi et al (1982) used a new adhesive resin on acid-etched cavities; no bacterial ingrowth occurred after 60 days. In unetched cavities filled with the same material, bacterial penetration occurred but it was much less pronounced than in conventional composite resins. There is preponderant evidence that such microleakage may be responsible for most of the pulp irritation. The microbial flora under composite resins produce the same inflammatory reactions in the pulp as that produced by dental plaque (Mjör and Tronstad, 1972; Bergenholtz and Lindhe, 1975; Mejare et al, 1979).

Amalgam, the most frequently used permanent restoration, exhibits leakage within the first few days (Hembree and Andrews, 1979). With the passage of time, leakage decreases around amalgam restorations, probably because of the formation of corrosion products that plug the amalgam-tooth interface.

Loiselle et al (1969) have pointed out that in vivo studies are needed to assess marginal leakage of restorations more realistically. Their studies indicated that assessments of microleakage around restoration margins may not be as severe in vivo as in vitro. The presence of dental plaque and the influence of pulpal hydrostatic pressure are other variables that could influence results (Steuver et al, 1971). On the other hand, McCurdy et al (1974) measured microleakage in vivo around restorations placed in monkey teeth. After feeding the animals food tagged with a radioisotope and topically applying the isotope solution to the restored teeth, they found that the results of subsequent radioautographs compared favorably with those of in vitro studies. They concluded that in vitro microleakage tests were useful for screening of dental restorative materials or adhesive systems. In order to assess microleakage, neutron activation analysis (Meyer et al, 1974; Douglas et al, 1980), electrochemical conduction techniques (Jacobsen and Fraunhoffer, 1975), scanning electron microscopy (SEM; Schoen, 1978), spectrophotometric dye-recovery methods (Douglas and Zakariasen, 1981), and reverse diffusion techniques (Vasudev, 1981) are being employed. In SEM studies, replicas of the tooth surfaces can be evaluated and repeated at selected intervals to assess changes, thereby avoiding tissue damage. Other methods of measuring changes in the restoration-dentin interface will undoubtedly be developed in the future.

MARGINAL PERCOLATION

Nelson et al (1952) demonstrated that leakage at the margins of the filling materials occurs when the teeth are subjected to alternate cooling and warming. The leakage is due to differences between the coefficients of expansion of the tooth and the filling materials, and the resultant ingress and egress of the fluids is called percolation. As a result of marginal percolation, bacteria can gain entry into the tooth through the aperture between the margins of the cavity preparation and the restoration. The temperature of a restoration within the mouth may range from about 9°C. (from drinking ice water at 4°C.) to about 52°C. (from drinking very hot coffee at 60°C.). With some filling materials a marginal space of about $10\,\mu$ may develop from such a temperature change. A gap of this size is well below the limit of visibility ($50\,\mu$) but larger than the diameters of common bacteria found in the mouth. Roydhouse and Paxon (1970) have pointed out that the change in relationship of restorations, cavity floors and margins depends more on the rate than on the range of temperature change.

Swartz and Phillips (1960) and Going et al (1960) have demonstrated by the use of radioactive tracers that much of this marginal percolation can be controlled or reduced by the use of rosin varnishes applied to the margins of cavities before filling. Therefore, the use of rosin varnishes in the cavity prior to the filling of teeth with amalgam or silicates has been recommended. According to Qvist (1983), thermal cycling is not the major cause of marginal percolation. Instead, he found that masticatory stress had a major influence on the marginal adaptation of composite restorations.

EVALUATION OF ALL FILLING MATERIALS

All studies have confirmed that leakage of restorative material causes pulp inflammation. Thus, to evaluate testing methods for pulp reactions properly, a distinction must be made between inflammatory pulp reactions due to restorative materials and those due to bacterial ingrowth. Specifications for pulpal filling materials with respect to their toxicity for the pulp are being developed. Comparable methodology and uniform criteria for assessment of the toxicity of filling materials must be formulated.

From an evaluation of all the filling materials, it can be concluded that none meet all of the physical, esthetic, and biologic requirements. No filling material is available that is safe from all points of view.

Therefore, it is recommended that varnishes be placed on the cavity walls after they are first lined with calcium hydroxide. Zinc phosphate or zinc oxide-eugenol cement should be placed before the teeth are filled with amalgam or silicates. A mixture of calcium hydroxide, zinc oxide, and polyacrylic acid has been shown to have good adhesion, good mechanical properties, and compatible pulpal properties for lining cavities (Negm et al, 1979). The evaluation of the best material to use under certain circumstances must be based on the judgment of the operator. He must take into account the age of the patient, the depth of the restoration, the periodontal condition, the occlusion, the esthetic requirement, and his own operative skill.

BIBLIOGRAPHY

Abraham GC, Baum L: International implantation of pins into the dental pulp. J Southern Cal Dent A 40:914, 1972

Arvidson K, Wróblewski R: Migration of metallic ions from screwposts into dentin and surrounding tissues. Scand J Dent Res 861:200, 1978

Bassiouny MA, Grant AA: A visible light-cured composite restorative: Clinical open assessment. Brit Dent J 145:327, 1978

Bergenholtz G: Effect of bacterial products on inflammatory reactions in the dental pulp. Scand J Dent Res 85:122, 1977

Bergenholtz G, Lindhe J: Effect of soluble plaque factors on inflammatory reactions in the dental pulp. Scand J Dent Res 83:153, 1975

Bowen RL: Development of an adhesive restorative material. In Adhesive Restorative Dental Materials-II. Public Health Service Publication No 1494, p 229. Washington, DC, US Government Printing Office, 1966

Bowen RL, Barton JA, Jr, Mullineaux AL; Composite restorative materials. In Dickson G, Cassel JM (eds): Dental Materials Research. National Bureau of Standards Spec Pub 354, p 93. US Government Printing Office, Washington, DC, 1972

Brännström M, Nordenvall K-J: Bacterial penetration, pulpal reaction and the inner surface of concise enamel bond. Composite fillings in etched and unetched cavities. J Dent Res 57:3, 1978

Brännström M, Nyborg H: The presence of bacteria in cavities filled with silicate cement and composite resin material. Sven Tandlak-Tidskr 64:149, 1971

Burke JH, Cermak A: Internal resorption following gold-foil insertion. Report of two cases. Oral Surg 32:938, 1971

Chandler HH, Bowen RL, Paffenbarger GC, Mullineaux AL: Clinical investigation of a radiopaque composite material. JADA 81:935, 1970

Council on Dental Materials, Instruments, and Equipment. Status report on microfilled composite resins. JADA 105:488, 1982

Craig RG: Selected properties of dental composites. J Dent Res 58:1544, 1979

Dickey DM, El-Kafrawy AH, Mitchell DF: Clinical and microscopic pulp response to a composite restorative material. JADA 88:106, 1974

Dickey DM, El-Kafrawy AH, Mitchell DF: Clinical and microscopic pulp response to a composite restorative material. JADA 88:108, 1974

Dolph RW: Intentional implanting of pins into dental pulp. Dent Clin N Am 14:73, 1970 (Jan)

Dolven RC: Measurement of cavity lining, using ultraviolet and reflected light, and the effect of the liner on marginal penetration, evaluated with Ca^{45}. J Dent Res 45:12, 1966

Douglas WH, Chen CJ, Craig RG: Neutron activation analysis of microleakage around a hydrophobic composite restorative. J Dent Res 59:1507, 1980

Douglas WH, Craig RG, Chen C-J: Visible light initiated hydrophobic composite from fluoromethacrylate. J Dent Res (Special Issue) 57:250, abst #703, 1978

Douglas WH, Zakariasen KL: Volumetric assessment of apical leakage utilizing a spectrophotometric dye-recovery method. IADR Progr and Abst 60:512, 1981

Eliasson ST: Compatibility of composite resins with pulp insulating materials. J Dent Res 58:397, 1979 (abstract No 1225)

Eriksen HM, Leidal TI: Monkey pulpal response to composite resin restorations in cavities treated with various cleansing agents. Scand J Dent Res 87:309, 1979

Fan PL, Leinfelder KF: High copper-content amalgam alloys. Council on Dental Materials, Instruments, and Equipment. JADA 105:1077, 1982

Fisher M: Experimental investigations of the tightness of fit of filling materials commonly used in dentistry. Schweiz Mschr Zahnkeilk 59:595, 1949

Frykholm KO: On mercury from dental amalgam: Its toxic and allergic effects and some comments on occupational hygiene. Acta Odont Scand 15 [Supp 22], 1957

Fusayama T, Nakamura M, Kurosaki N, Iwaku M: Non-pressure adhesion to a new adhesive restorative resin. J Dent Res 58:1364, 1979

Going RE: Marginal penetration of dental restorations as studied by dyes and radioactive isotopes. Master's thesis, University of Illinois, 1959

Going RE: Microleakage around dental restorations: a summarizing review. JADA 84:1349, 1972

Going RE: Reducing marginal leakage: A review of materials and techniques. JADA 99:646, 1979

Going RE, Massler M, Dute HL: Marginal penetration of dental restorations by different radioactive isotopes. J Dent Res 39:273, 1960

Grajower R, Shaharbani S, Kaufman E: Temperature rise in pulp chamber during fabrication of temporary self-curing resin crowns. J Prosth Dent 41:535, 1979

Granath L-E: Studies on microleakage with restorative materials. III. In vitro experiments on the sealing of 9 brands of silver amalgam. Acta Odont Scand 29:65, 1971

Grieve AR: Marginal adaptation of amalgam in relation to the finish of cavity margins. Brit Dent J 130:239, 1971

Hals E, Høyer Andreassen B, Bie T: Histopathology of natural caries around silver amalgam fillings. Caries Res 8:343, 1974

Halse A: Metals in dentinal tubules beneath amalgam fillings in human teeth. Arch Oral Biol 20:87, 1975

Heida T, Yao K, Koharo O: The improvement of restorative composite resin applicable to deciduous tooth. Japan. J. Pedo., 16 (part 1): 56, 1978

Hembree JH, Andrews JT: Microleakage for corrosion resistant amalgam alloys: Laboratory study. J Dent Res 58:397, 1979

Heys D, Cox CF, Heys RJ, Loesche WJ, Avery JK: Histopathologic and bacterial evaluations of conventional and new copper amalgam. J Oral Pathol 8:65, 1979

Heys RJ, Heys DR, Cox CF, Avery JK: Histopathologic evaluation of three ultraviolet-activated composite resins on monkey pulps. J Oral Pathol 6:317, 1977

Inokoshi S, Iwaku M, Fusayama T: Pulpal response to a new adhesive restorative resin. J Dent Res 61:1014, 1982

Jacobsen PH, Von Fraunhofer JA: Assessment of microleakage using a conductometric technique. J Dent Res 54:41, 1975

Jennings RE, Ranley DM: Autoradiographic study of ^{32}P penetration into enamel and dentin during acid etching. J Dent Child 39:69, 1972

Jerman AC: Silver amalgam restorative material with stannous fluoride. JADA 80:787, 1970

Johnson RH, Christensen GJ, Stigers RW, Laswell HR: Pulpal irritation due to the phosphoric acid component of silicate cement. Oral Surg 29:447, 1970

Jørgensen KD: Amalgams in dentistry. In Dickson G, Cassel JM (eds): Dental Materials Research. National Bureau of Standards Spec Pub 354. US Government Printing Office, Washington, DC, 1972

Jørgensen KD, Esbensen AL: Gravimetric determination of the corrosion of dental amalgams. Tandlaegebladet 77:162, 1973

Jørgensen KD, Wakumoto S: Occlusal amalgam fillings: Marginal defects and secondary caries. Odont T 76:43, 1968

El-Kafrawy AH, Mitchell DF: Pulp reactions to open cavities later restored with silicate cement. J Dent Res 42:874, 1963

Kurosaki N, Fusayama T: Penetration of elements from amalgam into dentin. J Dent Res 52:309, 1973

Langeland K, Dogon LI, Langeland LK: Pulp protection requirements for two composite resin restorative materials. Aust Dent J 15:349, 1970

Langeland LK, Guttuso J, Jerome DR, Langeland K: Histologic and clinical comparison of addent with silicate cements and cold-curing materials. JADA 72:373, 1966

Langeland K, Langeland LK: Pulp reactions to crown preparation, impression, temporary crown fixation, and permanent cementation. J Prosth Dent 15:129, 1965

Lee HJ, Jr, Orlowski JA, Scheidt GC, Lee JR: Effects of acid etchants on dentin. J Dent Res 52:1228, 1973

Lee HL, Swartz ML: Sealing of developmental pits and fissures. J Dent Res 50:133, 1971

Leirskar J: On the mechanism of cytotoxicity of silver and copper amalgams in a cell culture system. Scand J Dent Res 82:74, 1974

Loiselle RJ, Goldberg AF, Gross RL, Stuever CH, Jr: Marginal microleakage — an in vivo assessment. JADA 78:758, 1969

McCurdy CR, Swartz ML, Phillips RW, Rhodes BF: A comparison of in vivo and in vitro microleakage of dental restorations. JADA 88:592, 1974

Massler M, Barber TK: Action of amalgam on dentin. JADA 47:415, 1953

Mateer RS, Reitz CD: Galvanic degradation of amalgam restorations. J Dent Res 51:1546, 1972

Mejàre B, Mejàre I, Edwardsson S: Bacteria beneath composite restorations — a culturing and histobacteriological study. Acta Odont Scand 37:267, 1979

Meyer JM, Dennison JB, Craig RG: Improved method of neutron activation analysis for microleakage studies. J Dent Res 53:356, 1974

Meyers CL, Stanley HR, Heyde JB, Chamberlain J: Primate pulpal response to ultraviolet light-polymerized direct-bonding material systems. J Dent Res 55:1118, 1976

Mjör IA: The effect of calcium hydroxide, zinc-oxide-eugenol and amalgam on the pulp. Odont T 71:94, 1963

Mjör IA, Eriksen HM, Haugen E, Skogedal O: Biologic assessment of copper-containing amalgams. Int Dent J 27:333, 1977

Mjör IA, Pindborg JJ: Histology of the Human Tooth, p 11. Copenhagen, Munksgaard, 1973

Mjör IA, Tronstad L: Experimentally induced pulpitis, Oral Surg 34:102, 1972

Möller B, Granath LE: Reaction of the human dental pulp to silver amalgam restorations. The effect of insertion of amalgam of high plasticity in deep cavities. Acta Odont Scand 31:187, 1973

Mondelli J, Ishikiriama A, Galan J: Marginal microleakage of dental cements. J Prosthet Dent 40:632, 1978

Mortensen DW, Boucher NE, Jr, Ryge G: A method of testing for marginal leakage of dental restorations with bacteria. J Dent Res 44:58, 1965

Negm MM, Combe EE, Grant AA: New cements for lining and pulp capping. Brit Dent J 147:272, 1979

Phillips RW, Gilmore HW, Swartz ML, Schenker SI:

Adaption of restorations in vivo as assessed by Ca^{45} JADA 62:23, 1961

Pohto M, Scheinen A: Vital microscopy of the pulp in the rat incisor. VII. Reactions to silicate cements. Suom Hammaslääk Toim 63:178, 1967

Prosser HJ, Groffman DM, Wilson AD: The effect of composition on the erosion properties of calcium hydroxide cements. J Dent Res 61:1431, 1982

Qvist V: The effect of mastication on marginal adaptation of composite restorations in vivo. J Dent Res 62:904, 1983

Qvist V: Pulp reactions in human teeth to tooth-colored filling materials. Scand J Dent Res 83:54, 1975

Roydhouse RH: Silicate cements and pulpal degeneration. JADA 62:670, 1961

Roydhouse RH, Paxon PR: Thermal changes in dimension of restorative cavities. J Dent Res 49:567, 1970

Rud J, Omnell K-Å: Root fractures due to corrosion. Scand J Dent Res 78:397, 1970

Schoen FJ, et al: Objective evaluation of surface microreplication by dental impression materials. J Dent Res 57:283, 1978

Skogedal O, Eriksen HM: Pulpal reactions to surface-sealed silicate cement and composite resin restorations. Scand J Dent Res 84:381, 1976

Skogedal O, Mjör I: Pulpal response to dental amalgams. Scand J Dent Res 87:346, 1979

Souganidis DJ, Athanassouli TMN, Papastathopoulos DS: A study of in vivo fluoride uptake by dental tissues from fluoride-containing silver amalgams. J Dent Res 60:105, 1981

Special Report: Report of the committee on scientific investigation of the American Academy of Restorative Dentistry. J Prosth Dent 43:663, 1980

Stanley HR, Bowen RL, Folia J: Compatibility of various materials with oral tissues. II. Pulp responses to composite ingredients. J Dent Res 58:1507, 1979

Stanley HR, Going RE, Chauncey HH: Human pulp response to acid pretreatment of dentin and composite restoration. JADA 91:817, 1975

Stanley HR, Swerdlow H, Stanwich L, Suarez C: A comparison of the biological effects of filling materials with recommendation for pulp protection. J Am Acad Gold Foil Oper 12:56, 1969

Steuver CH, Goldberg AF, Gross RL: The effect of pulpal tissues on microleakage around dental restorations. Oral Surg 31:568, 1971

Stoner GE, Senti SE, Gileadi E: Effect of sodium fluoride and stannous fluoride on the rate of corrosion of dental amalgams. J Dent Res 50:1647, 1971

Suzuki M, Goto G, Jordon RE: Pulpal response to pin placement. JADA 87:636, 1973

Swartz ML, Phillips RW: Permeability of cavity liners to certain agents. J Dent Res 39:1232, 1960

Swartz ML, Phillips RW, Chamberlain N: Continued studies on the permeability of cavity liners. J Dent Res 41:66, 1962

Swerdlow H, Stanley HR: Response of human dental pulp to amalgam restorations. Oral Surg 15:499, 1962

Takahashi K: A study of the cytotoxic action of gold-copper alloy by means of tissue culture. J Jap Soc for Dent Apparat Materials 16(35):79, 1975

Thomas JJ, Stanley HR, Gilmore HW: Effects of gold foil condensation on human dental pulp. JADA 78:788, 1969

Thye RP: A comparison of the marginal penetration of direct filling golds using Ca^{45}. Am Acad Gold Foil Oper 10:12, 1967

Tobias M, Cataldo E, Shieve FR, Clark ER: Pulp reaction to a resin-bonded quartz composite material. J Dent Res 52:1281, 1973

Tobias RS, Plant CG, Browne RM: Reduction in pulpal inflammation beneath surface-sealed silicates. Int Endo J 15:173, 1982

Updegraff DM, Chiang RWH, Joos RW: Antibacterial activity of dental restorative materials. J Dent Res 50:382, 1971

Valcke CF, Cleaton-Jones PE, Austin JC, Pain E, Viura E: The pulpal response to a direct filling resin without an inorganic filler—Isopast. J Oral Rehab 7:1, 1980

Vasudev VB: A simple method of quantitating microleakage in dental restorations: Dental amalgams, pp 33–35. Master's thesis, University of Florida, 1981

Wing G, Lyell JS: The marginal seal of amalgam restorations. Austral Dent J 11:81, 1966

Zach L, Cohen G: Pulp response to externally applied heat. Oral Surg 19:515, 1965

12
PULPITIS FROM OPERATIVE PROCEDURES

ODONTOBLASTS

Each odontoblast is a chemical factory of its own. The cell manufactures or synthesizes enzymes and other proteins. The proteins are synthesized in the rough endoplasmic reticulum (rER) and released into the cisternae, where some glycosylation occurs. As the protein passes through the Golgi apparatus, extensive glycosylation is achieved. The proteins are then secreted through the odontoblastic cell membrane. The principal components of the membrane are lipids (approximately half of the mass) and proteins (the balance; Capaldi, 1974). A small quantity of carbohydrates is also present. It is generally assumed that the matrix of the membrane is composed of lipid molecules arranged in a bimolecular leaflet (Bretscher, 1973).

According to Capaldi, proteins and glycoproteins in the cell membrane not only contribute to the structural integrity of the membrane, but also play a variety of other roles. They can act as enzymes and function as pumps to move materials into and out of cells.

The odontoblasts form a syncytium and contact each other. Under normal circumstances, this continuous, uninterrupted contact between odontoblasts gives the odontoblastic layer a fence-stake arrangement, called palisading (Fig. 12-1). As a result of the continuous contact of the odontoblasts, the protoplasm of the nuclei at the predentin border gives the appearance of being an intact membrane and simulates, although it is not actually, a basement membrane. It stains hyperchromatically and is known as the pulpodentinal membrane (Fig. 12-1).

Odontoblastic Damage

In operative procedures involving the dentin, the protoplasmic processes of the odontoblasts are irritated. Hence, the first cells usually involved in the inflammatory process in the pulp are the odontoblasts. Changes occur within the odontoblastic cell that are related to changes in osmotic pressure, because of an increase in metabolites within the cell.

Cutting of the dentin results in loss of cytoplasmic continuity of the odontoblasts. Alterations of the fine structures within the body of the odontoblasts result. The membranes of the endoplasmic reticulum fragment and the mitochrondria degenerate. Proteins are denatured, resulting in structural changes of the cell membrane (Searls, 1967).

If the cell membrane is damaged, permeabil-

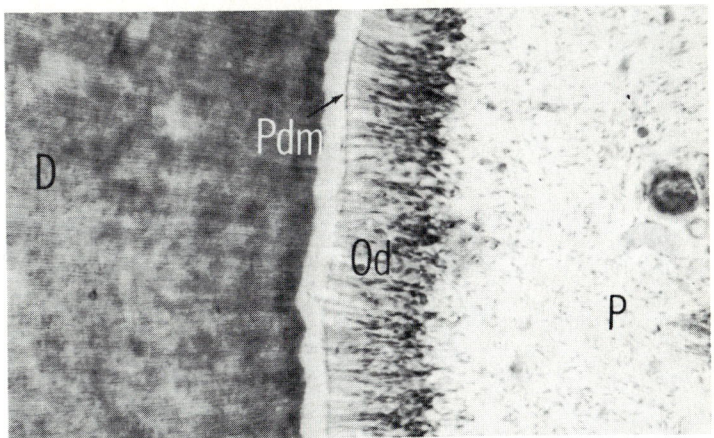

FIG. 12-1 Palisading of the odontoblasts. The odontoblasts (Od) are arranged in an orderly fashion, parallel with each other and in continuous contact. P, pulp; D, dentin; Pdm, pulpodentinal membrane. ×135. (Seltzer S, Bender IB: Early human pulp reactions to full crown preparations. JADA 59:912, 1959)

ity is altered. If a great amount of damage occurs, the nucleus is affected. The changes in structure result in liberation of cell products. Stewart (1965) has demonstrated in electron microscopic studies that there is an increase in odontoblastic cytoplasmic lipid granules following injury.

DISPLACEMENT OF ODONTOBLASTS

Another odontoblastic change that may occur after operative procedures is the displacement of the odontoblastic nuclei into the dentin. These are called aspirated, displaced, or ectopic odontoblasts (Fig. 12-2).

Pressure, both positive and negative, appears to be responsible for the odontoblastic displacement, but the process is not yet well understood (Stevenson, 1967; Eda and Saito, 1978). The odontoblasts are pushed or pulled into the dentin. When the odontoblastic processes are cut, they appear to react as an elastic band, and the nuclei are pulled into the dentin.

Several hypotheses have been offered for the displacement phenomenon. Stanley and Swerdlow (1958) claimed that inflammatory changes inside the pulp push the odontoblasts into the dentin. However, displaced nuclei are found in the dentin immediately after cavity preparation, before there has been time for inflammatory changes to have occurred.

Langeland (1957) postulated that the nuclei are pushed into the dentin when the dentin is dried. Also, odontoblastic nuclei are pushed into the dentin when a cavity is cut without moisture. Brännström (1960) found that odontoblastic nuclei were displaced into the dentinal tubules when cavities were exposed to a stream of air at room temperature for 30 seconds. On the other hand, Brännström (1961) also demonstrated odontoblastic displacement when the dentin of prepared cavities was subjected to water pressure of 2 kg/cm² for 3 minutes.

According to Brännström (1968), the displaced cells undergo autolysis within a short period of time (6 hours). Further displacement of other odontoblasts into the dentin may result from leaky restorations and an outward flow of dentinal fluid (Johnson et al, 1973). Berggren and Brännström (1965) estimated that the rate of fluid flow due to capillary attraction is about 4 mm/sec at a distance of 2 mm from the pulp.

Within a short time, the displaced odontoblastic nuclei having undergone autolysis are no longer visible within the dentinal tubules in tissue sections. An acceleration of reparative dentin formation occurs as a response to the odontoblastic injury. The degenerated nuclei in the predentin are mineralized.

It is apparent that more than one mechanism may be responsible for the passage of odontoblastic nuclei into the dentin.

POSTEXTRACTION CHANGES

When extracted teeth are examined histologically, care must be exercised to avoid misinterpretation of odontoblastic damage and pulp hemorrhage. When a tooth is extracted with forceps, the beaks of the forceps crush the cementum and the underlying dentin. Both the dentinal tubules and the odontoblasts are af-

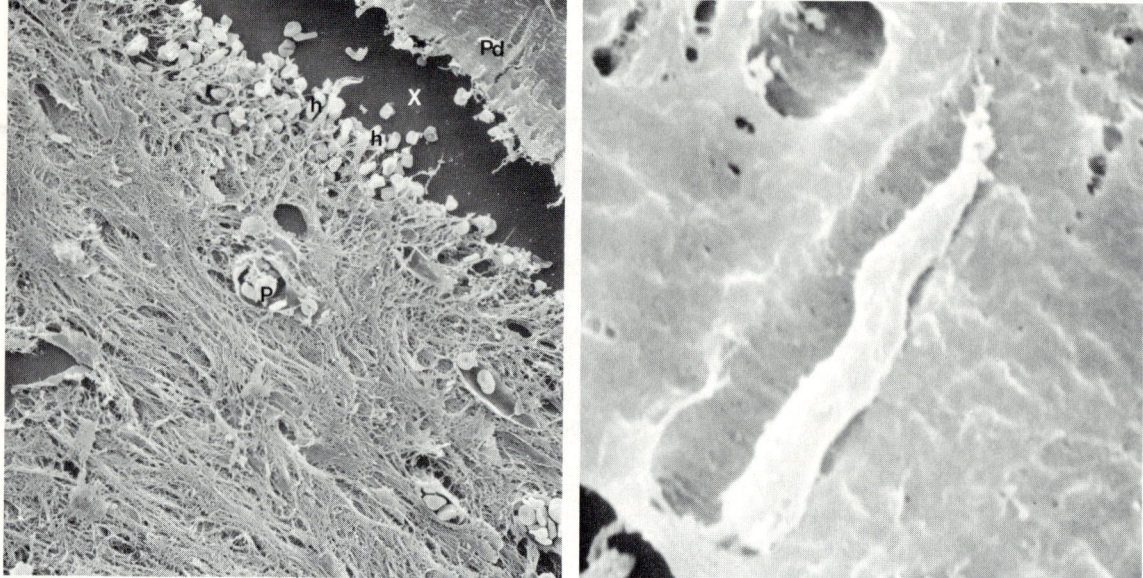

FIG. 12-2 *(Left)* Scanning electron micrograph of tissue section following cavity preparation. The odontoblastic layer of the pulp (P) has been separated from the predentin (Pd) at X. Hemorrhage (h) has resulted from the odontoblastic capillaries. ×500. *(Right)* Higher magnification of predentin from left photomicrograph showing displaced odontoblast in dentinal tubule. ×5000.

fected, and some disruption of the odontoblastic layer takes place. The odontoblasts are destroyed by the pressure, the odontoblastic layer is disturbed, and displaced nuclei are seen in the dentin (Corpron and Avery, 1971). Hemorrhage of the small capillaries in the odontoblastic layer may occur as a result of the pressure. Almost with mathematical precision, the odontoblasts that are damaged and displaced by the beaks of the forceps are those whose protoplasmic processes are in the crushed dentinal tubules. This indicates that pressure at the extreme end of the dentinal tubules is sufficient to damage the odontoblasts.

Postextraction operative procedures on teeth result in similar odontoblastic changes. If pressure from the forceps can damage and kill the odontoblasts, what is the effect of pressure from cavity cutting or cementing an inlay or taking an impression? This question is discussed in Chapter 9, Mechanical and Thermal Irritants.

The changes observed in inflammation of the other bodily connective tissues are found in inflammations of the dental pulp as a result of operative procedures. A similar sequence of events occurs.

ACUTE PULPITIS

Following damage to the odontoblasts from operative procedures, an acute partial pulpitis develops (Fig. 12-3). Such inflammation may be mild or severe in intensity, and the involvement of the pulp may be partial or, rarely, total. Clinically, pain (pulpalgia) may or may not be present. The acute pulpitis may be superimposed over a transitional stage or a chronic pulpitis* that was already present as a result of dental caries, or it may occur in a previously uninflamed pulp (Fig. 12-4).

Initiation of Inflammation. The breakdown products of the injured odontoblasts affect other odontoblasts, which, in turn, are injured or killed. The products that are liberated affect the underlying tissues, and the process of inflammation is initiated.

*See Chap. 17, Histologic Classification of Pulp Diseases.

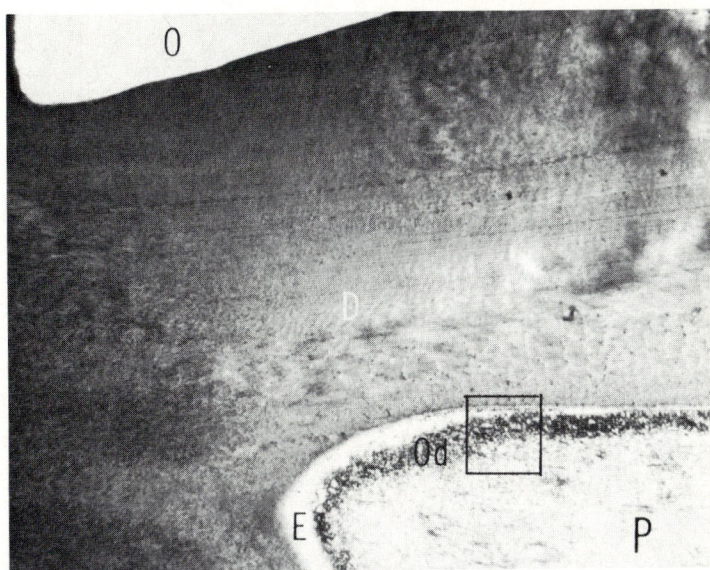

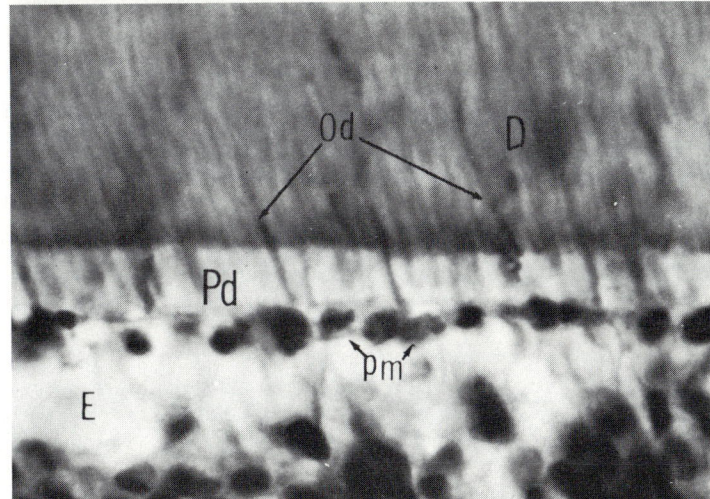

FIG. 12-3 Acute inflammation of the pulp. *(Top)* The pulp (P) underlying the region of the dentinal tubules involved by the operative procedure (O). Edema (E) has separated the odontoblasts (Od) from the dentin (D). ×54. *(Bottom)* Higher magnification of region outlined by rectangle in top photograph. Polymorphonuclear leukocytes (pm) are present along the predentin (Pd). The odontoblasts (Od) are displaced into the dentin (D). Fluid (E) is present. ×960.

VASCULAR CHANGES IN THE ODONTOBLASTIC LAYER

Characteristic changes are observed within the capillaries of the odontoblastic layer. These are typical of the dynamic changes that occur in inflammation elsewhere in the body. Odontoblastic cell damage causes a release of vasoactive inflammatory substances such as histamine, bradykinin, serotonin, prostaglandins, and leukotrienes. These mediators increase vascular permeability, especially in the postcapillary venules. There is, first, a slowing of the bloodstream and, then, a dilatation of the blood vessels. The initial change, arteriolar dilatation, takes place in the subodontoblastic vascular plexus. This results in an increase in the number of perfused capillaries. Presently, in the odontoblastic layer, capillaries are observed that were always there but were not visible prior to inflammation. They become apparent because they become packed with red blood cells. Capillary pressure is elevated. This elevation, together with the increased permeability, is responsible for fluid filtration. The fluid is distributed between and among the odontoblasts

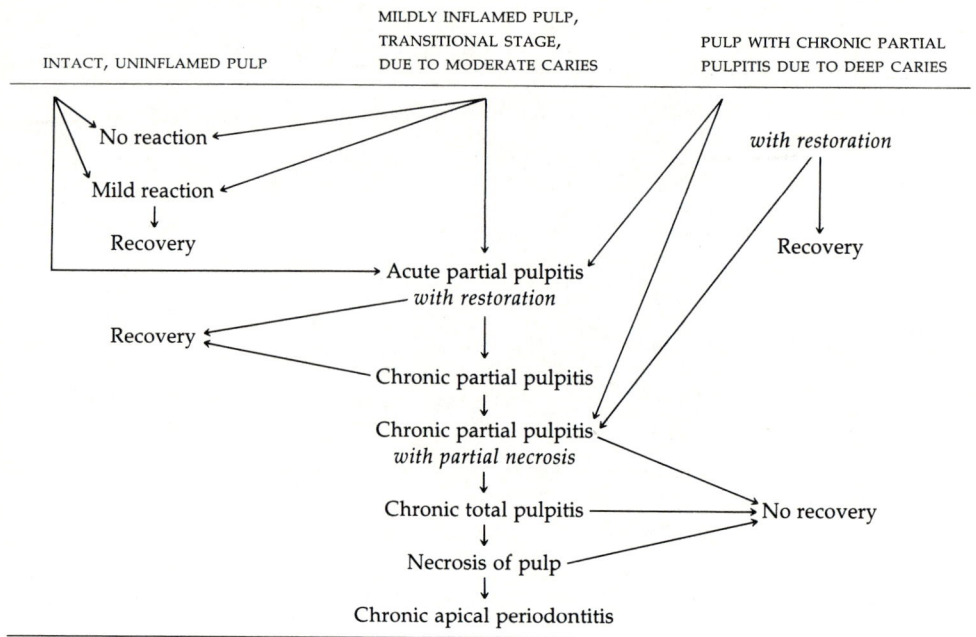

FIG. 12-4 Sequence of pulp reactions to irritation from operative procedures.

(Fig. 12-5). Leaking of fluid from the capillaries into the surrounding tissue (edema) follows. The increase in fluid filtration causes an elevation of tissue pressure, which, in turn, results in a rise in venous resistance, causing a stagnation of flow. Stasis, characterized by a standstill of blood flow, develops. According to Scheinin (1963), the stasis lasts for a relatively short time and is followed by thrombosis. As reported by Van Hassel (1973) and Tønder and Kvinnsland (1983), these local events, which occur in experimentally induced inflammation, will gradually spread circumferentially to the neighboring areas.

Filtrated fluid from the inflamed vessels is absorbed by the adjacent noninflamed microvessels. Since the pulp is encased in a rigid structure or a low-compliance environment, rapid elimination of filtered fluid is essential for the survival of the pulp.

Leaking of fluid from the capillaries into the surrounding tissue follows. Gradually, the odontoblasts are separated from the dentin and the underlying tissues by the accumulated fluid. A disruption of the pulpodentinal membrane is visible in tissue sections and in scanning electron micrographs (Fig. 12-6).

Hypothesis for the Pathophysiology of Pulpal Disorder (Fig. 12-7)

As a result of caries or operative procedures, many inflammatory agents or mediators are released from the inflamed area. These mediators are derived from the damaged cell membrane, from the blood vessels, platelets, or the sensory nerve endings. As examples, Ogart et al (1977) reported that tooth preparation caused a drastic increase in substance P levels in the feline pulp, and Araujo et al (1980) suggested that histamine and 5-hydroxytryptamine might be responsible for the initial stage of inflammation in the pulp.

Vascular reactivity is drastically reduced after tooth preparation. The healthy pulp is responsive to sympathetic nerve stimulation by vasoconstriction. However, during or immediately after tooth preparation, Ahlberg (1977) found that electrical stimulation of the sympathetic nerve caused no changes in pulpal blood flow, indicating an interference in vascular response.

The net result of the release of the inflammatory agents and the reduction of vascular reactivity is vasodilatation, i.e., a decrease in flow resistance in the afflicted area. The decrease in

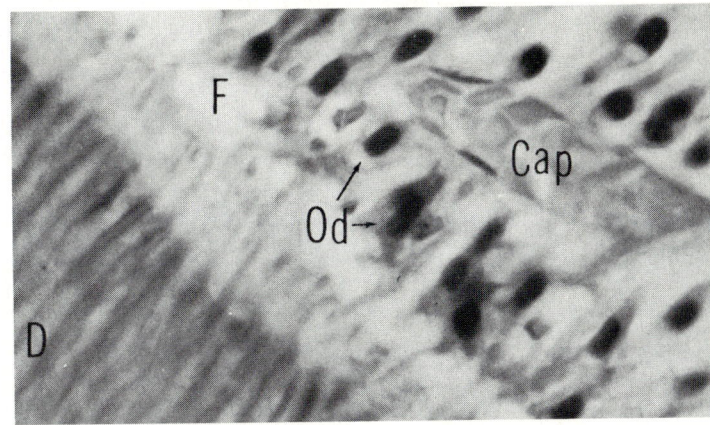

FIG. 12-5 Dilated capillary (Cap), with clumped red blood cells in the odontoblastic layer of the pulp. The odontoblasts (Od) are separated from the dentin by fluid (F). D, dentin. ×960.

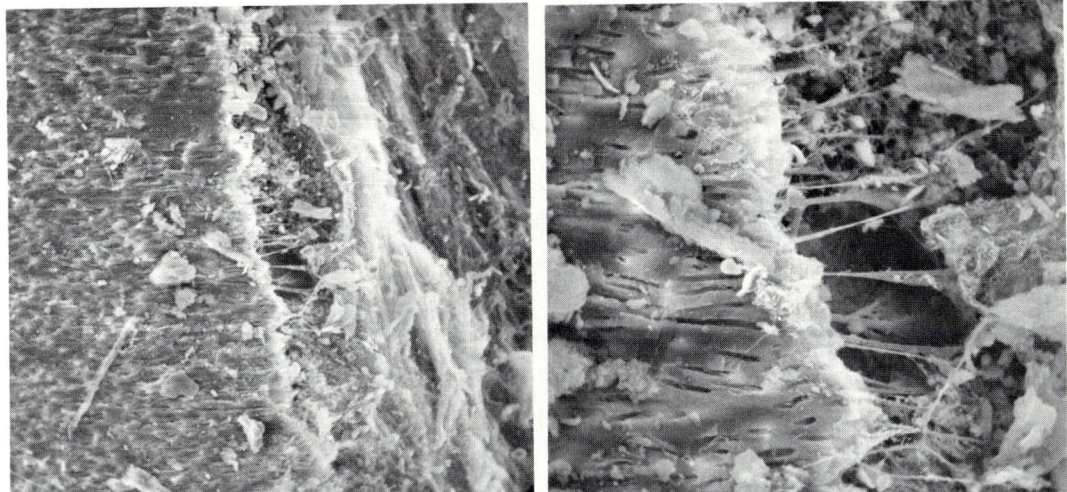

FIG. 12-6 *(Left)* Scanning electron micrograph of disruption of pulpodentinal membrane. ×180. *(Right)* Higher magnification, showing separation and destruction of odontoblasts. ×600.

flow resistance in the arteriolar bed causes an increase in blood flow through the capillary bed, concurrent with an elevation of the capillary pressure. Simultaneously, the vasodilation causes an increase in vascular permeability, resulting in leakage of various high molecular substances. The combined effect of the increases in the capillary pressure and flow and the vascular permeability is filtration into the extracellular space. The filtered materials are mostly high-molecular-weight substances that draw fluid outward, causing edema. In turn, an increase in pulp tissue pressure results.

It has been suggested that the pulp is compartmentalized (Bender, 1978; Nahri, 1978). Thus, a local increase in the tissue pressure occurs. When the tissue pressure is elevated so that the local venular pressure is exceeded, the flow resistance of the venules begins to increase. This increase in venular resistance has a deleterious effect on the local hemodynamics: The increase in venular resistance causes a decrease in blood flow because the drainage of blood is blocked. This sluggish flow will enhance red-cell aggregation, which in turn causes a drastic increase in blood viscosity. A vicious cycle begins. The increase in viscosity further decreases the blood flow, depriving the local area of oxygen. When

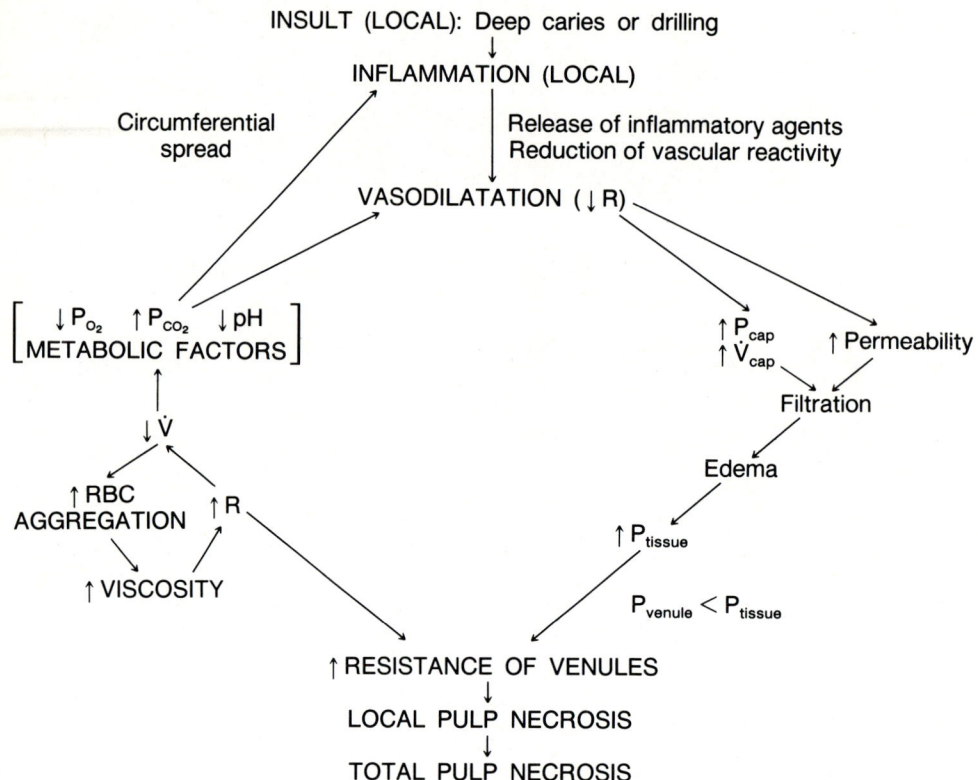

FIG. 12-7 The Pathophysiology of pulpal disorder. (Courtesy of Dr. S. Kim, Columbia University, New York)

the blood supply does not meet the tissue demands, the tissue becomes autoregulated by means of various metabolic factors, as described below, to re-establish blood flow.

The lack of blood flow to the affected area prompts a decrease in partial pressure of oxygen, an increase in partial pressure of carbon dioxide, and a low pH. These changes in local tissue metabolic factors stimulate vasodilation, thereby promoting inflammation in the adjacent tissue compartments. As shown by Van Hassel (1973), the spread of inflammation takes place circumferentially. Thus, the inflammatory action in a local area results in a local necrosis; following inflammation, this necrosis spreads circumferentially, eventually resulting in total pulp necrosis.

This hypothesis is based on many experimental results. However, there are many gaps in our understanding of each step in the process. These gaps must be filled in order to comprehend the pathophysiologic mechanism of pulp necrosis fully.

CHEMOTAXIS

A few hours after odontoblast displacement, margination of the leukocytes in the blood vessels occurs. Because of chemotaxis, the leukocytes emerge from the vessels and line the odontoblastic layer (Fig. 12-3), often separating the odontoblasts from the dentin (Fig. 12-8). The leukocytes are also found penetrating the underlying pulp tissue. When large numbers of leukocytes die, enzymes that digest tissue are liberated. Suppuration occurs and a small abscess may form in the pulp (Seltzer et al, 1977; Fig. 12-9). This occurs in the presence of a lower pH due to an accumulation of lactic acid.

Erythrocytes may be displaced into the dentinal tubules, resulting in a fall in the hydraulic conductance of dentin (Pashley et al, 1981). They may also escape into the tissue spaces (Fig. 12-10). The resultant hemorrhage may be of varying magnitude and may cause destruction of pulp tissue from pressure (Fig. 12-11).

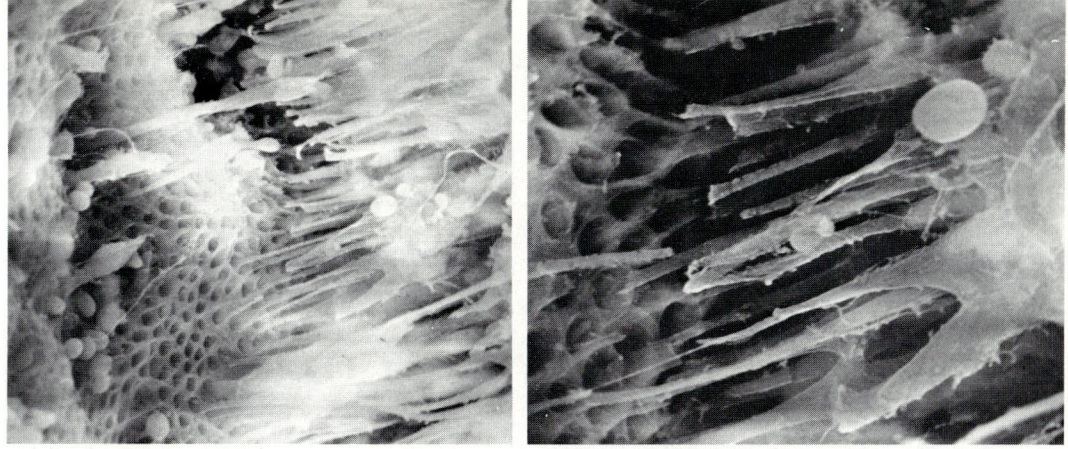

FIG. 12-8 *(Left)* Scanning electron micrograph of odontoblastic layer disrupted by leukocytes and erythrocytes. ×600. *(Right)* Higher magnification of disrupted odontoblasts. ×1800.

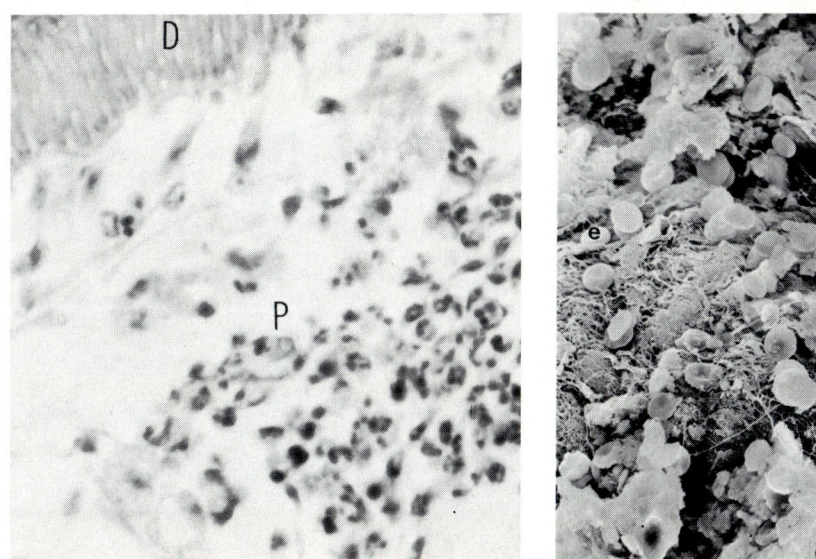

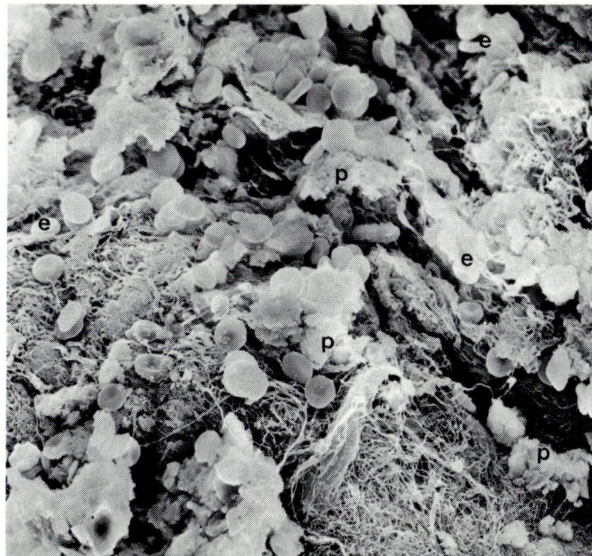

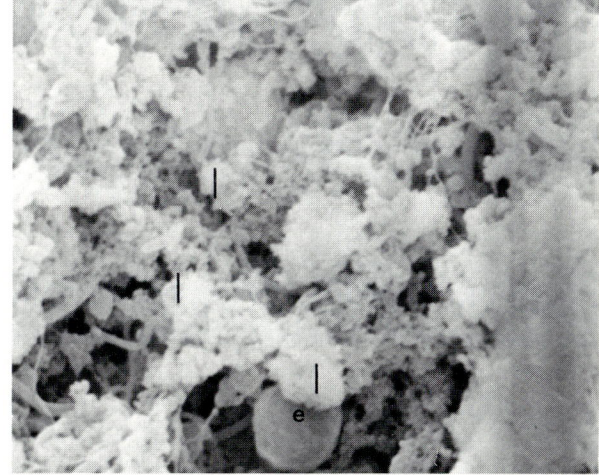

FIG. 12-9 *(Top left)* Suppuration in the pulp (P). A collection of polymorphonuclear leukocytes is present. Most of the pulp cells have undergone liquefaction necrosis. D, dentin. ×960. *(Top right)* Scanning electron micrograph of degranulating polys (p) and erythrocytes (e) in suppurative pulpitis. ×200. *(Bottom right)* Higher magnification of top right photomicrograph showing degranulation of polys, lysosomes (l), and erythrocytes (e). ×5000.

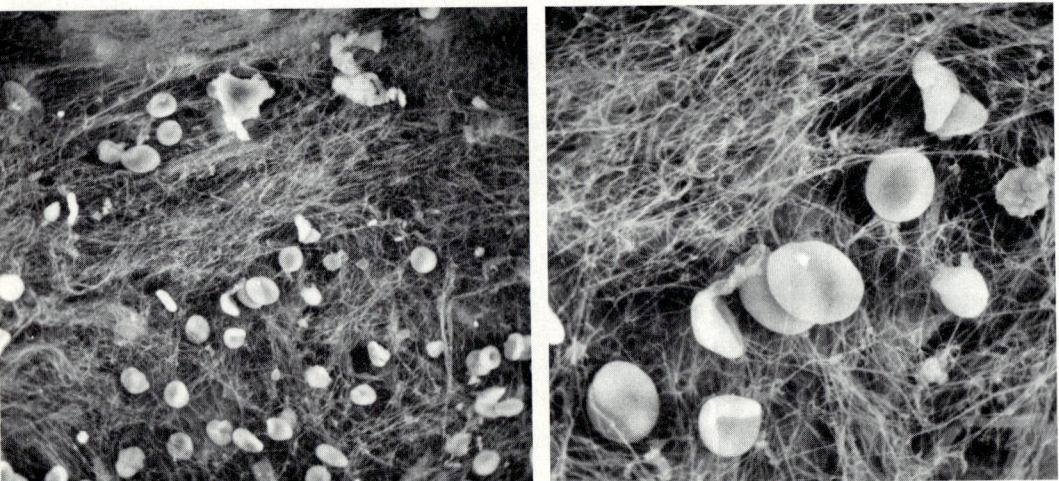

FIG. 12-10 *(Left)* Scanning electron micrograph of blood cells in deeper pulp tissue. ×600. *(Right)* Higher magnification of left photograph. ×1800.

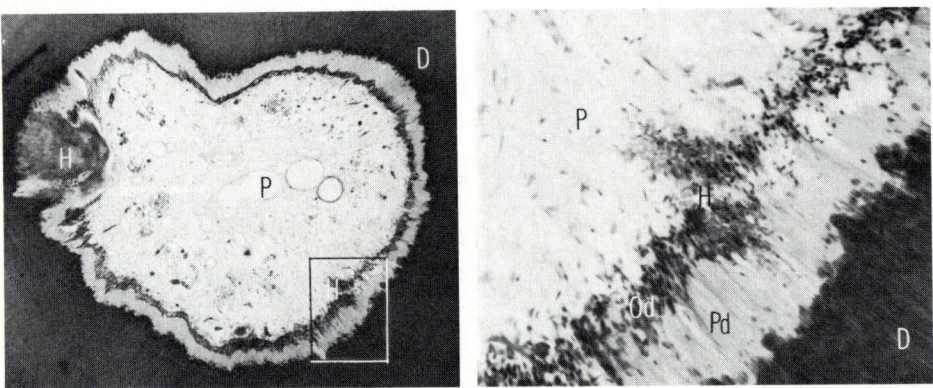

FIG. 12-11 Hemorrhage into the odontoblastic layer. *(Left)* Cross section of a lower bicuspid, following a crown preparation. Hemorrhages (H) into the pulp (P) have occurred. ×54. *(Right)* Higher magnification of region outlined by rectangle in photograph at left. Red blood cells (H) are scattered throughout the odontoblastic layer (Od) and the predentin (Pd). D, dentin. ×240. (Seltzer S, Bender IB: JADA 59:912, 1959)

As a result of disintegration of the extravasated erythrocytes, a brownish pigment may be present in the tissue spaces.

The effects of the inflammatory exudate on the odontoblastic layer are compression and death of the cells. The palisaded appearance of the odontoblastic layer is altered. When significant numbers of odontoblasts are killed, a reduction in size and width of the odontoblastic layer can be observed in tissue sections (Fig. 12-12).

CHRONIC PULPITIS

After approximately 1 week, the acute inflammation of the pulp subsides and chronic inflammation ensues. This is characterized by the presence of granulation tissue (Fig. 12-13). The inflammatory cells are those of the chronic series: lymphocytes, plasma cells, and macrophages. An increased number of mast cells has been reported in association with plasma cells

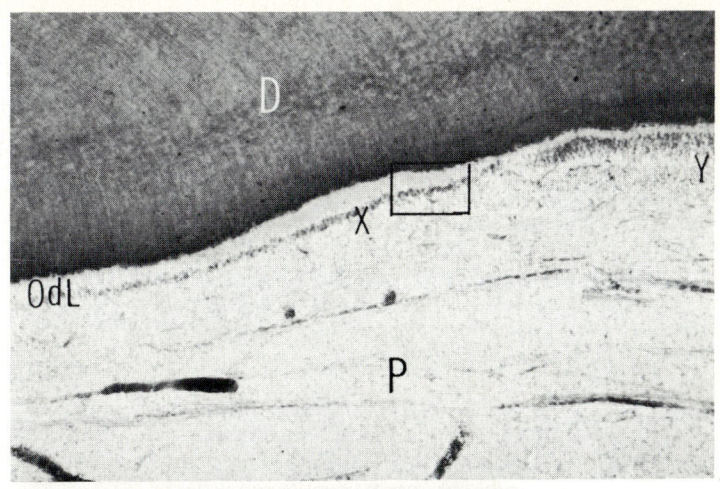

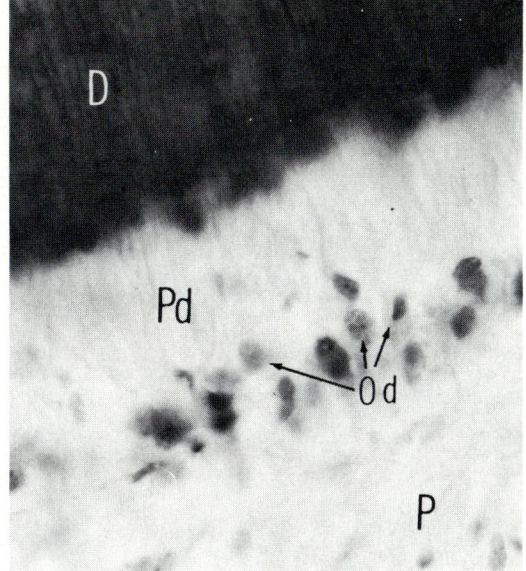

FIG. 12-12 Reparative dentin formation following operative injury. *(Top)* Under the region of the affected dentinal tubules (D), the odontoblastic layer (OdL) is thinner (region X) than it is under the unaffected tubules (region Y). P, pulp. ×54. *(Bottom)* Higher magnification of region outlined by rectangle in top picture. Odontoblasts (Od) have elaborated dentin matrix (Pd) which is collagenous. D, dentin; P, pulp. ×540.

FIG. 12-13 Granulation tissue (GT), invading the cell-free zone of the pulp (P). D, dentin. ×240. (Seltzer S: Reparative dentinogenesis. Oral Surg 12:595, 1959)

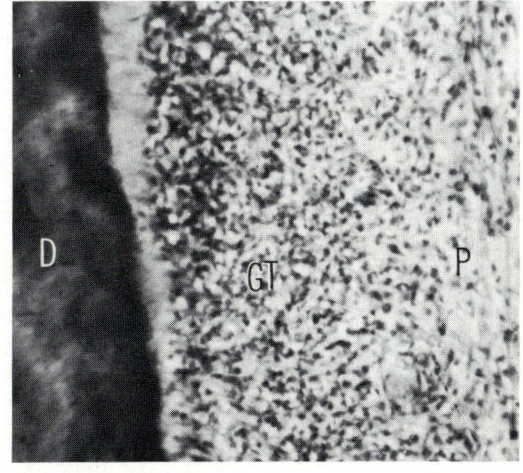

and lymphocytes (Zachrisson, 1971; Miller et al, 1978; Langeland, 1981). Chronic inflammatory cells may also be found in the cell-free zone, and they invade the odontoblastic layer (Seltzer et al, 1977; Fig. 12–13). Macrophages are large phagocytes with several functions, including digestion of bacteria, cellular debris, and antigen-antibody complexes (Fig. 12–14). They also play a role in processing antigens in the immune system.

Lymphocytes (Fig. 12–15), in addition to their role in the immunologic mechanism (see Chap. 7), have also been known as trephocytes (feeding or nutritive cells). They synthesize and store nucleoproteins and transport them to sites where other cells may use their components for growth and maintenance (Kelsall and Crabb, 1958). Concentration of proteins at the site of repair for an extended period of time is necessary for cell growth and differentiation.

FIG. 12-14 *(Top)* Scanning electron micrograph of inflamed pulp tissue containing macrophages. ×500. *(Bottom)* Higher magnification of macrophage in center of top photomicrograph engulfing bacteria and cellular debris. ×5000.

FIG. 12-15 *(Top)* Chronic inflammation of the pulp. Most of the cells are plasma cells (pc). Lymphocytes (l) also are present. f, fibroblast. ×960. *(Bottom)* Scanning electron micrograph of dissected plasma cell in tissue section. ×5000.

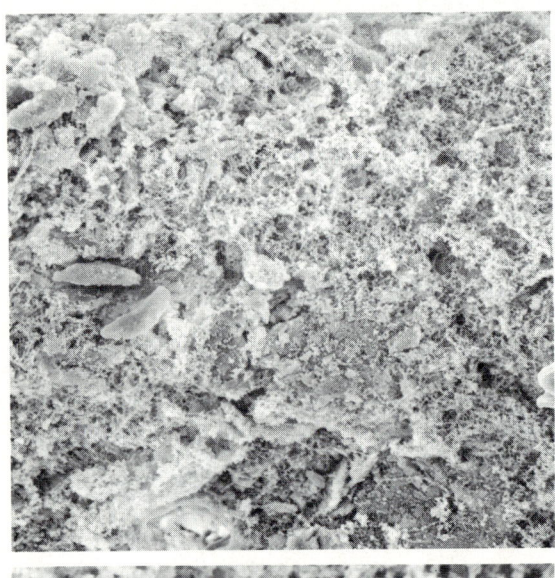
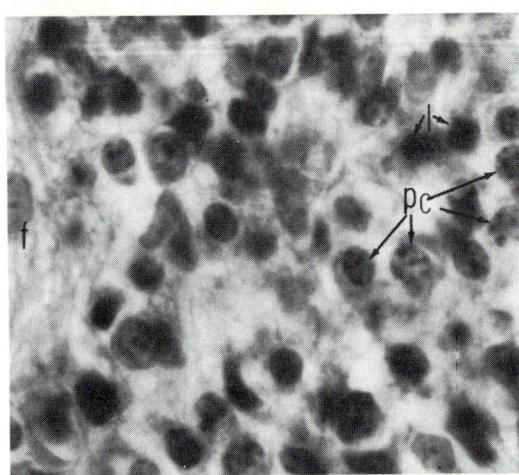
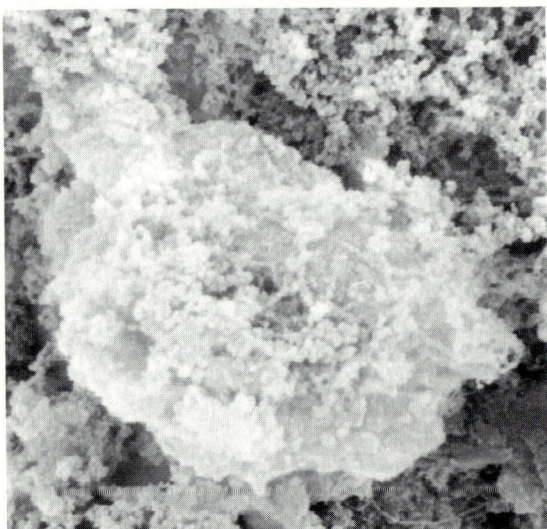
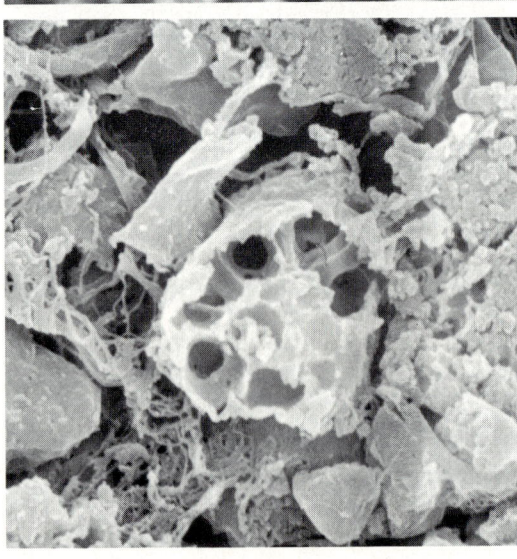

In chronic inflammation, plasma cells (Fig. 12–15) have the function of producing antibodies that neutralize antigens. Fluorescent antibody techniques have revealed the presence of immunoglobulins, primarily IgG, in most of the plasma cells of inflamed pulps (Honjo et al, 1968, 1970) — a finding suggestive of local antibody production in the dental pulp. The nuclei of plasma cells are rich in DNA. The plasma cells in chronic inflammation are believed to be converted from lymphocytes.

REPAIR

Repair is initiated when the chemical stimuli from the injured cells are elaborated and the critical concentration of the irritant is reduced. Healing or repair follows certain biologic principles, one of which is the establishment of drainage. Fibroplasia cannot take place in the presence of fluid; extravasated blood, pus, and excess cellular fluid must be removed before fibroblasts can proliferate. Concomitantly, with the drainage, pressure on the adjacent cells is relieved. Once the pressure is removed, cell migration begins. All cells in the process of repair move centripetally in the direction of pressure release.

At the periphery of the inflamed tissue, pulp injury is characterized by fibroblastic proliferation, inflammatory cell infiltration, and acid mucopolysaccharide accumulation, followed by collagen deposition and scar formation (reparative dentin). Granulation tissue that has invaded the cell-free zone (Fig. 12–13) begins to contract, possibly as a result of fibroblastic modulation (Majno et al, 1971).

During pulp repair, the injured odontoblasts may recover. Those that are destroyed are phagocytized, and other pulp mesenchymal cells are stimulated to differentiate into odontoblasts (Sveen and Hawes, 1968; Zach et al, 1969). They elaborate reparative dentin, sealing off the dead cells and tubules. Induction mechanisms for the conversion of pulp cells to odontoblasts exist. The enzyme alkaline phosphatase has been shown to stimulate such conversion, but the exact mechanism is unknown.

PREDENTIN CHANGES

Disturbance of the odontoblasts affects the elaboration of predentin, the collagenous material they extrude. As a result, changes in the width of the predentin occur. These changes may be toward either thinning or widening (Fig. 12–11). More predentin may be elaborated, or less, depending on the severity of the injury. The quality of the predentin is also changed. If a large quantity of matrix is elaborated quickly, an atubular, amorphous structure results. If a smaller quantity is elaborated slowly and more regularly, the reparative dentin appears more tubular and regular. Changes in mineralization of the dentin also occur, and the injury to the odontoblasts is registered permanently, since an alteration in mineralization results. Schour and Smith (1934) described this so-called calciotraumatic response, which they noted after injections of sodium fluoride in rats, as several alternating bands of hyperchromatically and hypochromatically staining dentin (Fig. 12–16). Osmanski and Yaeger (1964), using microradiography, and Grady and Yaeger (1965), using polarizing microscopy, subsequently found that the response consisted of two components; an external, hypermineralized and an internal, hypomineralized layer. The cells that line reparative dentin are cuboidal or flattened. Occasionally, no cells resembling odontoblasts are in evidence; however, since predentin continues to be elaborated, it may be assumed that other cells in the pulp, either fibroblasts or undifferentiated mesenchyme cells, have the potential for functioning as odontoblasts and elaborating collagen. This elaboration occurs during the reparative phase of dentinogenesis.

In chronic inflammation of the pulp, the pulp tends to become obliterated by elaboration of reparative dentin not only in the pulp chamber (Fig. 12–17) but also in the root canal.

MacCallum (1940) compared inflammation with a fire in a room in which a meeting is taking place. While the fire is raging, a number of firemen (leukocytes) attempt to extinguish it with water and chemicals (lymphocytes and plasma cells). As soon as the fire is extinguished in one region, carpenters and painters (fibroblasts) arrive. They repair, scrape, and paint the walls. Plumbers (endothelial cells) replace the pipes. By the time they finish, the room no longer looks as if a fire had taken place. This illustrates the concomitance of the processes of repair and those of inflammation.

However, repair does not always result. Persistence of irritation, such as occurs under caries or following the placement of a silicate restoration, causes the persistence of granulation tissue. Theoretically, the local immune response should retard and eventually eliminate the inflammatory process by neutralizing and elimi-

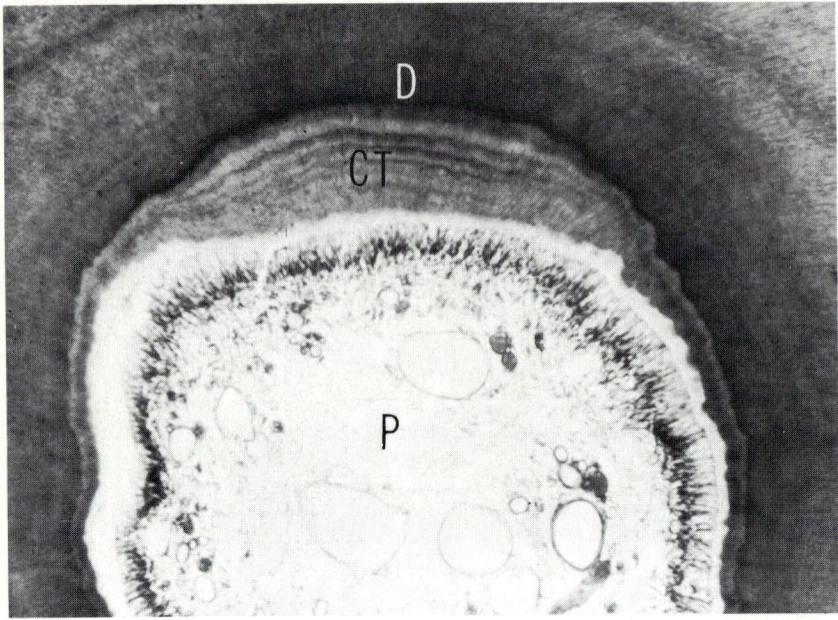

FIG. 12-16 Calciotraumatic response (CT). There are several alternating bands of hypochromatically and hyperchromatically staining dentin. P, pulp; D, dentin. ×96.

FIG. 12-17 Deposition of reparative dentin (Rd), as a result of injury to the pulp (p) and the persistence of chronic inflammation (Inf); 1 and 2 are zones of reparative dentin. D, primary dentin. ×100. (Seltzer S, Bender IB, Kaufman IJ: Oral Surg 14:856, 1961)

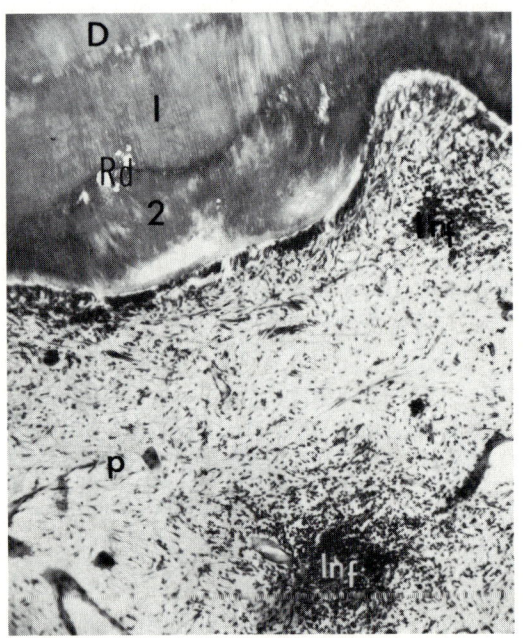

nating the etiologic factors. However, the immunologic mechanisms may contribute to the destructive phase of inflammation. Should the dominant immunoglobulin in the pulp lesion be IgG, there is a possibility of an Arthus-type reaction, after complement activation, owing to the local formation of immune complexes. On the other hand, if the dominant immunoglobulin is IgA, complement-fixing activity is low. Pulp destruction may then be the result of a shift in the production of IgG over IgA, causing perpetuation and aggravation of the inflammatory process (Brandtzaeg, 1973). Proteolytic and other enzymes, present in lysosomes of the chronic inflammatory cells, become active. Collagen fibers are degraded and ground substance is depolymerized. The broken down material is phagocytized by fibroblasts and macrophages (Fig. 12-14). Macrophage proliferation is directly proportional to the toxicity of the material they engulf (Salthouse et al, 1973).

In extensive inflammation, the lymphatic vessels in the core of the lesion shut down, resulting in retention of the interstitial fluid and breakdown products. These tend to increase intrapulpal pressure (Bernick, 1977). Eventually, the pulp may become necrotic. Thus, a variety of antigens may cause variable pulp reactions.

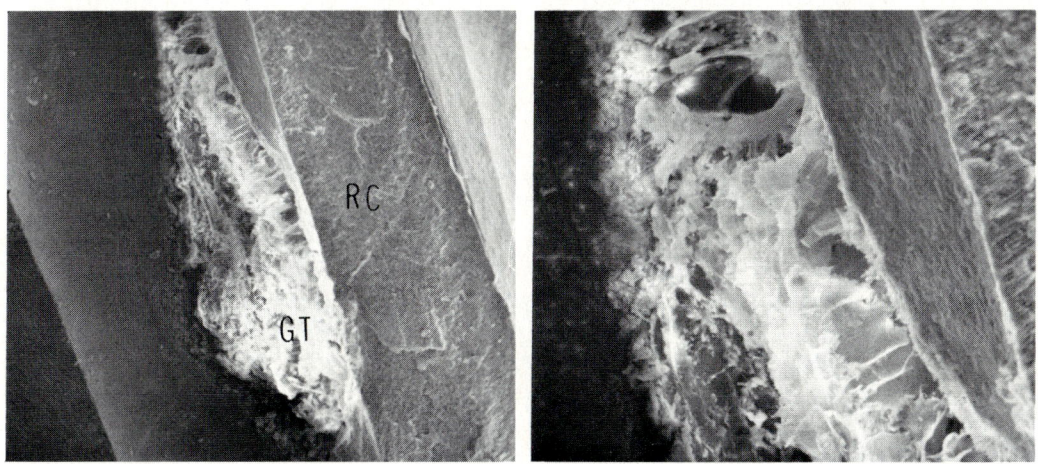

FIG. 12-18 Scanning electron micrographs of internal resorption resulting from chronic pulp inflammation. *(Left)* Resorbed area to left of root canal (RC), containing granulation tissue (GT). ×60. *(Right)* Higher magnification of figure at left, showing surface of inflamed tissue. ×180.

FIG. 12-19 *(Left)* Resorption (r) of dentin (D), caused by chronic inflammation of the pulp (P). *(Right)* Higher magnification of a region of resorption (Howship's lacunae) of the dentin (D). o, osteoclasts; P, pulp. ×240. (Seltzer S, Bender IB, Ziontz M: Oral Surg 16:846, 1963)

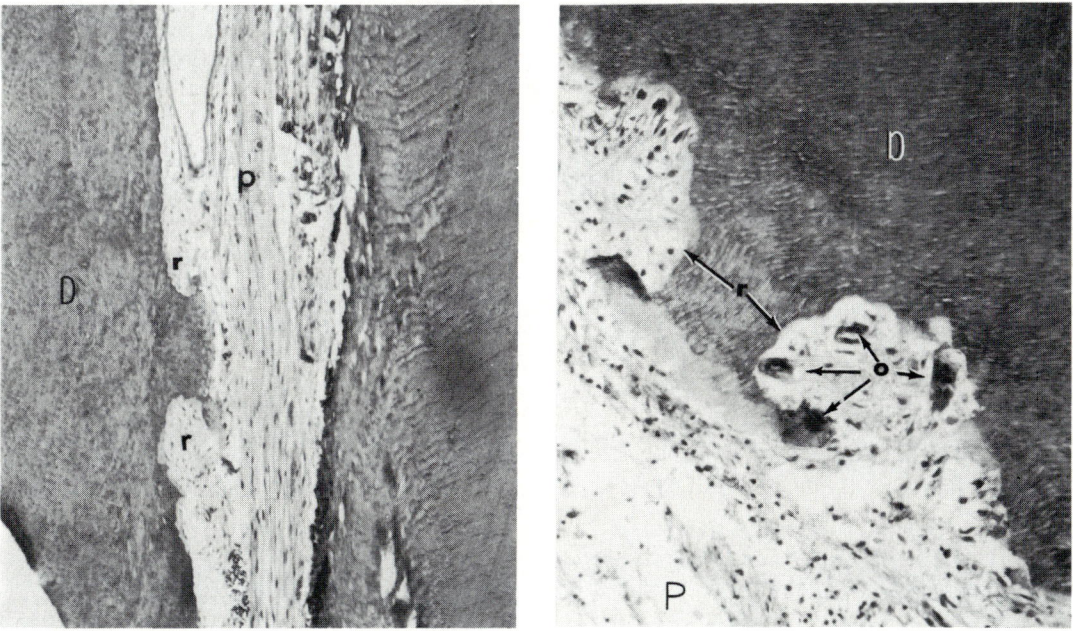

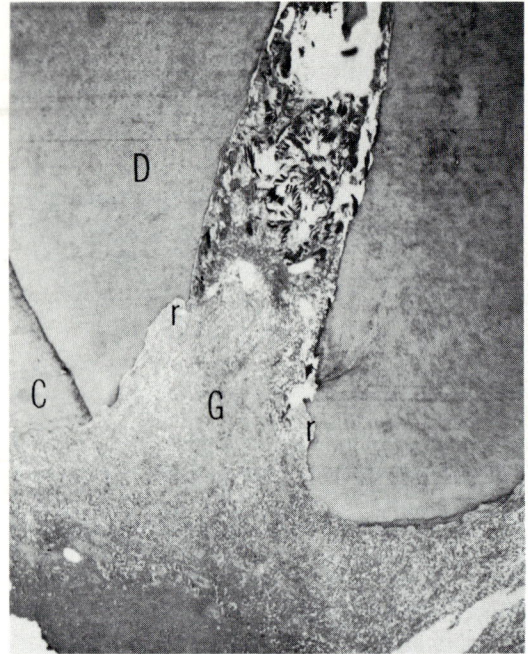

FIG. 12-20 Resorption of root apex. As a result of chronic total pulpitis, granulomatous tissue (G) has caused resorption (r) of the dentin (D) and the cementum (C) at the apex of the tooth. The apical foramen is widened. ×54.

ENZYMES IN PULP INFLAMMATION

Enzymes involved in energy (adenosine-5'-triphosphate; ATP) and anaerobic glycolysis (lactate dehydrogenase, LDH; malate dehydrogenase; MDH) have been studied in the pulp by Le Bell and Larmas (1979). They found that, as the pulp became inflamed, the ATP level remained the same, but the MDH activity was decreased. When pulps became necrotic, there was increased LDH activity and a concomitant decrease in ATP activity, indicating an increased rate of anaerobic glycolysis.

RESORPTION

Regions of resorption of the root canal walls are found in some teeth with chronically inflamed pulps (Fig. 12-18). In those teeth, baylike areas, often with osteoclasts present in the lacunae, are detected (Fig. 12-19). In some regions, the resorptions are being repaired by the deposition of cementum. In others, active resorption goes on. The granulation tissue at the apex of the tooth is invariably associated with resorption of the apical dentin and, often, the cementum, both in the root canal and along the sides of the root. The cementum and the dentin are resorbed to various depths. In some teeth the root apex is widened into a funnel-shaped area (Fig. 12-20). In others, the end of the root has a scalloped appearance. Within the granulation tissue of some pulps there are regions of liquefaction necrosis. In others, there is no evidence of necrosis of this type.

THE DYNAMICS OF PULP INFLAMMATION FOLLOWING OPERATIVE PROCEDURES

In a general way, pulp irritants cause an acute exudative response (acute inflammation). This may resolve when the irritant is mild, or the response may become proliferative if the irritation continues for a long time (chronic inflammation). Eventually, there may be repair or necrosis. The inflammation may be partial or total, depending on the amount of tissue involved (Fig. 12-21).

Pulp inflammation is not static, nor does it progress in an orderly way from one stage to another. Various phases of acute and chronic inflammation may be mixed together. In addition, acute inflammation in the pulp can become chronic and, conversely, chronic inflammations may, on occasion, become acute. Therefore, in tissue sections one may find both acute and chronic pulpitis present at the same time. Inflammation of the pulp may vary from acute to chronic and back to acute at various times, depending on circumstances. Therefore, although examination of an extracted tooth may show the pulp to be chronically inflamed, if the same

FIG. 12-21 Possible connective tissue reactions to irritants.

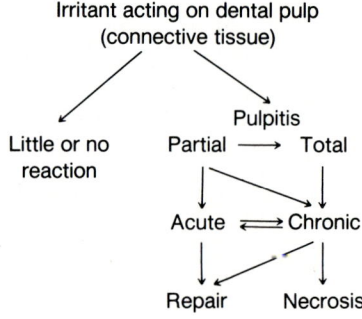

tooth had been extracted earlier, examination might have revealed it to be acutely inflamed.

As a rule, the acute partial pulpitis following operative procedures subsides and a chronic partial pulpitis ensues, with eventual resolution. Chronic inflammatory cells are found in the pulp under the cut dentinal tubules (Fig. 12–22), probably in the terminal stages of resolution of the pulp inflammation.

Chronic pulp inflammation under restorations may be partial, involving part or all of the coronal portion of the pulp, or the inflammation eventually may involve the entire pulp (chronic total pulpitis). There is no actual separation between chronic total pulpitis and the occurrence of apical pericementitis. The periapical tissues always become involved, once the entire pulp is affected, but they may also become inflamed in partial pulpitides.

Following operative procedures, pulps may remain chronically inflamed for months or even years. In cases of chronic, long-standing inflammation there are regions in the pulp where necrosis of the cells has occurred and mineralization has taken place. The mineralization may be diffuse or scattered or, eventually, may coalesce into large denticles that practically occlude the pulp chamber and/or the root canal (Fig. 12–23). The persistence of chronic pulpitis over long periods may explain why pulps that remain symptomless following operative procedures may eventually exhibit painful symptoms. The effect of additional operative procedures on such pulps is unknown, but it may be surmised that repair following an additional injury may not occur readily.

Acute Exacerbation of Chronic Pulpitis

The chronically inflamed pulp-periapical tissue complex may become acutely inflamed when another irritant temporarily overwhelms the defenses. The acute inflammation may produce liquefaction necrosis with severe pain. When drainage is established, the inflammation again becomes chronic. Thus, inflammation may change from chronic to acute and then to chronic again, at various times (Fig. 12–21).

CUMULATIVE EFFECTS OF IRRITANTS

As has been shown, the pulp may be injured by a number of irritating factors. The resultant inflammation may be mild or severe, depending on the intensity and duration of the irritation

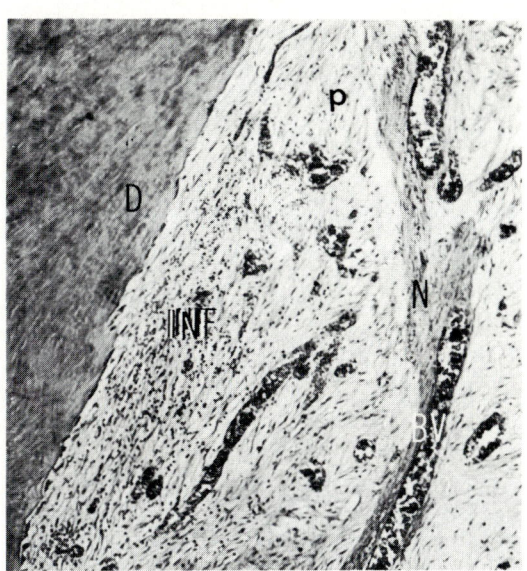

FIG. 12-22 Chronic partial pulpitis, following operative procedure. Buccolingual section of an upper canine restored with a silicate restoration. The odontoblastic layer of the pulp (p) subjacent to the cut dentinal tubules (D) is missing. A chronic partial pulpitis (INF) is present. BV, blood vessels; N, nerves. ×96. (Seltzer S, Bender IB, Ziontz M: Oral Surg 16:846, 1963)

FIG. 12-23 Diffuse mineralization (Ca) in the root canal. D, dentin. ×54.

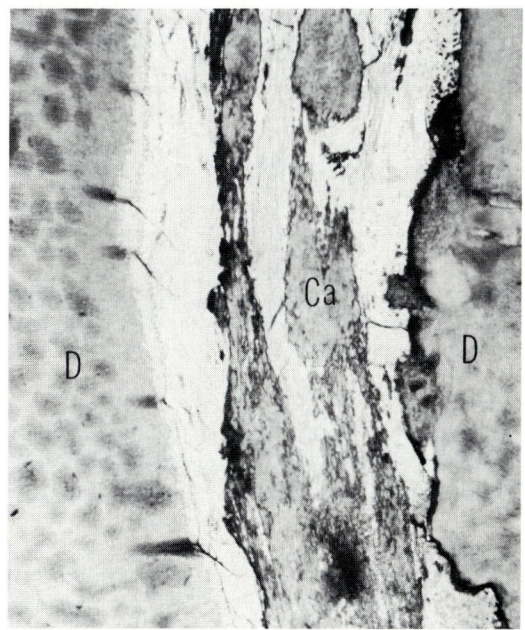

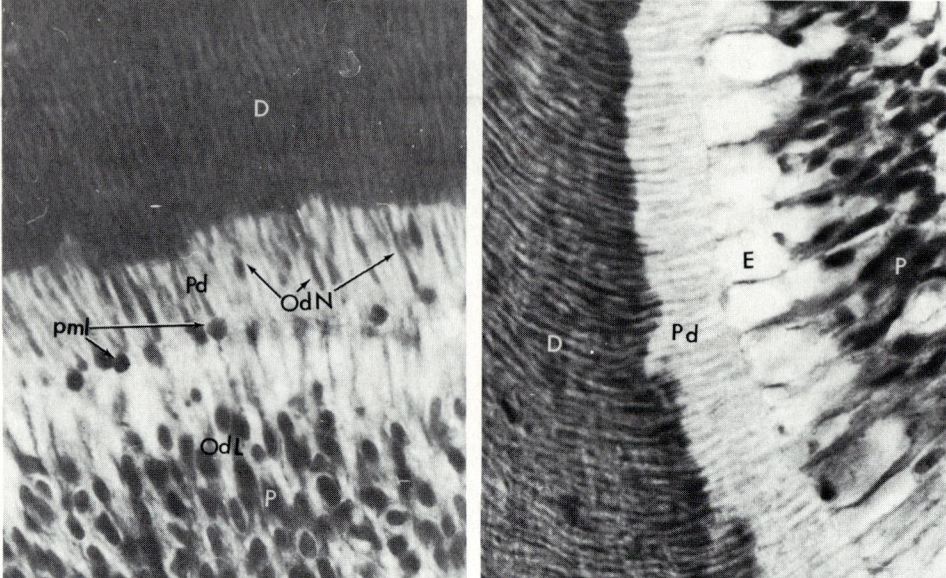

FIG. 12-24 Effects of pressure on the dentin. *(Left)* Pressure applied to a moderately deep preparation has caused displacement of the odontoblastic nuclei (OdN) into the predentin (Pd). Polymorphonuclear leukocytes (pml) have been attracted to the odontoblastic layer (OdL). D, dentin. ×450. *(Right)* After a shallow preparation of the dentin (D), the application of pressure has caused disruption of the odontoblastic layer of the pulp (P) by edema (E). D, dentin; Pd, predentin. ×450. (Seltzer S, Bender IB, Kaufman IJ: Oral Surg 14:327, 1961)

and the condition of the pulp tissue (i.e., resistance). When a number of irritants are applied to the pulp simultaneously or consecutively, the resultant inflammation is notably more severe. A number of our experiments that have led to this conclusion are described in the following sections.

Cavity Preparation and Pressure

Irritants were applied to prepared cavities in the teeth of dogs and monkeys. The animals were sacrificed at intervals, and the dental pulps were examined for evidence of histologic change. The degree of damage to the pulp was judged by such criteria as nuclear and cytoplasmic changes in the odontoblasts, altered arrangements of the odontoblasts, disruption of the pulpodentinal 'membrane,' vascular changes, changes in matrix formation and postoperative mineralization, formation of granulation tissue, and necrosis.

Deeper cavity preparations caused greater changes in the pulps. When the layer of dentin between the base of the cavity and the pulp was thick, it shielded the pulp from the irritants applied to the cavity. Next to the trauma from cutting of the cavity itself, the greatest damage to the pulp was caused by application of pressure (Fig. 12-24).

Application of pressure in shallow cavities was followed by changes in the odontoblastic layer of the same kind as those produced by the trauma of deep cavity preparation alone (Fig. 12-24). In general, application of one or more irritants to a shallow cavity preparation produced further changes, so that the total effect was similar to that of deep cavity preparation.

To summarize, pressure exerted on a relatively shallow cavity produces effects similar to those occurring after deep cavity preparation without added pressure. Pressure on a deep cavity preparation results in severe damage to the pulp.

A pulp exposure caused severe inflammatory changes in both the odontoblastic layer and the underlying pulp tissue. When the pulp was exposed in an otherwise shallow cavity and pressure was exerted, polymorphonuclear leukocytes heavily infiltrated the odontoblastic layer

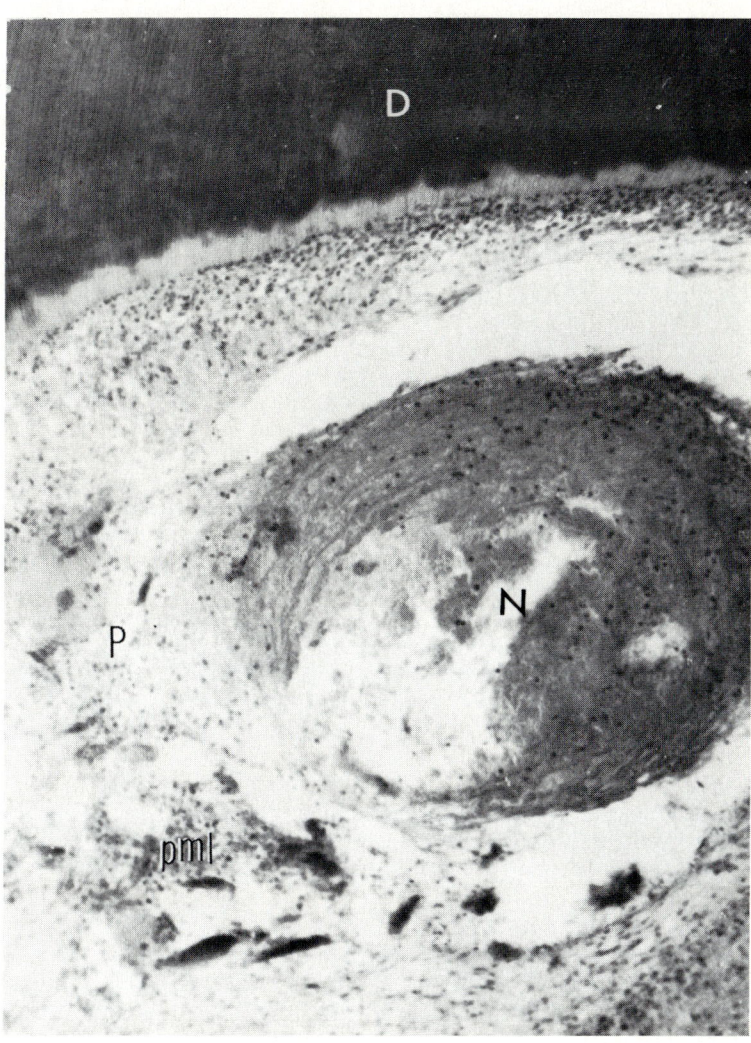

FIG. 12-25 Effects of pulp exposure and pressure. The central pulp tissue (P) is necrotic (N). The remainder of the pulp is infiltrated with polymorphonuclear leukocytes (pml). D, dentin. ×100. (Seltzer S, Bender IB, Kaufman IJ: Oral Surg 14:327, 1961)

and were found dispersed throughout the entire pulp. An acute pulpitis was produced (Fig. 12-25). Similarly, Horsted et al (1981) found that the pulp was more severely damaged when it was exposed, suffered hemorrhage, and was subjected to intrusion of dentin chips and capping material than when simple contact of the capping material with the wound surface occurred. If, in addition, drugs, bacteria, and pressure were applied, the bacteria could be found even on the odontoblastic layer of the opposite wall and scattered throughout the pulp. Pressure such as that exerted in modeling compound impressions on teeth with exposed pulps resulted in almost total destruction of the pulps by hemorrhage and edema (Fig. 12-25). The pulp succumbed quickly and violently.

Crown Preparation, Heat and Pressure

The pulps of dogs' teeth, subjected to full crown preparations similar to those made for human teeth, revealed significant inflammatory changes (Fig. 12-26, *left*). When pressure was applied to the dentin by means of a plasticine impression, the odontoblasts were sucked or pumped into the dentin in some areas (Fig. 12-26, *center*). In other teeth, impressions were taken with modeling compound at temperatures of 40°C to 45°C. The heat from the modeling compound impression caused a further in-

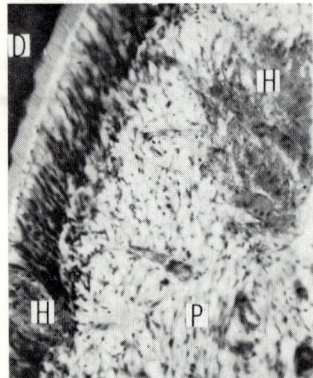 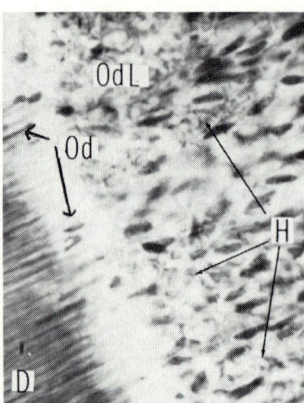 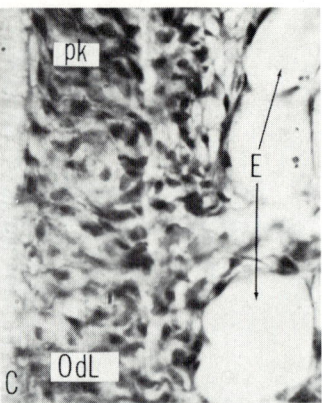

FIG. 12-26 Cumulative effects of irritants. *(Left)* Following full crown preparation at low speed, the pulp (P) of a dog molar has a large hemorrhage (H) in it. D, dentin. ×180. *(Center)* Pulp reaction to crown preparation and pressure with plasticine. In addition to hemorrhage (H), odontoblasts (Od) have been displaced into the dentin (D). The odontoblastic layer (OdL) is disrupted. ×600. *(Right)* Following full crown preparation and impression with modeling compound, the pulp is edematous (E). The odontoblastic layer (OdL) is disoriented and the odontoblastic nuclei are pyknotic (pk). ×600. (Seltzer S: Early pulp changes in the teeth of a dog following full crown preparations. J Dent Res 37:678, 1958. Copyright by the American Dental Association. Reproduced by permission)

crease in capillary permeability, as indicated by the presence of large quantities of plasma within the pulp tissue (Fig. 12-26, *right*). A large number of neutrophilic leukocytes were marginated along the blood vessel walls. These leukocytes were especially noticeable in the capillaries between the odontoblasts.

Thus, the combination of heat and pressure was responsible for inflammatory changes more severe than those produced by each irritant individually.

Drugs, Pressure, and Bacteria

Bacteria can penetrate the dentin by way of the dentinal tubules and reach the deep pulp tissue, as can be demonstrated both by histologic examination and by taking cultures. Pressure on the base of the cavity forced the bacteria through the dentinal tubules. Application of caustic cavity sterilizing agents or etchants facilitated entrance of the bacteria by rendering the tubules more permeable. When bacteria were placed on the dentin in either a shallow or a deep cavity and pressure was applied, a small number of bacteria could be observed in the odontoblastic layer.

If the pressure and other irritants are applied together, the inflammatory response is severe, the deep pulp tissue as well as the odontoblastic layer becomes involved, and the final result is likely to be complete necrosis of the pulp.

Caries, Operative Procedures, and Periodontal Lesions

Another illustration of the more deleterious effects of combinations of irritants on the pulp tissue may be obtained from our study of histologic findings in the pulps of periodontally involved teeth.

The effects of caries or operative procedures on the pulps of periodontally involved teeth and the effects of periodontal lesions on the pulps of operatively treated teeth were compared. The incidence of inflammatory reaction was greater in teeth subjected to both pulp irritants and periodontal irritants than in those subjected to operative procedures alone: 79% of teeth with both periodontal lesions and caries or restorations showed some degree of inflammation or necrosis, as compared with 61% of teeth with only periodontal lesions or only caries or restorations. This difference is statistically significant.

Reaction to New Irritations After Recovery from Previous Insult

When a pulp that has been subjected to various irritants and has recovered is exposed to further irritation, what is likely to occur? The answer to this question must be somewhat conjectural, inasmuch as the available experimental evidence does not lead to a definite conclusion. Examination of the tissue sections of many teeth that had been operated on disclosed that chronic inflammation persisted for long periods of time (measured in years). In addition, increased fibrosis, reduction in cell density, and increased mineralization and deposition of reparative dentin were evident. These phenomena tend to reduce the volume as well as the nutritional supply of the pulp. In effect, aging of the pulp tissue had occurred (Fig. 12–27). Subsequent operative procedures on the same tooth may not be well tolerated. The pulp no longer has the resistance of "young" tissue. When a previously filled tooth is operated on, the pulp may undergo degeneration, with ultimate necrosis. Care must be exercised in crown preparations of teeth with an abundance of deep restorations. The reparative potential of the pulp in a previously filled tooth is reduced. A common clinical experience is the development of pulpalgia in the tooth of a patient with a defective amalgam. Although the restoration may have been present for many years without symptoms, repair of a defective margin may now produce a painful pulpitis. The additional operative manipulations on a previously damaged pulp were responsible. Pulp capping or pulpotomy procedures are contra-

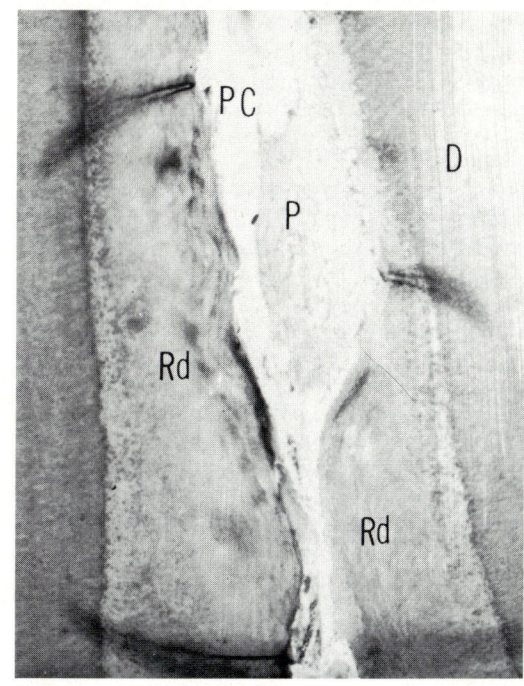

FIG. 12-27 Aging of dental pulp. As a result of reparative dentin formation (Rd), the pulp chamber (PC) is almost obliterated. The pulp (P) is reduced in volume, and only a small quantity remains. D, dentin. ×54.

FIG. 12-28 Factors that affect resolution of inflammation.

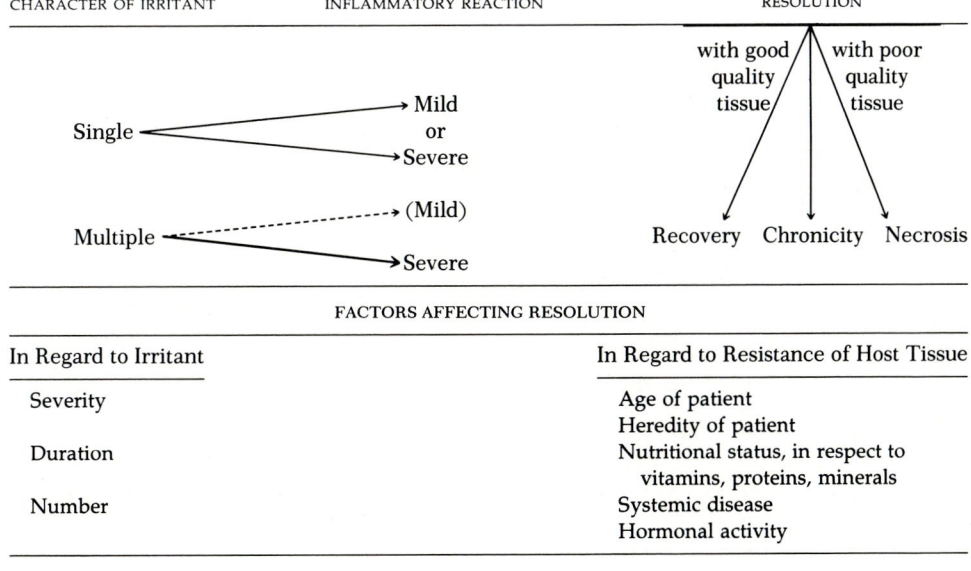

indicated in these circumstances. Endodontics or extraction must be performed. In many teeth, chronic inflammation apparently persists for long periods, resulting in dentinal resorptions and repair. In many periodontally involved teeth, atrophy of the pulp cells occurs, with eventual necrosis. The more severe the initial inflammatory reaction, the less the likelihood of complete repair. Should such teeth be subjected to new irritations, such as additional operative procedures, recovery would depend on the severity of the new irritant and the state of the pulp prior to the new injury as well as other local and systemic factors influencing the health of the connective tissues. Even an apparently mild irritation may call forth a violent reaction, thereby, precluding any chance for recovery.

The factors that influence the outcome are complex and variable, both in themselves and in their interactions. Moreover, it is often extremely difficult to identify these factors and define their roles, much less evaluate them. Therefore, the reaction of the pulp in a specific individual, even to a known irritant, cannot be predicted with certainty. Certain operative procedures provoke irreversible reactions in the pulp in some patients, whereas in others there is complete recovery.

The effects of irritants, the possible resolution, and the factors influencing both are presented in Fig. 12–28.

BIBLIOGRAPHY

Ahlberg KF, Edwall L: Influence of local insults on sympathetic vasoconstrictor control in the feline dental pulp. Acta Odont Scand 35:103, 1977

Araujo VC, Araujo NS, Mariano M: Altered vascular permeability in the dental pulp of traumatized rat teeth. Pathology 132:181, 1980

Bender IB: Factors influencing radiographic appearance of bony lesions. J Endodont 8:161, 1982

Bender IB: Pulp biology conference: A discussion. J Endodont 4:37, February 1978

Berggren G, Brännström M: The rate of flow in dentinal tubules due to capillary attraction. J Dent Res 44:408, 1965

Bernick S: Morphological changes to lymphatic vessels in pulpal inflammation. J Dent Res 56:841, 1977

Brännström M: Dentinal and pulpal response. I. Application of reduced pressure to exposed dentin. II. Application of an air stream to exposed dentin. Short observation period. III. Application of an air stream to exposed dentin. Long observation period. Acta Odont Scand 18:1, 17, 235, 1960

Brandtzaeg P: Immunology of inflammatory periodontal lesions. Internat Dent J 23:438, 1973

Bretscher M: Membrane structure: Some general principles. Science 181:622, 1973

Capaldi RA: A dynamic model of cell membranes. Sci Am 230:27, 1974

Corpron RE, Avery JK: Ultrastructure of odontoblasts in dentinal tubules. J Dent Res 50:511, 1971

Eda S, Saito T: Electron microscopy of cells displaced into the dentinal tubules due to dry cavity preparation. J Oral Pathol 7:326, 1978

Grady JE, Yaeger JA: Polarizing microscopy of abnormal dentine produced by injections of strontium or fluoride. Arch Oral Biol 10:175, 1965

Honjo H, Tsubakimoto K, Sumitani M: Homologous plasma proteins in the human dental pulp. J Osaka Dent Univ 2:147, 1968

Hørsted P, El Attar K, Langeland K: Capping of monkey pulps with Dycal and a ca-eugenol cement. Oral Surg 52:531, 1981

Johnson G, Olgart L, Brännström M: Outward fluid flow in dentin under a physiologic pressure gradient: Experiments in vitro. Oral Surg 35:238, 1973

Kelsall MA, Crabb ED: Lymphocytes and plasmacytes in nucleoprotein metabolism. Ann NY Acad Sci 72:293, 1958

Langeland K: Histologic evaluation of pulp reactions to operative procedures. Oral Surg 12:1235, 1357, 1959

Langeland K: Management of the inflamed pulp associated with deep carious lesion. J Endodont 7:169, 1981

Langeland K: Pulp response to caries and operative procedures. JDAS Africa 18:101, 1963

Langeland K: Tissue Changes in the Dental Pulp. Oslo, Oslo University Press, 1957

MacCallum WG: Textbook of Pathology, 7th Ed. Philadelphia, WB Saunders, 1940

Majno G, Gabbiani G, Hirschel BJ, Ryan GB, Statkov PR: Contraction of granulation tissue in vitro: Similarity to smooth muscle. Science 173:548, 1971

Miller GS, Sternberg RN, Piliers SJ, Rosenberg PA: Histologic identifications of mast cells in human dental pulp. Oral Surg 46:559, 1978

Nahri M: Activation of dental pulp nerves of the cat and the dog with hydrostatic pressure. Proceeding of the Finnish Dental Society, 74, [Suppl V], 1978

Olgart L, Gazelius B, Brodin E, Nilsson G: Release of substance P-like immunoreactivity from the dental pulp. Acta Physiol Scand 101:410 1977

Osmanski CP, Yaeger JA: Microradiography of rat incisor dentin during the development of the response to injected fluoride. Anat Rec 148:467, 1964

Pashley DH, Nelson R, Williams EC: Dentin hydraulic conductance: Changes produced by red blood cells. J Dent Res 60:1797, 1981

Salthouse TN, Matlaga BF, O'Leary RK: Microspectrophotometry of macrophage lysosomal enzyme activity: A measure of polymer implant tissue toxicity. Toxicol Appl Pharmacol 25:201, 1973

Schour I, Smith MC: The histologic changes in enamel and dentin of the rat incisor in acute and chronic experimental fluorosis. U Ariz Coll Agricult Exp Sta Tech Bull M 52, 1934

Searls JC: Light and electron microscope evaluation of changes induced in odontoblasts of the rat incisor by the high-speed drill. J Dent Res 46:1344, 1967

Seltzer S: Early pulp changes in the teeth of a dog following full crown preparations. J Dent Res 37:220, 1958

Seltzer S: Reparative dentinogenesis. Oral Surg 12:595, 1959

Seltzer S, Bender IB; Some influences affecting repair of the exposed pulps of dogs' teeth. J Dent Res 37:678, 1958

Seltzer S, Bender IB: Early human pulp reactions to full crown preparations. JADA 59:912, 1959

Seltzer S, Bender IB: Modification of operative procedures to avoid postoperative pulp inflammation. JADA 66:503, 1963

Seltzer S, Bender IB, Kaufman IJ: Histologic changes in dental pulps of dogs and monkeys following application of pressure, drugs, and microorganisms on prepared cavities. Oral Surg 14:327, 1961

Seltzer S, Bender IB, Kaufman IJ: Histologic changes in dental pulps of dogs and monkeys following application of pressure, drugs, and microorganisms on prepared cavities. II. Changes observable more than one month after application of traumatic agents. Oral Surg 14:856, 1961

Seltzer S, Bender IB, Ziontz M: The dynamics of pulp inflammation: Correlations between diagnostic data and actual histologic findings in the pulp. Oral Surg 16:846, 969, 1963

Seltzer S, Bender IB, Ziontz M: The interrelationship of pulp and periodontal disease. Oral Surg 16:1474, 1963

Seltzer S, Rainey E, Gluskin AH: Correlation of scanning electron microscope and light microscope findings in uninflamed and pathologically involved pulps. Oral Surg 43:910, 1977

Stanley HR, Swerdlow H: Aspiration of cells into dentinal tubules. Oral Surg 11:1007, 1958

Stevenson TS: Odontoblast aspiration and fluid movement in human dentine. Arch Oral Biol 12:1149, 1967

Stewart JM: The immediate response of odontoblasts to injury. Odont Tids 73:417, 1965

Sveen OB, Hawes RR: Differentiation of new odontoblasts and dentine bridge formation in rat molar teeth after tooth grinding. Arch Oral Biol 13:1399, 1968

Tönder KH, Kvinnsland I: Micropuncture measurements of interstitial fluid pressure in normal and inflamed dental pulp in cats. J Endodont, 9:105, 1983

Van Hassel HJ: Physiology of the human dental pulp. In Siskin M (ed): The Biology of the Human Dental Pulp, pp 16–24. St. Louis, Mosby, 1973

Zach L, Topal R, Cohen G: Pulpal repair following operative procedures. Oral Surg 28:587, 1969

Zachrisson BU: Mast cells in human dental pulp. Arch Oral Biol 16:555, 1971

13
RADIANT IRRITANTS

X-IRRADIATION

The basic cellular effect of ionizing radiation is interference with cell division. Chromatin material in tissues of all types irradiated with various doses of radiation becomes condensed. Small doses may not interefere with the cell division cycle but abnormalities may ultimately appear in some cells in later generations. At the ultrastructural level it has been found that radiation injury is mediated through the cell membrane system and the mitochondria; the underlying mechanism is the displacement of intracellular enzyme systems (Goldfeder, 1963).

Irradiation of the tissues of children with advanced protein-calorie malnutrition results in failure of cell division and the formation of structurally abnormal chromosomes (Evans et al, 1970).

Radiation damage to teeth depends on dose, source, and type of radiation, exposure factors, and stage of tooth development at the time of irradiation (West, 1973).

Irradiation of the anterior portion of the heads of experimental animals during the formative stages of tooth development causes damage to the developing teeth. The teeth are poorly formed or they may fail to develop at all. In the pulps of irradiated teeth, the odontoblasts are injured, and, instead of regular dentin, osteodentin and a dentinal niche is formed (Collett et al, 1966; Koppang, 1973). In time, the pulp cells become necrotic (Gartner et al, 1977; Khan et al, 1979). Rats fed on a purified diet and subjected to multiple sublethal doses of total body radiation developed severe periodontal lesions. In some, the cementum broke down and the uncovered dentinal tubules were invaded by bacteria. Root resorption followed, which eventually led to exfoliation of the involved teeth (Greulich and Ershoff, 1961). Markitziu et al (1974) and Horn et al (1975) found that fractionated doses of x-irradiation to the heads of rats produced more damage to the forming elements of the dental follicles of developing third molars than single doses. In higher animals such as the monkey, root end formation is inhibited after irradiation so that completely rootless teeth may erupt (Fig. 13–1).

In developing human teeth, the extent of the damage depends on the amount of radiation and the stage of tooth development at the time of irradiation (Poyton, 1968). Heavy doses at the earliest stage of development can cause complete failure of the tooth to develop; at the other extreme, mild doses can result in root end distortions and dilacerations. Between these two

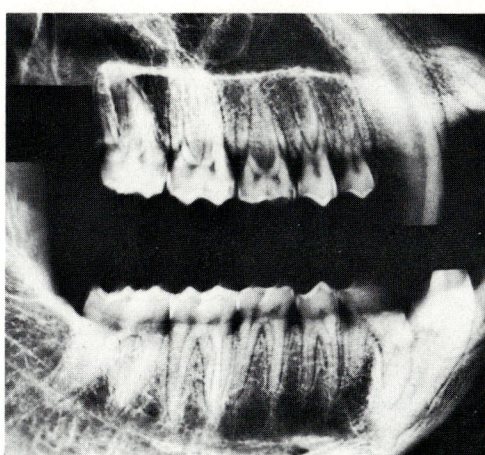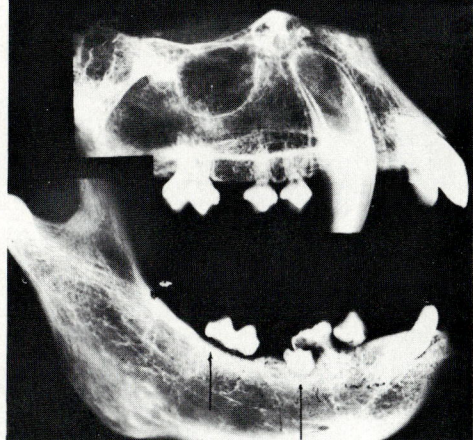

FIG. 13-1 Effects of irradiation on the teeth. (*Left*) The teeth of a normal, nonirradiated monkey. (*Right*) The teeth of a monkey, 39 months postirradiation, 5500 R. The teeth have been in occlusion for 18 months. Note rootless molar and bicuspids (arrows). (Gowgiel JM: Eruption of irradiation–produced rootless teeth in monkeys. J Dent Res 40:538, 1961. Copyright by the American Dental Association. Reproduced by permission)

extremes, various degrees of tooth malformation may result. Poyton has indicated that there is a decrease in mitotic activity of pulp cells. Circulatory disturbances in the tooth germ are manifested by the presence of dilated vessels, hemorrhages, and endothelial cell swelling. The odontoblasts fail to function normally and may elaborate abnormal dentin, and amelogenesis is retarded or ceases. In the later stages, fibrosis or atrophy of the pulp may occur (Poyton, 1968; Burke and Frame, 1979).

The pulps of fully formed human teeth may be affected in patients who are exposed to radiation therapy for malignant growth in the oral cavity or in the region of the neck. Relative to dosage, mature odontoblasts appear to be extremely radioresistant (Kimeldorf et al, 1963). However, in time, the pulp cells exposed to the ionizing radiation may become necrotic. The effects appear to be related to vascular damage and interference with mitosis of cells.

The periodontal ligament and cementum also exhibit changes following radiation therapy. Decreased vascularity and acellularity ensue in the ligament and the fibers become disoriented and thickened. Osteoradionecrosis, preceded by a periodontitis and periodontal infection, develops in many cases. The cementum manifests changes resulting in a severely compromised capacity for repair. Thus, periodontal treatment procedures, such as scaling and curettage of teeth within the radiation field, offer an unfavorable prognosis.

Severe root sensitivity following radiotherapy is often present in some patients. This complaint is ameliorated by burnishing the exposed surface with a 1% fluoride solution (Beumer et al, 1979).

The salivary glands are likewise affected by the cancericidal levels of radiation therapy. Progressive degeneration of the acinar elements of the salivary glands results in a reduction in salivary flow changes in the organic and inorganic constituents and pH (Anderson et al, 1981). These changes lead to an exceedingly high predisposition to dental caries and pulp involvement (Beumer et al, 1979). The reduced salivary flow causes an ultimate reduction in the lysozyme and immunoglobulin levels, resulting in a significant immunoprotein deficit (Brown et al, 1976a). High saliva agglutination titers against formalized cellular antigens of *Streptococcus* and *Lactobacillus* species were found by Brown et al (1981) in cancer patients before radiotherapy. After therapy, caries activity was directly related to the concentration of the saliva agglutination titers and IgA; the higher the titers, the lower the caries incidence. In addition, post-irradiation caries-active patients had higher serum IgD and IgG levels, compared to caries-inactive patients (Brown et al, 1978). A reduction of the immunologic mechanism can

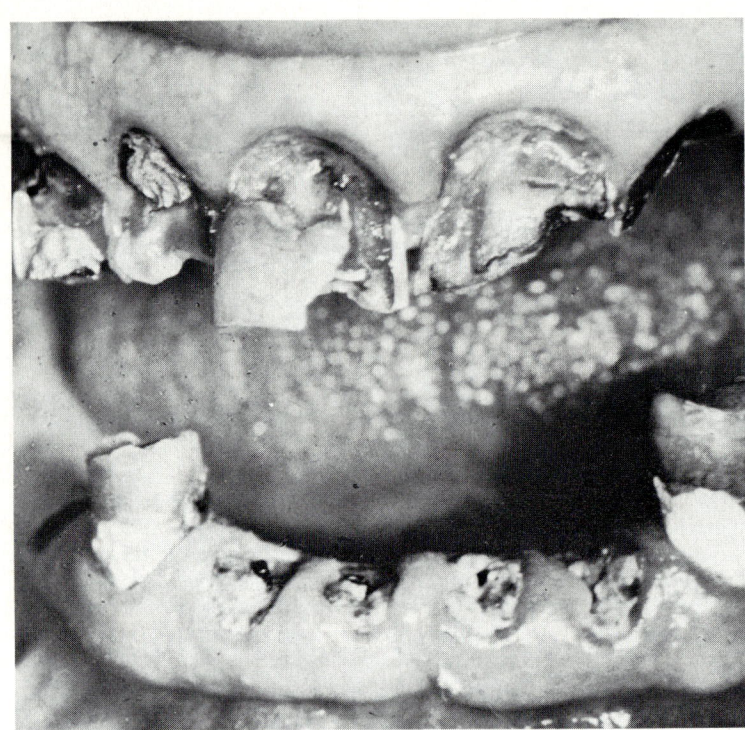

FIG. 13-2 The teeth of a patient who has received therapy of the neck.

lead to changes in the oral flora with increased incidence of caries (Brown et al, 1975) and, perhaps, to soft tissue and bone necrosis. The teeth become dry, brittle, and more prone to decay. In addition, there is loss of tooth structure in the cervical region resulting in a saucer-shaped lesion. Clinically, the carious lesions that appear after radiation therapy are somewhat different than those of ordinary smooth-surface dental caries and differ in location (Karmiol and Walsh, 1975). The lesions appear on all surfaces, including the incisal or occlusal edges—surfaces that are usually caries-free under normal clinical conditions. Crown fractures frequently occur in such teeth (Fig. 13-2). Therefore, prophylactic extraction of teeth within the radiation field has been advocated as a means of preventing osteoradionecrosis (Morrish et al, 1981). A program of strict oral hygiene and daily self-treatment with 0.4% stannous fluoride gel has been found effective for the prevention of postirradiation caries (Westcott et al, 1975). Comparative studies of patients irradiated before and after extractions have indicated that there was a significantly reduced incidence of osteoradionecrosis in the former group 2 years after radiation therapy. In the first group, an average interval of 25.3 days elapsed between extraction and initiation of radiation (Starke and Shannon, 1977).

According to Beumer et al (1979a), endodontic therapy on numerous infected or noninfected teeth within the radiation field has prevented bone infection or osteoradionecrosis. Thus, endodontic procedures, rather than extraction, often spare the patient the risk of bone necrosis.

The mode of radiation therapy is significant with respect to tissue effects. Radiation is administered to tumors either by an external source or by implanting radioactive substances within the tumor. In the former, the radiation beam must traverse tissue structures before reaching the target tissue, thereby exposing the salivary glands, periodontium, cementum, bone, and pulps to possible damage. However, when a source of radiation, such as a radon seed, is implanted in the tumor, the radiation is more confined. Such implantation seldom compromises salivary glands. Thus, xerostomia, radiation caries, and osteonecrosis are not significant problems in patients treated with interstitial radiation therapy. In such patients, postradiation extraction of teeth is not a high risk unless the teeth are close to the implant.

LASER BEAM

Laser, light amplification by stimulated emission of radiation, is a device that transforms waves in the ultraviolet, the visible, or the infrared spectrum into a very intense microbeam in which the waves are all in phase and very nearly nondivergent. Lasers employ a variety of methods and materials, e.g., gas, semiconductor diode injection, the usual one being the ruby crystal (solid state laser). The energy may be released continuously or in pulses. When the beam is directed at a target at close range, lasers are capable of mobilizing immense heat and power.

Since lasers are being used in therapy of conditions of the head and neck, the possible effects on the teeth and surrounding tissues become an important consideration.*

The effects of a laser beam on tooth structure have been studied by numerous investigators. Laser damage to pulps varies with the intensity of the energy and with the experimental animal. The pulps of rabbit teeth exposed to 20 joules were only slightly affected after 3 days. However, 40 joules produced degenerative changes in the cells, fibers, and ground substance of the pulp (Jesionowski, 1970). The solid state laser at 35 joules has been found to produce a craterlike cavitation on the surface of hamster teeth (Taylor et al, 1965). Below this was a zone with a roughened surface. The damage receded farther peripherally. Using electron probe microanalysis and polarized light microscopy, Kantola (1972a) found that changes in the mineral content of the enamel were induced by the laser. Various zones had altered contents of calcium and phosphorus, with the lowest content at the bottom of the crater. The dentin of the walls of the crater contained higher contents of calcium and phosphorus than those of untreated dentin (Kantola, 1972b). With higher energies (a 55-joule beam), the tooth surface alterations were found to be more extensive (Taylor et al, 1965). The pulps of the irradiated teeth were severely affected after 3 days, with greater damage caused by the higher energies. After 7 days, there was limited evidence of pulpal healing in the 25-joule group but none in the 55-joule group.

---

*For the reader interested in the medical applications of lasers and in their theory and operation, a number of references on these topics have been included in the bibliography at the end of this chapter.

A gas laser beam has been reported by Poyton (1968) to produce no changes in tooth surfaces. However, laser energy densities ranging from 60 to 250 joules/cm^2, which were sufficient to inhibit in vitro formation of incipient carieslike lesions, were found by Stern et al (1969) to cause limited and, in their view, reversible pulp changes in chimpanzee teeth.

In dogs' teeth, Adrian et al (1971) and Powell and Morton (1983) found no reaction in pulps that were laser irradiated at 1000 joules/cm^2. A moderate pulpal reaction occurred at 2300 joules/cm^2. Larger doses consistently produced pulp necrosis. Pulp damage was manifested by coagulation necrosis of the odontoblasts, edema, and occasional inflammatory cell infiltration. When applied to dogs' teeth, energy levels ranging from 20 to 90 joules/cm^2 produced no significant pulpal pathosis (Powell and Morton 1983). In contrast, Adrian (1977) found the pulps of monkey teeth exposed to 4494 to 6722 joules/cm^2 (two to three times more intense than the ruby laser exposure) became inflamed but not necrotic.

RADIUM

The uptake of radium into deciduous teeth from public water supplies has been studied by Samuels (1966). He found that the deciduous teeth take up radium in proportion to the radium exposure during tooth development. In the already formed teeth there was relatively little uptake of radium from the drinking water. Similarly, administration of high dosages of radium 226 to beagles produced no significant effect on dentin deposition (Taylor et al, 1969). However, radium is found in human dental tissues for many years after medical or occupational exposure. Rowland (1963) studied the teeth from three patients who died from radium poisoning and found that the dentin was radioactive. The dentin that had been formed after exposure had a significantly greater uptake of radium than the rest of the dentin.

The early lesions of radium intoxification include osteitis, osteomyelitis, and loss of teeth. Delayed dental effects consist of unusual carious lesions and spontaneous tooth fractures (Spiess and Mays, 1970; Sharpe, 1974). Both external and internal tooth resorptions occur (Reichert, 1982; Fig. 13–3). In addition, malignancies of the mastoid and paranasal sinuses may develop (Mays et al, 1968; Littman et al, 1978).

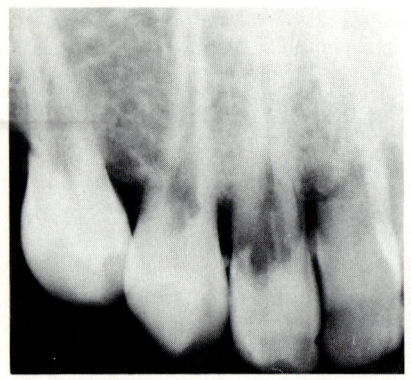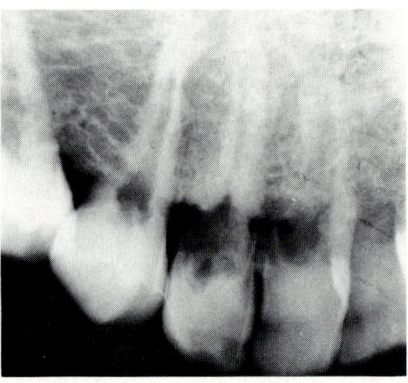

FIG. 13-3 (*Left*) Dental radiograph showing cervical internal–external radiolucencies that involve the maxillary right lateral incisor, canine, and premolar. (*Right*) After 5 years, the same teeth have undergone progressive resorption. (Reichart PA: ^{224}Ra–induced dental resorptions. Oral Surg 54:281, 1982)

STRONTIUM

The increase in radioactive fallout as a result of nuclear testing raised some questions about the effect of the accumulated ^{90}Sr on the teeth. Animal studies by Holgate (1959) and by Rosenthal and Harbor (1965) indicate that a single large dose of radiostrontium administered by injection, or a smaller dietary dose, is taken up rapidly by actively calcifying tissues, where it remains incorporated for a long time (half life of ^{90}Sr is 28 years). Both enamel and dentin incorporate strontium to the same degree as bone (Wolf et al, 1973). Thus, developing teeth incorporate the isotope; it is present, within less than 24 hours, in the odontoblastic layer and then in the dentin, where it remains. However, in another study (Cleall et al, 1962), low dosages were found to have caused minor damage to the teeth of older rats that were sacrificed some months after injection. Strontium-90 from radioactive fallout has been found to accumulate in the dentin of human deciduous teeth (Rosenthal et al, 1963).

In permanent teeth, although Lindemann (1967) found no ^{90}Sr accumulation, Starkey and Fletcher (1969) found a steady increase of the nucleotide in premolars extracted for orthodontic reasons in older age groups. The radioactivity of the crown was consistently lower than in the roots.

COBALT

Cobalt-60 irradiation, used for cancer therapy, has been shown to produce relatively little effect on dental pulps of experimental animals compared to conventional x-irradiation (Meyer et al, 1962, 1963). When the pulps of the erupted teeth were exposed to 1530 R, either at 200 kV of x-irradiation or of cobalt-60 radiation, there was some odontoblastic degeneration, but the alterations were not severe. Inflammatory infiltration was minimal, involving a small number of lymphocytes. Osteoradionecrosis did not occur in either group (Meyer et al, 1966). At higher fractionated doses of 7200 R, the odontoblasts and ameloblasts of rats' teeth were damaged and some pulps became inflamed and necrotic (Sweeney et al, 1977).

The pulps of monkey teeth, exposed to therapeutic doses of 3000 to 7000 R, from ^{60}Co, exhibited no degenerative changes on histologic examination. Moreover, no histologic differences were discernible between the pulp tissues of control teeth and those from teeth irradiated at any therapeutic dose level. All pulp tissues appeared normal and healthy (Hutton, 1974). In addition, the pulps of monkey teeth, which were restored with amalgam, composite resins, or gold crowns and then irradiated with 7600 R of ^{60}Co were not damaged (Nickens et al, 1977). Thus, ^{60}Co irradiation, in a dose range up to 7000 R, does not seem to have an adverse effect on the dental pulps of mature monkey teeth after 1 to 2 months.

In addition, no healing complications arose in the superficial oral tissues of animals after ^{60}Co irradiation. Negative effects of ^{60}Co irradiation on the healing potential of dog oral tissues have been demonstrated by Shearer (1967). Fractional ^{60}Co irradiation of mandibles of dogs, given at different time intervals up to 21 days, failed to produce any significant detrimental effects on the healing of extraction sites.

BIBLIOGRAPHY

Adkins KF: The effect of single doses of x-radiation on mandibular growth. Brit J Radiol 39:602, 1966

Adrian JC: Pulp effects of neodymium laser. A preliminary report. Oral Surg 44:301, 1977

Adrian JC, Bernier JL, Sprague WG: Laser and the dental pulp, JADA 83:113, 1971

Anderson MW, Izutsu KT, Rice JC: Parotid gland pathophysiology after mixed gamma and neutron irradiation of cancer patients. Oral Surg 52:495, 1981

Beumer J, Curtis T, Harrison RE: Radiation therapy of oral cavity: Sequelae and management, part 1. Head Neck Surg 1:301, 1979

Beumer J, Curtis T, Harrison RE: Radiation therapy of oral cavity: Sequelae and management, part 2. Head Neck Surg 1:392, 1979a

Brown LR, Dreizen S, Daly TE, Drane JB, Handler S, Riggin LJ, Johnston DA: Interrelations of oral microorganisms, immunoglobulins, and dental caries following radiotherapy. J Dent Res 57:882, 1978

Brown LR, Dreizen S, Handler S, Johnston DA: Effect of radiation-induced xerostomia on human oral microflora. J Dent Res 54:740, 1975

Brown LR, Dreizen S, Rider LJ, Johnston DA: The effect of radiation induced xerostomia on saliva and serum lysozyme and immunoglobulin levels. Oral Surg 41:83, 1976

Brown LR, O'Neill PA, Dreizen S, Handler SF, Riggan LJ, Perkins DH: Relationship between saliva and serum agglutination titers and post-irradiation caries activity in cancer patients. J Dent Res 60:10, 1981

Burke FJT, Frame JW: The effect of irradiation on developing teeth. Oral Surg 47:11, 1979

Cabrini RD, Itoiz ME, Caranza FA, Mayo J, Smolko EE: Histological and histochemical analysis of the effect on oral tissues and tooth germs of irradiation with a deuteron beam. Helv Odont Acta 11:124, 1967

Cleall JF, Buonocore MG, Fonts AR: Deposition of radioactive strontium in the developing enamel and dentin of the rat. J Dent Res 42:1480, 1963

Cleall JF, Fonts AR, Dale PP: Distribution and effects of strontium 90 and x-radiation on the teeth and surrounding structures of the rat. New York State Dent J 28:445, 1962

Collett WK, Watson JA, Wald N: Abscopal and direct effects on calcium mobilization, akaline phosphatase levels, and dentin formation following x-irradiation of either the rat incisor or the thyroid-parathyroid region. J Dent Res 45:1529, 1966

Evans HJ: In Jacobs PA, Price WH, Law P (eds); Human Population Cytogenetics, p 208. Baltimore, Williams and Wilkins, 1970

Gartner LP, Hiatt JL, Provenza DV: Effects of ionizing radiation on incisor development of the prenatal mouse. Acta Anat (Basel), 98:376, 1977

Goldfeder A: Cell structure and radiosensitivity. Trans NY Acad Sci 26:215, 1963

Gowgiel JM: Experimental radio-osteonecrosis of the jaws. J Dent Res 39:176, 1960

Gowgiel JM: Eruption of irradiation-produced rootless teeth in monkeys. J Dent Res 40:538, 1961

Greulich RC, Ershoff BH: Delayed effects of multiple sublethal doses of total body x-irradiation on the periodontium and teeth of mice. J Dent Res 40:1211, 1961

Holgate W: The incorporation and retention of 90 SR in the teeth. Brit Dent J 107:131, 1959

Horn Y, Markitziu A, and Ulmansky M: Effect of single versus fractionated doses of x-radiation on incisors in rats. J Dent Res 54:378, 1975

Hutton MF: Effect of Cobalt-60 radiation on the dental pulp of monkeys. J Dent Res 53:418, 1974

Jesionowski M: Investigation on the effect of laser radiation on the dental pulp in rabbits. Pol Med J 9:468, 1970

Kantola S: Laser-induced effects on tooth structure. IV. A study of changes in the calcium and phosphorus contents in dentine by electron probe microanalysis. Acta Odont Scand 30:463, 1972a

Kantola S: Laser-induced effects on tooth structure. V. Electron probe microanalysis and polarized light microscopy of dental enamel. Acta Odont Scand 30:475, 1972b

Karmiol M, Walsh RF: Dental caries after radiotherapy of the oral regions. JADA, 91:838, 1975

Khan MA, Gartner LP, Hiatt JL, Provenza DV: Sensitivity of mouse molar tooth germs to x-ray irradiation in vitro. J Biol Buccale 7:211, 1979

Kimeldorf DJ, Jones DC, Castanera TJ: The radiobiology of teeth (a review). Radiation Res 20:518 1963

Koppang HS: The radiosensitive stages of the rat incisor odontoblasts as demonstrated by autoradiography. Scand J Dent Res 81:303, 1973

Kowalik S: Post irradiation changes in dental tissues. Czas Stomat 19:1123, 1966

Lindemann J: Strontium 90 in teeth. Tandlaegebladet 71:731, 1967

Littman SM, Kirsh JE, Keane AT: Radium-induced malignant tumors of the mastoid and paranasal sinuses. Am J Roentgenol 131:773, 1978

Markitziu A, Horn Y, Ulmansky M: Effect of single versus fractionated doses of x-radiation on developing molars in rats. J Dent Res 53:637, 1974

Mays CW, Dougherty TF, Taylor GN, Lloyd RD, Stover BJ, Lee WSS, Christensen WR, Dougherty JH, Atherton DR: Radiation induced bone cancer in beagles. Second International Symposium, Delayed Effects of Bone Seeking Radionuclides. Salt Lake City, Utah, University of Utah Press, 1968

Meyer I, Shklar G, Turner J: A comparison of the effects of 200 kV radiation and cobalt-60 radiation in the jaws and dental structure of the white rat. Oral Surg 15:1098, 1962

Meyer I, Shklar G, Turner J: Effects of 200 kV radiation and cobalt-60 radiation on the oral mucosa, gingiva and alveolar bone of experimental animals. J Oral Surg Anesth Hosp Dent Serv 21:147, 1963

Meyer I, Shklar G, Turner J: Tissue healing and infection in experimental animals irradiated with cobalt-60 and orthovoltage. Oral Surg 21:333, 1966

Morrish RB, Chan E, Silverman S, Meyer J, Fu KK, and Greenspan D: Osteonecrosis in patients irradiated for head and neck carcinoma. Cancer 47:1980, 1981

Nickens GE, Patterson SS, El-Kafrawy AH, Hornback NB: Effect of cobalt-60 radiation on the pulp of restored teeth. JADA 94:701, 1977

Powell GL, Morton TH: Pulpal effects of continuous wave CO_2 lasers. J Dent Res AADR Abst #2, 62:170, 1983

Poyton HG: The effects of radiation on teeth. Oral Surg 26:639, 1968

Reichart PA: ^{224}Ra-induced dental resorptions. Report of a case. Oral Surg 54:281, 1982

Rosenthal HL, Gilster JE, Bird JT: Strontium-90 content of deciduous human incisors. Science 140:176, 1963

Rosenthal HL, Harbor NC: The absorption, retention, and distribution of strontium 90 from naturally contaminated food by female rabbits. J Dent Res 44:935, 1965

Rowland RE: Radium in human teeth. A quantitative autoradiographic study. Arch Oral Biol 8:13, 1963

Samuels LD: Uptake of radium-226 from drinking water into human deciduous teeth. Arch Oral Biol 11:581, 1966

Sharpe WD: Chronic radium intoxications: clinical and autopsy findings in long-term New Jersey survivors. Environ Res 8:243, 1974

Shearer HI: Effect of Cobalt-60 radiation on extraction healing in the mandibles of dogs. J Oral Surg 25:115, 1967

Spiess H: Late effects of ^{224}Ra injections in man. Health Phys 19:98, 1970

Starke EN, Shannon IL: How critical is the interval between extractions and irradiation in patients with head and neck malignancy? Oral Surg 43:333, 1977

Starkey WE, Fletcher W: The accumulation and retention of strontium-90 in human teeth in England and Wales—1959 to 1965. Arch Oral Biol 14:169, 1969

Stern RH, Renger HL, Howell FV: Laser effects on vital dental pulps. Brit Dent J 127:26, 1969

Stern RH, Sognnaes RF: Laser effect on dental hard tissues: A preliminary report. J Southern Cal Dent A 33:17, 1965

Sweeney WT, Elzay RP, Levitt SH: Histologic effect of fractionated doses of selectively applied ^{60}Co irradiation on the teeth of albino rats. J Dent Res 56:1403, 1977

Taylor GN, Rehfeld CE, Christensen WR, Jee WSS: Influence of ^{226}Ra and ^{239}Pu on the dental root canal of the dog. J Dent Res 48:924, 1969

Taylor R, Shklar G, Roeber F: The effects of laser radiation on teeth, dental pulp and oral mucosa of experimental animals. Oral Surg 19:786, 1965

West JL: Enamel hypoplasia of the deciduous incisor teeth of a calf. Am J Vet Res 34:839, 1973

Westcott, WB, Starcke EN, Shannon IL: Chemical protection against postirradiation dental caries. Oral Surg 40:709, 1975

Wolf N, Gedalia I, Yariv S, Zuckermann H: The strontium content of bones and teeth of human foetuses. Arch Oral Biol, 18:233, 1973

LASER

Belkahia A: Biological effects of laser beams in otolaryngology. Medical application approach. Ann Otolaryngol Chir Cervicofac 88:467, 1971

Bora B: Amazing Laser, Philadelphia, Franklin Institute, 1972

Brotherton M: Masers and Lasers: How They Work;What They Do. New York, McGraw–Hill, 1964.

Carroll, JM: Story of the Laser. New York, Dutton, 1970

Goldman L, Rockwell JR, Jr: Lasers in Medicine. New York, Gordon, 1971

Larsen E: Lasers Work Like This. Rockaway NY, Roy, 1973

Lytel Allen, Buckmaster: ABC's of Lasers, 3rd ed. Indianapolis, Sams, 1972

McGuff PE: Surgical Applications of Lasers. Springfield Ill, Charles C Thomas, 1966

Smith DL, et al: Laser welding of gold alloys. J Dent Res 51:161, 1972

Stern RH et al: Lased enamel: Ultrastructural observation of pulsed carbon dioxide laser effects. J Dent Res 51:455, 1972

Vahl J: Laser and its application in dentistry. Hippokrates 42:458, 1971

Wolbarsht ML: Laser Application in Medicine. Vol 1, 1971; Vol 2, 1974

14
PULP CAPPING AND PULPOTOMY

Pulp capping is the covering of an exposed pulp with a medicated dressing in an attempt to preserve vitality. Pulpotomy is the removal of the coronal portion of the pulp and the covering of the remaining pulp stump with a medicated dressing in order to maintain the vitality of the radicular pulp tissue.

Pulp capping has been employed after carious pulp exposures, mechanical exposure of the pulp during operative procedures, and traumatic exposures resulting from tooth fractures. Many investigators have reported a high incidence of clinical success with this procedure. However, when histologic examinations of teeth with capped pulps have been made, the success rate has not been so dramatically high. The histologic examinations have revealed chronically inflamed pulps after capping, even though clinical results, as measured by absence of pain, soreness to percussion, reactions to vitality tests, and negative radiographic findings, are usually satisfactory.

A significant proliferation of periapical fibroblasts, osteoblasts, and cementoblasts has been shown to follow pulp exposure in the teeth of young rats within 1 hour (Stahl et al, 1969). This elevated activity was associated with active connective tissue remodeling at the apex within a 30-day experimental period. As a result of such proliferative activity, apical closure usually ensued even though the pulp capping procedure may prove to have been unsuccessful (Torneck et al, 1973; Ravn, 1973). In older rats, proliferative fibroblastic activity was present but was significantly lower (Stahl et al, 1970). Thus, with advancing age, the chances for successful pulp capping diminish because of the normal aging of the dental pulp. Older pulps may be fibrotic and reduced in volume and may have increased calcific deposits. Pulp capping may also be employed for carious exposures in deciduous teeth that will be shed within a short time. When the deciduous teeth are expected to remain for a number of years, pulpotomy is the treatment of choice.

INDICATIONS FOR PULP CAPPING

Pulp capping is indicated mainly for mechanical exposures in young teeth, in which the vascular supply is greatest, especially those with incompletely formed root ends.

INDICATIONS FOR PULPOTOMY

When the pulps of young teeth have been exposed by dental caries, pulpotomy, rather than pulp capping, is indicated as an intermediate treatment. The infected, inflamed coronal pulp tissue is removed, thereby enabling the underlying uninflamed pulp tissue to remain uninvolved. Pulpotomy is especially indicated in permanent teeth with incompletely formed root ends (Ehrmann, 1981; Russo et al, 1982). Excellent clinical results with a partial pulpotomy technique have also been obtained by Cvek (1978) on young teeth with pulp exposures resulting from traumatic crown fractures. Confirmation of healing was subsequently obtained by Cvek and Lundberg (1983), who examined the pulps of 21 teeth for which pulpotomies had been performed 12 to 95 months before. The histologic findings revealed few inflammatory changes. In patients with a history of rheumatic heart disease, pulpotomy is a safe procedure. Beechen et al (1956) found that bacteremia was not produced by the pulpotomy operation. The remaining pulp tissue should be kept vital long enough to complete the formation of the root (Krakow et al, 1977). When root formation has been completed, vital pulp extirpation can be performed. Pulpotomy procedures are also highly successful in deciduous teeth and are preferable to complete endodontic procedures in deciduous teeth with chronic pulpitis. However, there is some evidence of a slightly increased prevalence of rotation and enamel surface defects of the subsequently erupted permanent successors after pulpotomy. Messer et al (1980) attributed these increases to the toxic effects of the medicaments used. If complete necrosis of the pulp has occurred, pulpotomy is valueless and should not be performed.

PHYSICAL PHENOMENA ASSOCIATED WITH MECHANICAL PULP EXPOSURES

When a dental pulp is exposed mechanically, a number of physical phenomena occur in the coronal pulp tissue that influence the subsequent reactions and prognosis. After surgical removal of the coronal portion of the pulp in a pulpotomy, the radicular portion of the pulp is similarly affected. The phenomena involved are:

Heat. The closer a cavity preparation is to the pulp, the greater is the likelihood of heat injury. Dentin is an effective insulator; as more and more dentin is removed, heat damage to the underlying pulp tissue becomes more likely unless adequate cooling has been employed. Excessive drilling in pulpotomy procedures also produces heat damage to the radicular pulp tissue unless proper precautions are observed.

Pressure. When the pulp is exposed, pressure is transmitted directly to the pulp by the bur or hand instrument. Pressure is damaging; the greater the pressure, the less favorable the prognosis.

Pulp tissue pressure is also increased intrinsically by pulp exposure. Stenvik et al (1972) found that mechanical exposures of the pulps of monkey teeth resulted in increases in tissue pressure, from an average initial pressure of 16 mm Hg, to 50 to 60 mm Hg. Such increases were accompanied by inflammatory responses. The pressures dropped below the initial values when the pulp tissues at the exposure site became necrotic.

Crushing of Pulp Tissue. Pulp tissue is inevitably contused by the exposure or surgical removal of a portion of the pulp. When pulp cells are crushed, some of them will die. The breakdown products of the dead or injured cells are irritants that cause an inflammatory response (Fig. 14–1).

Hemorrhage. Exposure of the pulp invariably results in some hemorrhage from the capillaries in the odontoblastic layer and, sometimes, the underlying pulp tissue (Luostarinen, 1971). Microcinematographic studies of rats' teeth indicate that, following pulp exposure, stasis also occurs in the adjacent capillaries, followed by thrombosis in the regional arterioles. The circulation in the remainder of the pulp appears to be normal (Laurichesse and Santoro, 1972). Despite the hemorrhage, successful repair after pulp capping may still occur (Brännström et al, 1979). In pulpotomy, the hemorrhage takes place in the radicular pulp tissue. The amount of hemorrhage depends on the number of blood vessels opened and the extent of the injury. The accumulated extravasated blood cells also cause some destruction of the underlying tissues by pressure.

Intrusion of Dentin Chips. As a result of exposure or pulpotomy, dentin debris (chips) from the grinding of the dentin is pushed into the remaining pulp tissue (Fig. 14–2). In addition, decalcified dentin and microorganisms may be forced into the pulp tissue (Patterson, 1976; Watts, 1979). The reactions of the underlying pulp will vary with the numbers, virulence, and pathogenicity of the microorganisms, as well as

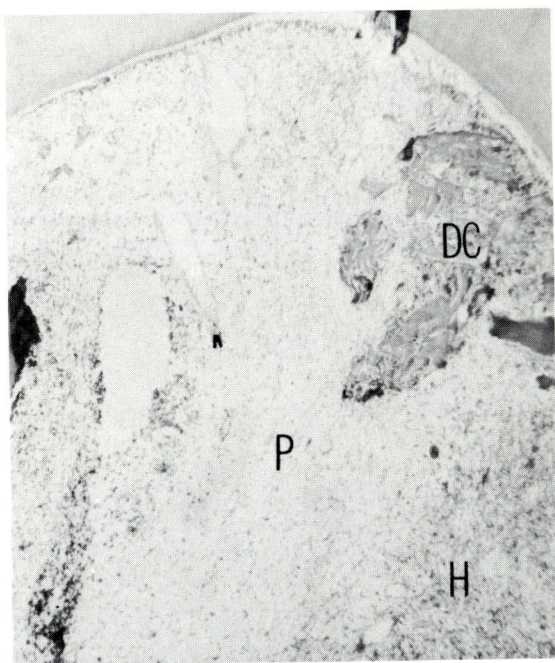

FIG. 14-2 Damage to pulp tissue, following mechanical exposure. Dentin chips (DC) and hemorrhage (H) are present in the pulp (P) under the region of the exposure. ×54.

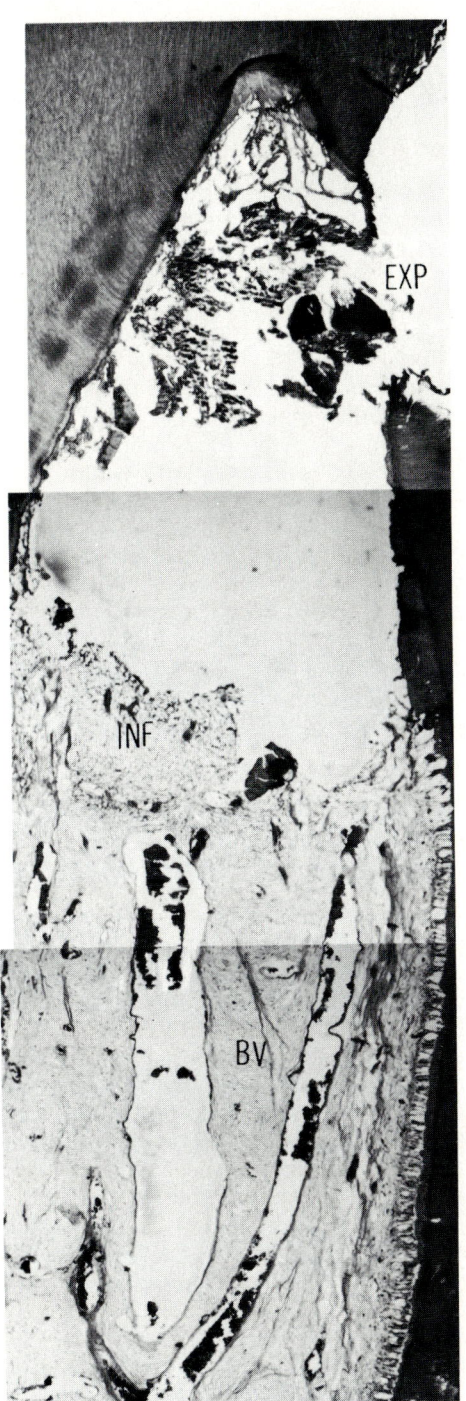

FIG. 14-1 Composite photomicrograph of a mechanically exposed pulp (EXP). The coronal pulp tissue has been crushed. The blood vessels (BV) of the underlying pulp tissue are dilated, and a region of chronic inflammation (INF) is present. ×54.

the resultant effects of all the other factors influencing repair of connective tissues.

FACTORS THAT AFFECT OUTCOME OF PULP CAPPING OR PULPOTOMY

The following factors must be considered in deciding whether or not to cap a mechanically exposed pulp:

The size of the exposure has a bearing on the eventual outcome. The larger the area of exposure, the less favorable the prognosis, because of the greater damage from the crushing of tissue and hemorrhage; these factors cause a more severe inflammatory reaction. Profuse hemorrhage may interfere with successful resolution, because more tissue is destroyed by compression.

Location of the exposure can influence the prognosis. When a pulp capping material, such as calcium hydroxide, is placed at a level at which the calcific deposit will produce a bridge, the two portions of the pulp can be separated. The blood supply to the vital pulp portion above the bridge of dentin may be choked off, resulting in the development of an intrapulpal abscess or necrosis (Stanley and Lundy, 1972; Hørsted et al, 1981). Such a complication often occurs in pulp exposures from root decay or class V cavities in single, narrow-rooted teeth. However, the repair of both buccal and occlusal pulp exposures in dogs' teeth that were capped with calcium hydroxide powder was equally favorable (Pereira and Stanley, 1981).

Exposure to saliva influences the end result. Short periods of exposure are not as harmful as long periods. However, microorganisms do not readily gain a foothold in healthy pulp tissue. Vital pulps of rats, dogs, and humans, when exposed to saliva, resisted the penetration of bacteria (Brännström et al, 1979; Watts and Paterson, 1982). Cvek et al (1982) found that when monkey pulps were exposed by either crown fracture or grinding, the depth of the inflammatory changes was related to time. The depth of inflammation increased gradually from 3 to 168 hours, but did not exceed 2.2 mm (mean, 1.6 mm). In contrast, exposure of the pulps to saliva following cavity preparations significantly increased the inflammatory reactions as deep as 8.2 mm (mean, 4.4 mm). The longer the time of exposure, the greater the likelihood that the microorganisms will gain a foothold in the injured tissue and cause a pulpitis (Obersztyn et al, 1968; Magnusson, 1970; Armstrong et al, 1979; Cox et al, 1982).

Marginal leakage is another important factor to be considered in pulp repair following pulp capping and pulpotomy. If the restoration leaks, inflammation persists and repair cannot occur (Cox et al, 1983). The end result is likely to be pulp necrosis. Thus, zinc phosphate cements should not be employed as intermediate fillings. Rather, an amalgam restoration should be placed over the base at the same sitting during which the pulp capping or pulpotomy is performed.

Systemic Factors

Hormonal disturbances influence pulp repair. For example, patients on prolonged cortisone therapy are poor risks for pulp capping, since cortisone interferes with the normal inflammatory response. If infection is present, it may become rampant, since cortisone interferes with phagocytosis. Cortisone also delays granulation tissue formation which is a necessary precursor to repair.

Nutritional deficiencies affect repair of teeth with capped pulps. Vitamin C, especially, is important for repair; it is needed for fibroplasia and the formation of ground substance. It is also necessary for the proper elaboration of collagen (Passmore, 1977).

Systemic diseases of some types interfere with repair of connective tissues. Among these are anemias, liver diseases, colitis, diabetes, and other diseases affecting alimentation or absorption of nutrients.

Antimetabolites, such as methotrexate, used for cancer chemotherapy, cause immunosuppression. The induced cytopenia interferes with the effectiveness of the inflammatory response. Kolzet et al (1979) found that administration of nonlethal doses of methotrexate to rats compromised the healing of pulp exposures.

Age and Status of the Pulp

Healing of pulp exposures in the teeth of old rats has been shown by Stahl et al (1970) and Luostarinen (1971) to be inferior to that of young rats. The pulps of the older rats tended to become necrotic despite dentin bridge formation, whereas the pulps of young rats tended to remain vital. Previously noncarious teeth are better risks for pulp capping than carious teeth because, in the latter, aging processes are accelerated. Similarly, teeth that have been exposed to previous operative manipulations are poorer risks for successful capping than are unaffected teeth. Periodontally involved teeth are poor risks for pulp capping because of the diminution of the blood supply to their pulps. Pulp capping in the teeth of adults likewise has less likelihood of success (Kapur et al, 1964), even though a limited number may be successful (Haskell et al, 1978). Especially in crown and bridge procedures, pulp capping and pulpotomy are contraindicted, since other irritants will be superimposed on an already injured pulp. These extra irritants are chemicals, pressure, and further manipulation.

Pulp capping should be discouraged for carious pulp exposures. The presence of infection as a factor in the repair of cariously exposed

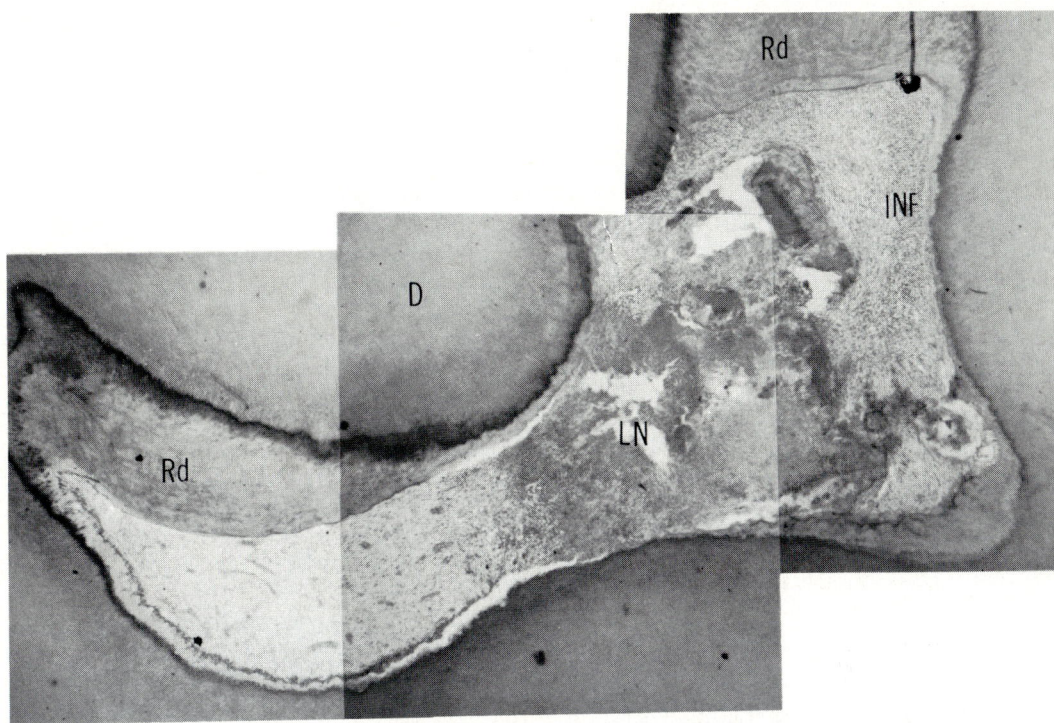
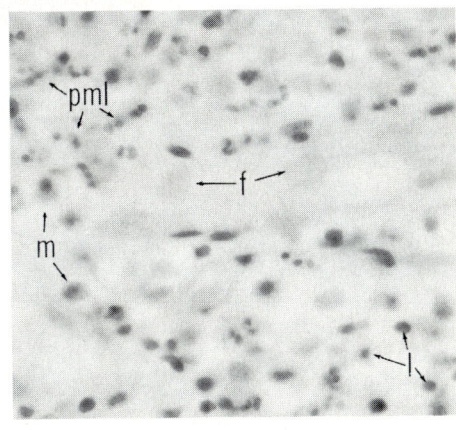

FIG. 14-3 Capping of a pulp exposed by caries. *(Top)* The coronal pulp tissue is chronically inflamed (INF), and a region of liquefaction necrosis (LN) is present, as a result of the carious lesion. Reparative dentin (Rd) has been elaborated in reaction to the decay. Pulp capping resulted in pain and swelling. ×54. *(Bottom)* Inflammatory cells in the pulp (higher magnification): pml, polymorphonuclear leukocytes; l, lymphocytes; m, macrophages; f, fibroblasts. ×960.

pulps cannot be ignored. Cariously exposed pulps are either infected or damaged by the products of the microorganisms or the defence cells. Kakehashi et al (1965) have shown that exposed pulps healed in germ-free animals, whereas pulp necrosis ensued in the exposed pulps of control animals. In most teeth with deep caries, the pulps are chronically inflamed, either partially or totally. Many have small regions of liquefaction necrosis within them (Fig. 14-3). Frequently, the operator is unaware of the status of the pulp from macroscopic examination. The odds are against successful repair in carious exposures in the presence of so much tissue destruction. Thus, pulpotomy in youngsters and total pulp extirpation and endodontic treatment in adults are preferable.

Coronal pulp tissue is much more cellular and less fibrous than apical pulp tissue. Pulpotomy operations in the teeth of adults are fraught with hazard because, in removing the coronal pulp tissue, the greatest portion of the cellular substance in the pulp, the tissue that has the greatest number of undifferentiated mesenchymal cells, is removed. The likelihood of repair becomes lessened. However, biologic variations occur. For example, Masterton (1966) reported that pulpotomy was successful in a small number of cariously involved posterior teeth in patients 25 to 42 years of age, for periods ranging from 25 to 70 months. Nonetheless, as a general rule, pulpotomies should not be performed in cariously exposed teeth of adults.

HISTOPATHOLOGY

After mechanical exposure or pulpotomy, an acute inflammation occurs in the pulp at the site of the exposure, but the remainder of the pulp is usually unaffected.

The underlying blood vessels dilate, edema occurs, and polymorphonuclear leukocytes (polys) accumulate at the site of injury. Within a few days, an acute abscess may develop in the region of the exposure. The severity of the reaction depends on the amount of initial tissue damage.

FIG. 14-4 Acute inflammation, following mechanical pulp exposure. *(Top, left)* Under the region of the exposure (Exp) an acute abscess (Abs) has developed. ×54. *(Bottom, left)* Higher magnification of inflammatory cells in the pulp (P). They are mainly polymorphonuclear leukocytes. D, dentin. ×960. *(Top, right)* Scanning electron micrograph of inflammatory cells, predominantly polymorphonuclear leukocytes, at margin of abscess seen at top left. ×500. *(Bottom, right)* Higher magnification of top right photomicrograph showing degranulating polys (P). Lysosomes (arrows) are dispersed. ×5000.

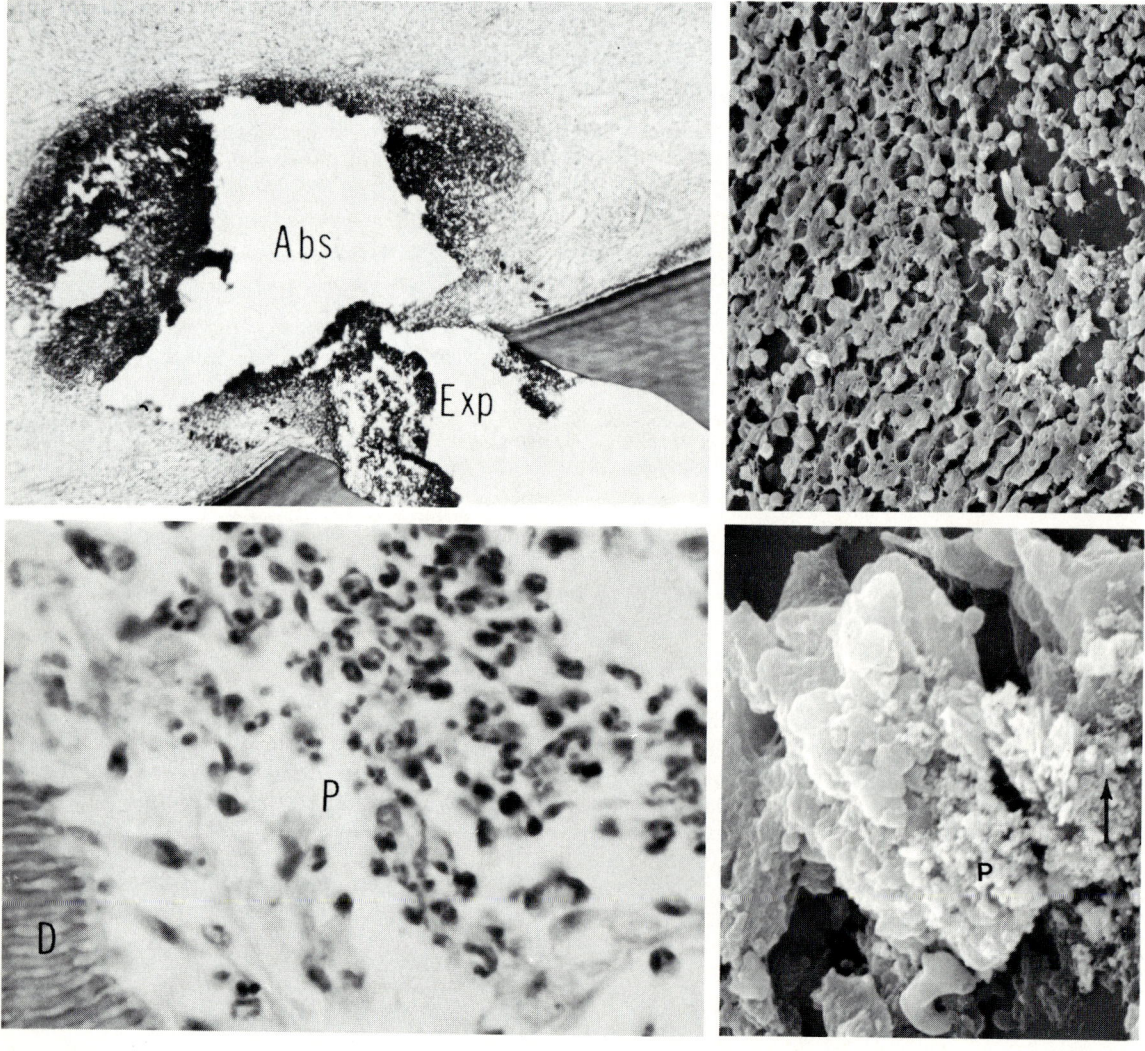

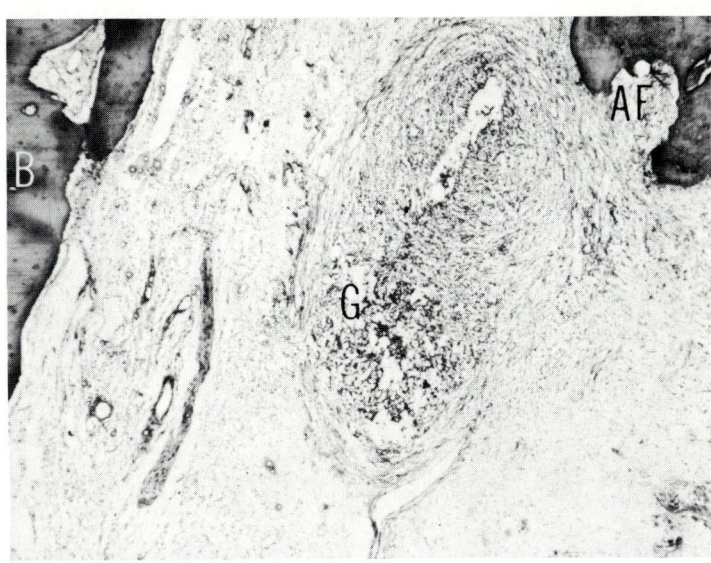

FIG. 14-5 Periapical granuloma (G), 90 days after pulp exposure. Most of the coronal pulp tissue is necrotic. The periapical tissue around the apical foramen (AF) is chronically inflamed. B, bone. ×54.

In the teeth of dogs and monkeys, we have noted that after mechanical pulp exposures from operative procedures, dentin chips burred from the dentinal wall are pushed into the pulp. Hemorrhage of varying magnitude also occurs. One week later, a collection of inflammatory cells, mainly polys, is present. Frequently, an acute abscess is found in the center of the pulp, surrounded by intact tissue that is infiltrated by inflammatory cells (Fig. 14-4). One month after a large mechanical exposure, the remainder of the pulp may be found to have been replaced by granulation tissue. Examination of the wall of the dentin opposite to the exposure site reveals dentinal resorption. Ninety days later, the pulp, in most instances, is still chronically inflamed or has become necrotic, and a granuloma has developed apically (Fig. 14-5).

However, in human teeth, repair can occur after pulp exposure. The prognosis for healing is much better for mechanical exposures of the pulp than it is for carious exposures, because the pulpitis that develops after mechanical exposure usually is not complicated by previous inflammation and infection. When treated, the acute inflammation is modified to a chronic inflammation, and repair may then occur. Repair depends on the amount of tissue destruction, the amount of hemorrhage, the patient's age (and, hence, the blood supply of the tissue), the resistance of the host, and other factors that influence the ability of the injured pulp connective tissue to repair itself.

When the pulp is injured as a result of exposure, the undifferentiated mesenchymal cells or, according to Fitzgerald (1979), fibroblasts adjacent to the exposure undergo proliferative activity. During the repair phase, differentiation of some of these cells into bone- or dentin-producing cells occurs, and hard tissue is elaborated. The studies of Inoue et al (1981) suggest that the presence of numerous blood vessels, with resultant increased oxygen tension, significantly enhances differentiation. One indication of repair is the formation of a "bridge" of reparative dentin over the exposed pulp. The pulp under this bridge should remain relatively normal (Fig. 14-6).

Occasionally, however, in spite of bridge formation, the remainder of the pulp remains chronically inflamed and eventually succumbs (Fig. 14-7). In almost one third of the teeth treated, internal resorption has been reported to follow pulpotomy and treatment with calcium hydroxide. In others, complete mineralization occurs, obliterating the remaining pulp tissue (Fig. 14-8). Eventually, the mineralization may occlude the canal to such an extent that there would be difficulties in instrumentation should future endodontics be necessary. For this reason, extirpation of the remaining pulp tissue should be performed as soon as root formation is completed. This procedure may prevent internal resorption, and it also stops the mineralization process that appears to continue in teeth treated with calcium hydroxide.

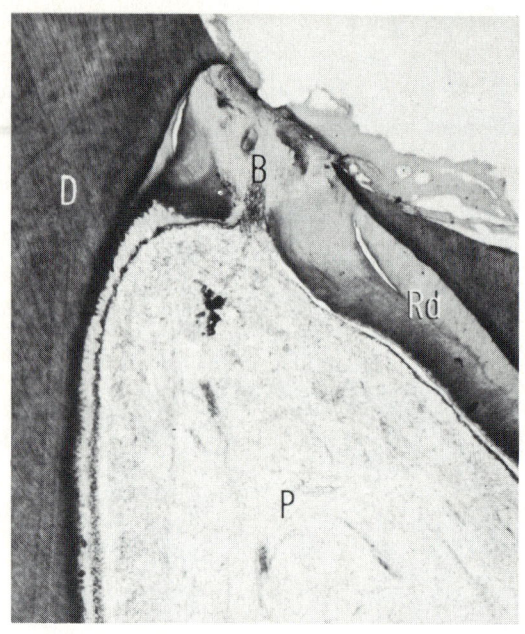

FIG. 14-6 The pulp (P) has recovered after exposure. A "bridge" (B), composed of reparative dentin (Rd), has formed over the region of the exposure. D, dentin. ×54.

FIG. 14-7 Inflammation of pulp under "bridge." In spite of bridge formation (B), the pulp (P) is chronically inflamed (INF). DC, dentin chips. ×100. (Seltzer S, Bender IB: J Dent Res 37:678, 1958. Copyright by the American Dental Association. Reproduced by permission)

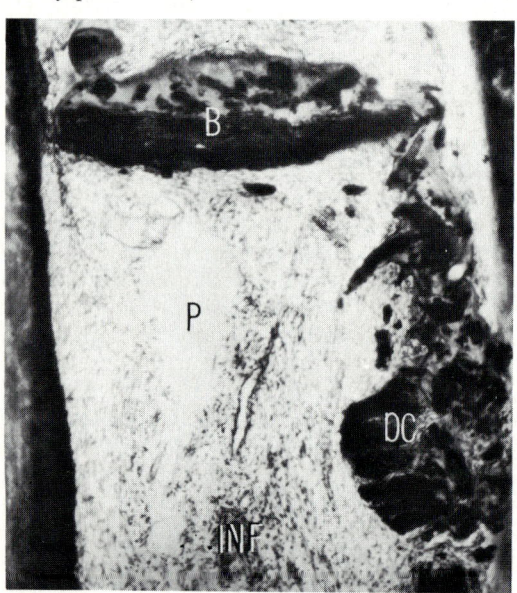

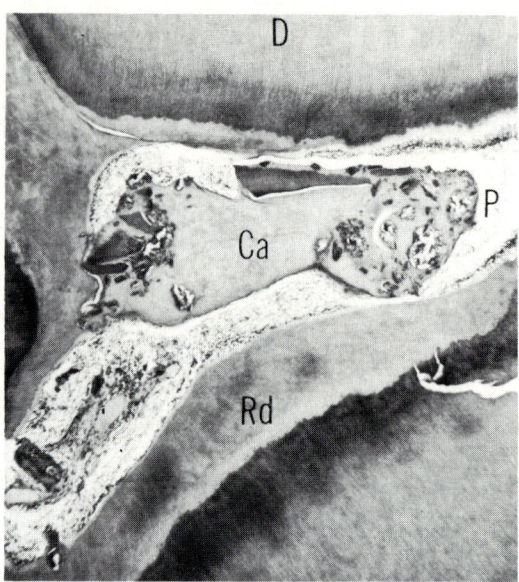

FIG. 14-8 Calcification under calcium hydroxide. Eight months after the application of calcium hydroxide to an exposed pulp (P), calcification (Ca) has continued, almost obliterating the pulp. D, dentin; Rd, reparative dentin. ×54.

The formation of reparative dentin is part of the repair process that occurs whenever there is pulp injury. Whenever inflammation takes place, repair accompanies it. Within a few weeks, the acute inflammation becomes chronic, exudate is resorbed, and, eventually, repair is complete in successful cases.

Reactions also occur around the dentin chips that have been pushed into the pulp as a result of the exposure. Fibroblasts or undifferentiated mesenchymal cells are attracted to these chips and begin elaborating dentin matrix. As more and more matrix is elaborated, many chips may be welded together, forming a dentin bridge (Fig. 14-7). According to Hørsted et al (1981), in areas of severe inflammation, pulp fibroblasts elaborate hard tissue without tubules; in areas of mild inflammation, the hard tissue produced by neighboring odontoblasts contains varying numbers of dentinal tubules. However, although the formation of a bridge affords protection against the irritation of applied filling materials (Holland et al, 1979), it does not guarantee success, nor does its absence presage failure (Tainter et al, 1981). Infrequently, successful pulp capping or pulpotomy may result without the formation of dentin over the exposure (Sayegh, 1969; Weiss and Bjorvatn, 1970).

DRUGS IN PULP CAPPING AND PULPOTOMY

There has been too much emphasis on drugs employed in pulp capping and pulpotomy rather than on diagnosis. Successful pulp capping has been reported to occur with the use of hosts of individual medicaments as well as combinations of antiseptics, caustics, anti-inflammatory agents, antibiotics, and enzymes. In 1883, Hunter reported on the successful use (98%) of English sparrow droppings mixed with sorghum molasses for pulp capping.* The basis for the

---

* Dr. F. A. Hunter, in the Missouri Association, said: I am very glad indeed that this subject was so enlarged upon the program as to include the capping and treatment of exposed pulps. I have spent a great deal of time experimenting upon the subject, and with a most marked degree of success. I do not hesitate to say, and I say it boldly and without fear of contradiction that, by my method, I have succeeded in saving every exposed pulp that has come my way; yes, even though the pulp may be suppurating and the pus welling up in volumes, I shall save it. I can save even *remnants* of pulps, be they never so small.

Some years ago—I can't just recall how long; at any rate it was about the time of the introduction in our city of the English sparrow, I began experimenting with a capping. It is so good and efficacious that your patients will bless you; you become happy in consequence, they leave your office showering down upon you the highest encomiums, and—never come back again. Some one remarked during the course of the discussion, not to make pressure upon the pulp. Now, I say that pressure is the very element upon which a great deal of the success depends. Drive your capping down as hard as you can, and, as Siddal says, "You have the pulp in a tight place." Now, as to the composition and mixing of my infallible capping. It ———
 VOICE: Write it on the board.
 DR. HUNTER: That is probably best, as many, no doubt, will wish to experiment for themselves, and here it is:

 ℞ Sorgum Molassum, 1 pint.
  Droppum English Sparrow, 1 pound.

Mix into a stiff plastic mass and apply. I must confess that though my success has been fully equal to 98 per cent of all cases with this capping, I have never experimented with chickens. I have no doubt but that their droppings are equally advantageous. Dr. Hunter here took his seat amid storms of applause.
 (Saving Pulps, A Queer Process, Dental Items of Interest, p 352 January 1883.)
 (*Authors' Note:* Dr. Hunter's formula seems to fit well with our present concern with conservation of new materials, not to mention recycling.)

use of many drugs is that they kill microorganisms, with little cognizance of the adverse effects of these drugs on the pulp tissue. Many of the drugs that kill microorganisms also kill tissue cells. The use of medicaments or medicated cements or capping materials cannot alter the fact that the tissue is damaged, sometimes severely, by the hemorrhage. In addition, when the pulp is exposed, the instrument causing the exposure creates tissue damage. In experimental pulpotomies, in which extreme care is taken to avoid tissue damage, excessive hemorrhage, and irritating drugs, Granath and Hagman (1971) have shown that the pulps withstand the procedure well. However, with more severe trauma, the tissue reacts with inflammation. If the irritant is severe and more pulp tissue is destroyed, as occurs in a large exposure, a severe inflammatory response results and an acute abscess develops.

When an acutely abscessed pulp is capped, what happens to the pus? By pressure, it destroys other pulp tissue. Eventually, it may be resorbed and repair may occur. However, in many instances, chronic inflammation persists and the rest of the pulp is converted into granulation tissue. The pulp may then be partially mineralized, internal resorption may occur, or total pulp necrosis may result.

Calcium Hydroxide

Calcium hydroxide has been the drug of choice for use in pulp capping and pulpotomy. It has antibacterial activity (Fisher and McCabe, 1978; Brännström et al, 1979) and appears to work efficiently, but the exact mechanism is not understood. Although suspensions of calcium hydroxide are highly alkaline, other compounds, such as ammonium hydroxide at the same pH, cause liquefaction necrosis of the pulp when placed on exposed pulp tissue. The calcium ions delivered to the site of the exposure by the calcium hydroxide suspension are not utilized in the repair of the exposure, according to some investigators. Sciaky and Pisanti (1960) and Attalla and Noujaim (1969) have shown, by means of radioautographs, that the calcium ions present in the dentin bridge that is formed during repair come from the systemic circulation. The applied calcium hydroxide (which, in their experiments, contained radioactive calcium) did not enter into the formation of the bridge. On the other hand, Holland et al (1982) found large carbonate granulations in pulps that were capped with barium or strontium hydroxide, as well as calcium hydroxide; the granulations were birefringent to polarized light. Their experiments suggested that the calcium in the granulations observed in the calcium hydroxide group came not from the bloodstream but from the capping material. The differences in the findings of the various investigators may be due to differences in the solubility of various calcium hydroxide products. Some of these may release Ca^{2+} slowly due to the presence of other binding components (Shubich et al, 1978).

The mechanism for the induction of dentin formation and repair under calcium hydroxide may be that it causes a superficial coagulation necrosis of the pulp tissue on which it is placed (Schröder and Granath, 1971). The necrosis is apparently initiated by damage to the blood vessels. The initial damage from calcium hydroxide occurs in the capillaries closest to the region of the capping. In their studies with the electron microscope, Kukletová and Svejda (1972) found that the appearance of the endothelial cells of the capillaries may range from normal to swollen, with increased vacuoles and the formation of vesicles. In severe damage, thrombi may be formed. However, after 7 days, inflammation was not found.

Because of its pH (approximately 11), calcium hydroxide helps to keep the immediate region in a state of alkalinity, which is necessary for bone or dentin formation. Under this region of calcium hydroxide-induced coagulation necrosis, which is saturated with calcium ions, cells from the underlying pulp tissue differentiate into odontoblasts, which then begin to elaborate matrix (Chen, 1978). The matrix is composed of acid mucopolysaccharides and glycoproteins (Fonseca and Gendelman, 1972). The calcium ions deposited in the matrix come from the systemic circulation. Thus, the role of calcium hydroxide is similar to that of dentin chips that have been pushed into the pulp as a result of exposure.

The injured pulp tissues of rats and dogs, which had been capped with calcium hydroxide, were studied with light and electron microscopes by Harrop and Mackay (1968) and by Ichikawa (1976). They reported that the underlying pulp cells underwent mitoses and proliferated into the wound. An extensive network of collagen fibrils formed between the cells. By the third day, in undecalcified sections, small clusters of crystals were observed in intimate relationships to the collagen fibrils. Progressive deposition of the crystals resulted in large expanses of calcified material. Demineralized sections revealed that the matrix was composed of collagen, resembling that of mature dentin. According to Ichikawa (1976), the dentin bridge is composed entirely of osteodentin and the cells adjacent to the bridge are similar to osteoblasts. Schröder and Granath (1972) examined the coronal surface structure of calcium hydroxide-induced bridges with both the light and the scanning electron microscope. They found tubular openings surrounded by collagen bundles similar to those found in normal predentin.

Caution must be exercised when calcium hydroxide is used for pulp capping or pulpotomy. Powdered calcium hydroxide used alone over a pulpotomy wound has been found to be highly irritating (Eleazer et al, 1981).

The calcium hydroxide used clinically should be chemically pure and fresh and should contain no irritating additives. On prolonged standing, calcium hydroxide reacts with atmospheric carbon dioxide to form calcium carbonate. As such, it is no longer effective. Calcium carbonate may react with the phosphoric acid of cement bases and silicates to yield carbon dioxide, which has been shown by Pohto and Scheinin (1967) to cause emboli in the capillaries of the dental pulp.

A number of commercially available hard-setting calcium hydroxide cements have been tested on the exposed pulps of both experimental animals and humans. The results are contradictory and depend on the formulation (Stanley and Lundy, 1972; Tronstad, 1974; Pitt Ford, 1980; Heys et al, 1980). For example, it has also been shown that a resin catalyst mixed with calcium hydroxide caused marked pathosis in the pulp, eventuating in necrosis (Sela et al, 1973). According to Fisher and McCabe (1978), the irritating catalyst contained a mixture of paraffin oil with a salicylate.

Weiss and Bjorvatn (1970) and Frankl (1972) have reported that calcium hydroxide in water or a base combined with metacresyl acetate induced bridge formation with regular reparative dentin and without pulp inflammation. However, similar results have been obtained without the addition of the metacresyl acetate (Pereira et al, 1980).

There are two undesirable side effects of calcium hydroxide: one is the possibility of eventual complete calcification of the tissue in the root canal. Should this occur, subsequent endodontic therapy, if needed, becomes a difficult—and, often, impossible—procedure. A second adverse effect of pulp capping with calcium hydroxide is the persistence of induced inflammation, eventually causing internal resorption.

Calcium hydroxide should not be used to treat existing pulpitis. It has no curative effect for inflammation and has no anodyne effect, since it does not reduce nerve impulse activity (Trowbridge et al, 1982). The osteogenic potential of calcium hydroxide has been demonstrated in experiments on lower animals by Mitchell and Shankwalker (1958), Yoshiki et al (1960) and Binnie and Mitchell (1973). However, their results were not confirmed by Rasmussen and Mjör (1971).

Undoubtedly, there are other induction devices for the formation of a dentin bridge over an exposed pulp.

Tricalcium Phosphate

Another calcium-containing compound, tricalcium phosphate (Synthos*) has been reported to be nonirritating to connective tissue. When implanted into bone, it stimulated new bone formation (Bhaskar et al, 1971). Heller et al (1975) tested tricalcium phosphate as a pulp capping agent in monkey teeth and found it nonirritating. Furthermore, it induced hard tissue formation. However, Boone and El-Kafrawy (1979) reported that despite inducing dentin formation around the ceramic in exposed monkey pulps, most of the pulps were inflamed and necrotic. They attributed these changes to bacterial contamination and advised against its use as a pulp capping agent.

Dentin Shavings

When placed on exposed pulps of experimental animals, lyophilized and sterilized dentin shavings or filings, either autologous (autogeneic) or homologous (allogeneic), have been shown to act as seeding agents for the formation of reparative dentin (Obersztyn, 1966; Anneroth and Bang; 1972). The induction of hard tissue formation by dentin is apparently caused by a noncollagenous portion of the matrix (Bang and Johannessen, 1972; Bang, 1973; Inoue, 1981).

Enzymes and Matrix Components

In our experiments, the enzyme alkaline phosphatase, when applied locally to exposed pulps, was found to stimulate the differentiation of other pulp cells into odontoblastlike cells, which then elaborated dentin matrix (Fig. 14–9). Similar results were not obtained with acid phosphatase, but matrix was found to develop around dentin chips without the use of any intervening drugs (Fig. 14–10).

Moss (1960) was able to induce heterotopic bone formation in the calvaria of rats by use of despeciated calves' bone paste. He subsequently identified the active agent as a fraction of chondroitin sulfate. Burger et al (1961) noted that bone repair was accelerated in calvarial wounds of rats which were implanted with chondroitin-treated demineralized bone. They postulated that chondroitin sulfate, or a complex of chondroitin sulfate with a protein, acted as an induction factor for the formation of new bone. We tried pastes containing chondroitin sulfate on pulp exposures but were unable to discern any stimulatory effect on dentin formation with this glycosaminoglycan (Fig. 14–11). However, matrix formation did occur when chondroitin sulfate was mixed with alkaline phosphatase (Fig. 14–12). In parallel experiments, Johansson et al (1963) also found that collagen and chondroitin sulfate were not stimulatory for dentin bridge formation when applied as capping agents to amputated pulps of rat molars.

However, it must be re-emphasized that pulps may not recover completely from the effects of exposure and capping, in spite of dentin bridge formation. Chronic inflammation may persist for long periods, occasionally causing internal resorption of the dentinal wall of the root canal (Magnusson, 1970). Eventually, partial and then total necrosis of the pulp ensues. Similarly, the presence of a dentin bridge in teeth with pulpotomy does not necessarily mean that complete repair has occurred. The underlying pulp tissue may remain chronically inflamed and, eventually, undergo complete necrosis. However, the pulpotomy may appear to be successful, as measured by negative radiographic findings, the comfort of the patient, and the absence of pain.

Collagen Preparations

Enriched collagen gels have been reported to enhance wound healing by promoting fibroblastic proliferation (Shoshan and Finklestein, 1970). There is also a reduction in inflammation and stimulation of hard tissue formation when foreign bodies are coated with collagen (Yaffe et al, 1982). When used as a pulp capping or pulpotomy agent, both collagen-calcium phosphate gel (Nevins, 1976) and native enriched collagen solution (Bimstein and Sho-

* Miter, Inc., Worthington, Ohio

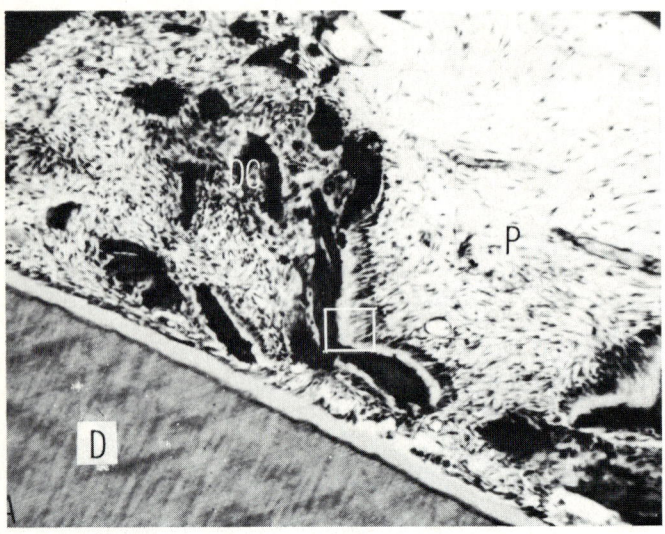

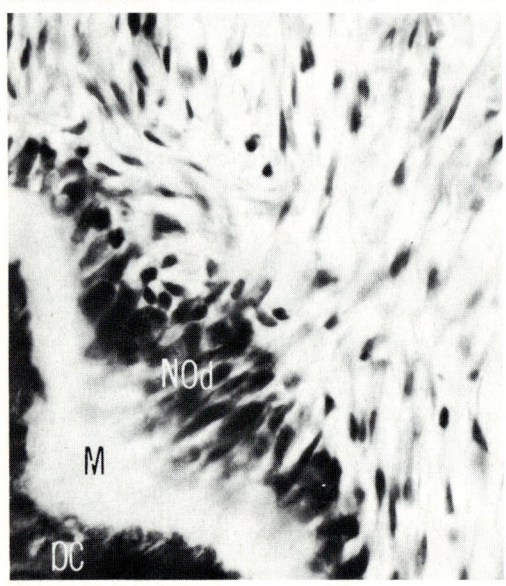

FIG. 14-9 The effect of alkaline phosphatase. *(Top)* Dentin chips (DC) have been pushed into the pulp (P), as a result of an exposure. Alkaline phosphatase was applied to the pulp. ×135. *(Bottom)* Higher magnification of region outlined by rectangle in top photograph. New odontoblasts (NOd) are present around a dentin chip (DC) and dentin matrix (M) is being elaborated. ×540.

shan, 1981) have been reported to produce successful results. However, native collagen, as a heterograft material, has been found antigenic (Carmichael et al, 1974). Carmichael et al attempted to alter the antigenicity of collagen by modifying it with enzymes. When applied to exposed dogs' pulps, such altered collagen failed to induce a mineralized dentinal bridge and caused pulp inflammation. Subsequently, several other types of collagen preparations, namely wet collagen sponges and fabrics, were found by Dick and Carmichael (1980) to be better than the collagen gel preparations, but they nonetheless produced pulp inflammation.

Glucocorticoids

Corticosteroids have been incorporated in pulp-capping materials with a view toward reducing pain and pulp inflammation. However, as with other new drugs and techniques, many of the claims made for the beneficial effects of corticosteroid pulp capping have now been invalidated. Topically applied corticosteroids do appear to inhibit or reduce pain (Hansen, 1969;

Shovelton et al, 1971; Schroeder, 1972). Several reports appear to indicate that pulp capping with corticosteroids reduces pulp inflammation (Barker and Lockett, 1972; Barker, 1975). However, according to Langeland and Langeland (1968) the reduction of inflammation is more apparent than real. Some reports indicate that, under corticosteroids, degeneration of the inflamed pulp eventually takes place (Hansen, 1963; Everett and Kirk, 1969; Barker and Ehrmann, 1969; Compton and Mitchell, 1970; Paterson, 1976). According to some reports, reparative dentin formation is inhibited under corticosteroid pulp cappings (Baume, 1964; Fiore-Donno and Baume, 1966; Barker and Lockett, 1972). Only when steroids are combined with calcium hydroxide does dentinal bridging occur at the exposure site (Fiore-Donno and Baume, 1962; Schroeder, 1972). Other investigators (Soto-Feine and Tchernichin, 1982) have questioned whether glucocorticoids could impair reparative dentinogenesis, since they could find no glucocorticoid receptors in the odontoblasts. In the uninflamed pulps of the teeth of laboratory animals and humans, the application of steroids over pulp exposures is neither helpful nor harmful (Kakehashi et al, 1969; Barker and Ehrmann, 1969).

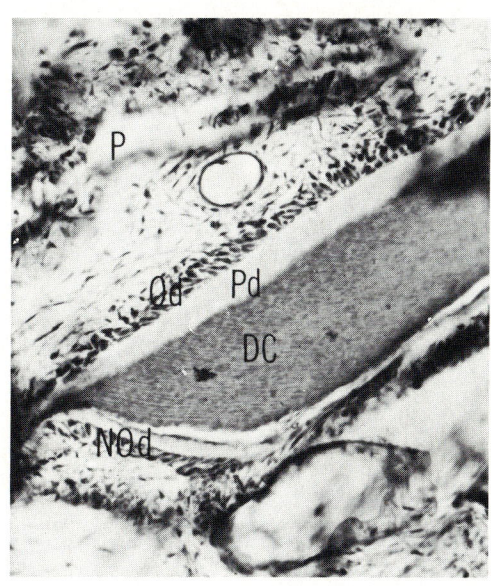

FIG. 14-10 New odontoblasts (NOd) have developed around dentin chip (DC), which has been pushed into the pulp (P) following a pulp exposure. No drugs were placed on the exposed pulp. Pre-existing odontoblasts (Od) and predentin (Pd) are also shown. ×180. (Seltzer S: Oral Surg 12:595, 1959)

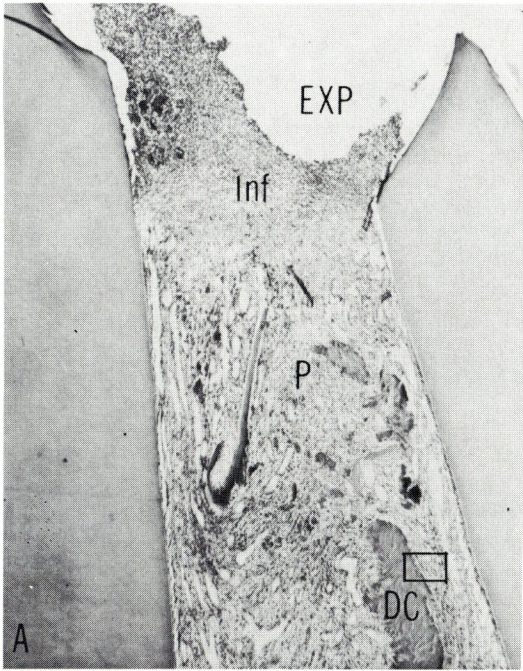

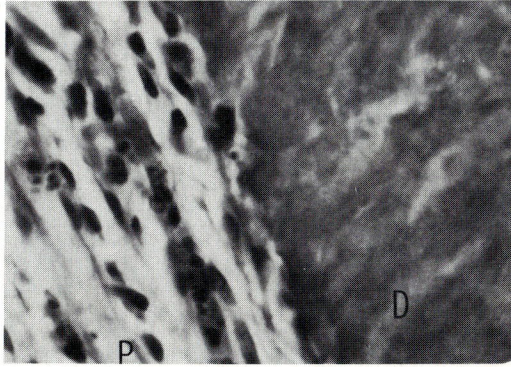

FIG. 14-11 Effect of chondroitin sulfate on pulp exposure. *(Left)* The pulp (P) underlying the exposure (EXP) to which chondroitin sulfate was applied is acutely inflamed (Inf). No matrix activity is discernible around dentin chip (DC). ×54. *(Right)* Higher magnification of region outlined by rectangle in picture at left. No new odontoblasts or matrix are present around the dentin chips (D). The pulp (P) is inflamed. ×960.

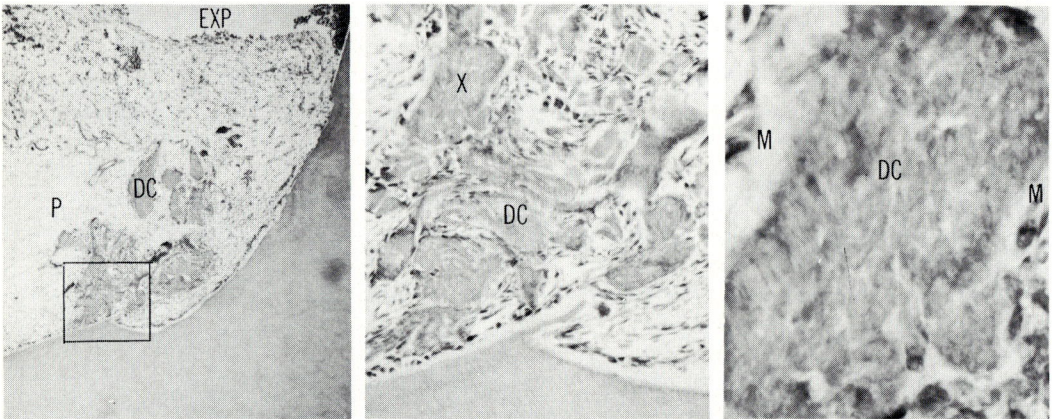

FIG. 14-12 Pulp reaction to chondroitin sulfate and alkaline phosphatase. *(Left)* After pulp exposure (EXP) and medicament application, dentin chips (DC) are pushed into the pulp (P). ×54. *(Center)* Higher magnification of dentin chips (DC) in region outlined at left. The chips are welded together by dentin matrix. ×240. *(Right)* Higher magnification of dentin chip (DC) in region X in center picture. M, dentin matrix, on the periphery. ×960.

Thus, the value of the use of steroids for pulp capping is open to question. Other antiseptics, such as camphorated parachlorophenol, antibiotics, and metacresyl acetate, when added to corticosteroids, produce the same questionable benefits, and there is no evidence that results are better than those obtained with calcium hydroxide alone. Moreover, local application of antibacterial agents with anti-inflammatory steroids has been found valueless (Meyers et al, 1978).

Formaldehyde Preparations

Formocresol (Buckley's formula) consists of formaldehyde, 19% and cresol, 35%, in a vehicle of 15% glycerin in water.* It and other formaldehyde-containing pastes have been advocated for pulpotomy procedures in both primary (Berger, 1972; Morawa et al 1975) and permanent (Trask, 1972; Starkey, 1978) teeth. However, the reports on efficacy are contradictory. In human primary teeth, Magnusson (1978) found that the pulp contained inflammatory cells and a high incidence of internal resorption. The use of such medicaments on the pulps of permanent teeth is not recommended.

The pulp reactions of young permanent monkey molars following pulpotomies and the application of Formocresol were studied by Kelley et al (1973) and Armstrong et al (1979). Despite the persistence of inflammation, Kelley et al considered their results favorable. Armstrong et al found that bridging and calcific metamorphosis of the pulp eventually occurred.

Formocresol is highly toxic to cells. At full strength, it depresses the respiratory activities of fibroblasts and matrix synthesis (Loos and Han, 1971). Polyvinyl sponge implants containing full-strength Formocresol caused fixation of fibroblasts and adjacent cells. The cells did not recover, and the sponges had been sloughed by 21 days later (Straffon and Han, 1970). When diluted to concentrations ranging from one fifth to one one-hundred twenty-fifth of the normal concentration, the fixation effect was reduced. The connective tissue cells showed the usual signs of degeneration. The matrix was swollen, with disorganization of the fibrous components, and there was infiltration of inflammatory cells. Although recovery occurred, the rate of recovery was progressively slower with sponges treated with concentrations of one one-hundred twenty-fifth through one fifth. The incorporation of proline-^{3}H into the secretory proteins of hamster fibroblasts was severely depressed by a one-fiftieth dilution of Formocresol (Straffon and Han, 1968). They concluded that Formocresol, when used in full concentration, thoroughly fixes the tissue, blocking the synthesis of connective tissue proteins and ribonucleic acids and suppressing the respiratory enzymes.

* Accepted Dental Therapeutics, 35th ed, p 217. Chicago, American Dental Association, 1973-74.

A 1:5 dilution of Formocresol also markedly suppressed lactic dehydrogenase activity (Cunningham et al, 1982). These respiratory enzymes are more fragile than hydrolytic enzymes, such as alkaline phosphatase, when pulp tissue is exposed to tissue fixatives (Mejàre et al, 1976).

Similar cytotoxic effects were produced by a one-fifth concentration, but there was recovery and stimulation of RNA synthesis after 2 weeks.

At weaker concentrations, Formocresol does not fix the tissue, but might create signs of cellular degeneration. The effects of minimal doses of Formocresol on the connective tissues of rats were studied by Powell et al (1973). They placed cotton pellets medicated with Formocresol into polyethylene tubes and implanted the tubes into the subcutaneous tissues in the backs of the rats. Microscopic sections revealed severe tissue destruction for as long as 14 days. The reaction subsided with time and, after 30 days, the tissues had recovered. Langeland et al (1971) found that Formocresol did not fix cells but caused them to degenerate. The necrotic cells were demarcated by a zone of tissue with impaired cellular activity resulting from circulatory disturbances. Varying degrees of inflammation were induced in the subjacent tissues. Hørsted et al (1982) performed pulpotomies in monkey teeth and treated them with N_2, a formaldehyde-containing preparation. They reported that, after 1 month to 2 years, histologic examinations revealed the presence of particles of cement in the residual pulp and periapical ligament. The particles were seen in vessels, macrophages, and multinucleated foreign body giant cells. Studies by Myers et al (1978) and by Chiniwalla and Rapp (1982) of the vasculature of monkey deciduous teeth after pulpotomy indicated that the microcirculation was compromised. Chiniwalla and Rapp found that a one-fifth concentration of Formocresol caused a reduction in the number of blood vessels beneath the pulp amputation site. However, in the remainder of the pulp, the vascular architecture was intact after 84 days.

Human clinical studies have shown that Formocresol treatment caused severe inflammatory reactions or necrosis of the pulp (Rølling et al, 1976; Rølling and Lambjerg-Hansen, 1978).

Furthermore, it is possible that when pulp tissue is treated with formaldehyde, the damaged tissue components may be rendered antigenic and induce autoantibody formation. However, the evidence is somewhat contradictory.

The immunologic responses vary in different experimental animals. Rats sensitized with formalin-treated pulp extracts developed homologous antibodies that were hemagglutinating throughout the sensitizing period; passive cutaneous anaphylaxis was elicited only during the early stages (Nishida et al, 1971).

Humoral and cell-mediated immune responses to dog pulp tissue treated with high concentrations of Formocresol have been detected by Block et al (1977–1978). On the other hand, Van Mullen et al (1983) found that Formocresol provoked a weak allergic response in guinea pigs which had been presensitized with either formaldehyde or cresol; cell-mediated immunologic responses were absent in guinea pigs that had not been presensitized (Simon et al, 1982). Longwill et al (1982) found significant lymphocyte transformation responses in 25 to 40 children who had received various types of pulpotomies. However, the responses were not specifically related to the use of Formocresol. Furthermore, Rølling and Thullin (1976) and Marshall and Creamer (1982) have offered clinical evidence that hypersensitivity reactions were not induced in human patients receiving Formocresol-treated pulpotomies.

In animals, the formaldehyde has been found extensively distributed in the dentin, pulp, periodontal ligament, and bone. Labeled formaldehyde has also been detected in the systemic circulation and in numerous organs of dogs and monkeys (Myers et al, 1978; Block et al, 1983).

In the light of the foregoing discussion, the use of formaldehyde-containing pastes on pulp tissue is controversial.

Glutaraldehyde

Glutaraldehyde is a protein cross-linking agent used as a tissue fixative. It apparently has limited diffusion through dentin and cementum ('s-Gravenmade, 1975; Dankert et al, 1976). On the connective tissues of rabbits and rats, acid glutaraldehyde produced moderate to severe inflammation (Martin, 1978). However, Kopel et al (1980) found that glutaraldehyde pulpotomies in human primary teeth yielded results superior to pulpotomies treated with Formocresol.

Ten percent glutaraldehyde solution has been found to cause a significant reduction in protein solubility (Nelson et al, 1979).

As with formaldehyde, treatment of protein with glutaraldehyde suppresses the activity of respiratory enzymes (Cunningham et al, 1982)

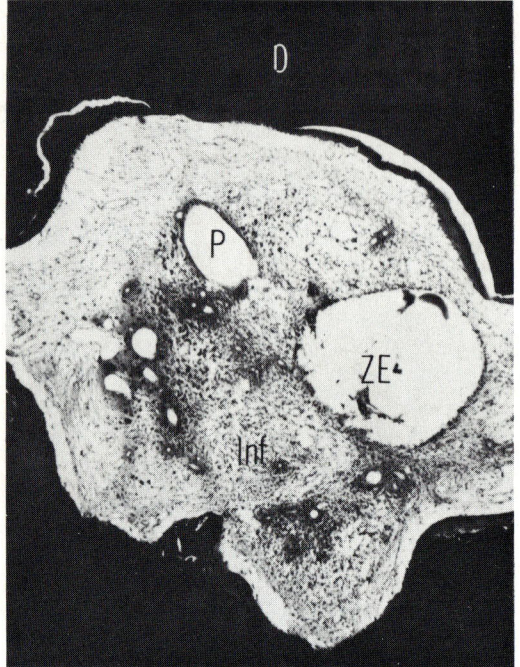

FIG. 14-13 The effect of zinc oxide-eugenol on pulp exposure. Cross section of dog molar. Nine months after pulp capping with a zinc oxide-eugenol paste (ZE), the pulp (P) is chronically inflamed (Inf). D, dentin. ×54.

and renders tissue immunogenic (Deng and Beutner, 1974).

Glutaraldehyde-fixed autologous tissue, when implanted subcutaneously, produces little acute reaction. However, in the long term, an immune response is evoked (Thoden Van Velzen and van den Hooft, 1977; Wesselink et al, 1977).

Polycarboxylate Cements

Polycarboxylate cements have also been advocated for pulp capping. Reports suggest that this material, although initially irritating, is well tolerated by the pulp (Negm et al, 1981). However, the induction of calcified bridges has not been reported to occur (Safer et al, 1972; McWalter et al, 1973, 1976; El-Kafrawy et al, 1974). Whether or not calcified bridges are needed is open to question.

Antibiotics

Various antibiotics, such as tetracyclines, neomycin, penicillin, cephalothins, and vancomycin, have been incorporated in pulp capping cements, presumably to reduce or eliminate pulp infections. Reports as to efficacy vary, depending on the antibiotic tested. In some cases, the pulps reacted with little inflammation and partial to complete dentin bridging (Obersztyn et al, 1968; Baker and Mitchell, 1969; Gardner et al, 1971). In most instances, the antibiotic was found to be ineffective in either reducing inflammation or stimulating hard tissue deposition (Sekine et al, 1960; McWalter et al, 1973, 1976). A dangerous sequel to the use of locally applied antibiotics is the possible induction of a hypersensitivity reaction. A tritium-labeled antibiotic was found in the blood plasma 10 minutes after it had been applied to the injured pulp tissues of rats (Page et al, 1973).

When specific antigens were applied to the dentin of immunized monkeys, Bergenholtz et al (1977) found that extensive pulp damage was induced. In addition, immunologic sensitization through pulp canals has been demonstrated by Barnes and Langeland (1966) and Okada et al (1967). In such cases, the cure may be worse than the disease.

Cyanoacrylates

Tissue adhesives or cyanoacrylates have been used for pulp capping in experimental animals with apparent success. The butyl forms appear to be well tolerated by the host tissues, and they have hemostatic and bacteriostatic properties (Wade, 1969; Berkman et al, 1971). Bhaskar et al (1969, 1972) and Berkman et al (1971) have tested isobutyl cyanoacrylate on exposed pulps in the teeth of rats and miniature pigs as well as human teeth. In contrast with calcium hydroxide, which produced a superficial zone of necrosis, the pulp tissue directly under isobutyl cyanoacrylate retained its vitality, and less pulp inflammation was evoked. On the other hand, Nixon and Hannah (1972) found severe inflammation after 4 to 14 weeks in all 32 of the pulps of dogs' teeth capped with N-butyl cyanoacrylate. Also, dentin formation was inhibited, so that no dentinal bridges were formed over the exposure sites.

Zinc Oxide-Eugenol

The results of the use of zinc oxide-eugenol for pulp capping and pulpotomy are a matter of controversy. Some investigators have claimed excellent results (Obersztyn et al, 1968; Ravn and Svarrer, 1968; Weiss and Bjorvatn, 1970); others have found that zinc oxide-eugenol, when placed directly over a pulp exposure, does not

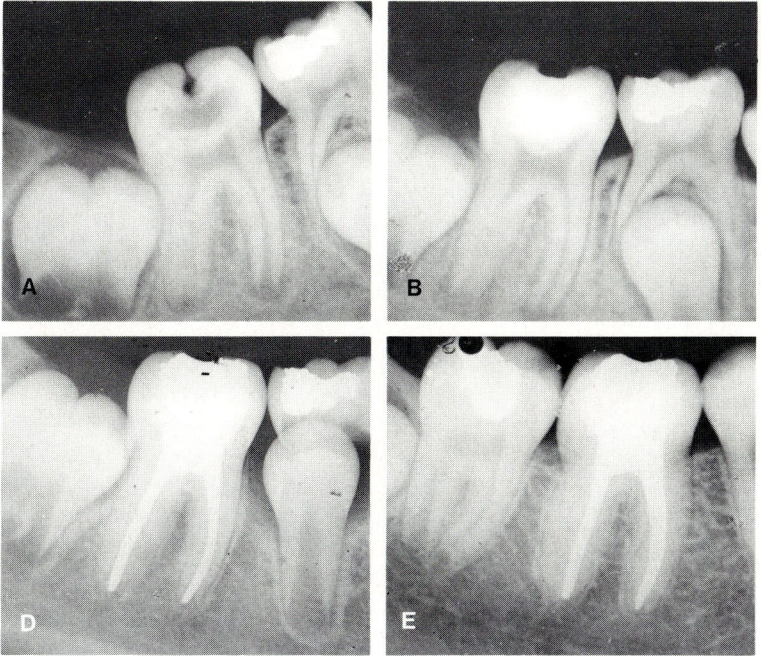

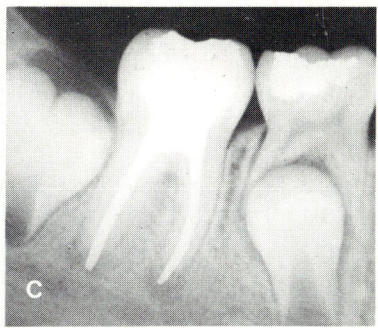

FIG. 14-14 Completed root end formation without the use of medicaments. *(A)* Radiograph of large carious lesion with pulp exposure. *(B)* Six months after pulpotomy procedure, the pulp has become necrotic. Both apexes are resorbed, with widening of the apical foramina. *(C)* One year after treatment. *(D)* Six years later, healing is complete with restoration of the lamina dura. *(E)* Eight years later.

have the same beneficial effect as is obtained when it is used in deep cavities with unexposed pulps. Chronic inflammation persists for extended periods of time (Fig. 14–13), possibly causing internal resorption (Magnusson, 1971; Nixon and Hannah, 1972; Goerig et al, 1980). The disparity in results of various investigators may be due to variations in the type of eugenol used in the mixture. Webb and Bussell (1981) have compared the responses of rat connective tissue to zinc oxide-eugenol mixtures made with either commerical or purified eugenol. Both mixtures were inflammatory, but the commercial mixture increased the inflammatory response.

Bridging of the exposure site under zinc oxide-eugenol is inhibited (Weiss and Bjorvatn, 1970; Nixon and Hannah, 1972). After pulpotomy, similar inhibition of reparative dentin formation has been reported to occur under a zinc oxide-eugenol cement containing *o*-ethoxybenzoic acid (Roberts et al, 1973). However, Tronstad and Mjör (1972) have found that zinc oxide-eugenol capping of monkey pulps in which pulpitis was experimentally induced gave more favorable results than capping with calcium hydroxide.

Pastes made with other oxides, such as magnesium oxide, have been found to be injurious to the pulp when placed over pulp exposures. Healing and hard tissue formation were not promoted (Kitagawa et al, 1968).

APEXIFICATION PROCEDURES

Various procedures and drugs have been used to treat vital and pulpless teeth with incompleted root formation. Among these procedures are routine endodontic therapy, including root canal debridement and overfilling the canal with root canal filling materials. Apical curettage is then performed. Such a procedure is not advocated, inasmuch as further root formation is stopped and, besides, the child is subjected to a needless surgical experience. Instead the inflamed or necrotic pulp tissue should be removed by thorough debridement. To induce root end closure, the use of various medicated root canal dressings has been advocated. Among these are Tricresol and Formalin (Cooke and Rowbotham, 1964), antibiotic pastes (Ball, 1964) and calcium hydroxide pastes (Frank, 1966; Steiner et al, 1968; Van Hassel and Natkin, 1970; Heithersay, 1970; Dylewski, 1971; Cvek, 1972; Ham et al, 1972); tricalcium phosphate (Koenigs et al, 1975; Roberts and Brilliant, 1975); and collagen-calcium phosphate gel (Nevins et al, 1976).

Histologic studies indicate that formation of hard tissue resembling bone or cementum is induced at the apex. Similar results were obtained by Torneck and Smith (1970) without the use of any medicaments, despite the presence of an inflammatory response; however, when inflammation persisted, formation of hard tissue decreased and the tissue appeared bonelike.

The root canal should be filled in the usual manner, either immediately after the placement of the dressing (Binnie and Rowe, 1973), or after the completion of root end formation (Fig. 14–14).

In infected root canals, root end development is irregular and the root length finally attained appears to be shorter than that of adjacent normal teeth (Torneck and Smith, 1970; Steiner and Van Hassel, 1971).

BIBLIOGRAPHY

Anneroth G, Bang G: The effect of allogeneic demineralized dentin as a pulp capping agent in Java monkeys. Odont Revy, 23:315, 1972

Armstrong RL, Patterson SS, Kafrawy AH, Feltman EM: Comparison of Dycal and formocresol pulpotomies in young permanent teeth in monkeys. Oral Surg 48:160, 1979

Attalla MN, Noujaim AA: Role of calcium hydroxide in the formation of reparative dentin. J Canad Dent A 35:267, 1969

Baker GR, Mitchell DF: Topical antibiotic treatment of infected dental pulps of monkeys. J Dent Res 48:351, 1969

Ball JS: Apical-root formation in a non-vital immature permanent incisor. Brit Dent J 116:166, 1964

Bang G: Induction of heterotopic bone formation by demineralized dentin: An experimental model in guinea pigs. Scand J Dent Res 81:240, 1973

Bang G, Johannessen JV: The effect of proteolytic enzymes on the induction of heterotopic bone formation by demineralized dentin in guinea pigs. J Oral Path 1:221, 1972

Barker BCW: Conservative treatment of cariously exposed vital pulps in posterior teeth with a glucocorticosteroid-antibiotic compound. J Brit Endo Soc 8:5, 1975

Barker BCW, Ehrmann EH: Human pulp reactions to a glucocorticosteroid-antibiotic compound. Austral Dent J 14:104, 1969

Barker BCW, Lockett BC: Reaction of dog pulp and periapical tissue to two glucocorticosteroid preparations. Oral Surg 33:249, 1972

Barnes GW, Langeland K: Antibody formation in primates following introduction of antigens into the root canal. J Dent Res 45:1111, 1966

Baume LJ: Survey of dentine biology. Brit Dent J 116:254, 1964

Beechen II, Laston DJ, Garbarino VE: Transitory bacteremia as related to the operation of vital pulpotomy. Oral Surg 9:902, 1956

Bergenholtz G, Ahlstedt S, Lindhe J: Experimental pulpitis in immunized monkeys. Scand J Dent Res 85:396, 1977

Berger JE: A review of the erroneously labelled mummification technics of pulpal therapy. Oral Surg 34:131, 1972

Berkman MD, Cucolo FA, Levin MP, Brunelle LJ: Pulpal response to isobutyl cyanoacrylate in human teeth. JADA 83:140, 1971

Bhaskar SN, Beasley JD, Ward JP, Cutright DE: Human pulp capping with isobutyl cyanoacrylate. J Dent Res 51:58, 1972

Bhaskar SN, Brady JM, Getter L, Grower MF, Driskell T: Biodegradable ceramic implants in bone: Electron and light microscopic analysis. Oral Surg 32:336, 1971

Bhaskar SN, Cutright DE, Boyers RC, Margetis PM: Pulp capping with isobutyl cyanoacrylate. JADA 79:640, 1969

Bimstein E, Shoshan S: Enhanced healing of tooth-pulp wounds in the dog by enriched collagen solution as a capping agent. Arch Oral Biol 26:97, 1981

Binnie WH, Mitchell DF: Induced calcification in the subdermal tissues of the rat. J Dent Res 52:1087, 1973

Binnie WH, Rowe AHR: A histolocial study of the periapical tissues of incompletely formed pulpless teeth filled with calcium hydroxide. J Dent Res 52:1110, 1973

Block RM, Lewis RD, Hirsch J, Coffey J, Langeland K: Systemic distribution of (^{14}C)-labeled paraformaldehyde incorporated within formocresol following pulpotomies in dogs. J Endodont 9:176, 1983

Block RM, Lewis RD, Sheats JB, Burke SH: Antibody formation to dog pulp tissue altered by formocresol within the root canal. Oral Surg 45:282, 1978

Block RM, Lewis RD, Sheats JB, Burke SH: Antibody formation to dog pulp tissue altered by N2-type paste within the root canal. J Endodont 3:309, 1976

Block RM, Lewis RD, Sheats JB, Burke SH: Antibody formation to dog pulp tissue altered by eugenol via the root canal. J Endodont 4:53, 1978

Block RM, Lewis RD, Sheats JB, Fawley J: Cell-mediated immune response to dog pulp tissue altered by formocresol within the root canal. J Endodont 3:424, 1977a

Block RM, Lewis RD, Sheats JB, Fawley J: Cell-mediated immune response to dog pulp tissue altered by 6.5% paraformaldehyde via the root canal. J Endodont 4:346, 1977

Boone ME, Kafrawy AH: Pulp reaction to a tricalcium phosphate ceramic capping agent. Oral Surg 47:369, 1979

Brännström M, Nyborg H, Strömberg T: Experiments with pulp capping. Oral Surg 48:347, 1979

Burger M, Sherman BS, Sobel AE: Acceleration of bone repair by chondroitin sulfate treatment of implants. School of aerospace medicine, USAF Aerospace Med. Center (ATC), Brooks Air Force Base, Texas. Report 61–63, July, 1961

Carmichael DJ, Dick HM, Dodd CM: Histologic effects of antigenically altered collagen as a heterograft for mammalian pulp exposures. Arch Oral Biol 19:1121, 1974

Chen C-H: An experimental study on healing of pulp wound following pulpotomy in dogs by autoradiography with tritiated thymidine. Shikwa Gakuho 78:287, 1978

Chiniwalla NP, Rapp R: The effect of pulpotomy using Formocresol on blood vessel architecture in primary anterior teeth of Macaca rhesus monkeys. J Endodont 8:205, 1982

Compton DE, Mitchell DF: Pharmacologic treatment of painful pulpitis: A five-year report. J Dent Res 49:183, 1970

Cooke C, Rowbotham JC: Root canal therapy in non-vital teeth with open apices. Brit Dent J 108:147, 1960

Cox CF, Bergenholtz G, Fitzgerald M, Heys DR, Heys RJ, Avery JK, Baker JA: Capping of the dental pulp mechanically exposed to the oral microflora—a 5 week observation of wound healing in the monkey. J Oral Pathol 11:327, 1982

Cox CF, Bergenholtz G, Syed SA, Heys DR, Fitzgerald M: A 13–15 month observation of wound healing. AADR Abst #730, J Dent Res 62:250, 1983

Cunningham KW, Lazzeri EP, Ranly DM: The effect of formocresol and glutaraldehyde on certain enzymes in bovine dental pulp. Oral Surg 54:100, 1982

Cvek M: Treatment of non-vital permanent incisors with calcium hydroxide: Odont Revy 23:27, 1972

Cvek M, Cleaton-Jones PE, Astin JC, Andreasen JO: Pulp reactions to exposure after experimental crown fractures or grinding in adult monkeys. J Endodont 8:391, 1982

Cvek M: A clinical report on partial pulpotomy and capping with calcium hydroxide in permanent incisors with complicated crown fracture. J Endodont 4:232, 1978

Cvek M, Lundberg M: Histological appearance of pulps after exposure by a crown fracture, partial pulpotomy, and clinical diagnosis of healing. J Endodont 9:8, 1983

Dankert J, 's-Gravenmade EJ, Wemes JC: Diffusion of formocresol and glutaraldehyde through dentin and cementum. J Endodont 2:42, 1976

Deng JS, Beutner EH: Effect of formaldehyde, glutaraldehyde and sucrose on the tissue antigenicity. Int Arch Allergy 47:567, 1974

Dick HM, Carmichael DJ: Reconstituted antigen-poor collagen preparations as potential pulp-capping agents. J Endodont 6:641, 1980

Doyle WA, McDonald RE, Mitchell DF: Formocresol versus calcium hydroxide in pulpotomy. J Dent Child 29:86, 1962

Dylewski JJ: Apical closure of non-vital teeth. Oral Surg 32:82, 1971

Ehrmann EH: Pulpotomies in traumatized and carious permanent teeth using a corticosteroid-antibiotic preparation. Int Endo J 14:149, 1981

Eleazer P, Bolanos O, Sinai I, Martin J, Seltzer S: The effect of unbound powdered materials on dog dental pulps. J Endodont 7:462, 1981

Everett AD, Kirk EE: Reaction of dental pulp to Ledermix cements. Dent Pract (Bristol) 19:348, 1969

Fiore-Donno G, Baume LJ: Effects of capping compounds containing corticosteroids on the human dental pulp. Helvet Odont Acta 6:23, 1962

Fiore-Donno G, Baume LJ: Clinical and histological response of human pulp to direct application of triamcinolone-dimethylchlor-tetracycline. J Canad Dent A 32:527, 1966

Fisher FJ, McCabe JF: Calcium hydroxide base materials. Brit Dent J 144:341, 1978

Fitzgerald M: Cellular mechanics of dentinal bridge repair using 3 H-thymidine. J Dent Res 58 (Spec. Iss. D):2198, 1979

Fonseca MM, Gendelman H: The role played by acid mucopolysaccharides in scar formation in the human dental pulp after administration of calcium hydroxide. Bull Group Int Rech Sci Stomat 15:185, 1972

Frank AL: Therapy for the divergent pulpless tooth by continued apical formation. JADA 72:87, 1966

Frankl SN: Pulp therapy in pedodontics. Oral Surg 34:293, 1972

Gardner DE, Mitchell DF, McDonald RE: Treatment of pulps of monkeys with vancomycin and calcium hydroxide. J Dent Res 50:1273, 1971

Goerig AC, Payne TF, del Rio CE: The pulpal response to ZOE with stock eugenol versus ZOE with purified eugenol. Oral Surg 50:557, 1980

Granath L-E, Hagman G: Experimental pulpotomy in human bicuspids with reference to cutting procedure. Acta Odont Scand 29:155, 1971

's-Gravenmade EJ: Some biochemical considerations of fixation in endodontics. J Endodont 1:233, 1975

Ham JW, Patterson SS, Mitchell DF: Induced apical closure of immature pulpless teeth in monkeys. Oral Surg 33:438, 1972

Hansen H: Pulp capping with corticoid-containing materials. Odont Tidskr 77:223, 1969

Harrop TJ, MacKay B: Electron microscopic observations on healing in dental pulp in the rat. Arch Oral Biol 13:365, 1968

Haskell EW, Stanley HR, Chellemi J, Stringfellow H: Direct pulp capping treatments: A long-term follow-up. JADA 97:607, 1978

Heithersay GS: Stimulation of root formation in incompletely developed pulpless teeth. Oral Surg 29:620, 1970

Heller AL, Koenigs JF, Brilliant JD, Melfi RC, Driskell TD: Direct pulp capping of permanent teeth in primates using a resorbable form of tricalcium phosphate ceramic. J Endodont 1:95, 1975

Heys DR, Heys RJ, Cox CF, Avery JK: The response of four calcium hydroxides on monkey pulps. J Oral Pathol 9:372, 1980

Holland R, Pinheiro CE, de Mello W, Nery MJ, de Souza V: Histochemical analysis of the dogs' dental pulp after pulp capping with calcium, barium, and strontium hydroxides. J Endodont 8:444, 1982

Holland R, de Souza V, de Mello W, Bernabé PFE, Otoboni Filho JA: Permeability of the hard tissue bridge formed after pulpotomy with calcium hydroxide: A histologic study. JADA, 99:472, 1979

Hørsted P, El Attar EK, Langeland K: Capping of monkey pulps with Dycal and a Ca-eugenol cement. Oral Surg 52:531, 1981

Hørsted P, Hansen JC, Langeland K: Studies on N_2 cement in man and monkey — cement lead content, lead blood level, and histologic findings. J Endodont 8:341, 1982

Hunter FA: Saving pulps. A queer process. Dent Items Int 5:352, 1883

Ichikawa T: Light and electron microscope studies of the dentin bridge formation following vital pulpotomy in dog's teeth. Shikwa Gakuho 76:391, 1976

Inoue T, Sasaki A, Shimono M, Yamamura T: Bone morphogenesis induced by implantation of dentin and cortical bone matrices. Bull Tokyo Dent Coll 22:213, 1981

Johansson BI, Persson I, Manera P: Histologic effects of collagen and chondroitin sulfate as capping agents in amputated rat molar pulps. Arch Oral Biol 8:503, 1963

El-Kafrawy AH, Dickey DM, Mitchell DF, Phillips RW: Pulp reaction to a polycarboxylate cement in monkeys. J Dent Res 53:15, 1974

Kakehashi S, Stanley HR, Fitzgerald R: The effects of surgical exposure of dental pulps in germ-free and conventional laboratory rats. Oral Surg 20:340, 1965

Kakehashi S, Stanley HR, Fitzgerald R: The exposed germ-free pulp: Effects of topical corticosteroid medication and restoration. Oral Surg 27:60, 1969

Kelley MA, Bugg JL, Jr, Skjonsby HS: Histologic evaluation of Formocresol and Oxpara pulpotomies in rhesus monkeys. JADA 86:123, 1973

Kitagawa M, Morikawa H, Ban H, Narita M, Ban M, Sekine N: A clinicopathologic study of the vital pulpotomy with magnesium oxide paste. Shikwa Gakuho 68:144, 1968

Koenigs JF, Heller AL, Brilliant JD, Melfi RC, Driskell TD: Induced apical closure of permanent teeth in adult primates using a resorbable form of tricalcium phosphate ceramic. J Endodont 1:263, 1975

Kolzet DJ, Shklar G, Krakow AA, Grøn P: Pulpal responses to operative procedures in rats receiving systemic methotrexate. Oral Surg 48:467, 1979

Kopel HM, Bernick S, Zachrisson E, DeRomero SA: The effects of glutaraldehyde on primary pulp tissue following coronal amputation: An in vivo histologic study. J Dent Child 47:425, 1980

Krakow AA, Berk H, Grøn P: Therapeutic induction of root formation in the exposed incompletely formed tooth with vital pulp. Oral Surg 43:755, 1977

Kukletová M, Svejda J: Ultrastructure of blood vessels in damaged pulps. Bull Group Int Rech Sci Stomat 13:445, 1972

Langeland K, Dowden WE, Tronstad L, Langeland LK: Human pulp changes of iatrogenic origin. Oral Surg 32:943, 1971

Langeland K, Langeland LK: Indirect capping and the treatment of deep carious lesions. Internat Dent J 18:326, 1968

Laurichesse JM, Santoro JP: The microcirculation of the dental pulp. I. Techniques of intravital microscopy. Rev Odontostomatol 19:297, 1972

Lawson BF, Mitchell DF: Pharmacologic treatment of painful pulpitis. A preliminary, controlled, double-blind study. Oral Surg 17:47, 1964

Lin L, Langeland K: Light and electron microscopic study of teeth with carious pulp exposures. Oral Surg 51:292, 1981

Longwill DG, Marshall FJ, Creamer HR: Reactivity of human lymphocytes to pulp antigens. J Endodont 8:27, 1982

Loos PJ, Han SS: An enzyme histochemical study of the effect of various concentrations of Formocresol on connective tissues. Oral Surg 31:571, 1971

Luostarinen V: Dental pulp response to trauma. An experimental study. Suom Hammaslääk Toim 67:Suppl. 11, 1971

McWalter GM, El-Kafrawy AH, Mitchell DF: Long-term study of pulp capping in monkeys with three agents. JADA 93:105, 1976

McWalter GM, El-Kafrawy AH, Mitchell DF: Pulp capping in monkeys with a calcium hydroxide compound, an antibiotic, and a polycarboxylate cement. Oral Surg 36:90, 1973

Magnusson B: Attempts to predict prognosis of pulpotomy in primary molars. Scand J Dent Res 78:232, 1970

Magnusson BO: Therapeutic pulpotomies in primary molars with the formocresol technique. Acta Odont Scand 36:157, 1978

Magnusson BO: Therapeutic pulpotomy in primary molars—clinical and histological follow-up. I. Calcium hydroxide paste as wound dressing. Odont Revy 21:425, 1970

Magnusson BO: Therapeutic pulpotomy in primary molars—clinical and histological follow-up. II. Zinc oxide-eugenol as wound dressing. Odont Revy 22:45, 1971

Marshall J, Creamer KR: Reactivity of human lymphocytes to pulp antigens. J Endodont 8:27, 1982

Martin HM: Connective tissue reactions to acid glutaraldehyde. Oral Surg 46:433, 1978

Masterton JB: The healing of wounds of the dental pulp of man. A clinical and histological study. Brit Dent J 120:213, 1966

Mejàre I, Hasselgren G, Hammerström LE: Effect of formaldehyde-containing drugs on human dental pulp evaluated by an enzyme histochemical technique. Scand J Dent Res 84:29, 1976

Messer LB, Cline JT, Korf NW: Long term effects of primary molar pulpotomies on succedaneous bicuspids. J Dent Res 59:116, 1980

Meyers EH, Jawetz E, Goldfein A: Review of Medical Pharmacology, p 364. Los Altos, California, Lange Medical Publications, 1978

Mitchell DF, Shankwalker GB: Osteogenic potential of calcium hydroxide and other materials in soft tissue and bone wounds. J Dent Res 37:1157, 1958

Morawa AP, Stratton LH, Han SS, Copron RE: Clinical evaluation of pulpotomies using dilute formocresol. J Dent Child 42:360, 1975

Moss ML: Experimental induction of osteogenesis. In Calcification in Biological Systems, p 323. Washington, American Ass Adv Sci Publ No 64, 1960

Myers DR, Shoaf HK, Dirkson TR, Pashley DH, Whitford GM, Reynolds KE: Distribution of ^{14}C-formaldehyde after pulpotomy with formocresol. JADA 96:805, 1978

Negm HM, Combe EC, Grant AA: Reaction of the exposed pulps to new cements containing calcium hydroxide. Oral Surg 51:190, 1981

Nelson JR, Lazzari EP, Ranly DM, Madden RM: Biochemical effects of tissue fixatives on bovine pulp. J Endodont 5:139, 1979

Nevins AJ, Findelstein F, Borden BG, Laporta R: Revitalization of pulpless open apex teeth in rhesus monkeys,

using collagen-calcium phosphate gel. J Endodont 2:159, 1976
Nishida O, Okada H, Kawagoe K, Tokunaga A, Tanihata H, Aono M, Yokomizo I: Investigation of homologous antibodies to an extract of rabbit dental pulp. Arch Oral Biol 16:739, 1971
Nixon GS, Hannah CMcD: N-butyl cyanoacrylate as a pulp capping agent. Brit Dent J 133:14, 1972
Obersztyn A, Jedrzcjczyk J, Smiechowska W: Application of lyophilized dentin chips, mixed with prednisolone and neomycin, on infected rat incisor pulp. J Dent Res 47:374, 1968
Okada H, Aono J, Yoshida J, Munemoto K, Nishida O, Yokimozo I: Experimental study on focal infection in rabbits by prolonged sensitization through dental pulp canals. Arch Oral Biol 12:1017, 1967
Page DO, Trump GN, Shaeffer LD: Pulpal studies. I. Passage of ^{3}H-tetracycline into circulatory system through rat molar pulps. Oral Surg 35:555, 1973
Passmore R: How vitamin C deficiency injures the body. Nutr Today, 12:6, 1977
Paterson RC: Bacterial contamination and the exposed pulp. Brit Dent J 140:231, 1976
Paterson RC: Corticosteroids and the exposed pulp. Brit Dent J 140:174, 1976
Pereira JC, Bramante CM, Berbert A, Mondelli J: Effect of calcium hyroxide in powder or in paste form on pulp-capping procedures: Histopathologic and radiographic analysis in dog's pulp. Oral Surg 50:176, 1980
Pereira JC, Stanley HR: Pulp capping: Influence of the exposure site on pulp healing—histologic and radiographic study in dogs' pulp. J Endodont 7:213, 1981
Pitt Ford TR: Pulpal response to MPC for capping exposures. Oral Surg 50:81, 1980
Pohto M, Scheinin A: Vital microscopy of the pulp in the rat incisor. 7. Reactions to silicate cements. Suom Hammaslaak Toim 63:178, 1967
Powell DL, Marshall FJ, Melfi RC: A histopathologic evaluation of tissue reactions to the minimum effective doses of some endodontic drugs. Oral Surg 36:261, 1973
Pruhs RJ, Olen GA, Sharma PS: Relationship between formocresol pulpotomies on primary teeth and enamel defects on their permanent successors. JADA 94:698, 1977
Rasmussen P, Mjör IA: Calcium hydroxide as an ectopic bone inductor in rats. Scand J Dent Res 79:24, 1971
Rayn JJ, Svarrer M: En klinisk-radiologisk efferundersøgelse af koronal vitalamputation: 200 primaere molarer, behandelt med zinkilte-eugenol som amputationspata. Tandlaegebladet 72:718, 1968
Roberts MW, Moffa JP, Hull JR, Lilly GE: An evaluation of a zinc oxide and eugenol cement containing o-ethoxybenzoic acid on the human deciduous dental pulp. Oral Surg 36:416, 1973
Roberts SC, Brilliant JD: Tricalcium phosphate as an adjuct to apical closure in pulpless permanent teeth. J Endodont 1:263, 1975
Rölling I, Hasselgren G, Tronstad L: Morphologic and enzyme histochemical observations of the pulp of human primary molars 3 to 5 years after formocresol treatment. Oral Surg 42:518, 1976
Rölling I, Lambjerg-Hansen H: Pulp condition of successfully formocresol-treated primary molars. Scand J Dent Res 86:267, 1978
Rölling I, Thullin H: Allergy tests against formaldehyde, cresol, and eugenol in children with formocresol pulpotomized primary teeth. Scand J Dent Res 84:345, 1976
Russo MC, Holland R, Souza V: Radiographic and histological evaluation of the treatment of inflamed dental pulps. Int Endo J 15:137, 1982
Safer DS, Avery JK, Cox CF: Histopathologic evaluation of the effects of new polycarboxylate cements on monkey pulps. Oral Surg 33:966, 1972
Sayegh FS: The dentinal bridge in pulp-involved teeth. Part 1. Oral Surg 28:579, 1969
Schroeder A: The problem of direct pulp capping. J Brit Endodont Soc 6:72, 1972
Schröder U, Granath L-E: Early reaction of intact human teeth to calcium hydroxide following experimental pulpotomy and its significance to the development of hard tissue barrier. Odont Rev (Malmo) 22:379, 1971
Schröder U, Granath L-E: Scanning electron microscopy of hard tissue barrier following experimental pulpotomy of intact human teeth and capping with calcium hydroxide. Odont Revy 23:211, 1972
Sciaky I, Pisanti S: Localization of calcium placed over amputated pulps in dogs' teeth. J Dent Res 39:1128, 1960
Sela J, Hirschfield Z, Ulmansky M: Reaction of the rat molar pulp to direct capping with the separate components of Hydrex. Oral Surg 35:118, 1973
Seltzer S, Bender IB: Some influences affecting repair of the exposed pulps of dogs' teeth. J Dent Res 37:678, 1958
Seltzer S, Bender IB, Kaufman IJ, Moodnik R: Alkaline phosphatase in reparative dentinogenesis. Oral Surg 15:859, 1962
Shoshan S, Finkelstein S: Acceleration of wound healing induced by enriched collagen solution. J Surg Res 10:485, 1970
Shovelton DS, Friend LA, Kirk EEJ, Rowe AHR: The efficacy of pulp capping materials. A comparative trial. Brit Dent J 130:385, 1971
Shubich I, Miklos FL, Rapp R, Draus FJ: Release of calcium ions from pulp-capping materials. J Endodont 4:242, 1978
Simon M, van Mullem PJ, Lamers AC: Formocresol: No allergic effect after root canal disinfection in non presensitized guinea pigs. J Endodont 15:269, 1982
Soto-Feine N, Tchernichin AN: Glucocorticoid receptors in dental pulp: A preliminary report. J Endod 8:136, 1982
Stahl SS, Weiss R, Tonna EA: Autoradiographic evaluation of periapical responses to pulpal injury. I. Young rats. Oral Surg 28:249, 1969
Stahl SS, Tonna EA, and Weiss R: Autoradiographic evaluation of periapical responses to pulpal injury. II. Mature rats. Oral Surg 29:270, 1970
Stanley HR, Lundy T: Dycal therapy for pulp exposures. Oral Surg 34:818, 1972
Starkey PE: The treatment of pulpally involved young permanent teeth. Quintessence Int 9:[Sect 2] (9), Report 1660, 1978
Steiner JC, Dow PR, Cathey GM: Inducing root end clo-

sure of non-vital permanent teeth. J Dent Child 35:47, 1968

Steiner JC, Van Hassel HJ: Experimental root apexification in primates. Oral Surg 31:409, 1971

Stenvik A, Iverson J, Mjör IA: Tissue pressure and histology of normal and inflamed tooth pulps in macaque monkeys. Arch Oral Biol 17:1501, 1972

Straffon LH, Han SS: The effect of Formocresol on hamster connective tissue cells, a histologic and quantitative radiographic study with proline-H^3. Arch Oral Biol 13:271, 1968

Straffon LH, Han SS: Effects of varying concentrations of Formocresol on RNA synthesis of connective tissue in sponge implants. Oral Surg 29:915, 1970

Taintor JF, Biesterfeld RC, Langeland K: Irritational or reparative dentin. A challenge of nomenclature. Oral Surg 51:442, 1981

Thoden van Velzen SK, Van den Hooff A: Long-term results of the implantation of glutaraldehyde-fixed tissue. Oral Surg 44:298, 1977

Torneck CD, Smith J: Biologic effects of endodontic procedures on developing incisor teeth. I. Effect of partial and total pulp removal. Oral Surg 30:258, 1970

Torneck C, Smith J, Grindale P: Biological effects of endodontic procedures on developing incisor teeth. II. Effect of pulp injury and oral contamination. Oral Surg 35:378, 1973

Trask PA: Formocresol pulpotomy on (young) permanent teeth. JADA 85:1316, 1972

Tronstad L: Reaction of the exposed pulp to Dycal treatment. Oral Surg 38:945, 1974

Tronstad L, Mjör IA: Capping of the inflamed pulp. Oral Surg 34:477, 1972

Trowbridge H, Edwall L, and Panopoulos P: Effect of zinc oxide-eugenol and calcium hydroxide on intradental nerve activity. J Endodont 8:403, 1982

Ulmánsky M, Sela J, Langer M, Yaari A: Response of pulpotomy wounds in normal human teeth to successively applied Ledermix and Calxyl. Arch Oral Biol 16:1393, 1971

Van Hassel HJ, Natkin E: Induction of root end closure. J Dent Child 37:57, 1970

van Mullem PJ, Simon M, Lamers AC: Formocresol: A root canal disinfectant provoking allergic skin reactions in presensitized guinea pigs. J Endodont 9:25, 1983

Wade GW: The cyanoacrylates (tissue adhesives): A survey of the literature. J Dist Columbia Dent Soc 44:141, 1969

Watts A: Bacterial contamination and the toxicity of silicate and zinc phosphate cements. Brit Dent J 146:7, 1979

Watts A, Paterson RC: Migration of materials and microorganisms in the dental pulp of dogs and rats. J Endodont 8:53, 1982

Webb JG, Bussell NE: A comparison of the inflammatory response produced by commercial eugenol and purified eugenol. J Dent Res 60:1724, 1981

Weiss MB, Bjorvatn K: Pulp capping in deciduous and newly erupted permanent teeth of monkeys. Oral Surg 29:769, 1970

Wesselink PR, Thoden van Velzen SK, Van den Hooff A: Tissue reaction to implantation of unfixed and glutaraldehyde-fixed heterologous tissue. J Endodont 3:299, 1977

Yaffe A, Ehrlich J, Shoshan S: One-year follow up for the use of collagen for biological anchoring of acrylic dental roots in the dog. Arch Oral Biol 27:999, 1982

15
THE INTERRELATIONSHIP OF PULP AND PERIODONTAL DISEASE

LATERAL AND ACCESSORY CANALS: ANATOMIC CONSIDERATIONS

The presence of lateral canals and their distribution in teeth have been demonstrated by numerous methods. Saunders (1957) used a microradiographic technique to visualize lateral canals in the pulp chamber floor in a vital human molar (Fig. 15-1); numerous blood vessels were shown coursing between the pulp and the periodontal ligament. Kramer (1951) studied the vasculature between pulp and periodontal ligament by perfusing teeth with India ink; the lateral canals were located in the midradicular region between the apex and the floor of the pulp chamber (Fig. 15-2). Radiographs taken by clinicians after the filling of root canals by diffusion or pressure techniques (Fig. 15-3) often demonstrate lateral canals in various regions of the roots and floors of pulp chambers.

Lateral and accessory canals are ubiquitous, and their distribution is readily observed in histologic specimens of anterior and posterior human teeth. Our data are from histologic studies of human, dog, and monkey teeth as well as numerous clinical cases. Examination of serial sections shows large numbers of lateral canals within the roots of posterior teeth and, occasionally, in anterior teeth. We have been able to trace the course of these canals from the pulp to the periodontal structures. Numerous accessory canals and foramina were also noted in the apical thirds of the roots (Fig. 15-4).

In molars, a great many accessory canals were seen, especially in the cementum "web" fusing the roots. In most instances, these canals were present in both the apical third and the coronal portions of the teeth. Lateral canals in profusion were seen in the furcation regions (Fig. 15-5) in some instances, coursing at different levels from the interradicular region of the tooth into the coronal portion of the pulp. In other instances, they traversed the root and entered the root canal. The tissue in the lateral canals was composed of capillaries, pulp cells, ground substance, and fibers and was confluent with the pulp tissue proper. In many teeth, the diameter of accessory foramina or lateral canals was extremely small, permitting only small-caliber vessels and their supporting stroma to pass. At some levels, the canals appeared to be obliterated; at others, remnants of pulp tissue were discernible. In a few teeth, the foramina on the periodontal side as well as the lumina of the lateral canals were narrowed by cementum dep-

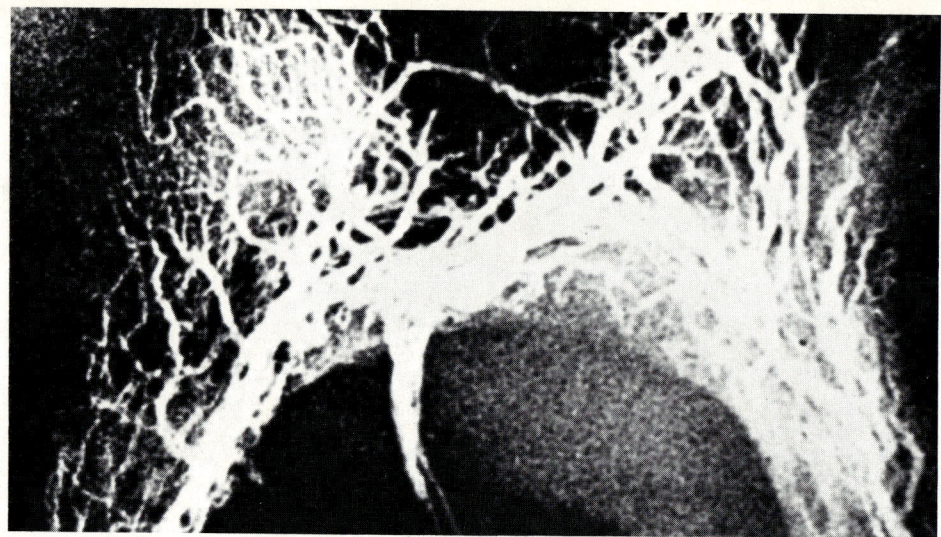

FIG. 15-1 Microradiograph showing the arrangement of blood vessels in the upper left second molar of a 22-year-old male. Note the vascular bridge extending across the pulp chamber and connecting the root canal vessels. Aberrant vessels are entering the pulp chamber near the bifurcation of the roots. (Saunders RL de CH: Microradiographic studies of human adult and fetal pulp vessels. In Cosslett VE, Engström A, Patee HH Jr (eds): X-ray Microscopy and Microradiography, pp 561–571. New York, Academic Press, 1957)

FIG. 15-2 *(A)* Buccal root of an upper first permanent molar. Six groups of vessels connect the root canal with the periodontal ligament. ×14.5. *(B)* Higher magnification of part of the specimen shown in *(A)*. In each case, the channel connecting the root canal (left) with the periodontal ligament contains a pair of vessels, one much larger than the other. The smaller vessels resemble arteries, the larger vessels veins. ×83. (Kramer IRH: Arch Oral Biol 2:177, 1960)

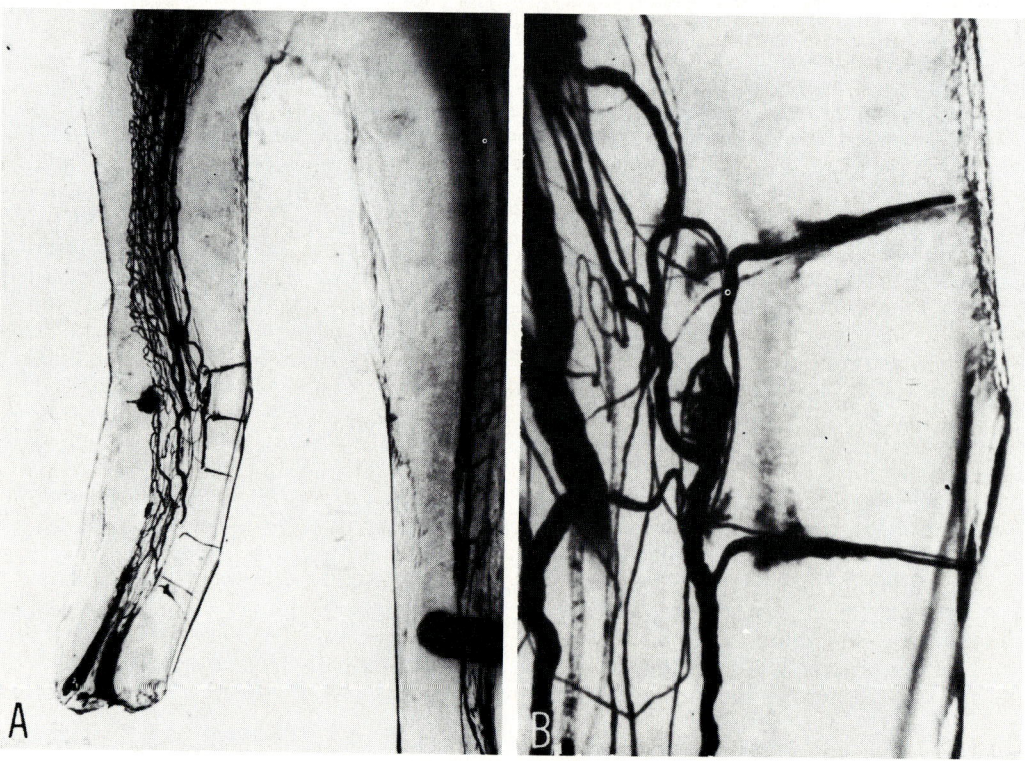

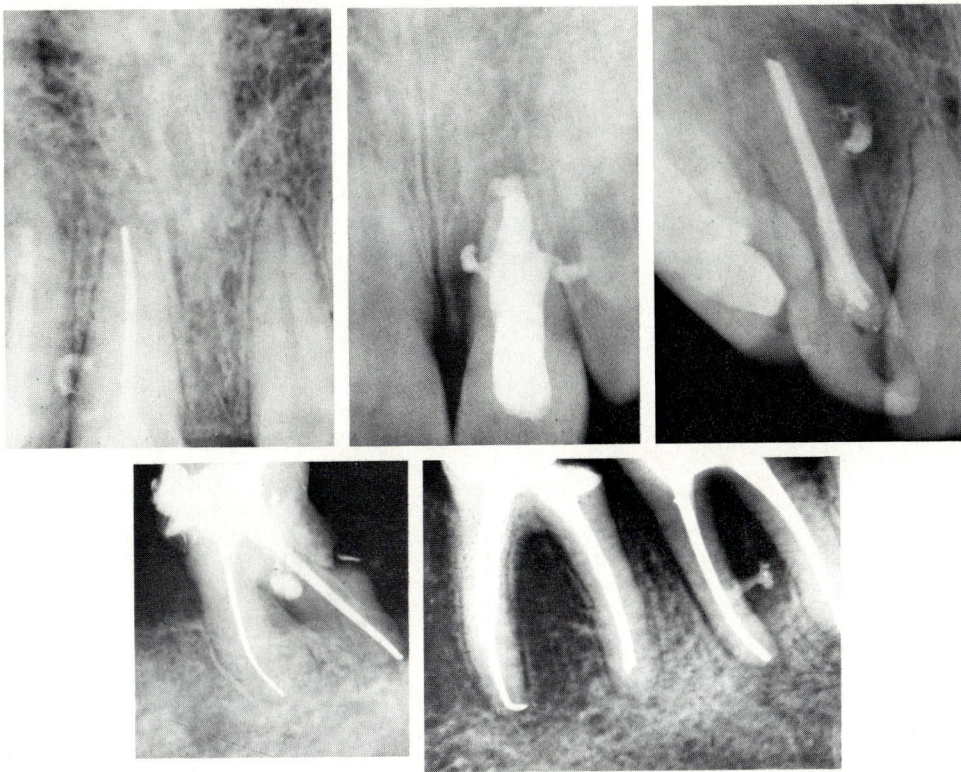

FIG. 15-3 *(Top)* Note location and distribution of lateral canals in some upper anterior teeth. *(Bottom)* Distribution of lateral canals in first molar and second molar, following root canal filling by pressure technique with cement.

osition. Many anomalies were observed in the size and shape of molar root canals, e.g., the palatal canal. Frequently, the canals fanned out toward the apex in a canoe-shaped arrangement. In some instances, chronic inflammation was found in one portion of the "canoe" and not in the remainder. Langeland et al (1974) observed inflammation in one root canal of molars and not in the other canals.

Blood Supply

The main blood supply of the pulp enters through the apical foramen or foramina. However, more than one blood vessel usually is present at the apex of a tooth (Fig. 15-4). In addition to the vessels entering the apical foramina, other vessels occasionally come into the pulp in the furcation areas (Fig. 15-5) and along the side of the root, at both the inner and the outer aspects (Fig. 15-2; Lowman et al, 1973). In molars, in which the roots are fused with cementum, vessels that course from one root canal to another are frequently present. Blood vessels from the periodontal ligament also may penetrate the cementum webbing and run to both canals. Perfusion of teeth with dyes, carbon particles, or radiopaque materials demonstrates the ramifying of blood vessels entering the pulp from many regions (Figs. 15-2 and 15-4). The intimate relationship between the periodontal vascular plexus and the pulpal blood vessels has been graphically demonstrated by Kramer (1960), Castelli and Dempster (1965), Carranza et al (1966) and Cutright and Bhaskar (1967, 1969). Besides vascular communication, connective tissue fibers run from the dental pulp to the periodontal ligament.

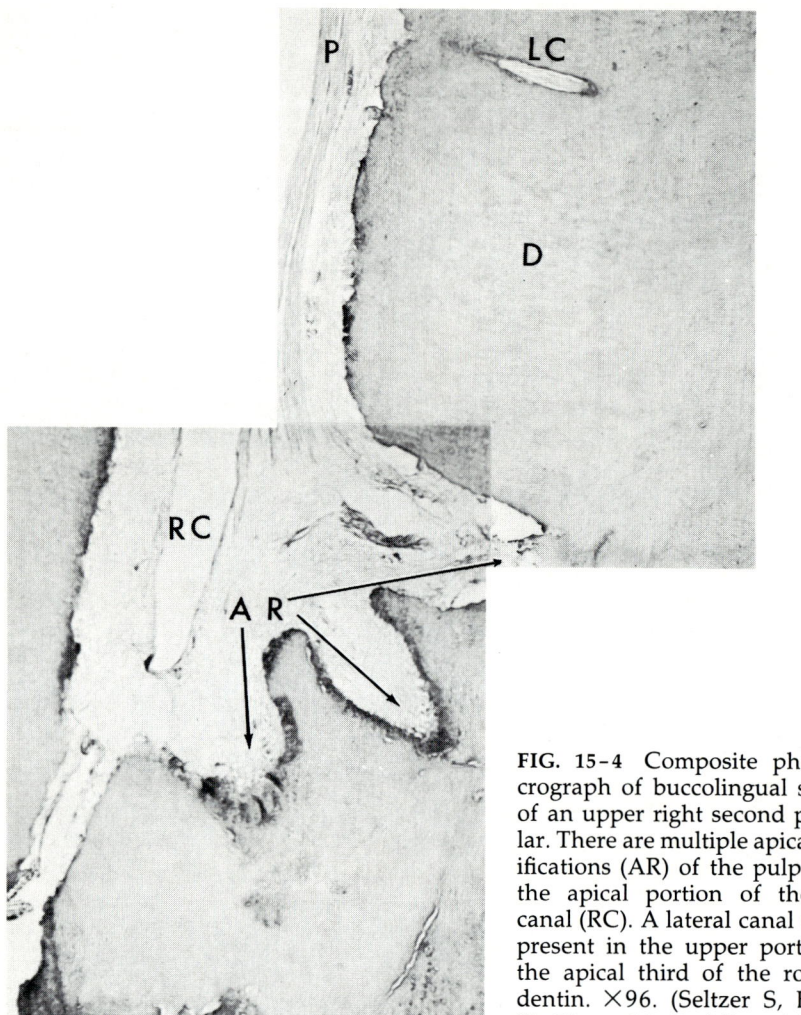

FIG. 15-4 Composite photomicrograph of buccolingual section of an upper right second premolar. There are multiple apical ramifications (AR) of the pulp (P) in the apical portion of the root canal (RC). A lateral canal (LC) is present in the upper portion of the apical third of the root. D, dentin. ×96. (Seltzer S, Bender IB, Ziontz M: Oral Surg 16:1474, 1963)

THE EFFECT OF PERIODONTAL DISEASE ON THE DENTAL PULP

A definite relationship appears to exist between the presence of periodontal lesions and the status of the pulp tissue. The effect of periodontal disease on the human dental pulp was reported first by Turner and Drew (1919), who showed that bacteria were present in periodontally involved teeth but absent in normal teeth. Cahn (1926, 1927) and later Sicher (1936) described the presence of communicating channels through the cementum and dentin, i.e., lateral canals, in a noncarious tooth with a focal area of chronic inflammation in the pulp at the level of the orifice of the lateral canal. They attributed the inflammatory pulp changes to ingress of toxins through these lateral canals.

In our histologic examinations of the pulps of 178 human teeth, intact, unaffected pulps were found in only a small number of teeth; many teeth showed distinct inflammatory and degenerative changes (Bender and Seltzer, 1972) (Table 15-1). However, the incidence of pulp inflammation was slightly higher, and the incidence of pulp degeneration was distinctly

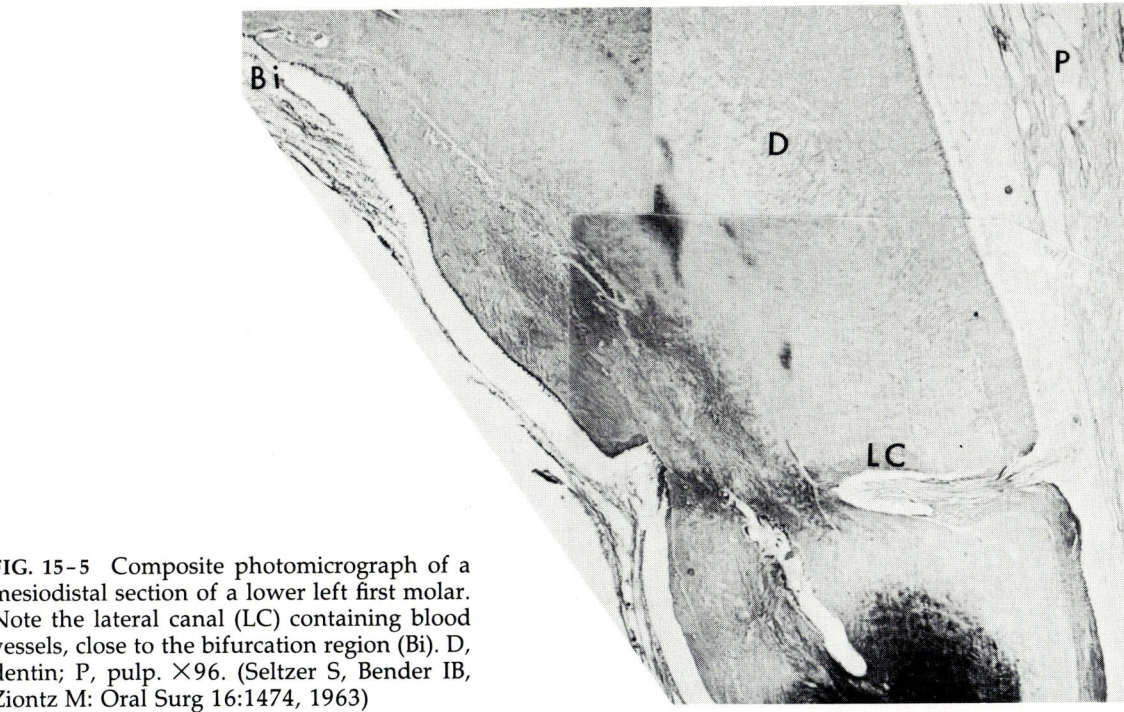

FIG. 15-5 Composite photomicrograph of a mesiodistal section of a lower left first molar. Note the lateral canal (LC) containing blood vessels, close to the bifurcation region (Bi). D, dentin; P, pulp. ×96. (Seltzer S, Bender IB, Ziontz M: Oral Surg 16:1474, 1963)

TABLE 15-1
Comparison of Histologic Status of Pulps in Periodontally and Nonperiodontally Involved Teeth

HISTOLOGIC DIAGNOSIS OF PULP	GROUP I NONPERIODONTALLY INVOLVED TEETH WITH CARIES, RESTORATIONS, OR BOTH		GROUP II PERIODONTALLY INVOLVED TEETH WITH CARIES, RESTORATIONS, OR BOTH		GROUP III WITH NO CARIES OR RESTORATIONS	
	Number of Teeth	Percentage	Number of Teeth	Percentage	Number of Teeth	Percentage
Intact, uninflamed	15	22	0	0	12	21
Pulposis*	7	10	11	20	18	32
Pulpitis	37	54	30	57	21	37
Total necrosis	9	13	12	23	6	10
Total	68		53		57	

* Pulposis: a term used to describe various stages of pulp atrophy and degeneration
(Bender IB, Seltzer S: The effect of periodontal disease on the pulp. Oral Surg 33:458, 1972)

308 | THE DENTAL PULP

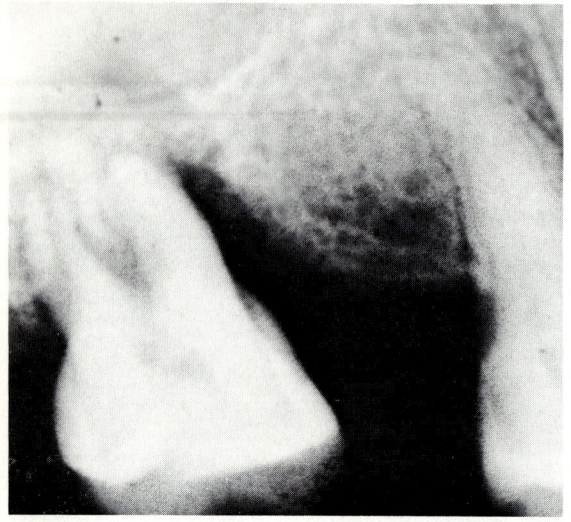
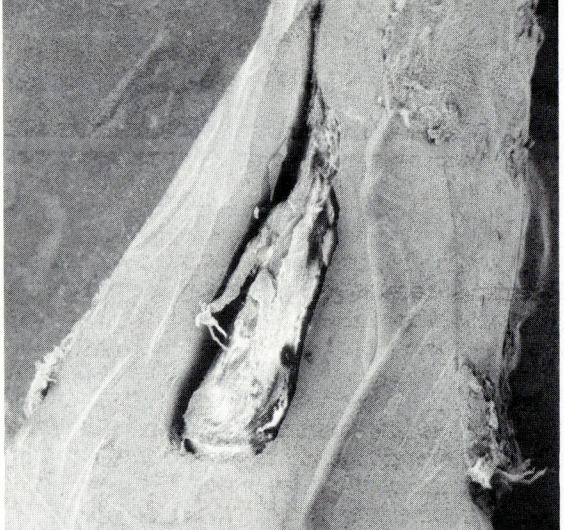
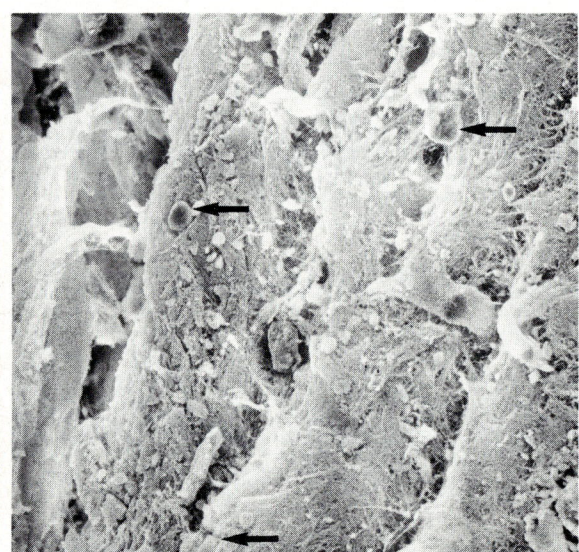

FIG. 15-6 *(Top)* Radiograph of periodontally involved upper left first molar. *(Bottom left)* Scanning electron micrograph showing fibrosis of coronal pulp tissue. ×10. *(Bottom right)* Higher magnification of pulp showing abundant collagen fibers and calcified cells (arrows). ×500.

greater in periodontally involved teeth. Such findings are in agreement with those of Rubach and Mitchell (1965); Mandi (1972); Langeland et al (1974); Bergenholtz (1977); and Okata et al (1979). The deleterious effects of periodontal disease on the pulp were not observed by other investigators (Sauerwein, 1955, 1956; Mazur and Massler, 1964; Czarnecki and Schilder, 1979). They found that pulps were not affected by periodontal disease. The disparity in the findings among the investigators may be attributed to variations in the incidence of teeth with lateral canals among different experimental animals and humans. Animal experiments have demonstrated that there is a scarcity of lateral canals in the teeth of rice rats (Hattler et al, 1977) and monkeys (Bergenholtz and Lindhe, 1978). This lack of communication between periodontal pockets and pulps may be related to the presence or absence of pulp pathosis.

The degenerative and inflammatory pulp changes that are associated with human periodontal disease are described in the following sections. The findings are based primarily on our observations but include those of other investigators.

ATROPHIC CHANGES (PULPOSIS)

Atrophic pulps are present in many periodontally involved teeth, the largest number in any specific diagnostic category. We found atrophic pulpal changes twice as often in periodontally involved teeth with caries, restorations, or both, (Group II, Table 15–1), and three times as often in periodontally involved teeth without caries, restorations, or both, (Group III, Table 15–1), compared with teeth without periodontal disease.

The atrophic pulps invariably had fewer than the normal number of cells in both the coronal and the radicular portions of the pulp. Collagen deposition was increased. Abundant dystrophic mineralizations were present throughout the pulp tissue (Fig. 15–6), often almost completely obliterating the coronal portions of the pulp and heavily infiltrating the fibrous tissue in the roots (Fig. 15–7). In addition, the root canals were excessively narrowed by the deposition of large quantities of reparative dentin along the dentinal walls, a finding corroborated by Lantelme et al (1976; Fig. 15–7). This dentin was highly irregular, having little or no tubular appearance. In some histologic sections, the canals appeared to be obliterated, but at other levels some remnants of the pulp tissue were seen. On x-ray examination, the canals appeared to be completely calcified in these instances. However, completely calcified canals were not usually found in histologic examinations.

Mechanism

The mechanism for the production of atrophy within the pulps appears to be interference with the blood supply through the lateral canals, both within the furcation regions and along the sides of the roots. The blood vessels supplying a small area of the pulp are involved by the periodontal lesion (Fig. 15–8). Loss of the blood supply to a small region of the pulp tissue leads to the death of the pulp cells supplied by the affected capillaries. Inasmuch as an immediate adequate collateral circulation is not available, there is insufficient nutriment and oxygen to satisfy the metabolic needs of the cells, and they die. In other words, a small area of infarction takes place, resulting in coagulation necrosis. The death of the cells and their subsequent calcification are natural sequelae to the deprivation of nourishment (Plačková and Vahl, 1974).

Presumably, periodontal lesions affect the pulp through this mechanism, inducing atrophic and other degenerative changes such as reduction in number of pulp cells, dystrophic calcification, fibrosis, reparative dentin formation, inflammation, and resorption. Stahl (1963) and Sinai and Soltanoff (1973) demonstrated similar effects, specifically the formation of huge quantities of reparative dentin in the pulp canals of rats, merely from gingival wounding by stripping the gingiva to the alveolar crest. Stahl (1966) also reported finding reparative dentin formation in the pulps of the teeth of cadaver specimens opposite periodontal pockets. Owing to impairment of nutrition, which is gradual and takes place over long periods, some pulp cells are deprived of the available blood supply, and, therefore, they die. However, death of the cells is so gradual that morphologic evidence sometimes appears to be lacking. The cells of the pulps of periodontally involved teeth appear to be smaller than normal, with greater collagen deposition than normal.

Possibly, some of the atrophic changes can be ascribed to the pressure atrophy that results from the mobility of periodontally involved teeth. The increased pressure from the movement of these teeth may affect the blood vessels of the main and lateral canals, thereby reducing the vascular supply to the pulpal tissue.

Histochemical studies have demonstrated the presence of greater amounts of enzymes, such as alkaline and acid phosphatases, 5-nucleotidase, glucose-6-phosphatase, and adenosine triphosphatase (ATPase), in the pulps of periodontally involved teeth than in those of normal teeth. Such increased concentrations of enzymes were found especially in the endothelium of the blood vessels (Brzezińska, 1968). Thus, periodontal disease may induce a more rapid aging process because of circulatory interference, with subsequent alterations in the nutritional status of the cells of the pulp.

Anatomic Anomalies

In molars containing enamel "pearls" many openings are found through which pulps could be affected (Fig. 15–9). Another anatomic anomaly that may affect the pulp is a developmental defect associated with an invagination or a vertical developmental radicular groove. These grooves are found in the central fossa area in the crowns of upper central and lateral teeth in the region of the cingulum (Simon et al, 1971; Hiatt, 1977). Such a groove can provide a nidus for progressive inflammation and can lead

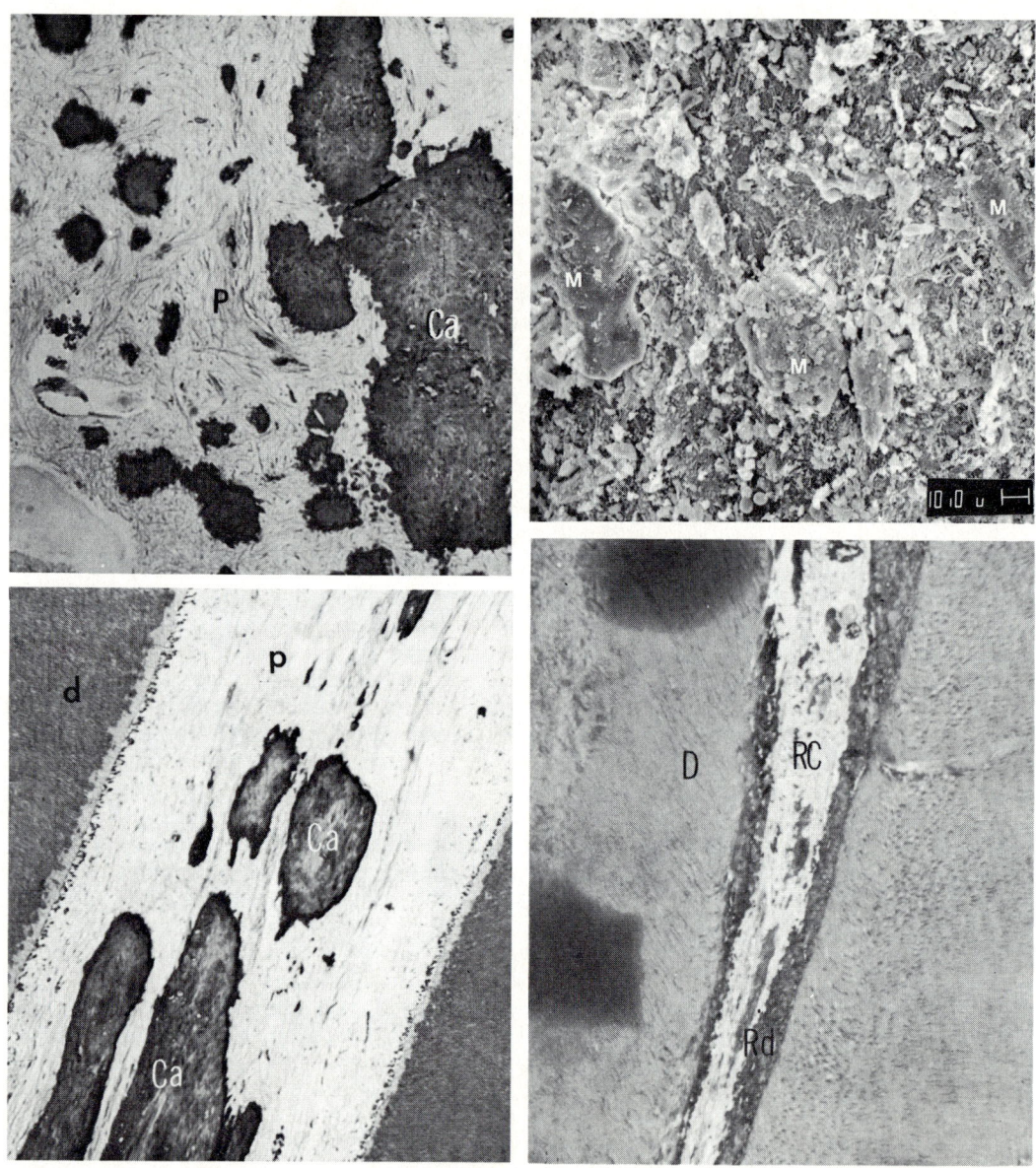

FIG. 15-7 *(Top, left)* Atrophic pulp due to periodontal disease. The coronal pulp (P) is atrophic. Note the abundant dystrophic mineralizations (Ca) throughout the pulp (P) tissue. ×96. *(Top, right)* Scanning electron micrograph of periodontally involved coronal pulp. Numerous mineralizations (M) are present. ×400. *(Bottom, left)* Dystrophic mineralizations (Ca) in the radicular pulp (P) of the same tooth. d, dentin. ×96. *(Bottom, right)* Narrowing of the root canal (RC) by deposition of reparative dentin (Rd). D, root dentin. ×96. (Seltzer S, Bender IB, Ziontz M: The interrelationship of pulp and periodontal disease. Oral Surg 16:1474, 1963)

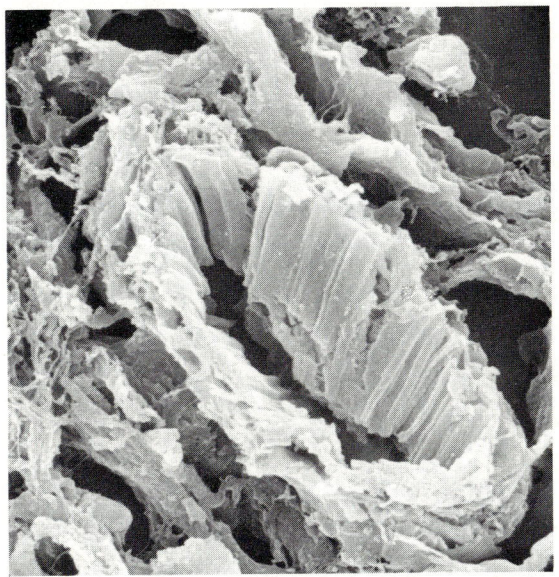

FIG. 15-8 Scanning electron micrograph of coronal pulp tissue section of periodontally involved tooth. A calcified blood vessel is present in the center. ×2000.

to an untreatable periodontal condition, ultimately affecting the pulp in the apical region or the region of lateral canals.

We found no constant relationship between the depth of the periodontal pocket, the extent of bone loss, or the extent of the periodontal disease, and the status of the pulp. In a number of teeth in which the roots were practically denuded of bone, either intact-uninflamed or atrophic pulps were found. We did find that reactions in the pulp appeared to be related to the presence of lateral and accessory canals. It seems likely, therefore, that pulp tissue can be affected by periodontal disease, but it does not necessarily follow that the pulp becomes involved just because periodontal disease exists. Rubach and Mitchell (1965) noted only 11 teeth with affected pulps in 74 periodontally involved teeth. However, the above observations indicate that periodontal lesions may produce a degenerative effect on the dental pulps of the involved teeth.

INFLAMMATORY CHANGES

In addition to atrophic changes, inflammatory lesions of varying intensity, including the transitional stage of inflammation, chronic pulpitis,

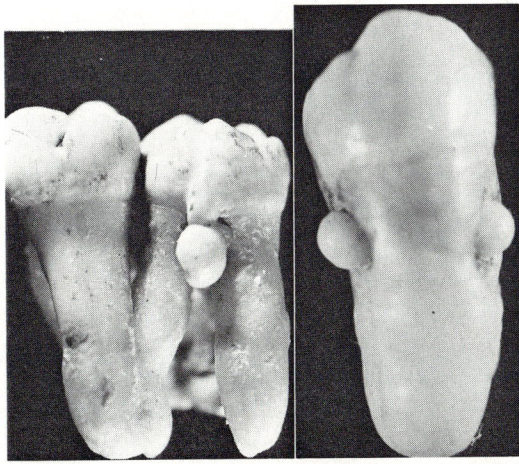
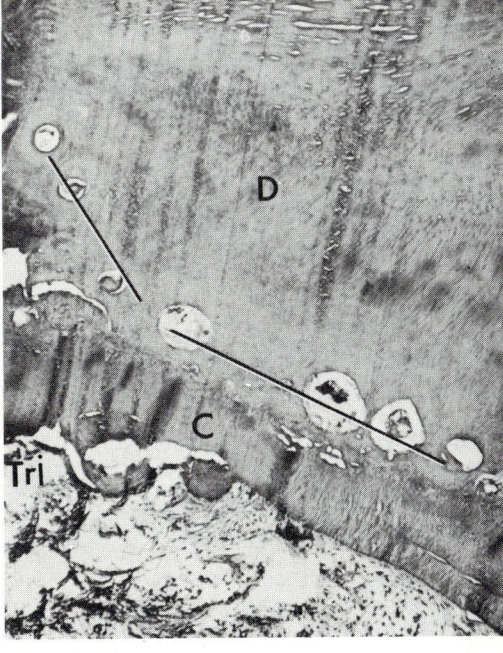

FIG. 15-9 (*Left*) Enamel pearls. (Cavanha AO: Enamel pearls. Oral Surg 19:373, 1965). (*Right*) Buccolingual section of an upper second molar containing enamel pearls. Near the trifurcation region (Tri) is a series of canals, indicated by solid lines. C, cementum; D, dentin. ×96. (Seltzer S, Bender IB, Ziontz M: Oral Surg 16:1474, 1963)

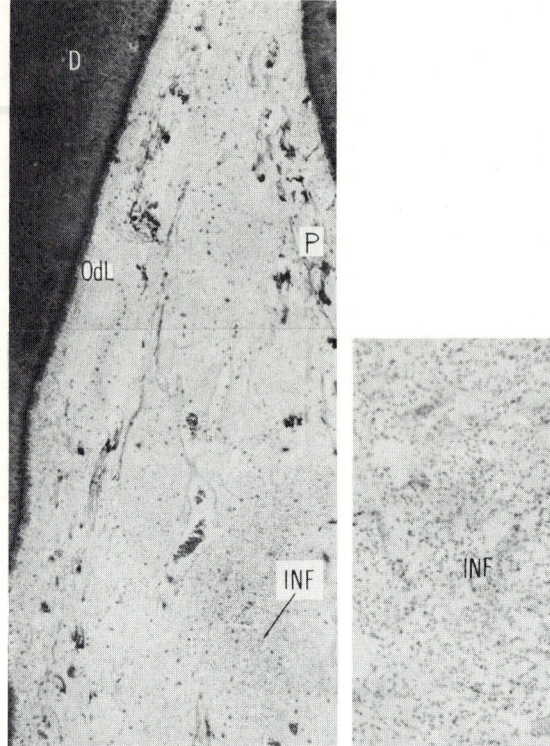

FIG. 15-10 Composite photomicrograph of a periodontally involved tooth that is free of caries. There have been no operative procedures. *(Left)* A region of chronic inflammation (INF) is present in the pulp (P). The odontoblastic layer (OdL) appears thinner. D, dentin. ×54. *(Right)* Higher magnification of region of chronic inflammation marked by arrow in picture at left. ×240.

partial (Fig. 15-10) and total, and necrosis (Fig. 15-11), were observed in all three groups. However, we found the percentage of teeth with total necrosis to be higher in Group II than in Groups I and III (see Table 15-1). In deep periodontal lesions, exposed lateral canals were frequently found along the sides of the roots. Such exposure interfered with the blood supply of the pulps. In the more advanced lesions, necrotic pulp tissue was discovered in the larger lateral canals that were exposed because of bone loss (Fig. 15-12).

On occasion, chronic inflammatory cells, consisting primarily of lymphocytes, were found in the radicular portion of the pulp at the level of a lateral canal communicating with the periodontal lesion. The inflammatory cell infiltration was light and chronic in nature. In serial section examinations, the coronal portion of the pulp was sometimes found to be free of inflammation.

The incidence of inflammatory reaction in teeth exposed to a combination of pulpal and periodontal irritants (Group II) was greater than in teeth with periodontal disease alone (Group III). Of the teeth in Group II, 80% showed pulp inflammation and necrosis, compared with 47% in Group III and 67% in Group I. The differences among the three groups are statistically significant. Thus, it appears that there is an interrelationship between caries, restorative procedures, or both, and periodontal lesions. Caries or restorative procedures can affect the pulps of periodontally involved teeth, and conversely, periodontal disease can affect pulps of teeth with caries or restorations.

RESORPTIONS

Resorptions of the sides of the roots are frequently found subjacent to the granulation tissue overlying the roots. When the periodontal lesions are deep, resorptions are found also within the root canals, often opposite lateral canals and at the apical foramina (Fig. 15-13).

TOXIC PRODUCTS

Inflammatory lesions in the pulp may also be responses to toxic products entering through canal openings that normally are covered with bone and periodontal ligament, but now are exposed to the oral fluids.

Pulp inflammation in periodontally involved teeth can occur from extension of the inflamed periodontal connective tissue. Just as products from inflamed pulpal tissue can cause periapical or interradicular inflammation, periodontal disease can cause a pulpitis. A retrograde or secondary pulpitis may be associated with periodontal disease (Fig. 15-11). In severe periodontal lesions, not only are apical granulomas and root resorptions produced through extension of the granulomatous tissue from the pocket, but also inflammatory cells can actually be detected infiltrating the apical pulp tissues. The coronal pulp tissue may, for a time, remain uninflamed.

In turn, inflamed or necrotic pulps, produced from periodontal lesions, are instrumental in perpetuating the periodontal lesion by elaborating toxic products that invade the periodontal

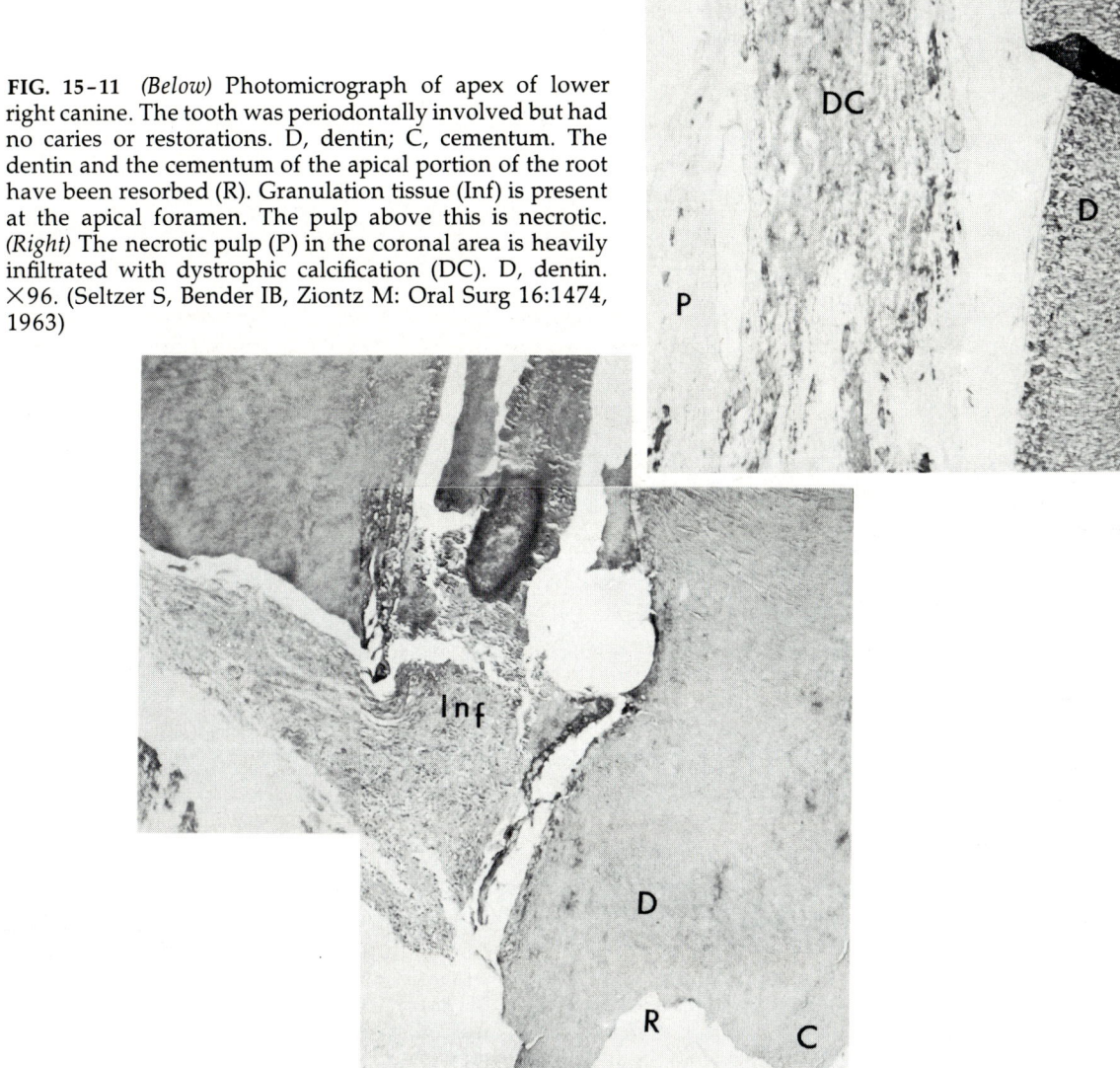

FIG. 15-11 *(Below)* Photomicrograph of apex of lower right canine. The tooth was periodontally involved but had no caries or restorations. D, dentin; C, cementum. The dentin and the cementum of the apical portion of the root have been resorbed (R). Granulation tissue (Inf) is present at the apical foramen. The pulp above this is necrotic. *(Right)* The necrotic pulp (P) in the coronal area is heavily infiltrated with dystrophic calcification (DC). D, dentin. ×96. (Seltzer S, Bender IB, Ziontz M: Oral Surg 16:1474, 1963)

tissues through the same lateral canals or other means of ingress. Thus, a vicious circle is established. In terms of treatment, it is difficult to visualize an effective cure without concurrent elimination of both the pulpal and the periodontal lesions.

Microorganisms

The microorganisms present in periodontal lesions may be capable of producing necrosis of cells and fiber degradation by action of their metabolic products, destructive enzymes, or other mechanisms. Such microorganisms, associated with periodontal lesions and root caries, have been found by Langeland et al (1974) to be capable of evoking an inflammatory reaction in the pulps of the involved teeth.

Toxic products from microorganisms in the oral cavity can also affect the pulp through denuded dentinal tubules. Mjör and Tronstad (1972) and Langeland et al (1974) have demonstrated that bacterial toxins produce an inflam-

314 | THE DENTAL PULP

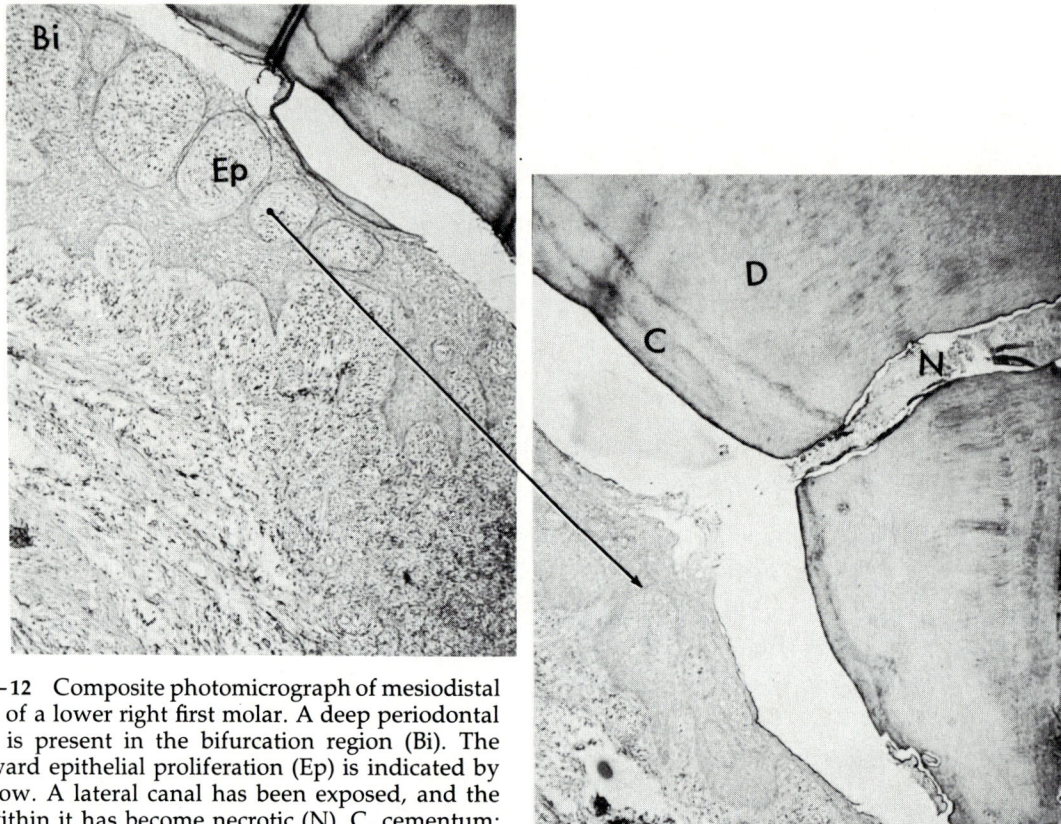

FIG. 15-12 Composite photomicrograph of mesiodistal section of a lower right first molar. A deep periodontal pocket is present in the bifurcation region (Bi). The downward epithelial proliferation (Ep) is indicated by the arrow. A lateral canal has been exposed, and the pulp within it has become necrotic (N). C, cementum; D, dentin. ×96. (Seltzer S, Bender IB, Ziontz M: Oral Surg 16:1474, 1963)

matory response in the pulp when dentinal tubules are exposed to the oral fluids.

Furthermore, Bergenholtz et al (1977) demonstrated that pulpitis may develop in the teeth of immunized monkeys after topical application of bovine serum albumin to the exposed dentin.

EFFECTS OF PERIODONTAL TREATMENT AND LOCAL MEDICATION

Deep Scaling

Deep scaling and curettage in periodontal treatment may possibly be instrumental in causing pulp damage. In laboratory animals, pulp damage from stripping of the gingivae from the alveolar crest was demonstrated by Stahl (1963). In beagles, more reparative dentin was formed after deep, rather than superficial, root planing (Selvig and Nilveus, 1983).

Both in vitro and in vivo experiments by Stallard (1968) showed that intact cementum acted as a barrier to the inward penetration of a dye (2% aqueous solution of trypan blue) into the dentin. Such protection is lost when cementum is removed by root planing. Studies on human teeth have revealed some odontoblastic damage from crushing of cementum, but a controlled investigation is needed. Sensitivity of the teeth after deep scaling and curettage may be due not only to denudation of the roots of the teeth but also to the production of inflammatory changes or hemorrhages in the pulps of the teeth. This process is similar to the induction of an acute inflammation in the pulp following deep cavity preparation in the crown of the tooth.

Deep scaling may sever blood vessels, especially in the furcation regions of molars. The consequent loss of blood supply to a small region of the pulp can produce a pain spasm and ultimately death of the pulp cells supplied by the

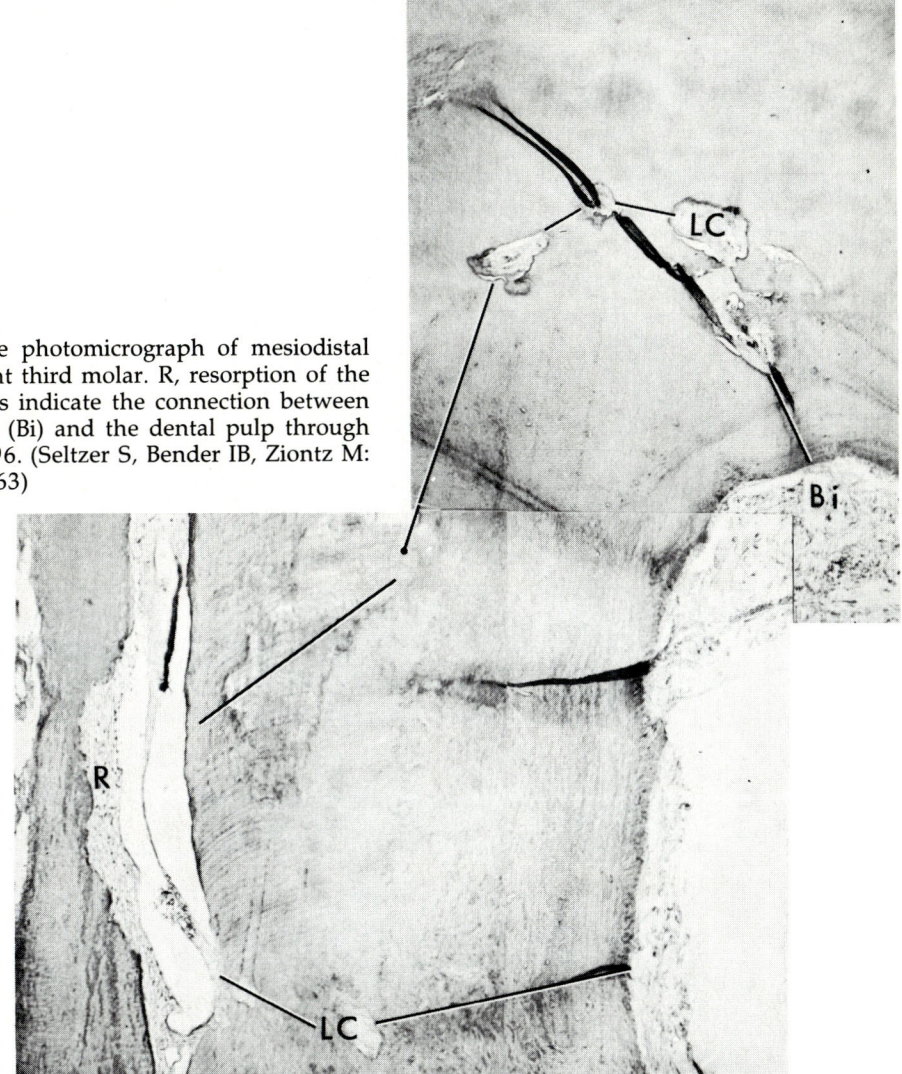

FIG. 15-13 Composite photomicrograph of mesiodistal section of a lower right third molar. R, resorption of the buccal root. Solid lines indicate the connection between the bifurcation region (Bi) and the dental pulp through lateral canals (LC). ×96. (Seltzer S, Bender IB, Ziontz M: Oral Surg 16:1474, 1963)

affected capillaries—a phenomenon comparable to a cardiac anginal attack. A small area of infarction develops in the pulp, followed by coagulation necrosis. Death of the cells, with subsequent calcification, is the usual sequel of blood deprivation.

However, not all periodontal curettements terminate in pulpal inflammation and necrosis. Evans* treated a periodontally involved molar with a deep pocket extending to the apex of the mesial root. Bone was transplanted to the curet-

* Evans R: Personal communication, 1972.

ted pocket. After 2 years, radiographs showed bone regeneration around the involved mesial root, with elimination of the periodontal pocket. Subsequently, the mesial root was resected *en bloc*, with the surrounding bone in place. Histologic studies showed bone regeneration around the periodontally involved root and all the transplanted bone appeared to be completely remodeled. One of the lateral canals in the apical third of the root was narrowed, and the foramen on the periodontal side showed deposition of cementum, suggesting that it was being obliterated. The coronal portion of the pulp was found

316 | THE DENTAL PULP

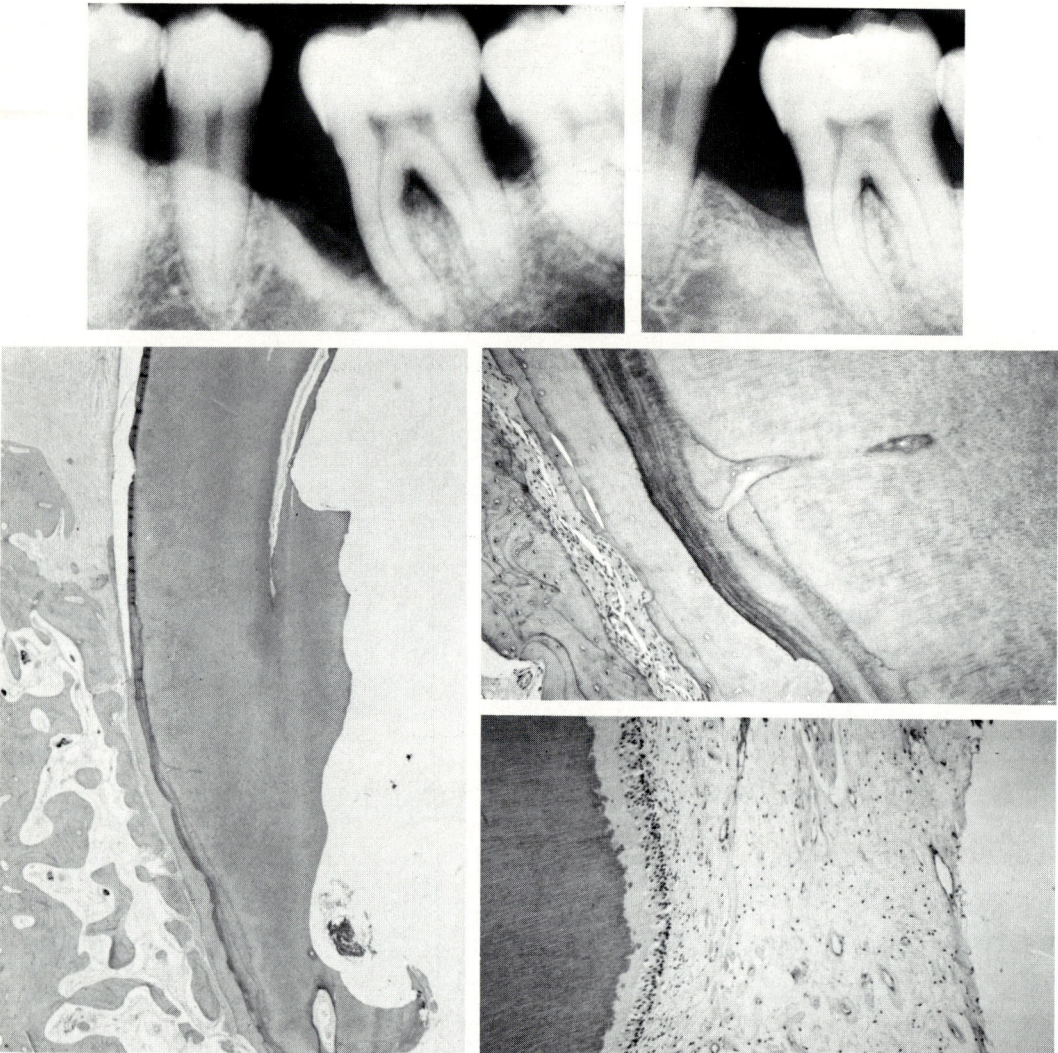

FIG. 15-14 *(Top, left)* Radiograph of lower right second molar. Periodontal lesion has persisted for 2 years following periodontal therapy. *(Top, right)* Treatment with bone transplant eliminated periodontal lesion. Radiograph shows evidence of healing 2 years after autogenous bone graft. No endodontic therapy was necessary. *(Bottom, left)* Resected root and surrounding bone, showing evidence of healing with new bone and cementum deposition. *(Right, center)* Deposition of cementum over orifice and obliteration of lateral canal. *(Right, bottom)* Section through coronal portion of pulp shows relatively normal pulp. (Courtesy of Dr. Richard Evans, Philadelphia) *(Top, left; top, right; bottom, left; and right, bottom* Bender IB, Seltzer S: Oral Surg 33:455, 1972)

to be relatively normal and the radicular portion displayed large calcific deposits (Fig. 15-14).

Thus, a productive response may occur in the pulps of periodontally involved teeth when the disease progresses slowly or there are fewer or narrower lateral canals. Cementum deposition appears to obliterate these canals, thereby retarding or preventing ingress of pulp irritants.

Local Medication

Local medication is another possible cause for injury and necrosis of pulp cells. The use of drugs such as formalin, zinc chloride, and sodium fluoride for desensitization of the necks of teeth, especially when root surfaces have been exposed by loss of bone and an epithelial downward proliferation, is potentially damaging. In these circumstances, irritating chemicals may enter the pulp tissue through accessory or lateral foramina, thereby causing injury to the pulp cells as well as the vessels that supply them with nutrients. For example, formalin, in relatively low concentrations, exerts a lethal effect on cells. Other substances may cause destruction of cells by derangement of osmotic equilibrium.

However, a few drugs used to treat hypersensitive dentin have been reported to induce dentinal sclerosis, with no adverse pulp effects (see Chap. 10, Chemical Irritants).

THE EFFECT OF PULP LESIONS ON PERIODONTAL LESIONS

Granulomas develop in the apical periodontal ligament following inflammation of the pulp from caries, trauma, or restorative procedures. In numerous microscopic studies, we found granulomas not only in the apical regions but also in any portion of the root or furcation area related to the location of lateral canals. Thus, any portion of the periodontium can become affected by pulp inflammation. The granulation tissue emanates from inflamed tissue in lateral canals and accessory foramina. This tissue is an extension of the chronic pulp inflammation.

Interradicular periodontal lesions can be initiated and perpetuated by inflamed or necrotic pulps. Such pulpitis-related bifurcation lesions have been induced experimentally in the teeth of cats, dogs, monkeys, and humans (Moss et al, 1965; Winter and Kramer, 1965, 1972; Seltzer et al, 1967). In extracted human teeth, granulomatous tissue occasionally is found attached to — and, obviously, emanating from — inflamed pulp tissue in lateral canals and accessory foramina. Inflammation of the periodontal ligament from severely inflamed pulp lesions and necrotic pulps can spread readily through these channels.

We have observed inflammation and epithelial proliferation, but no periodontal pocket formation, in the interradicular regions of dog and monkey molars after experimental pulp capping and root canal procedures. Comparative controls showed no inflammation. A periodontal lesion of this type may be considered a secondary periodontitis. On occasion, the apical granuloma may extend into the sulcular region, causing a sinus tract, also commonly known as a fistula. In a tooth with a carious exposure and chronic pulp inflammation, we have observed chronic inflammation in the periodontal ligament opposite the lateral canals of the bifurcation area (Fig. 15–15). This inflammatory lesion could be demonstrated only by serial section. In another tooth, bone necrosis developed in the furcation region of a lower first molar following the application of an arsenical dressing in the pulp chamber (Fig. 15–16).

Another mechanism by which the periodontal structures become involved was revealed by examination of teeth on which the interradicular bone remained attached to the roots after extraction. In teeth in which the periapical granulomas resulting from necrotic pulps were extensive, the granulomatous tissue was present all along the lateral aspects of the roots and had caused extensive resorptions (Fig. 15–15). In addition, the crest of the alveolar ridge was resorbed (Fig. 15–17). In some instances in which crestal bone resorption occurred, canals were not found in the furcation regions (although they may have been present).

Thus, extensive pulp lesions cause periodontal changes through the lateral and the accessory foramina and, also, through the crestal extension of the periapical granulomatous lesions. In such instances, periodontal treatment alone is not effective in eliminating the lesion. Only effective endodontic treatment will result in its eradication. In fact, the elimination of pulp disease through endodontic treatment may cause mobile teeth to tighten. In teeth with periapical involvements, endodontic treatment removes the inflammation not only of the periapical tissues but also in the region of the lateral canals and the accessory foramina. The resultant reduction of edema in the periodontal ligament and the subsequent bone elaboration, as the granuloma heals, cause the tooth to tighten. Inflammatory lesions in the bifurcation or trifurcation area will often disappear after endodontic treatment without any need for periodontal therapy.

CORRELATION OF PERIODONTAL INVOLVEMENT WITH PAIN

Incidence

Pain is felt in periodontally involved teeth that have no caries or restorations but less frequently than in periodontally involved teeth with caries or restorations. Atrophy or inflammation of the pulp is responsible for the highest incidence of

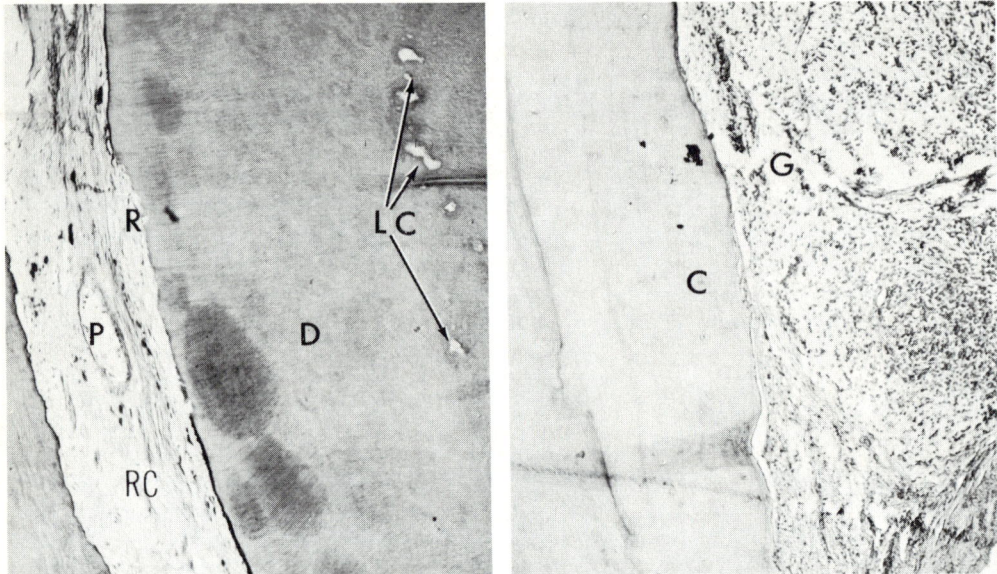

FIG. 15-15 Mesiodistal section of a lower right first molar. The pulp was exposed by caries. *(Left)* Chronic inflammation in the root canal (RC) has caused resorption (R) of the dentin (D). Lateral canals (LC) run from the pulp (P) to the periodontal ligament (demonstrable only in serial sections). *(Right)* The periodontal ligament opposite the lateral canals is chronically inflamed. Granulation tissue (G) is present along the cementum (C). ×96. (Seltzer S, Bender IB, Ziontz M: Oral Surg 16:1474, 1963)

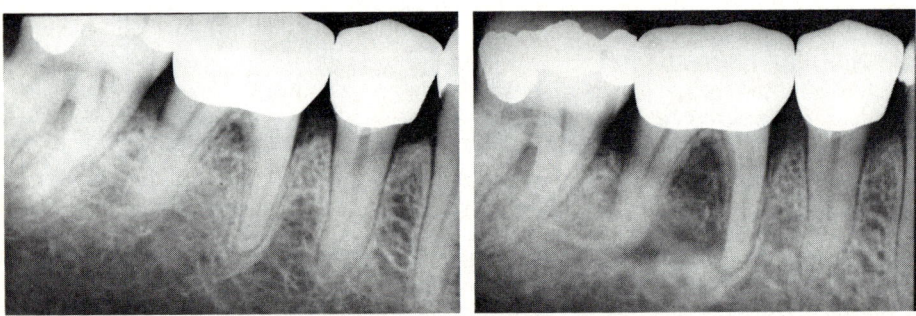

FIG. 15-16 *(Left)* Condition of bone of interradicular region prior to treatment. An arsenical paste was then inserted in the pulp chamber and left in place for 5 days. *(Right)* Note bone destruction 6 weeks after initial treatment with the arsenical paste.

pain in periodontally involved teeth. In our investigations, the incidence of pain in teeth with inflamed or atrophic pulps was approximately 37% if caries or restorations were present and periodontal lesions were absent. The superimposition of periodontal lesions appeared to increase the incidence of pain to 55%. In the teeth with periodontal disease but no caries or restorations, the incidence of pain was 40%.

Severity

The pain varies in degree—most often, from mild to moderate. In a few teeth with extensive periodontal pockets extending to the apex, pain may be severe. In these cases, the radiograph often reveals a region of rarefaction simulating a pulp-induced periapical lesion. The pockets can easily be probed with a root canal silver or gutta-

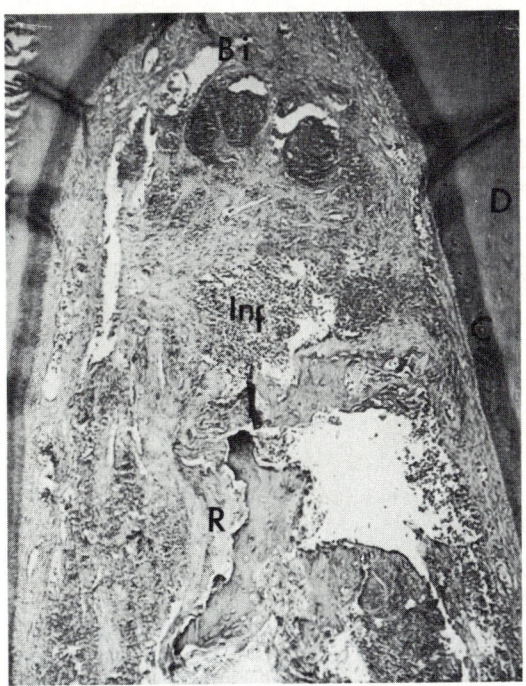

FIG. 15-17 Mesiodistal section of a lower right first molar. Note the presence of an extensive granuloma, resulting from pulp involvement. The inflammation (Inf) has spread to the bifurcation region (Bi), causing crestal bone resorption (R). D, dentin; C, cementum. ×96. (Seltzer S, Bender IB, Ziontz M: Oral Surg 16:1474, 1963)

percha cone, which goes directly to the radiographic lesion. Such teeth, on histologic examination, reveal the presence of inflammation in the apical portion of the pulp, with marked resorption of the apex and the inner surface of the root canal. The coronal portion of the pulp exhibits atrophic changes, with calcific deposits extending into the radicular portion of the pulp, but no evidence of inflammatory cells. The presence of pain and retrograde inflammation is a manifestation of a secondary pulpitis caused by the extension of the periodontal inflammation.

CORRELATION OF PERIODONTAL INVOLVEMENT WITH AGE

Periodontally involved teeth were found in all age categories. However, few teeth in the 1- to 20-year group were periodontally involved. The number of extracted teeth that had been periodontally involved increased with age, as would be expected.

CORRELATION OF PERIODONTAL LESIONS AND THERMAL RESPONSES

Reaction to Thermal Tests. In periodontally involved teeth, including those with and those without caries and restorations, normal responses to applied heat and cold are obtained from most teeth with intact-uninflamed pulps. In tests, half of the teeth with atrophic pulps react normally to heat and cold. Of the remaining teeth, many react abnormally to heat or cold or both, and a small number of teeth do not respond. The number of abnormal reactions to thermal tests increases sharply in all the inflammatory states, many teeth reacting abnormally to both heat and cold. There appears to be no correlation between the type of pulp inflammation and the response to a specific thermal test.

Many periodontally involved teeth respond normally to applied heat and cold. However, periodontally involved teeth with either necrotic pulps or totally inflamed pulps usually do not respond. Abnormal responses in periodontally involved teeth occur in those with atrophic pulps and with chronic partial pulpitis.

Subjective Symptoms. According to Mitchell (1960), in patients complaining of pulpalgia, about 15% of the toothaches were caused by gingival or periodontal disease. In our studies, among the patients complaining of pain, the largest number of those reporting increased pain from cold are patients with atrophic pulps. In most instances, patients complain of pain on application of both heat and cold. Patients whose pulps are intact-uninflamed, mildly inflamed, or necrotic (i.e., those whose pulps are not atrophied or severely inflamed) do not report increased pain in response to thermal stimuli. Thus, patients' complaints relating to pain on thermal stimuli cannot be used as an indicator of the pathologic state of the pulp in periodontally involved teeth.

THE PULPAL-PERIODONTAL SYNDROME

The etiology of a periodontal lesion can be either pulpal or periodontal. Furthermore, a particular aggregation of signs and symptoms, radio-

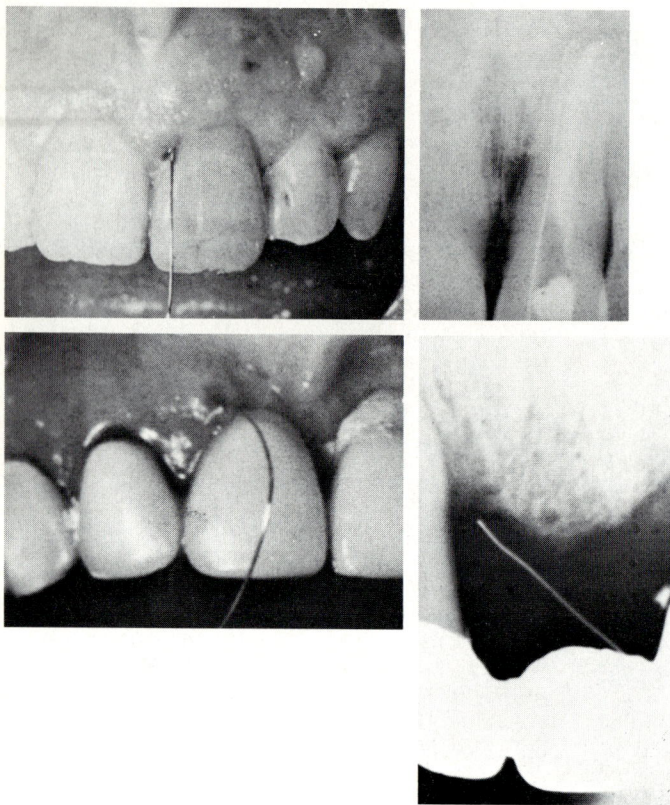

FIG. 15-18 *(Top, left)* Wire inserted in sinus tract through gingival sulcus. *(Top, right)* Radiograph shows wire traversing tract to periapical lesion. Sinus tracts of pulpal origin are common. *(Bottom, left)* Another case with wire inserted into sinus tract. *(Bottom, right)* Radiograph shows that the wire traversing sinus tract goes to crestal bone and the lesion is of periodontal origin. Periodontal lesions seldom exhibit sinus tracts. (Bender IB, Seltzer S: Oral Surg 33:458, 1972)

graphic findings, and test results, has led to the identification of a clinical entity, the pulpal-periodontal syndrome. This syndrome may be defined as one involving inflammation or degeneration of the pulp, with a clinical pocket of the same tooth, and it can be initiated by either pulpal or periodontal disease.

From the definition, every tooth with a periodontal pocket is potentially a case of pulpal-periodontal syndrome. This is particularly true in molar teeth—less so in single-rooted teeth, since lateral canals occur more frequently in molars.

Sequence of Therapy

In order to determine whether periodontal or endodontic treatment should be instituted first, it is necessary to determine whether the lesion is of pulpal or of periodontal origin. Therefore, in the presence of pulpal-periodontal syndrome, a differential diagnosis must be made. The criteria are clinical signs, symptoms, test results, and radiographic findings.

Pain. The presence of pain usually indicates endodontic involvement, especially if the pain is severe. Generally, severe pain is not encountered in periodontal disorders (Ross, 1972), although there are exceptions, such as periodontal abscesses, food impaction areas, necrotizing ulcerative gingivitis, and pain from clenching of the teeth. Mild to moderate pain occurs in both pulpal and periodontal disease, but to a lesser degree in the latter. It is the severity of the pain that is the differentiating factor between the two diseases.

Swelling. The location of swelling often aids in the differentiation between pulpal and periodontal lesions. In teeth with pulpal involvement, the swelling manifests itself in the mucobuccal fold, whereas in periodontal disease the swelling involves the region of the alveolar or palatal mucosa. Facial swellings, such as those resulting in closure of the eye or affecting other parts of the mandible or maxilla, are seldom observed in periodontal disease.

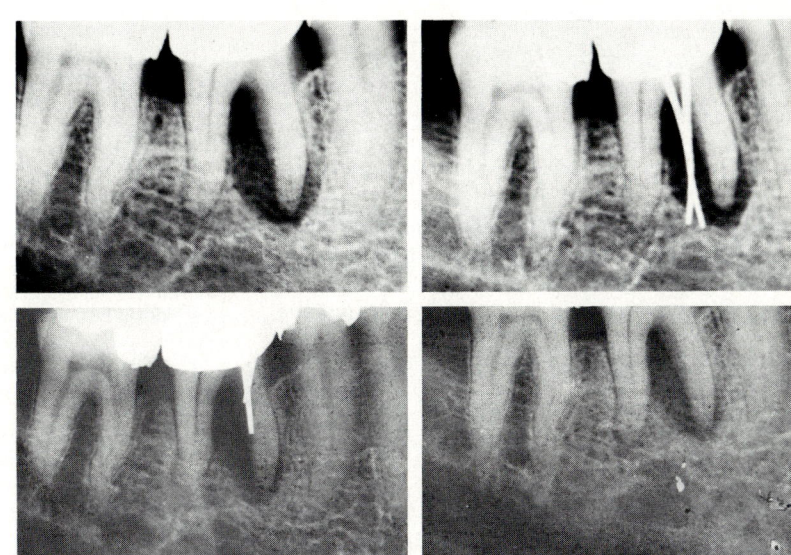

FIG. 15-19 (*Top, left* and *right*) Extensive lesion of periodontal origin. Numerous probes can be inserted through periodontal pocket. If this lesion were of endodontic origin, usually only one probe or wire could be inserted. (*Bottom, left* and *right*) Nine months after periodontal treatment there was a reduction in pocket depth, with bone regeneration. Pulp manifested vitality on drill test. (Bender IB, Seltzer S: Oral Surg 33:458, 1972)

Pulp Test Findings. Pulp testing, either electrical or thermal, or test drilling, is an **important** diagnostic criterion. If the patient complains of pain and the test produces a normal reaction indicating a vital pulp, periodontal treatment should be done first. On the other hand, if test findings are abnormal, with or without pain, endodontic treatment should be considered first.

Clinical Status of the Pulp. If no caries or if only a shallow restoration is present, periodontal measures should be considered first.

Sinus Tracts. Sinus tracts with openings on the mucosa are most often associated with endodontic problems. Occasionally, however, they may open into the sulcular region. Under such conditions, differentiation can be made by inserting a diagnostic wire into the sinus tract (Fig. 15-18). If the sinus tract is of endodontic origin, generally only one wire can be inserted, whereas if the lesion is of periodontal origin, multiple wires or diagnostic probes can be inserted (Fig. 15-19).

Radiographic Findings. Although the lesions may be similar, there are differences between endodontic and periodontal lesions radiographically. If the lesion is of periodontal origin, other teeth besides the one in question manifest involvement. A periapical lesion that does not communicate with the periodontal pocket is probably of endodontic origin. If a furcation lesion exists around one tooth, endodontic procedures should be employed first.

If endodontic procedures are performed initially and, following treatment, the pocket does not show evidence of healing, or there is no reduction in the size of the radiolucency, periodontal treatment should be instituted.

If, on the other hand, initial treatment was periodontal and radiographs subsequently showed no reduction in size of the lesion, or the pocket recurs or increases in size, or pain develops or persists, endodontic treatment is indicated.

Since there is no way of knowing beforehand whether the periodontal lesion has developed independently of the endodontic lesion, or vice versa, no combined therapy is indicated initially when only one tooth is involved. If generalized periodontal disease is present and there is a necrotic pulp, combined therapy may be required. Also, if a periodontal lesion is present on a single-rooted tooth and the pulp is necrotic, combined therapy may be employed.

In determining the diagnosis and sequence of treatment of the pulpal-periodontal syndrome, consideration should be given to proper total therapy. For example, a patient developed an interradicular lesion that did not heal (Fig. 15-14). A correct diagnosis was made; the lesion was of periodontal origin. However, subsequent periodontal treatment was inadequate. More comprehensive treatment, with the use of a bone transplant, produced resolution of the lesion. Thus, it was incorrect to assume that, since the lesion did not disappear following periodontal treatment, endodontic procedures should have been performed. In this case, had endodontic treatment been done subsequent to the periodontal therapy, the lesion still would not have healed. When healing does not occur after either endodontic or periodontal therapy, both the treatment and the diagnosis should be re-evaluated.

BIBLIOGRAPHY

Bender IB, Seltzer S: The effect of periodontal disease on the pulp. Oral Surg 33:458, 1972
Bergenholtz G, Ahlstedt S, Lindhe J: Experimental pulpitis in immunized monkeys. Scand J Dent Res 85:396, 1977
Bergenholtz G, Lindhe H: Effect of experimentally induced marginal periodontitis and periodontal scaling on the dental pulp. J Clin Periodontol 5:59, 1978
Brzezińska B: Obraz histologiczny miazgi zeba w przyzebicy ze szczególnym uwzglednieniem naczyń i nerwów. Czas Stomat 21:57, 1968
Cahn LR: Pathology of dental pulp. Dent Items of Interest 48:1, 1926
Cahn LR: A preliminary report on the dentinal-cemental communication with special reference to the abnormally large channels seen in pyorrhetic teeth. Dent Items of Interest 48:477, 1926
Cahn LR: Pathology of pulps found in pyorrhetic teeth. D Items Int 49:598, 1927
Carranza FA, Itoiz ME, Cabrini RL, Dotto CA: A study of periodontal vascularization in different laboratory animals. J Periodont Res 1:120, 1966
Castelli WA, Dempster WT: The periodontal vasculature and its responses to experimental pressures. JADA 70:890, 1965
Chilton NW: Periodontic endodontic relationships. A synthesis. In Siskin M (ed): Biology of the Human Dental Pulp. St. Louis, CV Mosby, 1973
Cutright DE, Bhaskar SN: A new method of demonstrating microvasculature. Oral Surg 24:442, 1967
Cutright DE, Bhaskar SN: Pulpal vasculature as demonstrated by a new method. Oral Surg 27:678, 1969
Czarnecki RT, Schilder H: A histologic evaluation of the human pulp in teeth with varying degrees of periodontal disease. J Endodont 5:242, 1979
Hattler AB, Snyder DW, Listgarten MA, Kemp W: The lack of pulpal pathosis in rice rats with the periodontal syndrome. Oral Surg 44:939, 1977
Hiatt WH: Pulpal periodontal disease. J Periodont 48:598, 1977
Kramer IRH: A technique for the injection of blood vessels in the dental pulp using extracted teeth. Anat Rec 11.91, 1951

Kramer IRH: Vascular architecture of the human dental pulp. Arch Oral Biol 2:177, 1960
Langeland K, Rodrigues H, Dowden W: Periodontal disease, bacteria, and pulpal histopathology. Oral Surg 37:257, 1974
Lantelme R, Handelman SL, Herbison RJ: Dentin formation in periodontally diseased teeth. J Dent Res 55:48, 1976
Lowman JV, Burke RS, Pelleu GB: Patent accessory canals: Incidence in molar furcation region. Oral Surg 36:580, 1973
Mandi FA: Histological study of the pulp changes caused by periodontal disease. J Brit Endo Soc 6:80, 1972
Mazur B, Massler M: Influence of periodontal disease on the dental pulp. Oral Surg 17:592, 1964
Mitchell DF, Tarplee RE: Painful pulpitis. Oral Surg 13:1360, 1960
Mitchell DF: Differential diagnosis of odontalgia. In Healey HJ (ed): Endodontics, Chap 1. St. Louis, CV Mosby, 1960
Mjör IA, Tronstad L: Experimentally induced pulpitis. Oral Surg 34:102, 1972
Moss SJ, Addelston H, Goldsmith ED: Histologic study of pulpal floor of deciduous molars. JADA 84:34, 1965
Okata T, Akiba K, Shima S, Maekawa S, Hada R, Kondo Y, Hashida K, Futaki S, Ito A, Asai Y: Clinicopathological studies on the pulp therapy, with special reference to histo-pathological changes of pulp and dentin due to exposure of roots of human vital teeth from endodontic viewpoint (preliminary report). Shikwa Gakuho 79:1707, 1979
Plačková A, Vahl J: Ultrastructure of mineralizations in the human pulp. Caries Res 8:172, 1974
Rubach WC, Mitchell DF: Periodontal disease, accessory canals and pulp pathosis. J Periodont 36:34, 1965
Rubach WC, Mitchell DF: Periodontal disease, age and pulp status. Oral Surg 19:482, 1965
Sauerwein E: Histopathology of the pulp in instances of periodontal disease. Deutsche Zahn-, Mund-, Kieferheilk 22:289, 1955 (Dent Abstr 1:467, 1956)
Saunders RL de CH: Microradiographic studies of human adult and fetal dental pulp vessels. In Cosslett VE, Engström A, Pattee HH Jr, (eds): X-ray Microscopy and Microradiography, pp 561–571. New York, Academic Press, 1957
Saunders RL de CH: Microangiographic studies of periodontic and dental pulp vessels in monkey and man. J Canad Dent A 33:245, 1967
Seltzer S, Bender IB, Nazimov H, Sinai I: Pulpitis-induced interradicular periodontal changes in experimental animals. J Periodontol 38:124, 1967
Seltzer S: Endodontology. New York, McGraw-Hill, 1971
Seltzer S, Bender IB, Ziontz M: The interrelationship of pulp and periodontal disease. Oral Surg 16:1474, 1963
Seltzer S, Bender IB, Ziontz M: The dynamics of inflammation: Correlations between diagnostic data and actual histologic findings in the pulp. Oral Surg 16:840; 16:969, 1963
Selvig KA, Nilveus R: Pulpal reactions to the application of citric acid to root-planed dentin in beagles. J Dent Res, AADR Abstr #693, 62:246, 1983
Sicher H: Über Pulpaerkrankungen als Folge von Paradontose. Z Stomat 34:819, 1936
Simon JH, Glick DH, Frank AL: Predictable endodontic

and periodontic failure as a result of radicular anomalies. Oral Surg 31:823, 1971

Simon JH, Glick DH, Frank AL: The relationship of endodontic-periodontic lesions. J Periodont 43:202, 1972

Sinai I, Soltanoff W: The transmission of pathologic changes between the pulp and the periodontal structures. Oral Surg 36:558, 1973

Stahl SS: Pulpal response to gingival injury in rats. Oral Surg 16:1116, 1963

Stahl SS: Pathogenesis of inflammatory lesions in pulp and periodontal tissues. Periodontics 4:190, 1966

Stallard RE: Periodontal disease and its relationship to pulpal pathology. Paradont Acad Rev 2:80, 1968

Stallard RE: Periodontic-endodontic relationships. In Siskin M (ed): Biology of the Human Dental Pulp. St. Louis, CV Mosby, 1973

Turner JG, Drew AH: Experimental inquiry into bacteriology of pyorrhea. Proc Roy Soc Med (Odontol) 12:104, 1919

Winter GB, Kramer IRH: Changes in periodontal membrane and bone following experimental pulpal injuries in deciduous molar teeth in kittens. Arch Oral Biol 10:279, 1965

Winter GB, Kramer IRH: Changes in periodontal membrane, bone and permanent teeth following experimental pulpal injury in deciduous molar teeth of monkeys (Macaca irus). Arch Oral Biol 17:1771, 1972

16
RETROGRESSIVE AND AGE CHANGES OF THE DENTAL PULP

The science of gerontology is receiving more attention as the life span of the individual increases. Comfort (1956) defined aging as a biologic process that causes increased susceptibility to disease.

Aging of human tissues is genetically controlled. It has often been said in jest that living to a ripe old age involves selection of the proper parents. Many theories about the causes of aging have been advanced. According to Shock (1960) and Curtis (1966), among these are the following:

The *wear and tear* theory simply postulates that the organism wears out with use. Each cell is endowed with specific amounts of vital substances, such as enzymes. When these substances are used up, they are not replaced. Cells from older patients have an impaired capacity to repair deoxyribonucleic acid (DNA; Staino-Coico et al, 1983). Eventually, death of the cells and the organism ensues. *Mathematical theories* have been postulated in which an empirical mortality curve fits into a formulated equation. The *cellular interaction theory* is based on the dependence of every part of the body on every other part. For example, all endocrine glands are interdependent for proper functioning. Individual cells in any organ are dependent on, and influenced by, their neighboring cells. The *collagen theory* postulates that collagen fibers form continuously at a slow rate and the collagen is eliminated slowly or not at all. As more and more collagen is elaborated, the cells of the tissues are gradually choked off. Tissue function is hampered and, eventually, cell death ensues. In the *waste product theory*, metabolic waste products are not readily excreted from the cells or intercellular fluids. Slowly, function is interfered with and, eventually, the organism is poisoned. In the *endocrine theory*, endocrine functions slowly decrease and cell metabolism is gradually affected adversely. The *calcium theory* suggests that aging is caused by a defect in calcium metabolism. According to Selye and Prioreschi (1960), large doses of either vitamin D or parathyroid hormone administered to rats causes mineralization of many soft tissues. Such changes resemble those seen in the tissues of the aged. Injury of a tissue results in its calcification (calciphylaxis), rendering the tissue nonfunctional. In the *somatic mutation theory*, it is postulated that the somatic cells of the body develop spontaneous mutations. As more and more cells mutate, an appreciable number of cells eventually become mutants. Almost all cell mutations are deleterious, and eventually the organs become inefficient and senescent. The *autoimmune theory* suggests that autoimmune reactions develop when some of the cells of the body synthesize proteins that differ immunologically from the other bodily proteins. These altered proteins cause immune and anaphylactic reactions within the body. Furthermore, lymphocytes from older patients have an impaired proliferative capacity when stimulated by mitogens (Staino-Coico et al, 1983). Thus, the immune system may be compromised in the elderly. *Circulatory deficiencies* result in deficient oxidation of cells, eventuating in cell death and replacement by collagen. With increase in collagen deposition, more capillaries are choked off, resulting in more anoxia. Mutations may also be induced in the endothelial cells of the capillary, leading to breakdown of part of the capillary and further deficiency in circulation.

Many of these theories can be applied to concepts concerning retrogressive and age changes in the dental pulp. Among the age changes that have been reported to occur in the pulp and dentin are:

Decrease in cellular components
Dentinal sclerosis
Decrease in number and quality of blood vessels and nerves
Reduction in size and volume of the pulp, owing to continued (secondary) dentin deposition and to reparative dentin formation
Increase in number and thickness of collagen fibers
Increase of pulp stones and dystrophic mineralizations

These, and other changes related to aging of the pulp, are discussed in this chapter.

DECREASE IN CELLULAR COMPONENTS

Fibroblasts

Aging effects a reduction in the number of cells of the pulp (Symons, 1967), possibly as a consequence of reduced circulation. The regression of older rat pulpal fibroblasts is characterized by their diminution in size and in the number of cytoplasmic structures associated with fibrogenesis. Most of the intracellular organelles of the older fibroblasts, such as rough-surfaced endoplasmic reticulum (rER) and mitochondria, are smaller. A Golgi complex is rarely found (Han, 1968). There is also a significant decrease in the number of regenerable cells (Pinzon et al, 1966). With increasing maturity, the pulpal fibroblasts exhibit a decreased oxygen uptake (Fisher et al, 1959). However, aging does not result in uniform alteration of the enzymes of the catabolic cycles, both aerobic and anaerobic, of the fibroblasts of the bovine dental pulp (Schwabe, 1969).

Odontoblasts

The odontoblasts appear to undergo degenerative changes with advancing age. Electronmicroscopic examinations reveal more vacuoles in older odontoblasts. Gradually, the odontoblasts atrophy and disappear over some or all areas of the dental pulp (Symons, 1967; Bhussry, 1968).

DENTINAL SCLEROSIS

The primary dentinal tubules are also affected by aging. Increases in peritubular dentin (Bradford, 1960; Harcourt, 1964) or increased deposit of apatite crystals (Takuma, 1967) occur. The dentinal tubules are ultimately occluded, a condition called sclerosis of dentin. Sclerosis of the dentinal tubules in the apical third of the root occurs consistently with aging (Fig. 16–1). The odontoblasts lining the sclerotic dentin become reduced in number and disappear. According to Miles (1972), such alterations are representative of a cell-mediated age change.

Sclerosis of the dentin is also initiated by dental caries. Dental caries elicits reactions within the primary dentinal tubules which tend to slow down the progress of the disease. The pulp defends itself against the lesion of caries quite efficiently. In response to advancing decay, the dentinal tubules of the primary dentin gradually become mineralized, provided that the odontoblasts remain vital. The distal extensions of Tomes' fibers, the protoplasmic processes of the odontoblasts within the dentinal tubules, form peritubular dentin. In electron microscopic examinations, it is seen that the peritubular matrix of dentin has a high degree of mineralization (see Chap. 2). This is in contrast to the remaining intertubular matrix, which is not as highly mineralized. The experiments of Young and Greulich (1963) furnished autoradiographic evidence that tritiated glycine may be found in the peritubular matrix 2 hours after injection. Since the dentin matrix is relatively stable, this possibly demonstrated the continuing appositional pattern of peritubular matrix. This process, sclerosis of the dentin, constitutes the initial defense

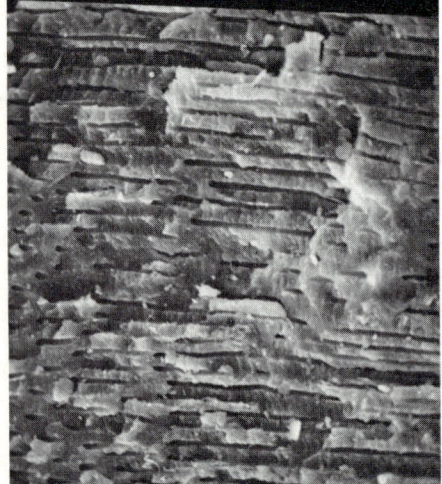

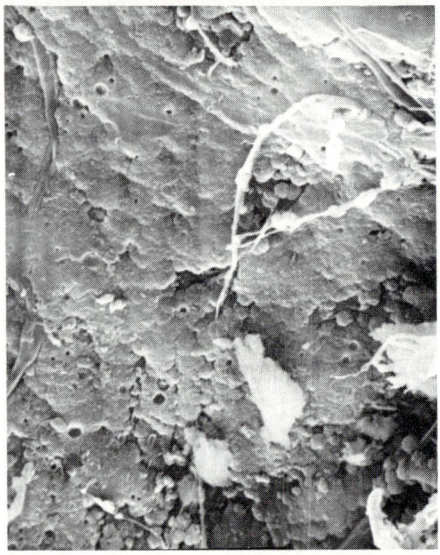

FIG. 16-1 Scanning electron micrographs of dentin, showing age changes. *(Top)* Regular dentin in midportion of tooth in middle-aged individual. ×600. *(Bottom)* Sclerotic dentin in apical portion of root. Note the amorphous character of the dentin, and the decrease in number and reduction in width of dentinal tubules. ×3000.

of the pulp against dental caries (Fig. 16-2). Bradford (1960) has pointed out that, where dead tracts form instead of sclerotic tubules, caries spreads more rapidly toward the pulp. This rapid carious penetration is more likely to occur in younger teeth. In older teeth, the caries is more likely to spread along the dentinoenamel junction, with less tendency to extend toward the pulp.

Sclerosis of the dentin also occurs in response to slow, external irritations such as abrasion, attrition, and erosion (Brännström and Garberoglio, 1980). In response to attrition, the sclerotic dentin is nonetheless permeable to dyes (Tronstad, 1978), since some dentinal tubules still remain open (Fig. 16-3). There appear to be two patterns of dentinal tubule mineralization: continuous growth of peritubular dentin and intratubular crystal deposition (Hawkinson and Eisenmann, 1983). Mendis and Darling (1979) found that, under attrition, peritubular dentin thickness increased by only 20%. The lumina of the occluded tubules were filled with large crystals. Under the attrited areas of monkey teeth, Haugen and Mjör (1975) found irregular secondary (reparative) dentin. Despite this, inflammatory reactions were found in about one third of the pulps of the attrited teeth.

Erosion is the loss of tooth structure by physicochemical influences and not by bacterial action. Under erosion, minerals are deposited within the dentinal tubules (sclerosis). Reparative dentin is formed at the interface between pulp and dentin (Isokawa et al, 1970, 1973).

Certain drugs such as calcium hydroxide and corticosteroids, when placed on the dentin after cavity preparation, also have been demonstrated by densitometric studies, microhardness tests, and electron micoroscopy to cause sclerosis (Mjör, 1960; Bergenholtz and Reit, 1980). Apparently, some remineralization also occurs when sedative dressings, such as zinc oxide-eugenol, are placed in carious cavities.

FIG. 16-2 Sclerosis of the primary dentin. Ground section. As a result of dental caries (C), sclerotic changes (SD) have occurred in the dentinal tubules.

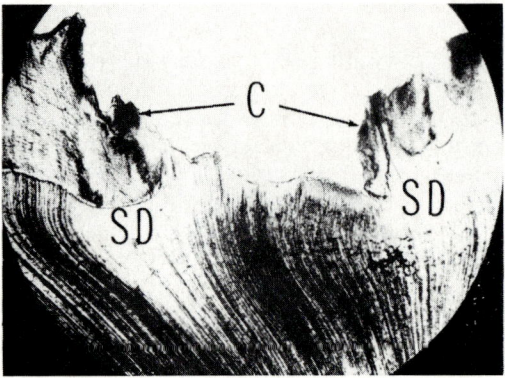

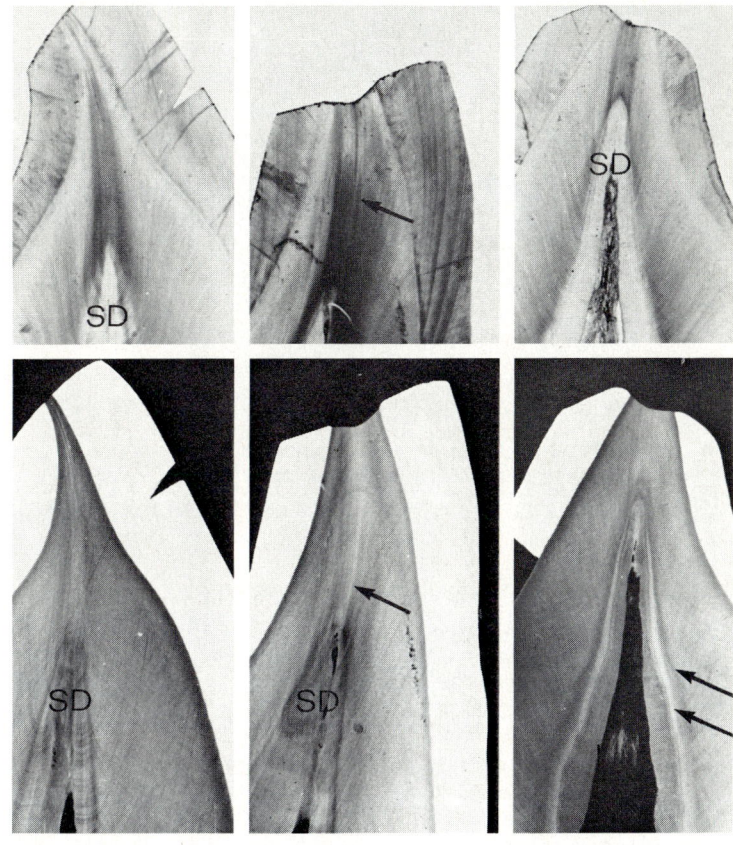

FIG. 16-3 Attrition of anterior teeth. *(Top)* Ground sections, in transmitted light: *(Left)* The incisal dentin is barely exposed by attrition in a tooth of a 50 year old. There is an opaque zone extending from the incisal tip of the dentin to the pulp horn. A translucent streak is discernible centrally in the opaque zone. The pulp horn is filled with translucent secondary dentin (SD). ×8. *(Center)* Incisor, from a 50 year old. Part of the opaque zone near the exposed surface is translucent. The mantle dentin has remained translucent after exposure to the mouth. The central streak (arrow) is opaque, with translucent borders. ×8. *(Right)* Canine from a 60 year old. The opaque zone occupies only the most central part of the incisal dentin, and the exposure of the dentin does not seem to have influenced its optical properties. Secondary dentin (SD) is also present outside the area of attrition. ×8. *(Bottom)* Microradiographs of the ground sections shown left, center, and right above. *(Left)* The radiopaque central streak is divided by a slit in the most incisal part and bordered by radiolucent bands. Mineral in the secondary dentin (SD) is unevenly distributed. ×8. *(Center)* A central area, extending from the exposed surface to the pulp horn, appears to be hypermineralized compared with the adjacent exposed dentin. The central streak (arrow) and the bordering dark bands are partly visible. ×8. *(Right)* An area of the incisal dentin is slightly hypermineralized. No changes in the mineralization of the adjacent exposed dentin are apparent. Arrows indicate the dark and light zones of the last formed primary dentin. ×8. (Tronstad L: Optical and microradiographic appearance of intact and worn human coronal dentine. Arch Oral Biol 17:847, 1972)

DEAD TRACTS IN THE PRIMARY DENTIN

When caries progresses rapidly, the odontoblasts degenerate. The dentinal tubules are no longer filled with living protoplasm, and "dead tracts" result. A similar occurrence follows fractures of the crowns of the teeth (with sudden exposure of the dentinal tubules), severe operative injuries, such as deep cavity cutting without coolant, and drug injuries, such as may be caused by the application of phenol, silver nitrate, or ionization to the base of the cavity preparation. The remaining vital odontoblasts or other pulp cells attempt to seal off the dead tracts by the elaboration of reparative dentin. The dead tracts are not necessarily devoid of protoplasm, and they are not as highly mineralized as sclerotic dentinal tubules. Apparently, caries progresses more rapidly in the presence of dead tracts.

DECREASE IN NUMBER AND QUALITY OF BLOOD VESSELS AND NERVES

Blood Vessels

Aging has an adverse effect on the number and quality of blood vessels supplying the dental pulp (Bennett et al, 1965). Blood vessels of aged

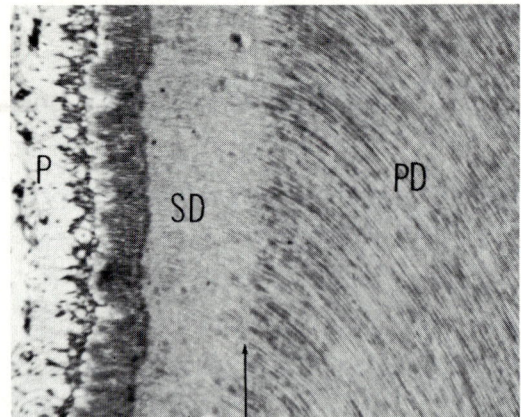

FIG. 16-4 The transition from primary dentin (PD) to secondary dentin (SD) is indicated by the arrow. P, pulp. ×54.

Nerves

Few studies have been made of the age changes of the nerves of human teeth. Armenio et al (1956); Bernick (1967); and Bernick and Nedelman (1975) have indicated that retrogressive changes occur, probably as a result of progressive mineralization of the radicular nerve sheath and the nerve itself. As a consequence, there is a reduction in the number of nerve branches in the coronal portion of the aged pulp (Bernick, 1967). Vacek and Plačková (1959) have noted that under caries the pulp nerve fibers become coarsened and irregular, and argyrophilic varicosities are formed.

FORMATION OF SECONDARY DENTIN

Continuous deposition of the dentin, which tends to reduce the volume of the dental pulp, takes place throughout life (Kawasaki et al, 1980). As a result of this deposition there is a tendency toward eventual pulp obliteration. As an individual ages, the tubules become less regular and more wavy and they change direction (Fig. 16-4). This indicates that changes are occurring in the odontoblasts, possibly as a result of continuous ionic exchange from the saliva. Such secondary dentin formation occurs in the absence of inflammation. It increases when a tooth is worn down through chewing, thereby exposing the dentin. The irritation is mild, yet is sufficient to stimulate the odontoblasts to elaborate dentin.

The pattern of dentin deposition varies somewhat among the different groups of teeth. In molars, dentin is deposited mainly on the floor of the pulp chamber, with less deposition on the occlusal and lateral walls (Sicher, 1962; Philippas, 1952, 1961). In upper anterior teeth, the greatest dentin deposition occurs on the lingual wall of the pulp chambers, as a result of masticating forces (Philippas and Applebaum, 1966, 1967, 1968), with subsequent deposition in the incisal tip and walls of the pulp chamber. In persons 71 years of age or older, the pulp canal has become almost obliterated. The additonally formed secondary dentin is highly irregular, with fewer dentinal tubules.

Thus, the pulp chamber "shrinks" in an occlusoradicular direction much more than it does mesiodistally. As a result, the horns of the pulp in molars are left behind. They also recede, but

pulps undergo arteriosclerotic changes, resulting in a diminished blood supply to the cells of the coronal portions of the pulps (Kindlová and Matěna, 1959; Saunders, 1967).

Comparisons of the pulpal blood vessels of noncarious teeth from younger people (less than 20 years of age) with those of older individuals (40 to 70 years of age) were made by Bernick (1967) and by Bernick and Nedelman (1975). The pulpal arterioles from young teeth typically consisted of endothelial layers abutting directly on a thin internal elastic membrane. The media consisted of one or two layers of muscle cells, and the adventitia contained collagenous and elastic fibers. PAS-stained sections showed a deep red stain of the internal elastic membrane, whereas the media and adventitia stained pink.

In contrast, the arterioles of the older pulps exhibited hyperplasia of the intima, resulting in a narrowing of the vessel lumen. The internal elastic membrane was masked by the deposition of a PAS-positive material. In some older pulps, there was also a hyperplasia of the elastic fibers together with deposition of PAS-positive material. Dystrophic changes in the media and adventitia were also noted. In some instances, deposition of fine mineral deposits was observed to have progressed to complete obliteration of both adventitia and media.

Blood vessels supplying the coronal pulp tissue were extensive and numerous in younger teeth. These blood vessels decreased in number in older teeth, regardless of whether or not the pulps exhibited mineralization.

not as much as the rest of the pulp tissue. Some filling-in of the pulp horns with collagen occurs. Care must be exercised during cavity preparation to avoid cutting the so-called recessional lines of the pulp. When a cavity is cut, even though bleeding is not evident, a minute exposure of the pulp may be present. There is less danger of such accidental exposure in older individuals.

FORMATION OF REPARATIVE DENTIN

The formation of reparative (irregular, secondary, tertiary, irritation) dentin* is an important mechanism in the defense against disease processes in the pulp. New dentin is constantly being formed throughout the life of the tooth. This dentin is more amorphous, less tubular and slightly less regular than primary dentin. However, when the pulp is injured more severely and the injury is accompanied by an inflammatory response, there is a rapid elaboration of reparative dentin.

Reparative dentin is found in all instances under the involved dentinal tubules in dental caries, restorations, abrasion, and attrition (Fig. 16–5). Exposure of the dentin to the oral environment leads to an increase in mineral content of the dentin. However, the mineralization of reparative dentin is uneven, as disclosed by microradiography (Tronstad, 1972). Hypomineralized, as well as hypermineralized, zones are present (Fig. 16–3). In some instances reparative dentin is found practically obliterating the coronal portion of the pulp, even in teeth in which the primary dentin has not been exposed.

If the odontoblasts are injured as a result of either dental caries or operative procedures, some may die (Fig. 16–6), and dentin that is formed subsequently is less regular. This dentin is known as reparative dentin. Under conditions of severe injury, such as burning of the dentin, many of the odontoblastic nuclei are displaced into the tubules. After an initial lag period, reparative dentin is formed. New dentin continues to be formed unless the pulp dies. This new dentinal tissue is elaborated by other pulp cells

---

* Dentin that has been formed as a result of injury of the pulp may also be called secondary, tertiary, or irritation dentin. However, this type of dentin is referred to here as reparative dentin because the adjective "reparative" describes its function. The name does not imply complete pulp repair.

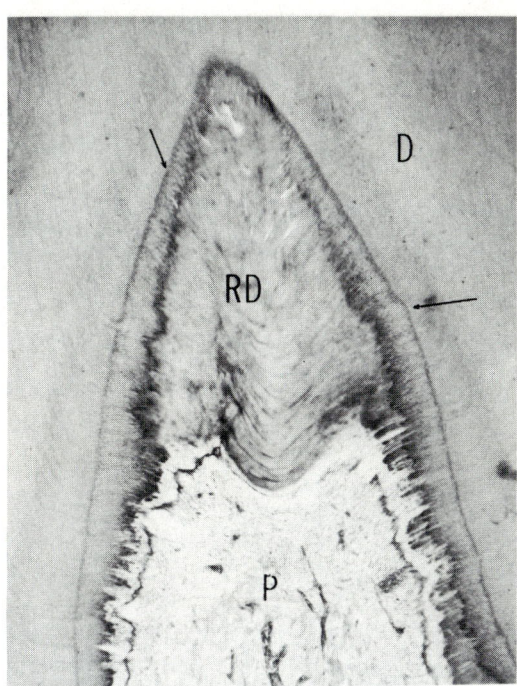

FIG. 16–5 Elaboration of reparative dentin (RD), from attrition. The original pulp space is marked by dark line (arrows). P, pulp; D, dentin. ×54.

which have been transformed into odontoblasts or cells like odontoblasts (Sveen and Hawes, 1968). According to Senzaki (1980), these new odontoblasts may be derived from perivascular cells. The reparative dentin is much more amorphous or irregular (Fig. 16–5).

Reparative Dentin Under Caries

The reparative dentin under dental caries is less abundant and much more regular than that found under restorations. The tubular structure is more readily discernible. The odontoblasts under the dentin are arranged in an orderly, palisaded fashion. Apparently, when functioning adequately, the pulp maintains an amount of dentin between itself and the advancing process of decay which is at least equal to the quantity of primary dentin lost because of the disease process. If caries is rampant, the reparative dentin is decayed as readily as primary dentin. Reparative dentin is marked off from the primary and the secondary dentin by a calciotraumatic response, so that the region where the odontoblasts had been present before recession stains hyperchromatically.

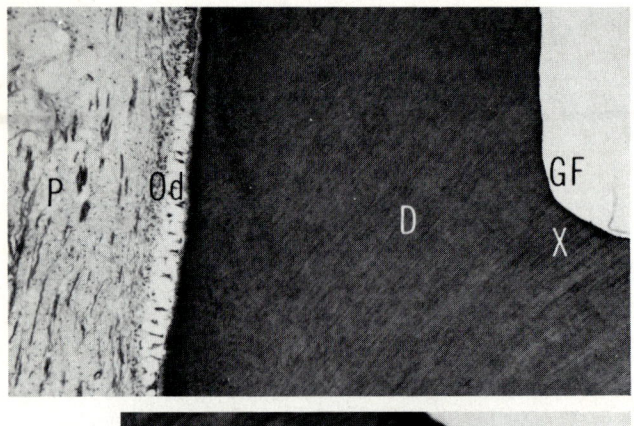
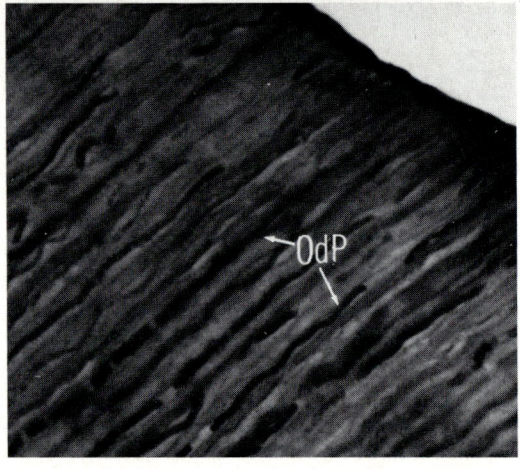

FIG. 16-6 *(Top)* As a result of cavity preparation and gold foil insertion (GF), the underlying odontoblasts (Od) have been destroyed. P, pulp; D, dentin. ×54. *(Bottom)* Higher magnification of region at X, above. The contents of the dentinal tubules (the odontoblastic processes—OdP) are disrupted. ×960.

Inflammatory cells (mainly macrophages and lymphocytes, with occasional polys) are found in the pulp, primarily in the region under the reparative dentin. A severe pulpitis may destroy the original odontoblastic layer.

Reparative Dentin Under Restorations

The reparative dentin under restorations is much more amorphous and irregular than the reparative dentin found in other conditions. The reparative dentin is also softer than the primary dentin in the same tooth (Cox et al, 1980).

The daily rate of reparative dentin formation after operative procedures varies with time. In monkey teeth, dentin has been reported to form at the rate of 2.9 μm to 4.0 μm daily (Fisher et al, 1970; Wennberg et al, 1982). In humans, the average daily reparative dentin formation has been reported to be 2.8 μm for deciduous (Goto and Machiola, 1972) and 1.5 μm for permanent (Stanley et al, 1966) teeth. The quantity of reparative dentin formed after operative procedures depends on the depth of the cavity (Fisher et al, 1970). In deep cavities, there may be a lag period in the onset of new predentin, followed by the elaboration of huge amounts under the cut dentinal tubules. The odontoblasts lining this dentin appear to be altered in structure. The regular, palisaded arrangement is changed. Instead of the columnar appearance typical of odontoblasts in the coronal portion of the uninflamed pulp, these odontoblasts appear flattened, like fibroblasts, and are reduced in number, the odontoblast layer sometimes being only one or two cells in depth. It is likely that most, if not all, of the original odontoblasts have died and have been replaced by other pulp cells. An intense calciotraumatic response, related to the operative procedures, is demonstrable in the dentin. Frequently, the pulp underlying the region of the cut dentinal tubules is infiltrated with chronic inflammatory cells in varying amounts

(Fig. 16–7). In some cases the density of the inflammatory cell infiltration justifies the diagnosis of chronic pulpitis. In other instances, the number of inflammatory cells remaining appears to indicate resolution of a pre-existing pulpitis, probably caused by the operative procedure. Occasionally, no inflammatory cells are found under the reparative dentin.

The presence of abundant amounts of reparative dentin, observed in many tissue sections, does not appear to be correlated with pulp-test readings. In some teeth delayed pulp-test readings are recorded; in others, the responses are very quick, that is, at the lowest point on the scale of the pulp tester.

The pulp test responses are apparently unrelated to dentin innervation, since Byers and Dong (1983) found that, in monkey teeth, the reparative dentin was poorly innervated.

Reparative Dentin in Root Canals

Reparative dentin is present in significant amounts in the root canals of all teeth that are chronically inflamed and especially in those that are periodontally involved. In both of these circumstances, the root canals are excessively narrowed and almost obliterated. However, complete obliteration of the root canal is rarely seen. There are always some viable tissue elements remaining within the root canal.

Formation of Dentin Matrix

The pulp cells secrete collagen precursors. These are probably nonfibrous, incomplete molecules which are secreted into the extracellular ground substance where polymerization to fibrils occurs. It is believed that a firmly bound collagen-mucopolysaccharide complex is formed. The collagen precursors found within the cells are nonsulfated amino-polysaccharides associated with protein. When they leave the cells, they become sulfated. Sulfation may play a part in the transformation of precursors into the characteristic matrix (predentin), but this has not been established.

Pulp cells other than odontoblasts are capable of elaborating dentin matrix. Alkaline phosphatase was applied to exposed dental pulp tissue (Seltzer and Bender, 1958). Fibroblasts became oriented around dentin chips which had been pushed into the pulp following exposure. Dentin matrix was formed abundantly in those pulps (Fig. 16–8). A small amount of matrix was also formed in exposed pulps that were not treated with enzymes. Thus, the pulpal connective tissue is a reservoir for the continuous supply of matrix-forming cells throughout the life of the dental pulp.

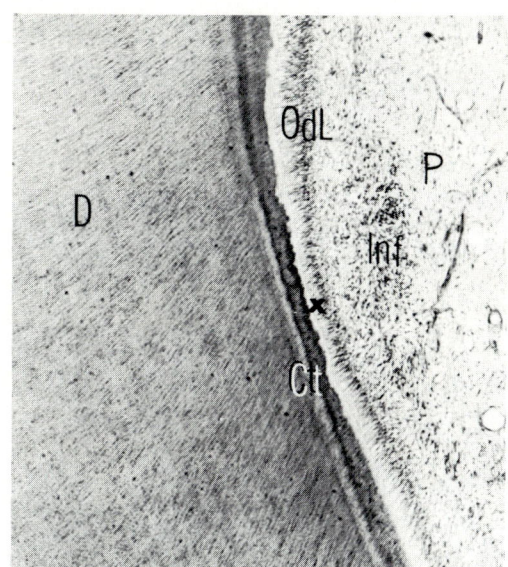

FIG. 16-7 Chronic inflammation (Inf) of the pulp (P) under reparative dentin. A calciotraumatic response (Ct) is evident in the dentin (D). The odontoblastic layer (OdL) is thinned at region x. ×54. (Seltzer S: Oral Surg 12:595, 1959)

Often, the cells that line reparative dentin are cuboidal or have the flattened appearance of fibroblasts rather than the columnar shape of odontoblasts. However, after the initial injury to the pulp, the fibroblasts or other mesenchymal cells hypertrophy and tend to assume a columnar shape. The elaboration of dentin matrix now appears to become their primary function. These cells are strongly basophilic, showing the presence of ribose nucleoproteins, which indicates that active synthesis of extracellular materials is going on. The elaboration of dentin matrix in layers proceeds continuously. Investigators have demonstrated in labeled carbon experiments that two dentin layers are present. The ^{14}C-labeled matrix layer is separated from the pulp by an increasingly thick layer of unlabeled matrix as the circulating ^{14}C decreases. Experiments with tritiated glycine also demonstrate the appositional secretion and the relative stability of dentin matrix.

All collagenous substances contain small amounts of carbohydrates, as well as two or

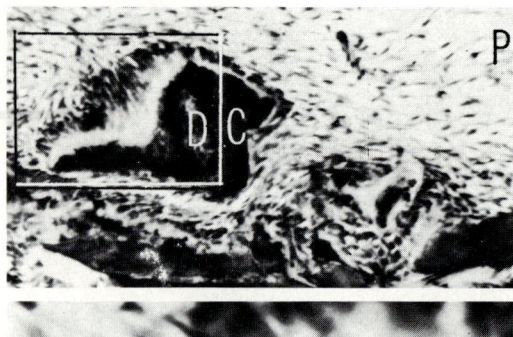
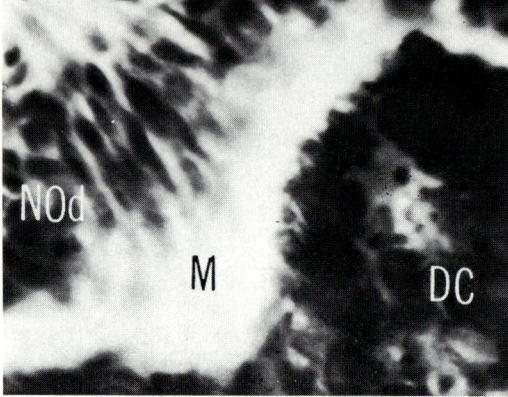

FIG. 16-8 *(Top)* Following a pulp exposure, dentin chips (DC) were pushed into the pulp (P). Then a suspension of alkaline phosphatase was applied. ×135. *(Bottom)* Higher magnification of region outlined by rectangle in top photograph. New odontoblasts (NOd) have differentiated from pulp cells, and they are elaborating dentin matrix (M) around a dentin chip (DC). ×540. (Seltzer S, Bender IB: Some influences affecting repair of the exposed pulps of dogs' teeth. J Dent Res 37:678, 1958. Copyright by the American Dental Association. Reproduced by permission)

three mucoproteins or mucopolysaccharide components.

The new odontoblasts or matrix-forming cells have many metachromatic cytoplasmic granules. These granules contain both protein and mucopolysaccharide, and they appear to contain alkaline phosphatase, among other enzymes. The alkaline phosphatase activity has been shown to be much greater in the odontoblasts than in other pulp cells. The increase of mucopolysaccharides during the repair of injury, the sulfation of the polysaccharides, the increase in alkaline phosphatase activity and/or the process of epitaxy apparently make the matrix capable of binding minerals, thus leading to mineralization.

Mineralization of the Matrix

Mineral salts are attracted to the collagen fibrils of dentin, which may be visualized as being coated with sulfated polysaccharides. Initially, there is an intense metachromasia, but, as mineralization takes place, metachromasia disappears—phenomena that coincide with the initial abundance of the administered radiosulfate in nonmineralized areas (predentin). Subsequently the sulfate-tagged substances disappear as the matrix becomes mineralized. However, the precise reason for the attraction of mineral salts to the matrix is not known. One theory is based on epitaxy: a nucleus of octacalcium phosphate or hydroxyapatite crystals is deposited in the interfibrillar cementing substances or on the fibrils. These nuclei grow by apposition. The dentin is formed by coalescence of these particles into spherical bodies called calcospherites (Fig. 16-9).

Mineralization may be an enzyme-controlled phenomenon. Regions of actively mineralizing dentin bordering on the predentin show the most intense esterase reaction histochemically. This is correlated with microradiographic findings. The enzyme alkaline phosphatase, which is elaborated by odontoblasts, may be involved in mineralization. It may split phosphoric esters so that free phosphate ions are liberated. These react with calcium ions to form a precipitate within the matrix. The enzyme probably assists in making the dentin matrix mineralizable.

There are regions in the dentin that are not as well mineralized; these are known as interglobular areas of dentin (Fig. 16-10).

EXPERIMENTAL DENTINOGENESIS

The process of reparative dentin formation has been graphically illustrated experimentally. Various calcium salts were placed on the exposed pulps of dogs' teeth to determine the effects on induction of dentin bridge formation. Calcium compounds such as calcium hydroxide, calcium carbonate, calcium chloride, and calcium phosphate were used. In addition, some exposed pulps were capped with an aqueous suspension of penicillin and some with an aqueous suspension of alkaline phosphatase (an enzyme associated with mineralization). As controls, some pulps were capped with sterile physiologic

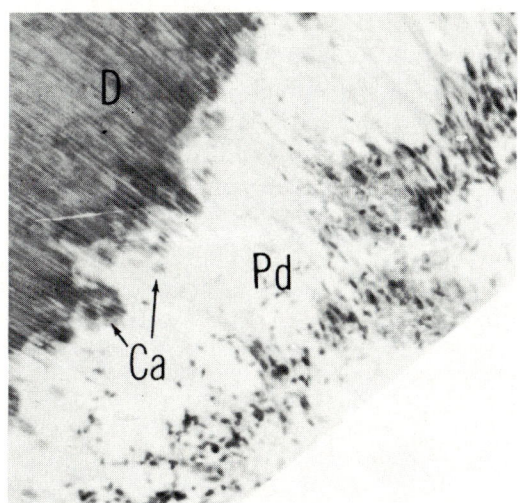

FIG. 16-9 Globular pattern of dentin calcification. There is coalescence of calcospherites (Ca) in the predentin (Pd) to form mature dentin (D). ×540. (Seltzer S, Bender, IB: JADA 59:915, 1959)

In all cases, after 3 days an abscess occurred in the pulp as a result of the exposure. Inflammation extended throughout the coronal portion of the pulp but usually terminated at the radicular portion. In most teeth, dentin chips were pushed into the pulp as a result of the exposure. Around these dentin chips some cellular activity was discernible in most of the teeth.

The reaction of the pulp to alkaline phosphatase was unusual. A new layer of odontoblasts formed around the dentin chips, and dentin was being elaborated. Dentin matrix was found on both sides of the chips, indicating recent elaboration (Fig. 16-8).

Thirty to ninety days later, the pulps of most of the teeth were either chronically inflamed or necrotic. Around some of the teeth, apical granulomata had formed.

saline solution. The animals were sacrificed at intervals of 3 to 90 days after the operative procedures.

With the exception of calcium hydroxide, the various salts tested were harmful to the pulp. Calcium hydroxide encouraged dentin bridging. However, bridging also occurred when physiologic saline solution was applied.

SUMMARY

The formation of reparative dentin seems to follow essentially the pattern of the formation of bone and other hard tissue. The matrix formers are connective tissue cells—the odontoblasts and the less differentiated fibroblasts. It seems reasonably certain that any mesenchymal pulp cell can assume the function of forming dentinoid, or predentin, and synthesize cytoplasmic granules (collagen precursors) that contain aminopolysaccharides associated with proteins.

FIG. 16-10 Interglobular areas of dentin. *(Left)* In coronal portion of tooth: D, dentin; IG, interglobular areas ×54. *(Right)* Higher magnification of interglobular area. The alternation of darker and lighter stained areas indicates differences in degree of mineralization. ×960.

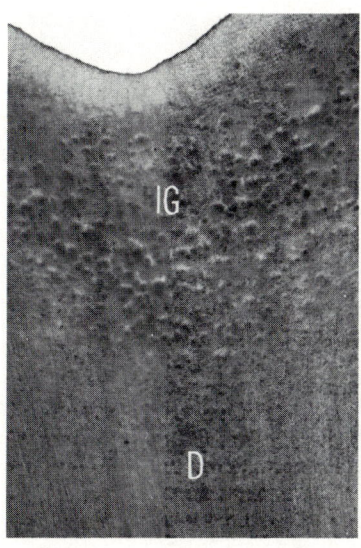
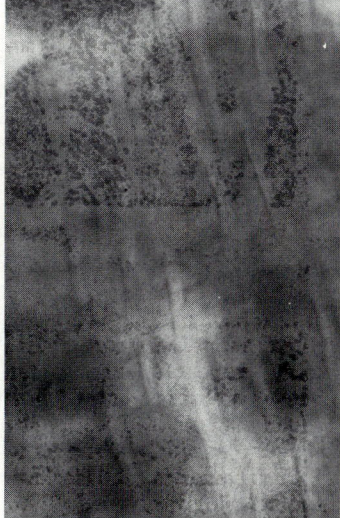

These granules are secreted extracellularly, and, during this process, they become sulfated. The collagen fibrils that make up the predentin are coated with a sleeve of the sulfated polysaccharides. Alkaline phosphatase appears to be involved in the process of matrix formation. Finally, mineral salts are attracted to the matrix and mineralization ensues, resulting in the formation of mature dentin.

CLINICAL CORRELATIONS

The formation of reparative dentin is an attempt by the pulp to wall off the injured odontoblasts. It is comparable with a scar that becomes mineralized. Thus, formation of large quantities of reparative dentin means that a great deal of damage has occurred. Once the reparative dentin has been elaborated there is no assurance that the pulp will remain uninflamed. In spite of reparative dentin formation, if severe pulp damage has occurred, the pulp still can become necrotic.

The deliberate induction of reparative dentin in order to protect the pulp against later damage — a method formerly advocated — is not biologically acceptable. Injury to the pulp should be avoided even though repair may occur, in order to avoid the aging that is an inevitable consequence of the reparative process.

Dentin chips play an important role in dentin bridge formation. Calcified material is needed for the apposition of dentin, just as bone is needed for bone apposition.

When bridging and successful repair have occurred in pulp capping with calcium hydroxide, mineralization does not always stop. After several years the entire pulp may become mineralized or obliterated. Even with an obliterated pulp, the possibility exists that an apical granuloma may develop. Similar obliteration of the pulp occurs in a tooth that has received a blow or after too rapid orthodontic tooth movement.

INTERFERENCE WITH MATRIX FORMATION AND MINERALIZATION

Interference with the formation of reparative dentin may occur under certain local and systemic conditions.

LOCAL FACTORS

Severe Pulp Inflammation

When pulp inflammation is severe, there may be interference with both the elaboration and the mineralization of the predentin. Then, no dentin is formed. For example, if a silicate is placed within a deep tooth cavity, a severe reaction occurs both in the odontoblastic layer and in the underlying pulp tissue. The odontoblasts may be killed, causing a lag or cessation in the formation of dentin (Fig. 16–11). In time, unless the entire pulp becomes necrotic, the pulp usually recovers, and then reparative dentin is formed. The quantity of dentin formed depends on the severity of the injury. The odontoblastic layer may be thinned after reparative dentin formation because some of the odontoblasts have died (Fig. 16–7). The remaining odontoblasts are still able to elaborate dentin. Sometimes, so much dentin is laid down that almost the entire pulp is obliterated. This is more likely to happen when a drug injury of the exposed pulp occurs, such as takes place under calcium hydroxide.

The rate of production of dentin alters the morphology of the odontoblasts, which, in turn, affects the structuring of the dentin. When the deposition of reparative dentin takes place at a regular rate, the odontoblasts remain palisaded and columnar. When a great deal of reparative dentin is elaborated, the odontoblasts flatten and look like fibroblasts. Conversely, when the cells are tall and columnar, tubular dentin, which is regular in appearance, is laid down. When the odontoblasts are flattened, amorphous dentin with irregular tubules is formed.

Operative Manipulations

Operative procedures involving the dentin cause degeneration of the odontoblasts. After the initial injury to the odontoblasts caused by cutting of a cavity or other operative procedures, certain subtle changes occur. The odontoblasts tend to swell and accumulate metabolites; they then liberate chemical mediators, which act as irritants to the underlying pulp, and an inflammatory response is initiated.

The injured odontoblasts may recover, but in all probability most undergo necrosis. Within a few weeks, cellular debris or the dead cells themselves are no longer visible, having been encased in new matrix (predentin) or calcified intercellular substance. The new matrix must come from the remaining odontoblasts or from odontoblastlike cells which have differentiated from other mesenchymal pulp cells or from fibroblasts which have the potentiality of elaborating dentin matrix (Sveen and Hawes, 1968).

Operations on the dentin, with resultant damage to the involved odontoblasts, cause temporary derangement in mineralization shown by the formation of a basophilic line. This has been defined as a calciotraumatic reaction. In a histologic section of a tooth that has been subjected to an operative procedure, a region that stains deep bluish (i.e., is basophilic) is found, followed by a region that stains less intensely (Fig. 16–12). This alteration may be associated with changes in both the orientation of collagen fibers and the ground substance of the dentinal matrix, thereby affecting subsequent mineralization (Eisenmann and Yaeger, 1969). The calciotraumatic response is a record within the dentin, showing that there was an interference with the mineralization of the dentinal matrix at the time of the cutting procedure.

Yeager (1963a,b) and Yeager et al (1963) studied the hypomineralized and the hypermineralized components of the dentin of rats' teeth after subcutaneous injections of sodium fluoride or strontium. He found that the hypomineralized component was caused by an inhibition of polysacchardie-collagen interaction, resulting in paucity of apatite nucleation sites and a more soluble organic matrix. The matrix contained a homogeneous interfibrillar material—presumably, nonfibrillar collagen. The failure of aggregation of collagen into its fibrillar form could account for the inhibition of mineralization. On the other hand, the hypermineralized component was caused by increase in the duration of matrix aggregation, with the formation of more nucleation sites, more numerous crystals and a less soluble organic matrix.

Ogawa et al (1981) found that injections of strontium chloride in rats produced two hypomineralized layers, external and internal. The external layer contained abundant, apparently normal collagen fibrils, whereas the internal layer contained few collagen fibrils, suggesting a disturbance in collagen synthesis. Quantities of proteoglycans were found in the hypomineralized layers.

Inasmuch as human reparative dentin is elaborated at the rate of 1 μ to 3 μ a day, it is possible to estimate, from the amount of reparative dentin formed, when the operation was performed.

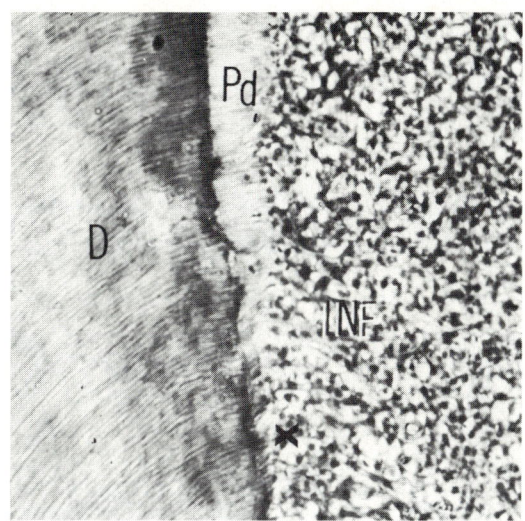

FIG. 16-11 Lag in reparative dentin formation, due to inflammation (INF) of the pulp. At region x no predentin is being elaborated. D, dentin; Pd, predentin, ×180. (Seltzer S: Oral Surg 12:595, 1959)

FIG. 16-12 An operative procedure in the dentin (D) is recorded by a calciotraumatic response (CT). The pulp (P) underlying the dentin has recovered. ×450.

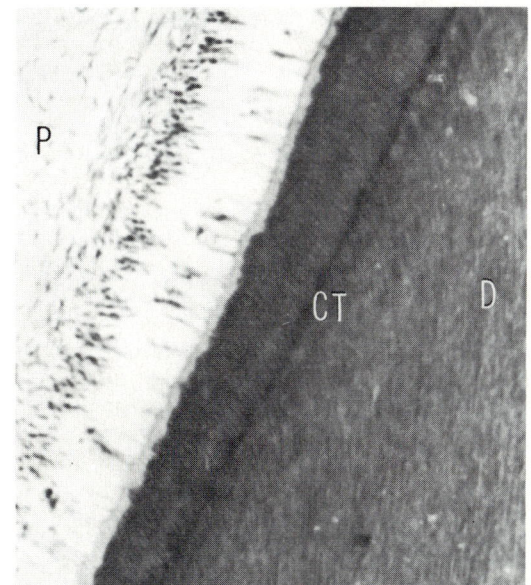

336 | THE DENTAL PULP

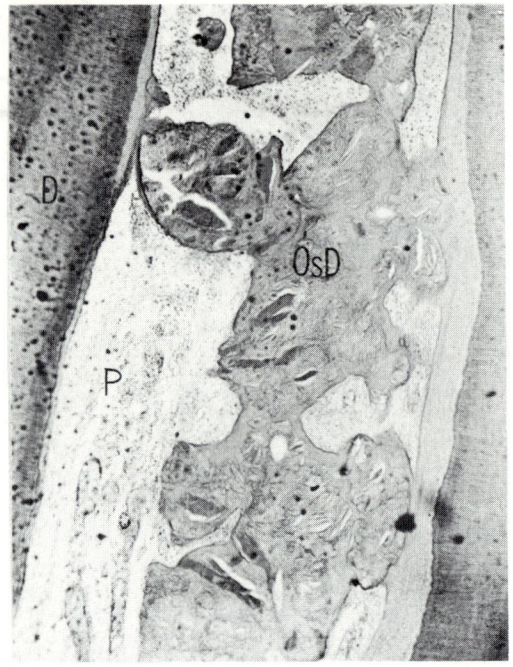

FIG. 16-13   As a result of severe injury, the pulp (P) has elaborated osteodentin (OsD). Pulp is inflamed. D, dentin. ×55. (Seltzer S: Oral Surg 12:595, 1959)

in massive amounts and tends to obliterate the coronal pulp chamber.

SYSTEMIC FACTORS

Neonatal

Temporary interferences with mineralization, such as those that occur at birth, result in incompletely mineralized dentin which appears as the so-called neonatal line (Fig. 16-14). This is found within the first permanent molar and some deciduous teeth. Dentin formation is interfered with not only by the actual process of birth but also by the abrupt change from the minimal metabolism of the fetus to the maximal metabolic participation of the newborn infant.

The neonatal line becomes wider if there is brain damage; hypoplastic enamel is found to coincide with the neonatal line in persons with cerebral palsy. The enamel hypoplasia indicates

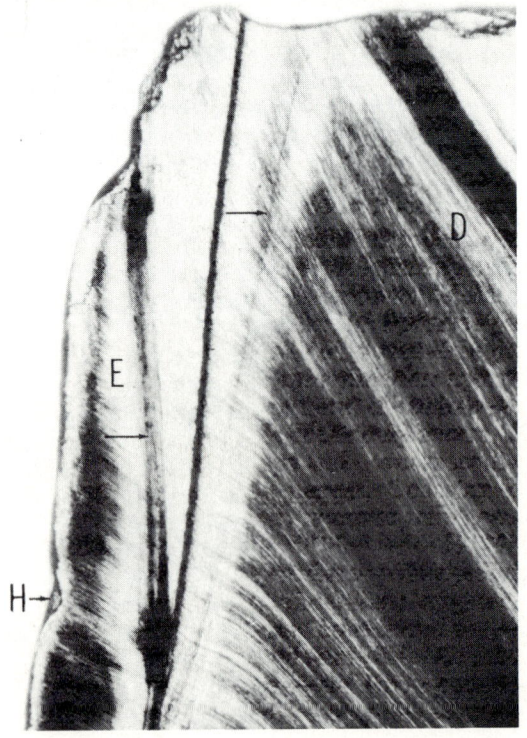

FIG. 16-14   Neonatal line. Ground section of deciduous molar in a patient with cerebral palsy. Arrows indicate neonatal lines in enamel (E) and dentin (D). A region of mild hypoplasia (H) is also evident. (Courtesy of Dr. Maury Massler, Chicago)

Histologically detectable reparative dentin begins to be elaborated shortly after the injury. In some of our experiments, reparative dentin was evident in tissue sections within 3 days of pulp exposure. Elaboration of reparative dentin matrix probably begins almost immediately after pulp injury.

Severe irritation may cause such rapid elaboration of matrix that the tubular structure may become lessened or tortuous, or even disappear. At times, cells or blood vessels may be surrounded and engulfed by the rapidly formed ground substance. The dentin thus formed is known as osteodentin because of its bonelike appearance. Heat cauterization of a pulp can cause the formation of osteodentin (Fig. 16-13). The pulp underlying reparative dentin may remain chronically inflamed, with eventual necrosis.

Ionizing Radiation

Irradiation of the heads of experimental animals causes degenerative changes in the odontoblasts and other pulp cells. As a result, the dentin that is formed is of the osteodentin type. It is formed

that there was interference with mineralization as a result of brain injury (McMillan and Kashgarian, 1961).

Fluorosis

Fluoride has a number of effects on dental hard tissues, such as reduction in volume of the unit cell, improvement of the crystallinity of hydroxyapatite and increase in the size of hydroxyapatite crystals (Furseth, 1971). Other possible actions include a reduction in molecular size of proteoglycans (Smalley and Embery, 1976) and a hastening of crystal growth concomitant to an inhibition of apatite nucleation (Fejershov et al, 1979).

Systemic administration of fluoride leads to its incorporation in all the hard tissues of the teeth (as well as bone) both pre- and post-eruption, with the formation of fluorapatite.

The effects of water-borne fluoride on the developing enamel and dentin of both rat and human teeth were studied by microradiography (Fejershov et al, 1979). Extensive hypomineralization of the enamel was produced. If the fluoride is administered while the ameloblasts are active, enamel fluorosis results.

In the dentin, fluorosis does not interfere with elaboration of matrix. However, mineralization is affected, resulting in irregular and widened predentin and poorly mineralized dentin. After single or multiple fluoride injections, both hyper- and hypomineralized zones are produced (Walton and Eisenmann, 1975; Fejershov et al, 1979). Apparently, fluoride interferes with the ability of the odontoblast to synthesize or transfer active sulfate into sulfated glycosaminoglycans (Embery and Smalley, 1980). However, the odontoblasts are not permanently damaged (Walton and Eisenmann, 1975).

Nutritional Influences

Both matrix formation and mineralization are influenced by various nutritional deficiencies and other nutritional factors. Shaw (1955) listed many nutritional factors that affect the bones and the teeth. With respect to dentin formation, the following seem to be significant.

Vitamin A Deficiency. In rats and guinea pigs, Vitamin A deficiency causes failure of the pulp cells to differentiate into odontoblasts. The characteristic alignment of the odontoblasts is lost. Thus, there is intereference with the elaboration of dentin matrix. Hence, dentin is formed irregularly and varies in quantity.

Vitamin C Deficiency. Ascorbic acid deficiency interferes with the formation of intercellular substances throughout the body. Wolbach and Howe (1925, 1926) and Boyle et al (1940) placed guinea pigs on a scorbutic diet. The odontoblasts failed to deposit normal predentin. They became atrophic and soon resembled nearby pulp cells. Eventually, they were completely disorganized. Therefore, dentin was laid down irregularly and at a greatly reduced rate. The dentinal tubules were arranged haphazardly. In severe deficiencies, deposition of dentin soon stopped entirely and the predentin became hypermineralized. Replacement dentin was of the osteodentin type. Dentin was elaborated so quickly that pulp cells were trapped in it.

Yale and associates (1959) injected radioactive ascorbic acid into scorbutic animals and found the tagged material in the odontoblasts and the predentin within a short time. Nakamura et al (1969) found that the level of alkaline phosphatase was markedly reduced in the dental tissues of scorbutic guinea pigs. In humans, such a deficiency of vitamin C is rarely found.

Vitamin D. Lack of vitamin D has been considered a nutritional disorder. However, vitamin D actually functions as a hormone. The hormonal activity is initiated by the action of sunlight on the skin, where previtamin D_3 is formed. D_3 is subsequently hydroxylated in the liver and then in the kidney to form the antirachitic metabolite $1,25(OH)_2 D_3$, calcitriol (Deluca, 1981). Vitamin D plays a role in the mineralization of dentin by controlling serum phosphorus and calcium levels (Engström, 1980; Kim et al, 1983).

Deficiency of vitamin D causes a disturbance in mineralization of the dentin. The formation of predentin is retarded and there is interference in mineralization due to an irregular deposition of inorganic salts.

Combinations of low–vitamin D and low-calcium diets also affect dentinogenesis in rats. The predentin width increases. These dentinal changes are related to increased phosphatase activity in the odontoblasts (Engström et al, 1977).

Excessive amounts of vitamin D can cause enamel hypoplasia, hypermineralization of enamel matrix, defective dentin formation, and mineralization of the pulp, possibly associated with increased acid phosphatase activity (Hammarstrom et al, 1973).

In vitamin D–depleted rats, the administra-

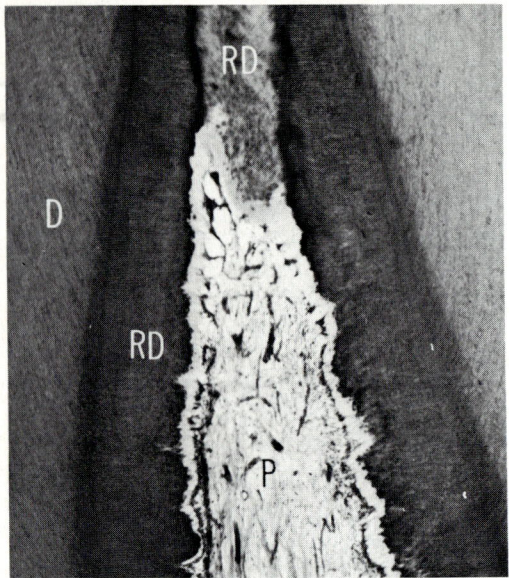

FIG. 16-15 Atrophy of the pulp. Atrophic pulp (P), as a result of aging. Reparative dentin (RD) formation has caused a reduction in the number of cells and an increase in collagen formation. ×54.

tion of toxic doses of 1,25-dihydroxycholecalciferol (the hormonal metabolite of vitamin D_3) caused premature aging of incisor pulp fibroblasts and odontoblasts, disturbances in the dentinal matrix, and osteodentin formation (Pitaru et al, 1982).

Hormones

All connective tissues are affected by hormones. Reparative dentinogenesis is specifically influenced, because of the effect of various hormones on the fibroblasts and the odontoblasts which are involved in the formation of the dentinal matrix. High dosages of parathyroid extract have been shown to produce hypomineralization of the newly formed dentinal matrix of rats' teeth (Yaeger and Eisenmann, 1963).

Progeria (Pituitary Senility). Aging processes are depicted graphically in the disease progeria. Album and Hope (1958) reported a case of a youngster suffering from this disease who showed all the semblances of aging. He had perivascular disease and a tendency toward arthritis. His skin became taut and his hair fell out. He became thin and emaciated. His teeth also were aged. The pulps of the teeth had a tendency toward fibrosis, with decreased cellular components. They had tremendous amounts of reparative dentin. The odontoblasts were flattened, like fibroblasts, and some mineralization was present in the blood vessels.

ATROPHY (PULPOSIS)

An atrophied pulp is one that has become smaller through some physiologic or pathologic process. Atrophy of the pulp occurs normally with advancing age (Fig. 16-15). As the individual gets older, there is a relative increase in the amount of collagen fibers in the pulp due to a decrease in the number of cells. Actually, the rate of collagen synthesis is lower in the pulps of older human teeth than in those of erupting teeth (Uitto, 1976). According to Bernick and Nedelman (1975), the prominence of fiber bundles in old pulps may partly be attributed to the persistence of the connective tissue sheaths in a narrowed pulp chamber. Zerlötti (1964) observed that, in addition to a decrease in the ratio of ground substance to collagen, aged pulps also exhibited an increase in resistance to proteolytic enzymes and decreases in collagen solubility, water content and chemical reactivity. This is a normal process which occurs throughout the life of the individual. The chronologic age of the individual is not necessarily indicative of the state of the pulp. In many comparatively young persons, large quantities of collagenous fibers and mineralization are found in the pulp, and there is a tendency toward the disappearance of the cells. Thus, even in young persons, aged pulps may be encountered. Conversely, highly cellular pulps have been found in older persons.

Atrophy from Caries and Operative Procedures

Atrophy may occur as a result of dental caries or operative procedures on the dentin. Under such circumstances, there is a reduction in the size and a decrease in the total number of cells. The pulps underlying large areas of reparative dentin appear in many instances to be atrophic, having fewer cells and more collagen fibers (Fig. 16-15). The remaining cells appear shrunken. The pulps seem to be "burned out," having suffered exhaustion atrophy. In some, coagulation necrosis seems to be imminent. There is an apparent increase in dystrophic mineralization scattered throughout both the coronal and the radicular portions. Mineralization is found in the walls of blood vessels and perineural sheaths as well as in unrelated regions. Apparently, atrophic or necrotic cells are instrumental in initiating mineral deposits, which then form nuclei for further addition of mineral salts.

Atrophy from Periodontal Disease

Atrophic pulps are found frequently in teeth with advanced periodontal disease. The cells are smaller in size and fewer in number, as a result of the impairment of the nutritional supply. (See Chap. 15, The Interrelationship of Pulp and Periodontal Disease.)

DYSTROPHIC MINERALIZATION

Aging

Dystrophic mineralization is found in varying amounts and degrees in most pulps. In some pulps in which there has been no caries or operative intervention, the coronal portions are relatively free of mineralization. However, even in those teeth, the apical portion of the pulp, especially in regions of collagen fibers, contains scattered mineralization. The presence of mineralization appears to be unrelated to any known condition or cause.

Ground substance alterations in the dental pulps apparently occur on aging and result in a decreased reactivity and predominance of highly aggregated, less soluble macromolecules (Zerlotti, 1969). Such changes may contribute to cellular degeneration and incrased dystrophic mineralization. The finding of increased mineralization as a result of aging was confirmed by Saunders (1967), Zackson (1969), and Bernick and Nedelman (1975). Such mineralizations suggest that circulatory disturbances may be the initiating factor.

Examination of pulp tissue with the electron

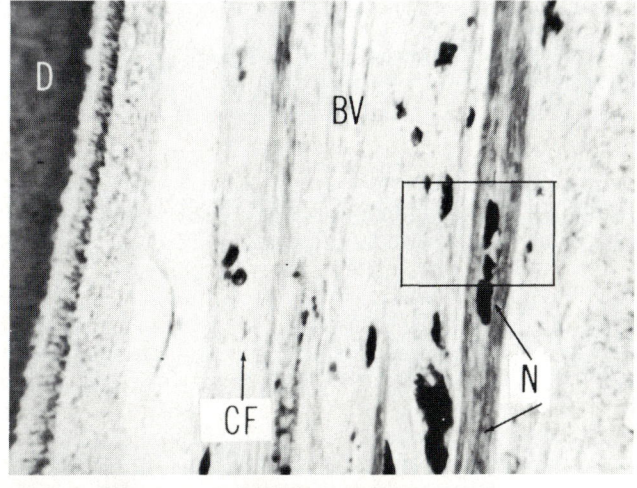

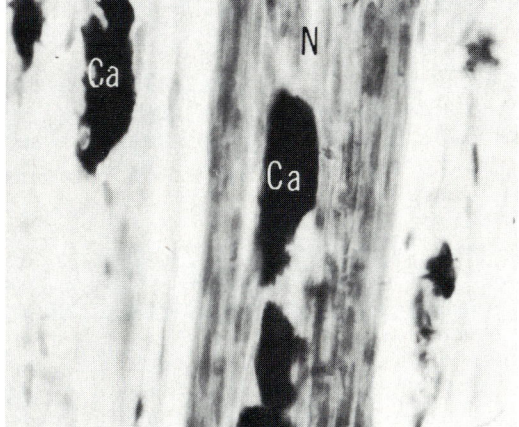

FIG. 16-16 *(Top)* Dystrophic calcifications in myelin sheath (N). CF, collagen fibers; BV, blood vessels; D, dentin. ×135. *(Bottom)* Higher magnification of region outlined by rectangle, above. Dystrophic mineralizations (CA) are seen on the myelinated nerve (N) and in the pulp tissue. ×540.

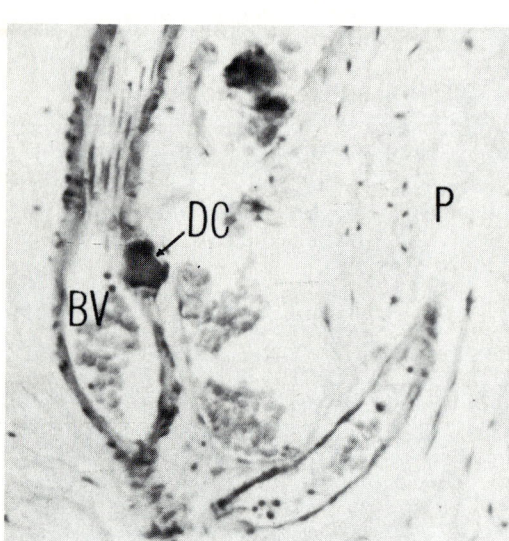 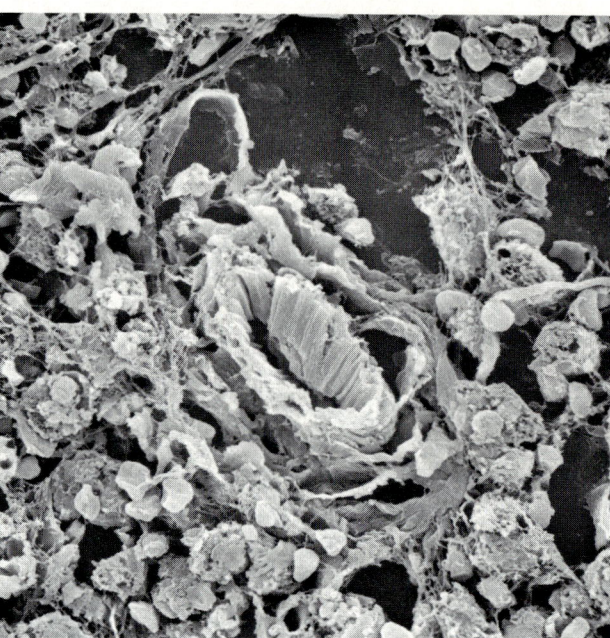

FIG. 16-17 *(Left)* Dystrophic mineralization (DC), beginning in wall of arteriole (BV) of the pulp (P). ×240. *(Right)* Scanning electron micrograph of tissue section, showing mineralized blood vessel in pulp. ×200.

microscope reveals the beginning of mineralization in the collagen fibrils long before the mineralizations can be seen by the light microscope.

Normally, mineralization takes place in a preformed organic matrix. However, Appleton and Williams (1973) have described small smooth-surfaced, spherical clusters either closely packed around collagen fibers or in the form of intracellular deposits in the fibroblasts. The crystallites were platelike or needlelike and diffuse and varied considerably in size. The diffraction pattern was typical of hydroxyapatite material. Some of the small, smooth-surfaced foci of mineralization did not appear to have any relationship to a specific matrix component. It appeared to them that the deposition of minerals in the pulp was coincident with the deposition of organic material other than, or in addition to, the collagen fibers already in the matrix.

Once a nucleus is deposited, further mineralization takes place by secretion. The exact reason for mineralization of pulp fibrils is unknown. The changes that enable mineralization of pulp fibrils seem to occur in the mucopolysaccharide content of the sheaths around the fibrils. It is believed that they become sulfated. Sulfated mucopolysaccharides appear to be involved in the attraction mechanism for mineralization, but other factors also are involved.

Mineralizations occasionally are seen in the myelin sheaths of nerves (Fig. 16-16). Their beginnings are also found in the vessel walls, as in arteriosclerosis (Fig. 16-17). Older, fibrotic pulps attract mineral salts more readily. A mineralized pulp, when extirpated, feels wooden and hard.

Dystrophic Mineralization Due to Caries and Periodontal Disease

Dystrophic mineralizations also apparently increase markedly as a result of disease processes such as caries and periodontal disease (Bernick, 1967; Sayegh and Reed, 1968; Hall, 1968). In teeth with caries and/or restorations, there is a significant increase in coronal dystrophic mineralization.

Teeth whose pulps are chronically inflamed contain dystrophic mineralizations in regions of previous liquefaction necrosis and, in varying amounts, in the remaining pulp tissue. Our SEM examinations of teeth with inflamed and/or degenerating pulps (Seltzer et al, 1977) revealed

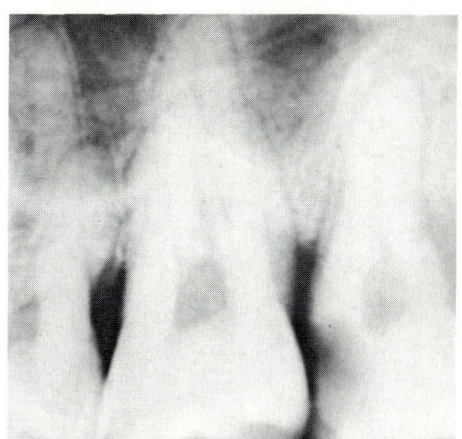

FIG. 16-18 *(Top)* Radiograph of upper right third molar, showing deep carious lesion. *(Bottom left)* Increase of fibrillar (dystrophic) mineralization (DysC) in the pulp (P) as a result of dental caries. D, dentin. ×54. *(Bottom right)* Scanning electron micrograph showing mineralized coronal pulp tissue from caries. ×200.

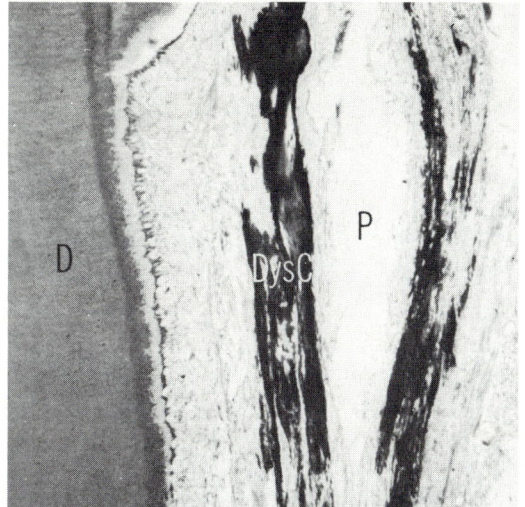
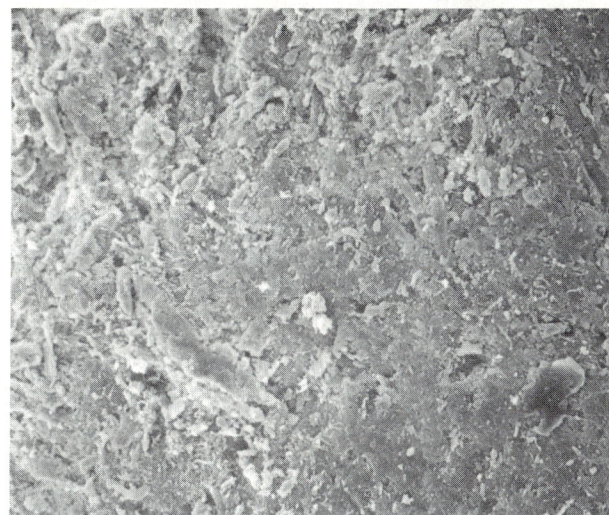

the presence of pathologic mineralizations (Fig. 16–18). Both cells and fibers are involved in the mineralizing process. The surfaces of the cells change; they become smooth and folded'. Accretion of surface minerals interferes with the interchange of nutrients through the cell membranes (Fig. 16–19, *left*). The cell contents then degenerate, resulting in a hollow interior (Fig. 16–19, *right*). Various cell types, including odontoblasts, fibroblasts, endothelial cells, and inflammatory cells, become mineralized (Fig. 16–20). The fibers initially assume a beaded appearance (Fig. 16–21, *left*). Minerals are found near these degenerating fibers. Eventually, the mineralizing fibers coalesce and become larger masses (Fig. 16–21, *right*).

There are several postulations for the formation of dystrophic mineralizations in the presence of inflammation. Irving (1963) has observed that sudanophilic material is present at connective tissue mineralization sites. Perhaps, lipids associated with collagen or lipoprotein complexes become exposed or altered in such a way as to play a role in crystal nucleation or in facilitating crystal growth. Another possibility is that inhibitors of mineralization, such as pyrophosphates (Fleisch, 1964), and diphosphonates (Fleisch and Russell, 1972), have been removed, thereby permitting mineralization. Finally, Granström's experiments (1982, 1983) have indicated that alkaline phosphatase in odontoblasts may function as a calcium pyrophosphatase, thereby stimulating Ca^{2+} uptake in rat pulps.

In teeth with periodontal disease, dystrophic mineralizations increase tremendously in both

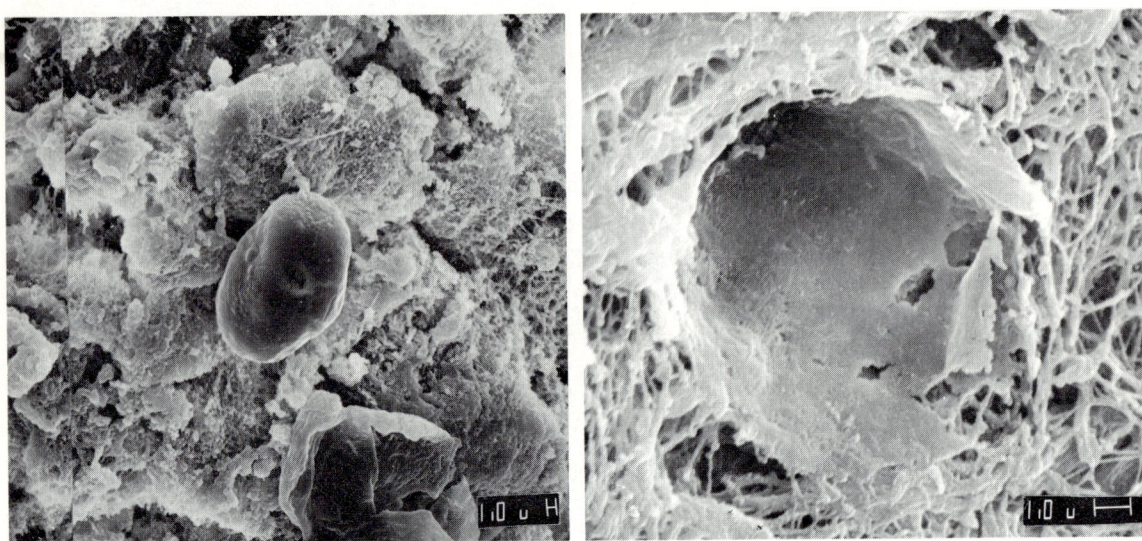

FIG. 16-19 *(Left)* Scanning electron micrograph of upper molar shown in Fig. 16-18 with chronic total pulpitis. Mineralized cell is seen in center. A broken mineralized cell is seen at bottom. ×1000. *(Right)* Scanning electron micrograph of tissue section of left frame showing dissected cell with hollow interior. ×5000.

FIG. 16-20 *(Left)* Tissue section showing incorporation of inflammatory cells (arrows) in mineralizing mass (M). ×500. *(Right)* Scanning electron micrograph showing cells being entrapped in mineralized mass. ×5000.

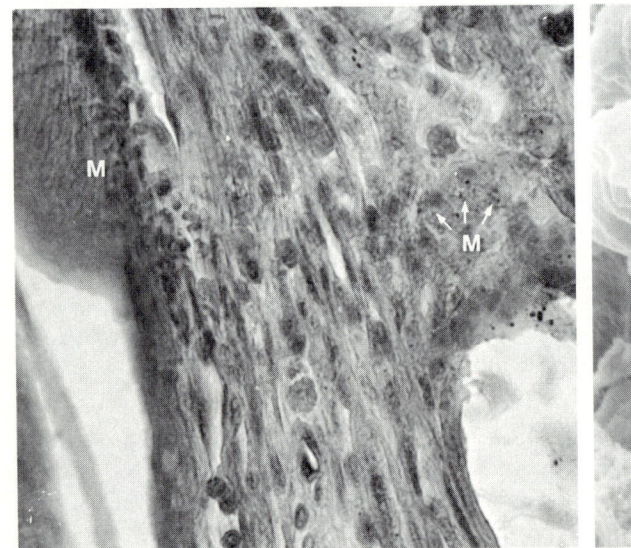
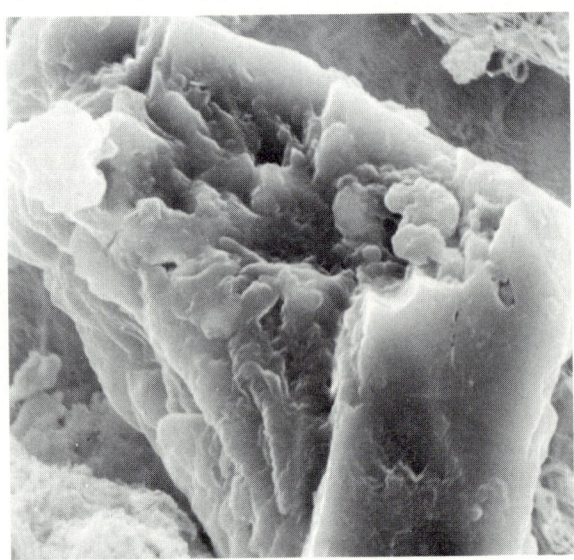

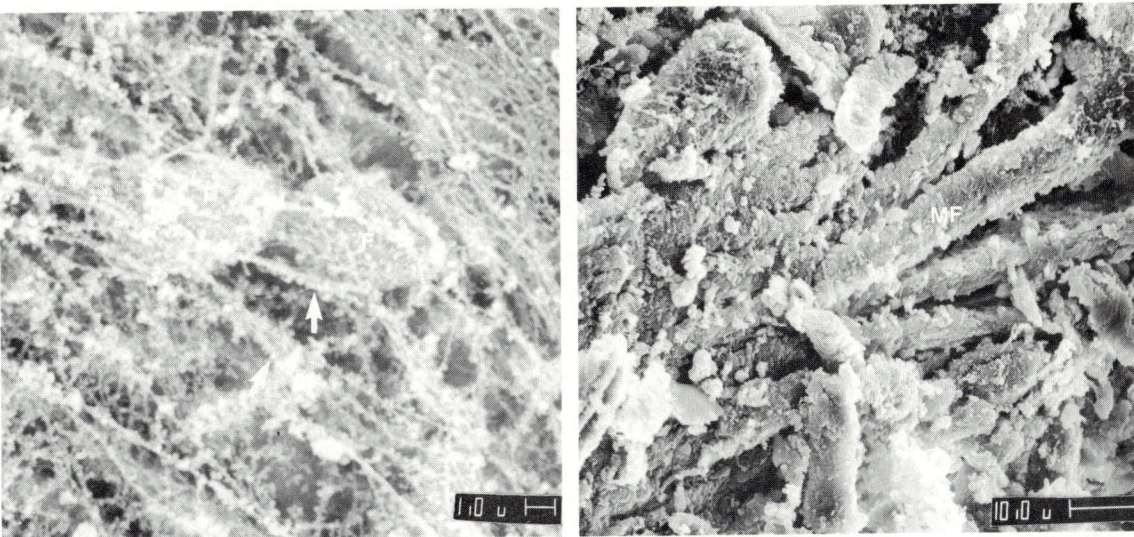

FIG. 16-21 *(Left)* Scanning electron micrograph of tooth with carious pulp. Fibers (arrow) have assumed a beaded appearance. Two fibroblasts (F) are seen in center. ×4000. *(Right)* Mineralizing fibers (MF) in floor of pulp chamber. ×200.

the coronal and the radicular portions of the pulp.

DENTICLES

The larger mineralizations are called denticles. These are large mineralized bodies which sometimes result from fusion of several smaller ones. Denticles can become extremely large, at times almost obliterating the pulp chamber or the root canal.

Denticles may be classified (1) structurally, (2) according to size, and (3) according to location.

Structure

From the standpoint of structure, there are true denticles and false denticles. The difference between the two is morphologic, not chemical.

A true denticle is supposed to be made up of dentin and is lined by odontoblasts. Generally, they are found in the apical portion of the tooth.

False denticles are formed from degenerating cells of the pulp that tend to mineralize. The mineralizing cells coalesce. Concentrically, thereafter, layer upon layer of mineral salts are laid down (Fig. 16-22). Matrix is laid down first, inasmuch as, whenever mineralization occurs, a matrix is first elaborated which attracts the mineral salts.

Size

According to size, there are fine, diffuse mineralizations, also known as fibrillar mineralizations, and denticles. The former are found more frequently in the root canals, but they may also be present in the coronal portion of the pulp (Fig. 16-18).

Location

According to location, denticles can be classified as (1) embedded or interstitial, (2) adherent and (3) free denticles.

Embedded denticles are formed originally in the pulp. Subsequently, dentin matrix is deposited and mineralization continues. Eventually, as more and more dentin is elaborated, the denticles may be completely embedded. Embedded denticles are found most frequently in the apical portion of the root (Fig. 16-23). They are of clinical significance during endodontic therapy because they can be dislodged during instrumentation and may block the apex of the tooth, thus causing difficulties in further treatment.

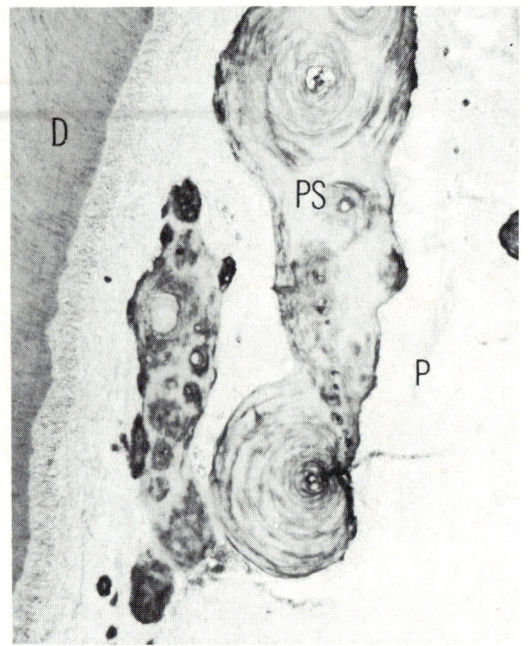

FIG. 16-22 False denticle. The denticle (PS) grows concentrically in the pulp (P). Denticles gradually enlarge by joining with others. D, dentin. ×54.

FIG. 16-23 Denticle at root apex. A portion of the large denticle (PS) is embedded, and another denticle already has been embedded (arrow). P, pulp; AF, apical foramen. ×54.

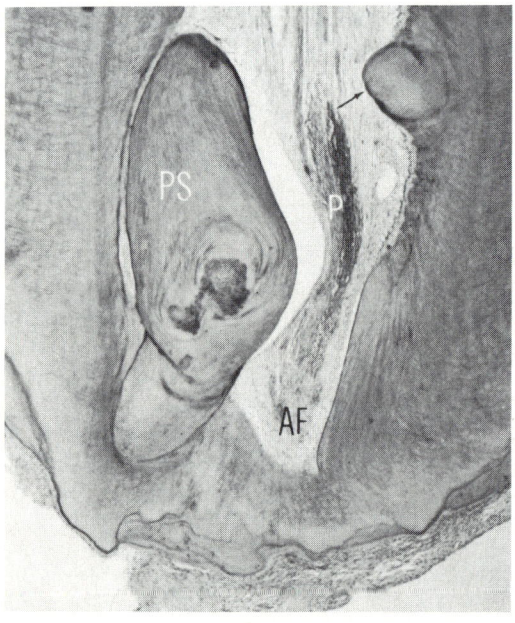

Blockage of the apical third of the root canal may be attributed mistakenly to the packing of debris. When large denticles are present, they may interfere with extirpation of the entire pulp or removal of the coronal portion of the pulp.

Adherent denticles are those that are attached to the dentin but are not completely embedded in it.

Free denticles are those that are found lying free in the pulp tissue. They are present in a large percentage of teeth and in fact are so prevalent that almost all pulps have some mineralization within them. They are present in young as well as in old people. There is a tendency for more and more denticles to be deposited with increased age.

Denticles have been found in teeth in utero, in teeth that have not yet erupted and in deciduous as well as permanent teeth. James (1958) found early mineralization of the pulp in 56% of young, permanent teeth extracted for orthodontic reasons. In a radiologic survey by Tamse et al (1982), 20.7% of 1380 teeth contained denticles and the incidence was greater in females than in males. However, they are not always detected in radiographs unless they are fairly large. There appears to be no correlation between the presence of denticles and other mineralization or disease processes in the body.

It is questionable whether pulpalgia should be attributed to denticles, although it is possible that as the denticle gets larger, it can create pressure against nerves in the vicinity. The presence of denticles may be either the cause or the result of atrophic pulp changes.

Occasionally, but not usually, inflammatory pulp responses are seen around denticles.

INCREASE IN NUMBER AND THICKNESS OF COLLAGEN FIBERS (FIBROSIS)

In intact-uninflamed pulps, collagen fibers are infrequent or absent in the coronal portions of posterior teeth that are free of caries and have not been operated on. In anterior teeth, the quantity of coronal collagen is significantly greater (Fig. 16-24). In the apical third of the root canal there is a gradual transition from the cellular pulp to a more collagenous, less cellular tissue in which blood vessels and nerves are present.

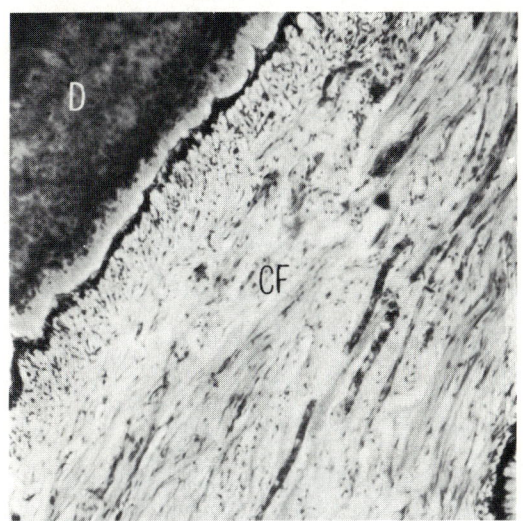

FIG. 16-24 Collagen fibers in anterior tooth. The collagen (CF) is of the bundle type. D, dentin. ×96.

CLINICAL CORRELATIONS OF INDUCED PULP AGING

The pulps of all teeth that have been subjected to extensive caries, abrasion, attrition, erosion or operative procedures, such as cavity and crown preparation and/or restoration, appear to have undergone retrogressive and atrophic changes. These changes are: diminution in the number of cells, increase in the amount of collagen fibers and profuse dystrophic mineralizations. The volumes of these pulps have been reduced by the formation of reparative dentin under the regions of the involved dentinal tubules, sometimes in massive amounts, tending to obliterate almost the entire coronal portion of the pulp. In regions where chornic inflammation has been present, the lumina of the root canals also have been narrowed.

The presence of peridontal lesions contributes to the aging of the dental pulp. In such pulps, many regions of atrophy, necrosis, mineralization and narrowing of the lumina of the root canals are found. It seems evident that external influences, either from the periodontal ligament of from disease processes affecting the odontoblasts, are instrumental in causing degenerative changes within dental pulps. These changes are somewhat compatible with the wear and tear theory of aging, which postulates that each stress to which an organism is subjected takes its toll, until, finally, the organism wears out.

Histologic examination reveals that, in older pulps there is a relative increase in the number of argyrophilic reticular fibers and in the number and thickness of collagen fibers as compared to young pulps (Bhussry, 1968). The relative increase is due to reduction in the volume of the pulp by the continuous deposition of secondary dentin. Moreover, actual increase in the number of collagen fibrils also occurs. Electronmicroscopic examination of the pulps of premolars and molars of normal persons aged 13 and 14 years and of those aged 56 to 62 years (Cahan, 1970) revealed that in the ground substance of the younger pulps there was a sparse distribution of collagen fibrils about 750Å in diameter. Collagen bundles were embedded in a denser ground substance. In the pulps of persons aged 56 to 62 years, there was a decided increase in the number of collagen fibrils. Near the collagen fibrils, bundles of unstriated small fibrils, about 150 Å in diameter, were noted.

Fibrosis in the coronal portion of the pulp increases under the influence of caries, abrasion, attrition and, markedly, after operative procedures, with a concurrent filling-in of the pulp horns with reparative dentin. There is a simultaneous reduction in the number of pulp cells. In chronically inflamed pulps, fibrosis is markedly increased and the blood vessels become prominent and vastly dilated.

FIG. 16-25 Scanning electron micrograph, showing region of odontoblasts (Od) of pulp (P) that have degenerated owing to poor fixation. ×600. In a histologic section, such a condition would appear like the section shown in Fig. 16-26.

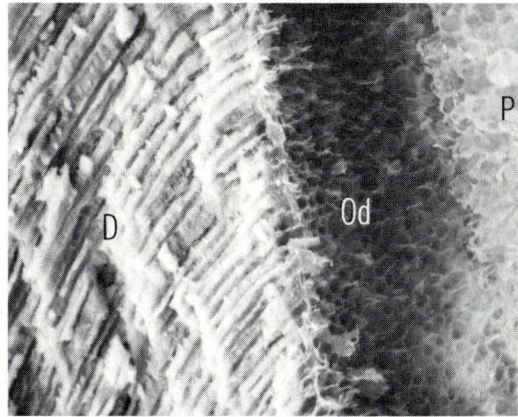

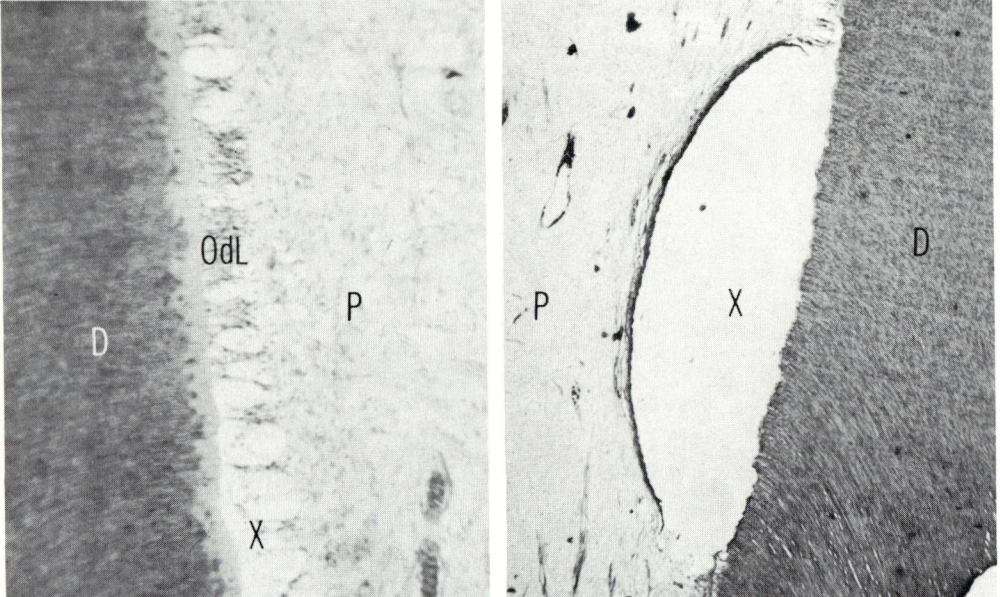

FIG. 16-26 Artifacts, due to poor fixation. *(Left)* "Vacuolization" of the odontoblastic layer (OdL) at X. ×135. *(Right)* "Blister" formation (X) in the pulp (P) under cut dentinal tubules (D). ×54.

As a result of all of these age changes, i.e., increase in fibers, decrease in cells and reduction of volume, there is probably an interference with the defense capacity of the pulp.

In general, aged tissue cannot defend itself as well against injury as can young tissue. For example, when a youngster fractures a limb, he usually recovers quickly, and, within a short period of time, he is functioning normally. However, a fracture in an older individual is more serious, and recovery is not as rapid. Complications may arise more readily, and function does not return as rapidly. Pains and aches may persist in older persons for longer periods. Thus, induced aging of the pulp by dental procedures should be avoided, in order to avoid impairment of the defence capacity of the pulp. The more injuries inflicted on the pulp through cavity cutting, drugs, pressure, impression taking, and so forth, the more the likelihood of pulp aging. Any injury which causes an inflammatory response to occur within the pulp will cause an aging process, i.e., more dentin will be elaborated, more mineralization will take place, and the volume of the pulp will be reduced. In spite of recovery, it is possible that subsequent injuries will not be so well tolerated, though this has not been proved experimentally.

ARTIFACTS

A number of conditions that have been described as indicative of pathologic or regressive changes are now believed to be artifacts attributable to poor fixation or errors in the processing of tissue (Fig. 16-25). Among these are "reticular atrophy," "vacuolization" of the odontoblastic layer, "blister formation," and "fatty degeneration" (Fig. 16-26). Another pulp change which may be due to imperfect or delayed fixation is the presence of an increased eosinophilia of the ground substance of the pulp, especially in the region of the pulp horns.

BIBLIOGRAPHY

Album MA, Hope JW: Progeria, report of case. Oral Surg 11:985, 1958
Anderson WAD: Pathology. St. Louis, CV Mosby, 1948
Appleton J, Williams MJR: Ultrastructural observations on the calcifications of human dental pulp. Calc Tiss Res 11:222, 1973
Bennett CG, Kelln EE, Biddington WR: Age changes of the vascular pattern of the human dental pulp. Arch Oral Biol 10:995, 1965
Bergenholtz G, Reit C: Reactions of the dental pulp to microbial provocation of calcium hydroxide treated dentin. Scand J Dent Res 88:187, 1980

Bernick S: Age changes in the blood supply to human teeth. J Dent Res 46:544, 1967a

Bernick S: Effect of aging on the nerve supply to human teeth. J Dent Res 46:694, 1967b

Bernick S, Nedelman C: Effect of aging on the human pulp. J Endodont 3:88, 1975

Bhussry BR: Modification of the dental pulp organ during development and aging. In Finn SB (ed): Biology of the Dental Pulp Organ, pp 146–165. University of Alabama Press, 1968

Boyle PE, Bessey OA, Howe PR: Rate of dentin formation in incisor teeth of guinea pigs on normal and on ascorbic acid-deficient diets. Arch Path 30:90, 1940

Bradford EW: The dentin, a barrier to caries. Brit Dent J 109:387, 1960

Brännström M, Garberoglio R: Occlusion of dentinal tubules under superficial attrited dentine. Swed Dent J 4:87, 1980

Byers MR, Dong WK: Autoradiographic location of sensory nerve endings in dentin of monkey teeth. Anat Rec 205:441, 1983

Cahan PM: Electron microscopic study of human dental pulp. J Dent Res 49:688, 1970 (abstr)

Comfort A: The Biology of Senescence. London, Routledge, 1956

Cox CF, Heys DR, Gibbons PK, Avery JK, Heys RJ: The effect of various restorative materials on the microhardness of reparative dentin. J Dent Res 59:109, 1980

Curtis HJ: Biological mechanisms underlying the aging process. Science 141:686, 1963

Curtis HJ: Biological Mechanisms of Aging. Springfield, Illinois, Charles C Thomas, 1966

Darlington GJ, Weksler ME: Increased sensitivity of lymphocytes from people over 65 to cell cycle arrest and chromosomal damage. Science 219:1335, 1983

Deluca HF: The vitamin D system: A view from basic science to the clinic. Clin Biochem 14:213, 1981

Eisenmann DR, Yaeger JA: Alterations in the formation of rat dentine and enamel induced by various ions. Arch Oral Biol 14:1045, 1969

Embery G, Smalley JW: The influence of fluoride on the uptake of radiosulfate by rat incisor odontoblasts in vitro. Arch Oral Biol 25:659, 1980

Engström C: Odontoblast metabolism in rats deficient in vitamin D and calcium. IV. Lysosomal and energy metabolic enzymes. J Oral Pathol 9:264, 1980

Engström C, Linde A, Magnusson B: Odontoblast metabolism in rats deficient in vitamin D and calcium. II. Changes in activities of alkaline phosphatases. J Oral Pathol 6:367, 1977

Fejershov O, Yaeger JA, Thylstrup A: Microradiography of the effect of acute and chronic administration of fluoride on human and rat dentine and enamel. Arch Oral Biol 24:123, 1979

Fischer FM, El-Kafrawy A, Mitchell DF: Studies of tertiary dentin in monkey teeth using vital dyes. J Dent Res 49:1537, 1970

Fleisch H: Role of nucleation and inhibition of calcification. Clin Orthop 32:170, 1964

Fleisch H, Russell RGG: A review of physiological and pharmacological effects of pyrophosphate and diphosphonates on bones and teeth. J Dent Res 51:325, 1972

Furseth R: Fluor og de hårde tannev. Norske Tannlaegeforen Tid 81:605, 1971

Goto G, Machiola Y: The rate of reparative dentine formation in the human teeth. Bull Tokyo Dent Coll 13:251, 1972

Granström G: Influence of bivalent cations, phosphate and complexing substances on inorganic pyrophosphate in the microsomal fraction of isolated rat odontoblasts. Arch Oral Biol 28:453, 1983

Granström G: Relationship of inorganic pyrophosphatase and p-nitrophenylphosphatase activities of alkaline phosphatase in the microsomal fraction of isolated odontoblasts. Scand J Dent Res 90:271, 1982

Hall DC: Pulpal calcifications—a pathological process? In Symons NBB (ed): Dentine and Pulp: Their Structure and Reactions, pp 269–274. Baltimore, Williams and Wilkins, 1968

Hammarstrom LE, Ramp WK, Toverud SU: Histochemistry of various acid phosphatases in developing bones and teeth in hypervitaminosis D in the rat. Arch Oral Biol 18:109, 1973

Han SS: The fine structure of cells and intercellular substances of the dental pulp. IN Finn SB (ed): Biology of the Dental Pulp Organ. pp 103–139. University of Alabama Press, 1968

Harcourt JK: Further observations on the peritubular translucent zone in human dentine. Austr Dent J 9:387, 1964

Haugen E, Mjör IA: Pulpal reactions to attrition. J Endodont 1:12, 1975

Hawkinson RW, Eisenmann DR: Electron microscopy of dentinal tubule sclerosis in the enamel-free region of the rat molar. Arch Oral Biol 28:409, 1983

Irving JT: The sudanophil material at sites of calcification. Arch Oral Biol 8:735, 1963

Isokawa S, Kubota K, Kuwajima K: Scanning electron microscope study of dentin exposed by contact facets and cervical abrasion. J Dent Res 52:170, 1973

Isokawa S, Toda Y, Ajisaka M, Inoue Y, Saito T, Tsuchida S: Scanning electron microscopic observation of the peritubular zone in dentin sclerosis. J Nihon Univ School Dent 12:105, 1970

Kawasaki K, Tanaka S, Ishikawa T: On the daily incremental lines in human dentine. Arch Oral Biol 24:939, 1980

Kim YS, Stumpf WE, Clark SA, Sar M, DeLuca HF: Target cells for 1,25-dihydroxyvitamin D_3 in developing rat incisor teeth. J Dent Res 62:58, 1983

Kindlová M, Matêna V: Blood circulation in the rodent teeth of the rat. Acta Anat (Basel) 37:163, 1959

Leaf A: Getting old. Sci Amer 229:45, 1973

Leblond CP, Bélanger LF, Greulich RC: Formation of bones and teeth as visualized by radioautography. Ann NY Acad Sci 60:631, 1955

McMillan RS, Kashgarian M: Relation of human abnormalities of structure and function to abnormalities of the dentition. I. Relation of hypoplasia of enamel to cerebral and ocular disorders. JADA 63:38, 1961

Mendis BRRM, Darling AI: Distribution with age and attrition of peritubular dentine in the crowns of human teeth. Arch Oral Biol 24:131, 1979

Miles AEW: "Sans teeth": changes in oral tissues with advancing age. President's address. Proc Roy Soc Med 65:801, 1972

Nakamura R, Tsunemitsu A, Matsumura T: Effect of adrenal cortical hormones and insulin on the alkaline phosphatase activity of alveolar bone in scorbutic guinea pigs. Arch Oral Biol 14:725, 1969

Ogawa Y, Ishida T, Yagi T: Ultramicroscopy of hypomineralized responses in rat incisor dentine to injected strontium. Arch Oral Biol 26:229, 1981

Philippas GG: Effects of function on healthy teeth: The evidence of ancient Athenian remains. JADA 45:443, 1952

Philippas GG: Influence of occlusal wear and age on formation of dentin and size of pulp chamber. J Dent Res 40:1186, 1961

Philippas GG, Applebaum E: Age factor in secondary dentin formation. J Dent Res 45:778, 1966

Philippas GG, Applebaum E: Age changes in the permanent upper lateral incisor. J Dent Res 46:1002, 1967

Philippas GG, Applebaum E: Age changes in the permanent upper canine teeth. J Dent Res 47:411, 1968

Pitaru S, Blaushild N, Noff D, Edelstein S: The effect of 1,25-dihydroxycholecalciferol on dental tissues in the rat. Arch Oral Biol 27:915, 1982

Saunders RL de CH: Vascular supply of the dental tissues, including lymphatics. In Miles AEW (ed): Structural and Chemical Organization of Teeth. Vol 1, p 235. New York, Academic Press, 1967

Sayegh FS, Reed AJ: Calcification in the dental pulp. Oral Surg 25:873, 1968

Schwabe C: Age dependent changes of certain peptide hydrolases and dehydrogenases in bovine dental pulp. J Dent Res 48:951, 1969

Seltzer S, Bender IB, Kaufman IJ, Moodnik R: Alkaline phosphatase in reparative dentinogenesis. Oral Surg 7:859, 1962

Seltzer S, Bender IB, Ziontz M: The dynamics of pulp inflammation: Correlations between diagnostic data and actual histologic findings in the pulp. Oral Surg 16:846, 969, 1963

Seltzer S, Bender IB, Ziontz M: The interrelationship of pulp and periodontal disease. Oral Surg 16:1474, 1963

Seltzer S, Rainey E, Gluskin AH: Correlation of scanning electron microscope and light microscope findings in uninflamed and pathologically involved human pulps. Oral Surg 43:910, 1977

Selye H, Prioreschi P: Stress theory of aging. In Shock NW (ed): Aging, Some Social and Biological Aspects. pp 261–272. Washington, DC, Am Ass Adv Sci 1960

Senzaki H: A histological study of reparative dentinogenesis in the rat incisor after colchicine administration. Archc Oral Biol 25:737, 1980

Shaw JH: Effect of nutritional factors on bones and teeth. Ann NY Acad Sci 60:733, 1955

Shock NW: Aging. Some Social and Biological Aspects. Washington, DC, Am Ass Adv Sci publ No 65, 1960

Sicher H: Orban's Oral Histology and Embryology, 5th ed, pp 121–127; 139–140. St. Louis, CV Mosby, 1962

Smalley JW, Embery G: Effect of fluoride on molecular size of proteoglycans in the rat incisor tooth. Arch Oral Biol 21:703, 1976

Staino-Coico L, Darzynkiewicz Z, Hefton JM, Dutkowski R, Stanley HR, White CL, McCray L: The rate of tertiary (reparative) dentine formation in the human tooth. Oral Surg 21:180, 1966

Sveen OB, Hawes RR: Differentiation of new odontoblasts and dentine bridge formation in rat molar teeth after tooth grinding. Arch Oral Biol 13:1399, 1968

Symons NBB: The microanatomy and histochemistry of dentinogenesis. In Miles AEW (ed): Structural and Chemical Organization of Teeth, Vol 1, pp 317–318. New York, Academic Press, 1967

Takuma S: Ultrastructure of dentinogenesis. In Miles AEW (ed): Structural and Chemical Organization of Teeth, Vol 1, p 364. New York, Academic Press, 1967

Tamse A, Kaffe I, Littner MM, Shani R: Statistical evaluation of radiologic survey of pulp stones. J Endodont 8:455, 1982

Tronstad L: Optical and microradiographic appearance of intact and worn human coronal dentine. Arch Oral Biol 17:847, 1972

Tronstad L: Vital staining of coronal dentin in monkey teeth. Oral Surg 45:612, 1978

Uitto V-J: Collagen biosynthesis in the dental pulp in vivo. Proc Finnish Dent Soc 72: Suppl #1, 1976

Vacek von ZD, Plačková A: Die Innervation der Zähne. Acta Anat 36:59, 1959

Walton RE, Eisenmann DR: Ultrastructural examination of dentine formation in rat incisors following multiple fluoride injections. Arch Oral Biol 20:485, 1975

Wennberg A, Mjör IA, Heide, S: Rate of formation of regular and irregular secondary dentin in monkey teeth. Oral Surg 54:232, 1982

Wolbach SB, Howe PR: The effect of the scorbutic state upon the production and maintenance of intercellular substances. Proc Soc Exp Biol Med 22:400, 1925

Wolbach SB, Howe PR: Intercellular substance in experimental scorbutus. Arch Path Lab Med 1:1, 1926

Yaeger JA: Microscopy of the response of rodent dentin to injected fluoride. Anat Rec 145:139, 1963a

Yaeger JA: Fine structure of the matrix of the response in rat incisor dentin to injected strontium. J Dent Res 42:1178, 1963b

Yaeger JA, Eisenmann DR: Response in rat incisor dentin to injected strontium, fluoride, and parathyroid extract. J Dent Res 42:1208, 1963

Yale SH, Jeffay H, Mohammed CI, Wach EC: Oral changes in normal and scorbutic guinea pigs injected with ascorbic acid I-C 14. J Dent Res 38:396, 1959

Young RW, Greulich RC: Distinctive autoradiographic patterns of glycine incorporation in rat enamel and dentine matrices. Arch Oral Biol 8:509, 1963

Zakson ML: Age specific changes of teeth in aged and senile persons. Stomatologiia (Moskva) 48:4:29, 1969

Zerlotti E: Histochemical study of the connective tissue of the dental pulp. Arch Oral Biol 9:149, 1964

Zerlotti E: Histochemical changes in the connective tissue of the dental pulp during inflammation. Oral Surg 27:664, 1969

17
HISTOLOGIC CLASSIFICATION OF PULP DISEASES

Numerous studies have shown that histologic diagnoses of pulp conditions cannot be made with assurance from a clinical standpoint (Hess, 1967; Baume, 1970; Hasler and Mitchell, 1970; Garfunkel et al, 1973). The clinician can make an educated guess as to the character of the pathologic lesions on the basis of symptoms and results of various tests. However, accurate pathologic diagnoses can be made only from examinations of histologic sections of the involved pulp tissues. For example, a physician may make a clinical diagnosis of a tumor mass and characterize it as benign or malignant. However, the exact diagnosis cannot be established without a biopsy. Similarly, a dentist may decide on the basis of clinical symptoms that a tooth has pulpitis of a certain type. However, the final diagnosis must be based on an analysis of the histologic section of the tooth. The importance of the correct diagnosis may be of only academic interest when subsequent endodontic procedures are employed, since the pulp will be extirpated in any event. However, more conservative procedures aimed at preservation of the vitality of the pulp or healing of pulp inflammations must be based on an accurate assessment of the status of the pulp if the therapy is to be effective. In this chapter and the ensuing chapters on Differential Diagnosis (Chap. 18) and Clinical Diagnosis (Chap. 19), an attempt is made to enable the clinician to make a rapprochement between histologic diagnosis and clinical signs, tests, and symptoms.

CLASSIFICATION

There is wide variation in the histologic appearance of normal pulps. In fact, so many variations exist that the classification "normal" does not reflect accurately the condition of the pulp. Pulps that exhibit no inflammatory signs may be classified more realistically as "intact-uninflamed" or "atrophic," depending on the presence or the absence of inflammatory cells and the relative abundance and appearance of fibroblasts, collagen fibers, dystrophic mineralization, and reparative dentin. In many uninflamed pulps, atrophic changes are discernible, sometimes unrelated but often related to previous operative interference or dental caries. Dystrophic mineralizations are present in many uninflamed pulps and in most teeth that are periodontally involved or have undergone operative manipulations.

Inflammatory cells are present in the pulps of most teeth with moderately deep caries and almost all teeth with deep-seated carious lesions.

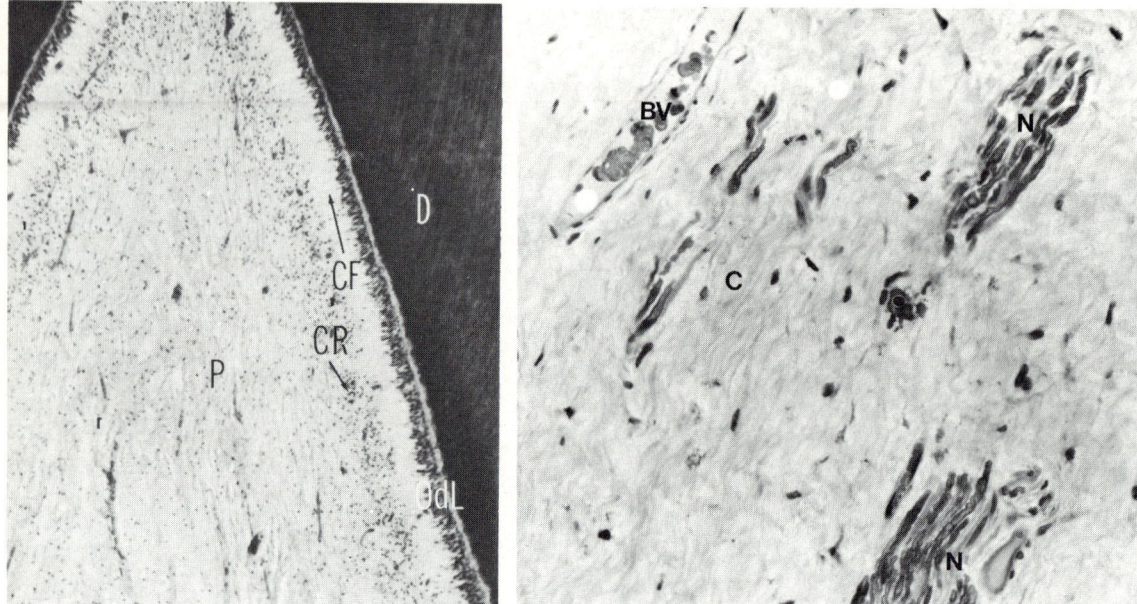

FIG. 17-1 *(Left)* Intact uninflamed pulp. Buccolingual section of an upper left canine. The pulp (P) is uninflamed. The odontoblastic layer (OdL) is orderly and palisaded. Note cell-rich (CR) and cell-free (CF) zones. D, dentin. ×96. *(Right)* Higher magnification of pulp showing nerves (N) and blood vessels (BV). C, collagen. ×875. (Courtesy of Dr. Calvin Leifer, Temple University, Philadelphia)

FIG. 17-2 Atrophic pulp. Buccolingual section of an upper canine. The pulp (P) is atrophic. The odontoblastic layer (OdL) is reduced in width. Note presence of dystrophic mineralizations (DC). Collagen fibers (CF) are increased and the number of cells is reduced. Compare with Fig. 17-1. ×96. (Seltzer S, Bender IB, Ziontz M: Oral Surg 16:846, 1963)

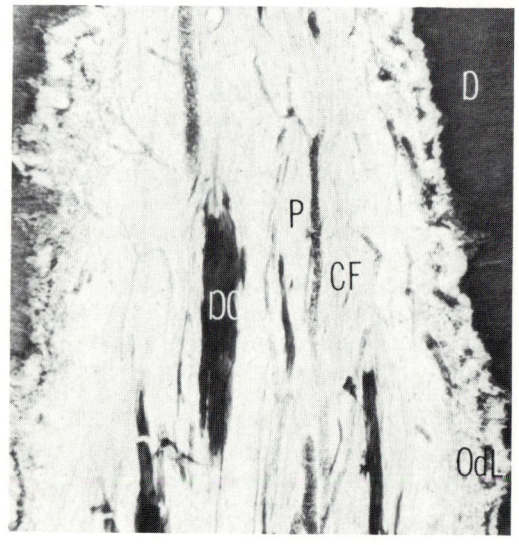

The number of these cells appears to be correlated with the depth of the lesion. In operatively manipulated teeth, the presence of inflammatory cells is relatively common.

The following classes of pulp conditions are discussed in this chapter:

Intact-uninflamed pulp
Atrophic pulp (pulposis)
Acute pulpitis
Intact pulp with scattered chronic inflammatory cells (transitional stage)
Chronic partial pulpitis
   With partial liquefaction necrosis
   With partial coagulation necrosis
Chronic total pulpitis
   With partial liquefaction necrosis
Total pulp necrosis

INTACT-UNINFLAMED PULP

Pulps in which the cells appear to be unaltered are classified as intact-uninflamed. A normal, palisaded odontoblastic layer is present (Fig. 17-1, *left*). The fibroblasts contain nuclei enclosed within a distinct nuclear membrane, and a structurally distinct cytoplasm. The chromatin stains a deep blue and is dispersed in a lacy network. Collagen fibers are absent or of minimal quantity. The blood vessels appear normal in caliber; however, in many instances, dilated vessels that appear to be unrelated to a disease process are found. This is compatible with Scheinin's observations (1963) that seemingly widened vessels filled with blood cells, as observed in histologic sections, do not indicate a hyperemic condition. The nerve bundles appear unaltered (Fig. 17–1, *right*).

ATROPHIC PULP (PULPOSIS)

Pulps that may be classified as atrophic appear to be smaller than usual. In some instances the pulp has shrunken to a fraction of its original volume (Fig. 17–2). In these instances, a large amount of reparative dentin is found to have filled the space that originally contained pulp tissue. In anterior teeth, the pulp chambers contain varying amounts of reparative dentin. In some, the coronal portion of the pulp from the incisal edge rootward is filled with reparative dentin, and the lumen of the root canal is narrowed. In posterior teeth, the horns of the pulp have receded and are replaced by reparative dentin. The root canals have been narrowed by the deposition of additional dentin (Fig. 17–3). There appears to be a decrease in the size of the cells, as well as a reduction in the number. In addition, in most of these pulps, there is an increase in the number and the distribution of collagen fibers. This appears to occur especially in anterior teeth, in which the collagen bundles become increasingly apparent in the coronal portion of the tooth. In posterior teeth, collagen bundles increase mainly in the root canal. With the increased number of collagen fibers, the blood vessels appear larger and wider (Fig. 17–4). The odontoblastic layer in these pulps is reduced in width, and the odontoblasts have a flattened, cuboidal appearance, rather than the columnar appearance typical of uninvolved pulps. Especially in those cases in which large quantities of reparative dentin have been elaborated, the cells of the pulp appear to have suffered exhaustion atrophy.

INTACT PULP WITH SCATTERED CHRONIC INFLAMATORY CELLS (TRANSITIONAL STAGE)

Pulps in which chronic inflammatory cells are detected, but are not present in sufficient quantity to be regarded as inflammatory exudate, are

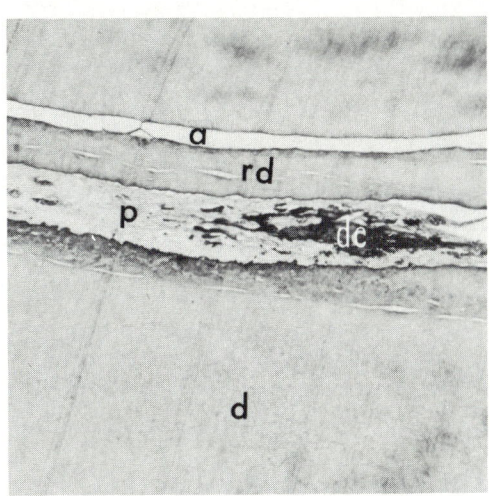

FIG. 17-3 Narrowing of the root canal. Longitudinal section of the distal canal of a lower left first molar. The pulp tissue (p) in the root canal is infiltrated with dystrophic mineralizations (dc). The root canal is narrowed by deposition of reparative dentin (rd). d, dentin. The space at (a) is an artifact. ×96. (Seltzer S, Bender IB, Ziontz M: Oral Surg 16:846, 1963)

FIG. 17-4 Apparent widening of blood vessels (BV) in atrophic pulp. D, dentin; Rd, reparative dentin. ×135.

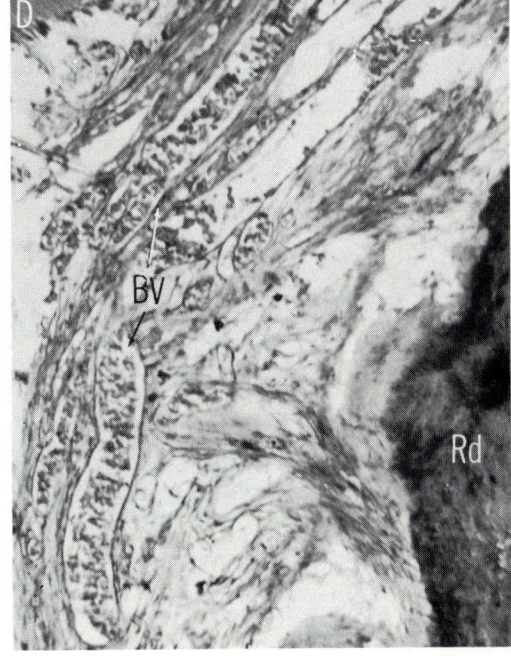

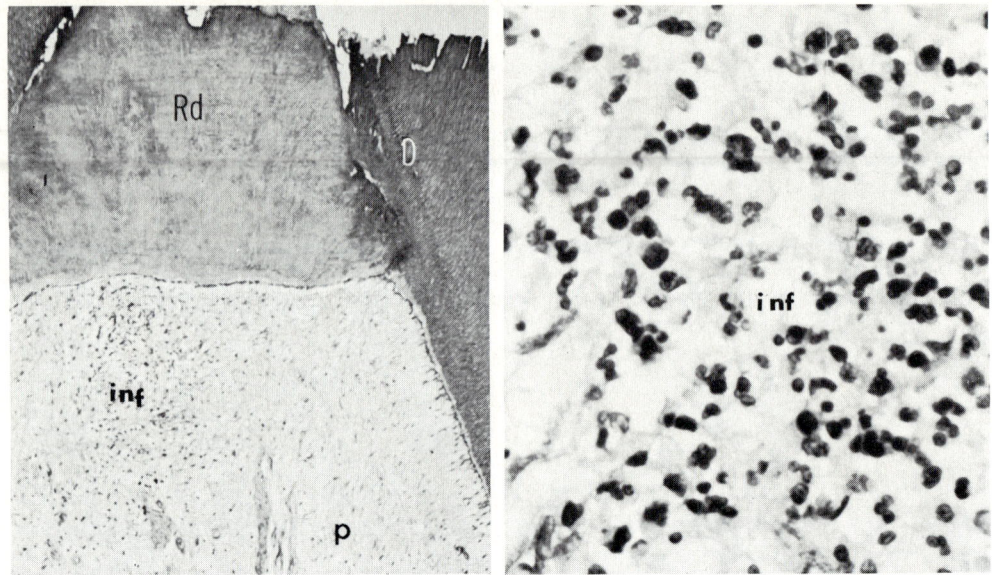

FIG. 17-5 Transitional stage. *(Left)* Buccolingual section of a lower first molar. A deep cavity was present, but the pulp was not exposed. The pulp (P) is intact but infiltrated by scattered chronic inflammatory cells (inf). Reparative dentin (Rd) has been elaborated. D, dentin. ×96. *(Right)* Higher magnification of zone of inflammatory cell infiltration (inf). Lymphocytes and macrophages predominate. ×540. (Seltzer S, Bender IB, Ziontz M: Oral Surg 16:846, 1963)

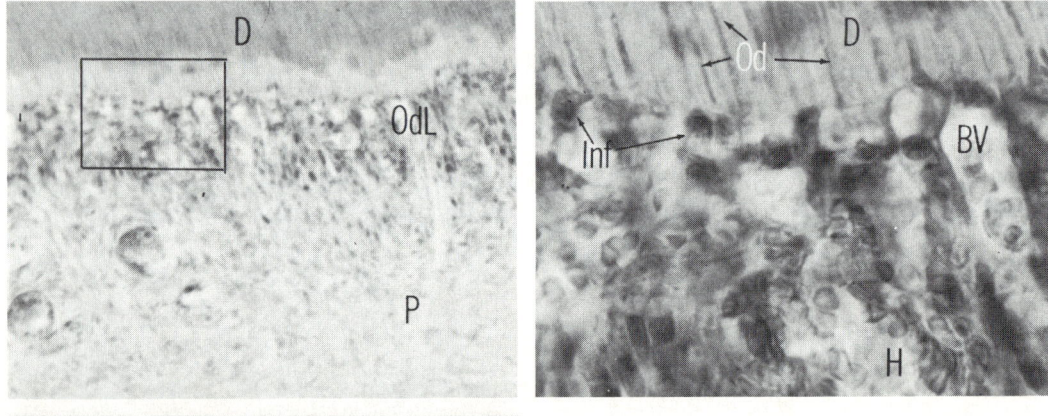

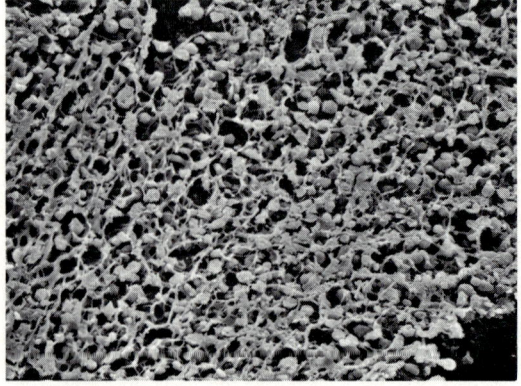

FIG. 17-6 Acute pulpitis. *(Top, left)* One week following high-speed cavity preparation of the dentin (D) without coolant, the odontoblastic layer (OdL) of the pulp (P) is infiltrated with inflammatory cells. ×240. *(Top, right)* Higher magnification of region outlined by rectangle in picture at left. Odontoblastic nuclei (Od) are displaced into the dentin (D). Inflammatory cells (Inf) are present at the predentin border. Blood vessels (BV) are dilated and hemorrhages (H) have occurred. ×960. *(Bottom)* Scanning electron micrograph of tissue section of acutely inflamed pulp infiltrated predominantly with polys. ×500.

classified as transitional stage pulps. In the pulps of most teeth with deep carious lesions, chronic inflammatory cells (for example, lymphocytes and macrophages) are found scattered throughout the portion of the pulp under the affected dentinal tubules (Fig. 17–5). The vessels in the region are dilated.

Inflammatory cells are found in teeth that have been subjected to operative procedures and have apparently recovered. Such cells are also found in the pulps of some teeth in which huge quantities of reparative dentin have been elaborated as a result of abrasion, attrition, caries, or periodontal disease. They do not constitute a typical inflammatory exudate, in which inflammatory cells are abundant, with concomitant edema and dilatation of blood vessels. Their presence in the pulp seems to be due to persistent low-grade irritation, such as may be caused by dental caries and/or periodontal disease.

ACUTE PULPITIS

Acute pulpitis* usually occurs as a sequel to various operative procedures (Fig. 17–6), including mechanical pulp exposures and pulpotomies. Also, acute pulpitides in various regions of the coronal and the radicular pulp tissue may result from exposure of lateral canals in periodontal disease and also following deep scaling and curettage in which the root cementum and/or the dentin is traumatized.

Following operative procedures, acute pulpitides are generally partial in extent, i.e., only that portion of the pulp that is subjacent to the involved dentinal tubules becomes inflamed. The extent of involvement may be somewhat greater in severe mechanical exposures in which a large amount of pulp tissue is damaged. After pulpotomies, the radicular portion of the pulp is acutely inflamed. Occasionally, the inflammation extends into the periapical-periodontal tissue.

A differentiation must be made between acute *symptoms* and acute *inflammation*. Most pulp inflammations that cause pain are chronic. The pulp has been inflamed for an extended period. When acute symptoms, such as pain and swelling develop, the inflammation is basically

---

* The term pulpitis commonly has been used by clinicians to refer to toothache. Actually, pain in the teeth may be caused by various factors and is not necessarily due to inflammation of the pulp (pulpitis). Instead, tooth pain should be referred to as pulpalgia — a term that describes the clinical entity, not the histopathologic diagnosis.

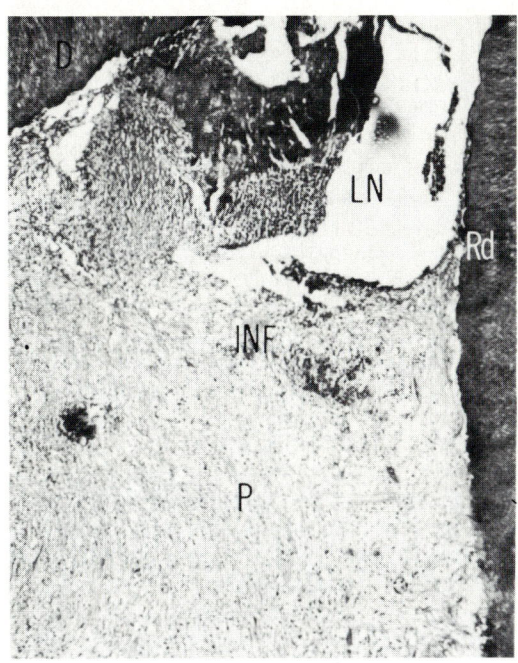

FIG. 17-7 Carious pulp exposure. The pulp (P) is chronically inflamed (INF), yet the patient had no symptoms. Under the region of the exposure, an area of liquefaction necrosis (LN) is present. D, dentin; Rd, reparative dentin. ×96. (Seltzer S, Bender IB, Ziontz M: Oral Surg 16:846, 1963)

chronic, but, as in all chronic inflammation, acute inflammatory responses may be overlaid on the pre-existing chronic disease process. A patient complaining of *acute* pain usually has *chronic* pulpitis. Acute pulpitis (histologic) rarely causes pain. Thus, when a pulp exposure develops as a result of dental caries, the pulp has been chronically inflamed for a long time. The lack of symptoms in many of these conditions is not necessarily indicative of the severity of the underlying inflammatory response (Fig. 17–7). Both acute and chronic inflammation are found. Frequently, the development of painful symptoms is related to blockage of the coronal orifice through which drainage of exudate occurs. Thus, when pain develops, the histologic condition may be referred to as an acute exacerbation of a chronic inflammation.

Acute inflammation may be found after more recent operative manipulations on teeth that had been prepared and filled previously. In such cases, chronic inflammation of the pulp has persisted for long periods under the restoration.

When a new operative procedure is performed on such a tooth, ensuing pain is related to an acute exacerbation of the previously existing chronic pulpitis. In a pulp that is acutely inflamed after an operative procedure, odontoblastic changes, dilated blood vessels, edema, polymorphonuclear leukocytes, macrophages, and erythrocytes are found around and under the odontoblastic layer. The extent of the inflammation is usually partial, involving a small region of the pulp subjacent to the cut dentinal tubules. The acute inflammation is of short duration, and it either disappears soon afterward or becomes chronic. A disturbance in dentin formation and mineralization of subsequently formed dentin matrix takes place because of the injury to the involved odontoblasts. This disturbance is visible as a calciotraumatic response in tissue sections. Reparative dentin is elaborated concurrently with the inflammatory response. The quantity and quality of the reparative dentin are related to the severity of the injury.

CHRONIC PULPITIS

Chronic pulpitis develops from deep dental caries, pulp exposures, operative procedures, deep periodontal lesions, and excessive orthodontic tooth movement.

When deep dental caries is untreated, the pulp gradually becomes chronically inflamed. The inflammation is confined to the coronal portion of the pulp initially (i.e., a chronic partial pulpitis). Eventually, however, the entire pulp and periapical-periodontal tissues become involved (i.e., chronic total pulpitis). In younger persons, in whom the blood supply to the pulp is maximal, the chronically inflamed exposed pulp tissue may be irritated by the rough edges of the cavity, and the proliferating granulomatous* tissue may grow out of the pulp chamber. The granulomatous tissue then simulates gingival tissue (chronic hyperplastic pulpitis). Such pulp polyps are innervated, but are not necessarily sensitive (Southam and Hodson, 1973). In older persons, hyperplasia following pulp exposure does not occur. The chronic pulpitis in these adults is referred to as ulcerative pulpitis, because the covering of the pulp (the dentin) has been removed by the carious process.

Chronic pulpitis that develops after operative manipulations or as a result of periodontal lesions or orthodontic tooth movement may be found in teeth with restorations. Although some of these restorations may be defective the quality of the restoration is, frequently, unrelated to the presence of the pulpitis. The chronic pulpitis has developed from an original acute pulpitis related to the operative procedure.

Chronic pulpitides of operative, periodontic, or orthodontic etiology may be partial or total, depending on the extent of the pulp involvement. Usually, the coronal pulp tissue underlying the region of the involved dentinal tubules is inflamed (i.e., chronic partial pulpitis). However, the inflammation may extend from the area of the initial injury into the deeper pulp tissues for some distance. Not infrequently, a small region of liquefaction necrosis develops within the inflamed pulp tissue (i.e., chronic partial pulpitis with partial liquefaction necrosis). Painful symptoms may, but do not necessarily, arise when this occurs (Fig. 17–7). Frequently, however, the inflammation involves the radicular pulp tissue (i.e., chronic total pulpitis). Invariably, regions of liquefaction necrosis are found in the totally inflamed pulps (i.e., chronic total pulpitis with partial liquefaction necrosis). Painful symptoms are associated commonly with this stage of pulpitis.

Chronic Partial Pulpitis

Pulps that contain tissue, exudate, or inflammatory cells characteristic of a chronic inflammatory response are classified under the heading chronic pulpitis. Granulomatous tissue, typical of chronic inflammatory states, is found in such pulps. There is a profuse number of new capillaries, as well as an increased number of fibroblasts and fibers. Cells of the chronic inflammatory series are present (Fig. 17–8). In most instances, the lesion is walled off by dense collagen fiber bundles. However, inflammatory cells are often found in regions distant from the site of the lesion. In this category are placed pulp inflammations confined to one small coronal region but do not extend beyond the coronal portion of the pulp. In some instances, regions of partial coagulation or liquefaction necrosis are also present (Fig. 17–9).

---

* The term granulomatous tissue in the pulp refers to a chronic, long-standing inflammation resulting from a persistent irritant. On the other hand, granulation tissue is that tissue which is a precursor to healing. Histologically, both appear similar in cellular content, but granulomatous tissue has a greater number of chronic inflammatory cells, and the granulations within it are surrounded by dense collagen fiber bundles.

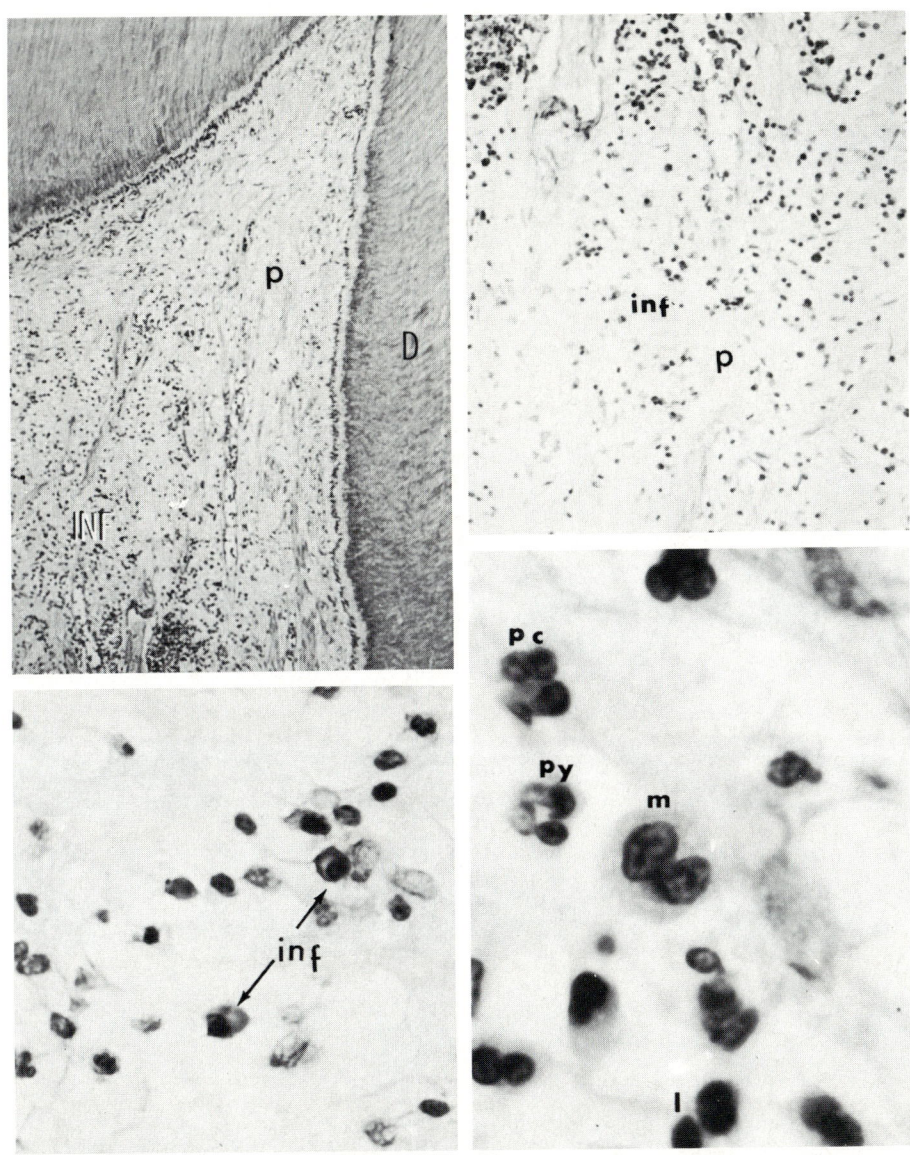

FIG. 17-8 Chronic partial pulpitis. *(Top, left)* Buccolingual section of a lower left second premolar. The pulp (P) is inflamed (INF). D, dentin. ×96. *(Top, right)* Higher magnification of the same pulp shown at left, going rootward. The density of inflammatory cells (inf) in the pulp (P) is lower. ×135. *(Bottom, left)* Higher magnification of inflammatory cells (inf). ×960. *(Bottom, right)* Types of inflammatory cells found in chronic partial pulpitis. m, Macrophages; Py, polymorphonuclear leukocytes; l, lymphocytes; pc, plasma cells. ×1100. (Seltzer S, Bender IB, Ziontz M: Oral Surg 16:846, 1963)

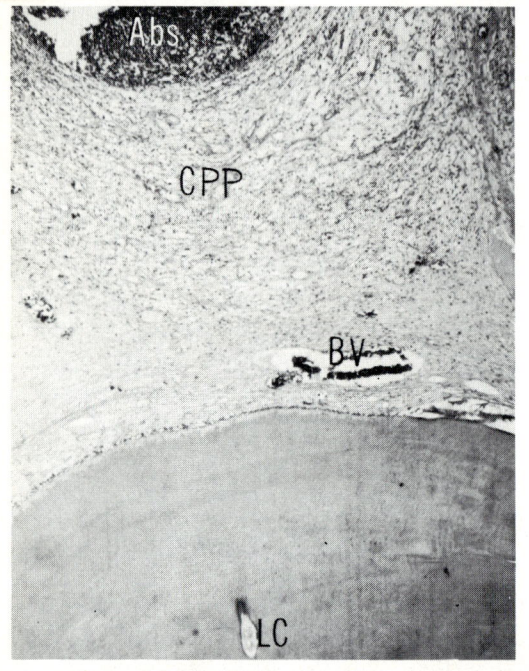

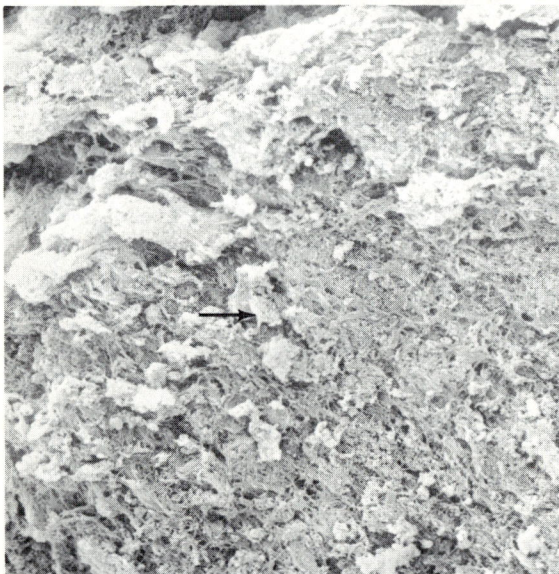

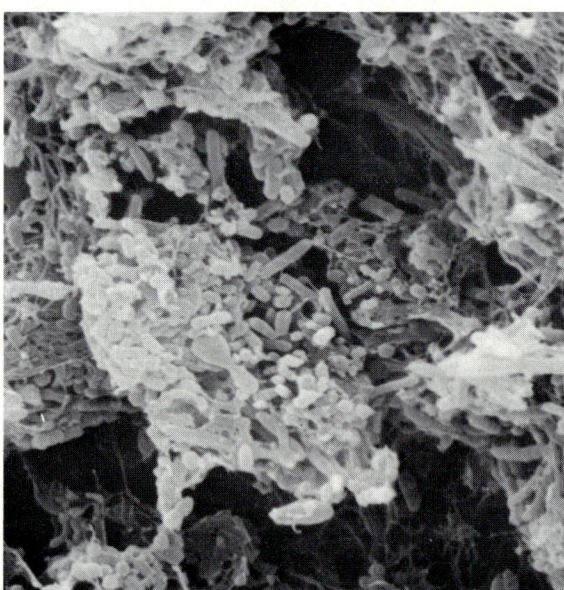

FIG. 17-9 *(Top)* Chronic partial pulpitis with partial liquefaction necrosis. Under a carious exposure, a region of liquefaction necrosis (Abs) is present. Beneath this, the pulp is chronically inflamed (CPP). BV, a dilated blood vessel in the floor of the pulp chamber. LC, a lateral canal, which extends from the periodontal ligament. ×54. *(Bottom, left)* Scanning electron micrograph of chronically inflamed pulp tissue under carious exposure. Inflammatory cells are prevalent. ×500. *(Bottom, right)* Higher magnification of bottom, left micrograph showing poly (arrow in bottom, left frame) engulfing bacteria. ×5000.

HISTOLOGIC CLASSIFICATION OF PULP DISEASES | 357

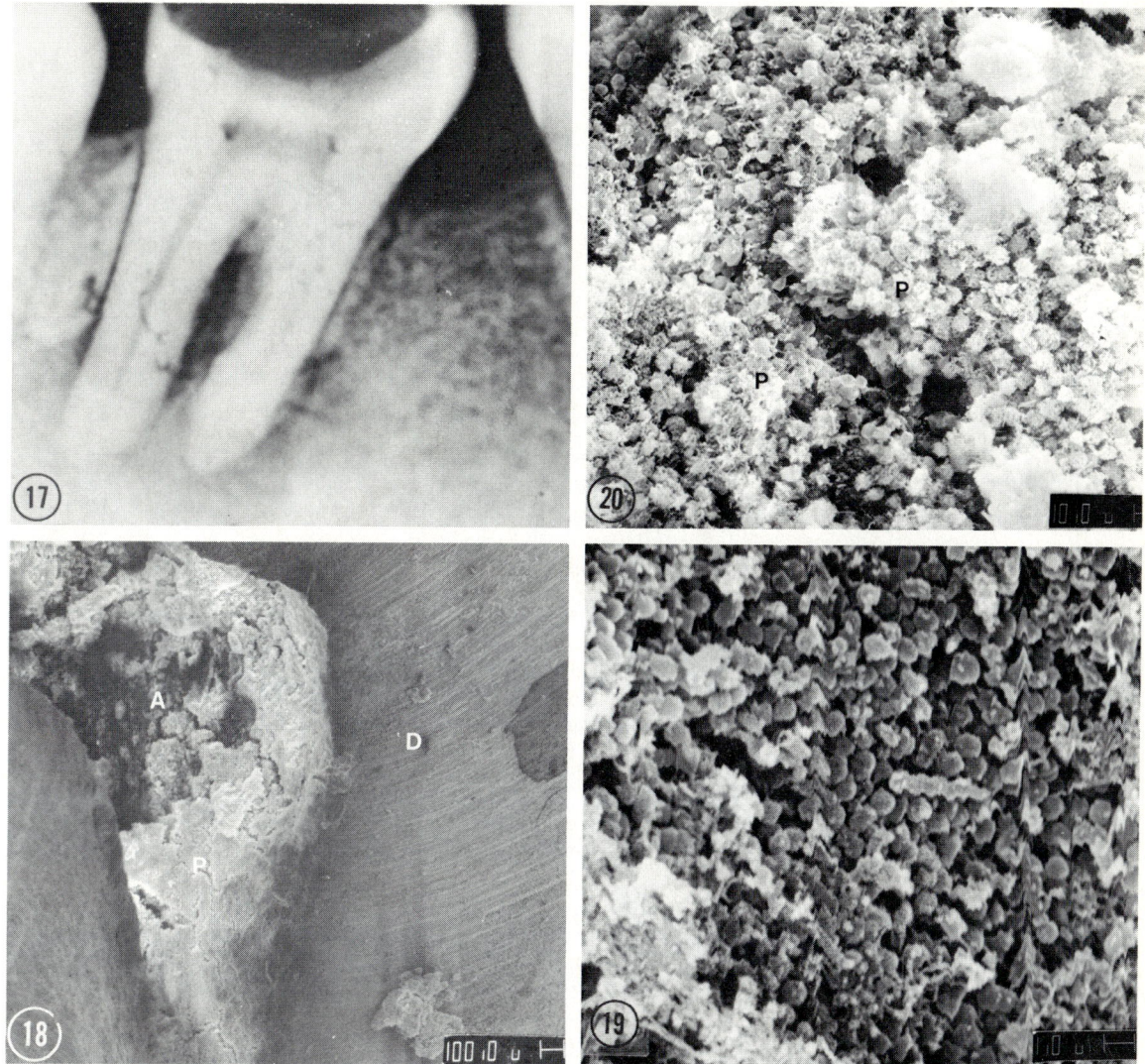

FIG. 17-10 *(Top, left)* Radiograph of lower left first molar of carious tooth. *(Bottom, left)* Scanning electron micrograph of coronal pulp (P) showing pulp abscess (A). D, dentin. ×30. *(Top, right)* Inflammatory cell infiltrate in mid-root area. P, polys. ×400. *(Bottom, right)* Bacteria in mid-root area. ×4000.

Chronic Total Pulpitis

When the entire pulp, including both the coronal and the radicular portions, is inflamed, it is classed as a chronic total pulpitis. In such teeth the inflammation has spread into the periodontal ligament. Coronally, an area of liquefaction or coagulation necrosis is always discerned (Fig. 17-10). The remainder of the pulp and the periapical tissues contain granulomatous tissue (Fig. 17-11).

NECROTIC PULP

Pulps of teeth in which the pulp cells have died as a result of coagulation or liquefaction are classed as necrotic. In coagulation necrosis, the protoplasm of the cells has become fixed and opaque. A coagulated cell mass is still recognizable histologically, but the intracellular detail has disappeared (Fig. 17-12). In liquefaction necrosis, the entire outline of the cell has disappeared, and around the liquefied area there is a

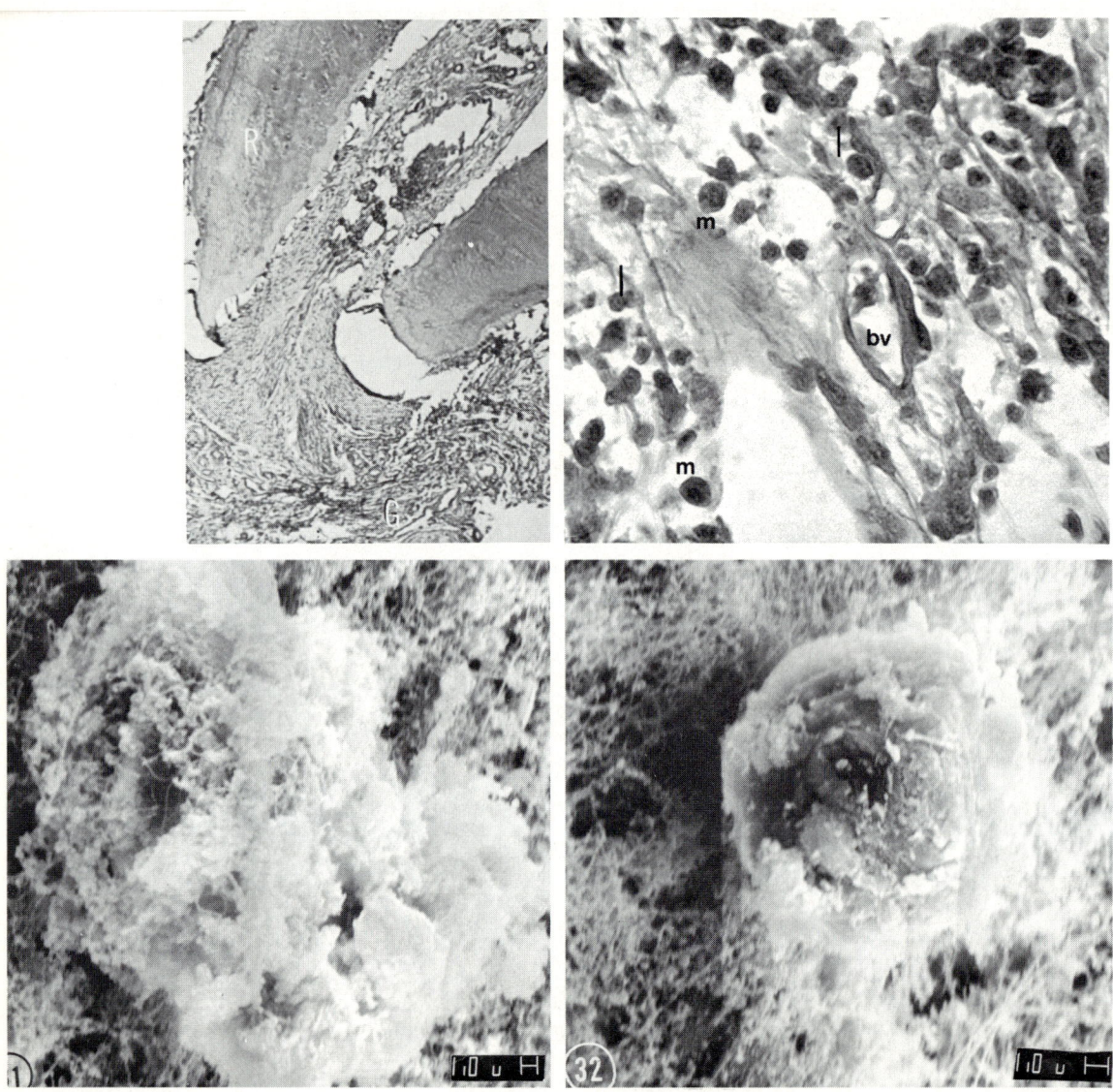

FIG. 17-11 Chronic total pulpitis. *(Top, left)* Buccolingual section of a lower right third molar. The pulp (P) was exposed by caries and is inflamed. A small granuloma (G) is attached to the root of the tooth (R). ×96. *(Top, right)* Chronic inflammatory infiltrate in apical third of pulp. m, macrophage; l, lymphocyte; bv, blood vessel. ×500. *(Bottom, left)* Scanning electron micrograph of macrophage in inflammatory infiltrate. ×2000. *(Bottom, right)* Lymphocyte in inflammatory infiltrate. ×3000. (Top, left Seltzer S, Bender IB, Ziontz M: Oral Surg 16:846, 1963)

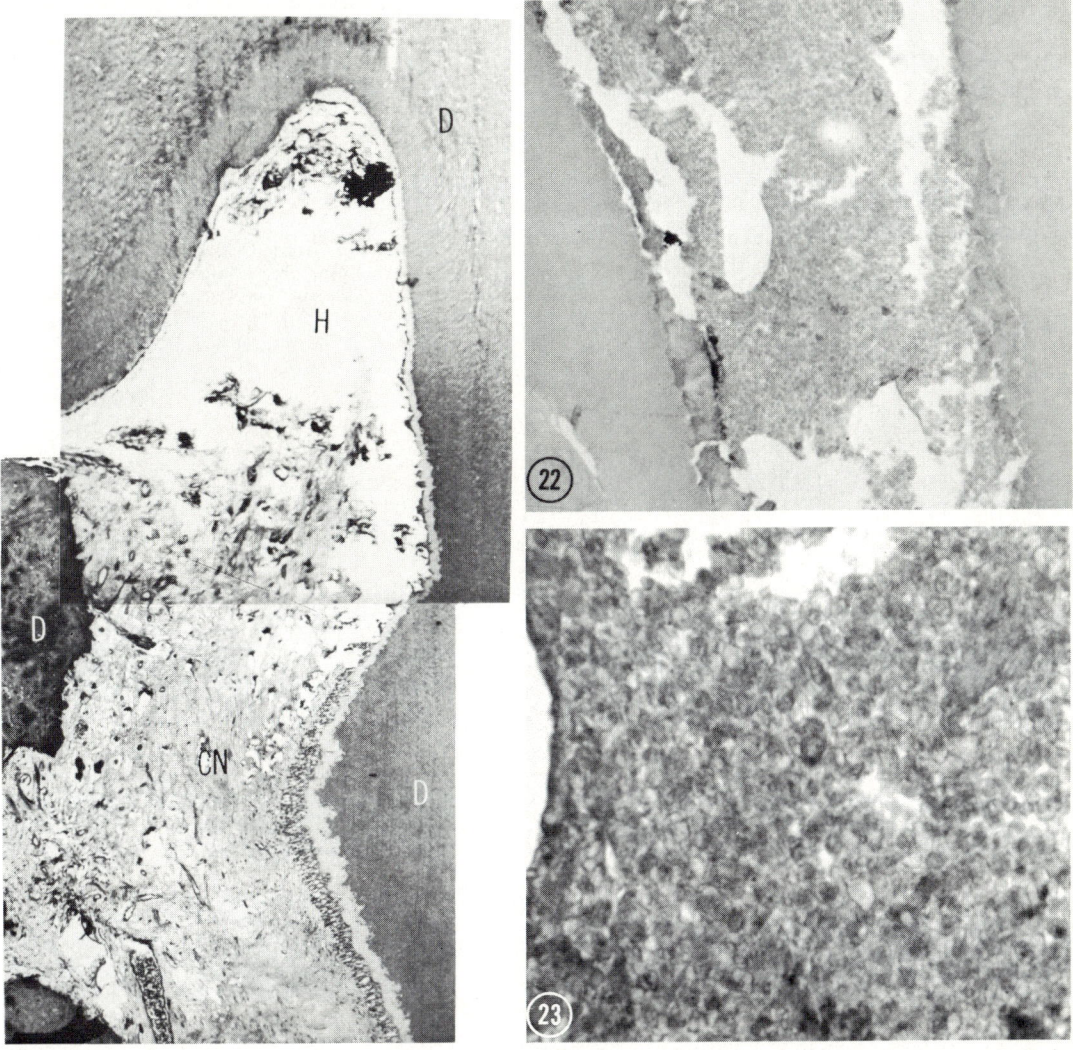

FIG. 17-12 *(Left)* Coagulation necrosis of the pulp. Composite photomicrograph of coronal portion of pulp in lower first molar. The pulp in the distal horn (H) is necrotic and only a space remains. The remaining pulp has undergone coagulation necrosis (CN). D, dentin. ×54. *(Top, right)* Degenerating inflammatory cells in mid-root area. ×175. *(Bottom, right)* Higher magnification of top right frame. ×500.

dense zone of polymorphonuclear leukocytes, both dead and dying, together with cells of the chronic inflammatory series (Fig. 17–11).

DIFFICULTIES IN CLASSIFICATION

It is sometimes difficult to classify the state of a pulp accurately, since various transitional stages are also encountered. Inflamed pulps invariably exhibit regions of atrophy. Thus, an overlapping of classification often occurs. However, when a pulp is chronically inflamed, even though regions of atrophy are detected, it is classified under chronic pulpitis.

No classification of pulp diseases is complete. Not only are there many overlappings, but diagnoses of tissue sections depend on complete examinations of all levels, some of which are often technically poor or even missing. Thus, pulp inflammation of various types sometimes may be diagnosed inaccurately, depending on the level at which the tissue section to be examined was taken. For example, at the periphery of a pulp lesion there may be an abundance of fibers and fibroblasts and a few scattered lymphocytes and plasma cells, apparently justifying a diagnosis of repair. Nearer the center of the lesion, many chronic inflammatory cells may be found, leading to a diagnosis of chronic pulpitis. Directly in the center, there may be an area of liquefaction necrosis, which would permit a diagnosis of pulp abscess. And, at the periphery, normal tissue could be found.

BIBLIOGRAPHY

Baume LJ: Diagnosis of diseases of the pulp. Oral Surg 29:102, 1970
Garfunkel A, Sela J, Ulmansky M: Dental pulp pathosis. Clinico-pathologic correlations based on 109 cases. Oral Surg 35:111, 1973
Hasler JF, Mitchell DF: Painless pulpitis. JADA 81:671, 1970
Hess JC: New conceptions of pathology and treatment of the pulp. Rev Franc Odontostomat 14:61, 1967
Scheinin A: Flow characteristics of the pulpal vessels. J Dent Res 42:488, 1963
Southam JC, Hodson JJ: Neurohistology of human dental pulp polyps. Arch Oral Biol 18:1255, 1973

18
DIFFERENTIAL DIAGNOSIS

From a clinical standpoint, the dentist is generally unable to make an accurate pathologic diagnosis of the state of the pulp. However, from analysis of the subjective symptoms, past dental history, and the objective findings, a probable categorization can be made.

The following information can be used to help to make a decision as to whether treatment of the dental pulp is likely to be successful or whether endodontic treatment or extraction is indicated: the intensity, duration, and previous history of pulpalgia; the presence of dental caries with or without pulp exposure; restorations; tooth color; swelling; periodontal disease; radiographic findings; results of thermal, percussion, palpation, anesthetic, and electric pulp tests; test drilling; and regions of referred pain.

Teeth with pulps in the histologic categories intact-uninflamed pulp, transitional stage, atrophic pulp, acute pulpitis, and chronic partial pulpitis without necrosis have a reasonable chance for resolution with conservative treatment (i.e., the pulps are treatable). The teeth whose pulps are in the remaining states, i.e., chronic partial pulpitis with partial necrosis, chronic total pulpitis, and total pulp necrosis, require endodontic treatment or extraction (i.e., the pulps are nontreatable). See Tables 19–1 and 19–2.

We hold this view despite earlier reports (Fry et al, 1960; Schroeder and Triadan, 1962; Lawson and Mitchell, 1964) that painful pulpitis may be treated successfully with glucocorticoids and antibiotics. Their evidence was suggestive but not conclusive. Furthermore, the relief of pulpalgia following the application of glucocorticoids indicates only that the pain symptom has been suppressed (Schroeder, 1979). Treatment with glucocorticoids does not imply inhibition or arrest of pulpal inflammation. More recent evidence has indicated that the reversal of chronic pulpitides, especially those in which liquefaction necrosis has occurred, is unlikely.

SUBJECTIVE FINDINGS

INTENSITY AND DURATION OF PULPALGIA

The intensity and duration of a toothache is a significant clue. If pulpalgia is absent or mild, the pulp of the tooth is likely to be in any one of the following conditions:

Intact-uninflamed pulp
Atrophic pulp
Transitional stage
Acute pulpitis

Chronic partial pulpitis (without necrosis)
   Hyperplastic pulpitis
Necrosis of pulp

With the exceptions of hyperplastic pulpitis and necrosis of the pulp, treatment along conservative lines directed toward pulp conservation is indicated, designated category A (Treatable). Hyperplastic pulpitis may be treated by pulpotomy when the root ends are incompletely formed. Otherwise, endodontic treatment or extraction is indicated.

When the pulpalgia is moderate to severe, the dental pulp is probably in one of the following states, designated Category B (Nontreatable):

Chronic partial pulpitis with partial necrosis
Chronic total pulpitis with partial necrosis
Total necrosis of pulp
Acute pulpitis superimposed on a chronic pulpitis

Teeth with pulps in any of these states require endodontic treatment or extraction.

PREVIOUS HISTORY OF PULPALGIA

A prior history of toothache is significant in terms of diagnosis. If there has been no previous history of pain, the chances are good that the condition of the pulp will be one of those listed in Category A, except hyperplastic pulpitis and necrosis of the pulp. Conversely, a previous episode of pain is good evidence that the pulp is severely inflamed or necrotic (Category B).

OBJECTIVE FINDINGS

The following objective findings are significant aids in pulp diagnosis.

Dental Caries. The depth of the cavity plus the presence or absence of pain is important. In a tooth with a deep cavity without painful symptomatology, the condition of the pulp is probably one of those in Category A. In a study of 300 teeth, Clark et al (1983) found that a history of pain alone was not a predictor of success or failure in the conservative treatment of deep carious lesions. However, absence of pain, in itself, cannot be considered a reliable criterion of the state of the pulp, since painless pulpitides are probably as common as the painful ones. Hasler and Mitchell (1970) found that, of 47 carious, asymptomatic teeth the pulps of 27 (58%) were inflamed; in 14 of the 27 teeth, the pulps were exposed. These teeth reacted positively to electric vitality tests and were indistinguishable from those without pulp exposures. Thus, other diagnostic pulp procedures should be performed.

Conversely, the pulp of a tooth with deep dental caries associated with pain generally is in one of the stages in Category B. This classification helps to determine the correct therapy. Teeth in Category A may be treated successfully with sedative dressings or indirect or direct pulp cappings (Fig. 18–1). There is greater assurance of successful resolution than there is for teeth in Category B, except in teeth in which the pulp is necrotic. The presence of necrosis must be determined by other tests. In teeth with necrotic pulps, endodontics or extraction is recommended.

Extensive Restorations. The presence of extensive restorations in teeth is an important diagnostic finding. Pain in a tooth with a large restoration is good evidence that the pulp is in Category B. Teeth with extensive restorations are prime suspects when the patient has pulpalgia but is unable to point to the exact tooth. In the absence of pain, the category may be A1, 2, 3, or 5 (intact-uninflamed pulp, atrophic pulp, transitional stage, or chronic partial pulpitis without necrosis).

Pulp Exposure. A carious pulp exposure automatically places the pulp of the tooth in one of the stages listed under Category B. Hence, treatment must be endodontic or exodontic. Mechanical or traumatic pulp exposures are probably in Category A4 (acute pulpitis). More conservative treatment can be considered for the teeth with mechanical exposures.

Swelling. The swelling of pulp tissue itself is an indication of hyperplastic pulpitis (Category A).* Swelling of the mucosa over the apical region of the tooth invariably is associated with a pulp in Category B (Fig. 18–2)—either chronic total pulpitis with necrosis or total pulp necrosis. Usually, some liquefaction necrosis is present. Treatment must be designed for evacuation of the pus.

---

* This is true only if pulpotomy can be performed; otherwise Category B.

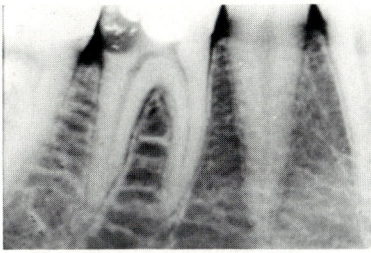 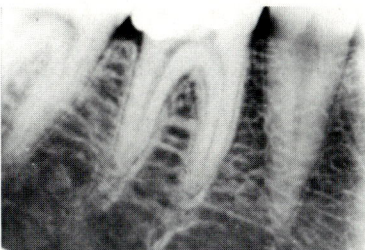 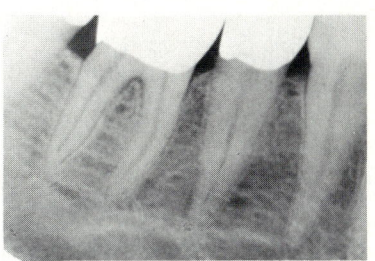

FIG. 18-1 Indirect pulp capping. *(Left)* Deep carious lesion. Patient was symptom-free with normal response to pulp tests. Complete removal of decay would have resulted in pulp exposure. Instead, gross caries was removed and a zinc oxide-eugenol dressing was applied. *(Middle)* Six months later, the tooth was still asymptomatic and pulp vital. *(Right)* Thirty years later, tooth is still asymptomatic and pulp still vital.

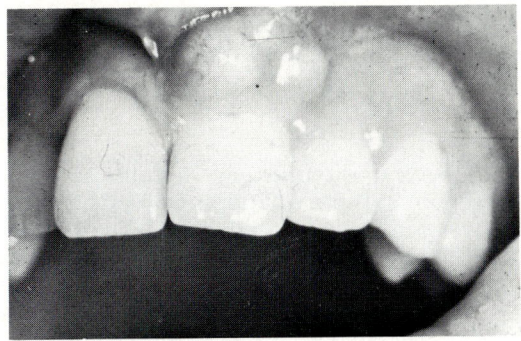

FIG. 18-2 Swelling of the mucosa over the upper left central incisor. This indicates that the pulp of the tooth is untreatable (Category B).

Sinus Tract. The presence of a sinus tract indicates that the pulp of the tooth has undergone partial or total necrosis (Category B). Endodontic treatment or extraction is indicated. Occasionally, the origin of the sinus tract is doubtful. The use of a 0.01 gauge stainless-steel orthodontic wire or gutta-percha cone is helpful in determining which tooth is responsible. The wire is inserted into the orifice of the sinus tract and twisted until it penetrates to the base of the bone. A radiograph is then taken. The wire frequently goes directly to the offending tooth (Fig. 18-3).

Periodontal Disease. The presence of periodontal disease in a tooth that is free of pain or has sensitivity to thermal changes points to a pulp diagnosis compatible with Category A2 (atrophic pulp). However, when pain is present, the chances for the presence of more advanced pulp pathosis increase (Fig. 18-4). The category is then B. In the latter case, combined endodontic and periodontic treatment or extraction is indicated if pain is severe.

OTHER DIAGNOSTIC AIDS

Other diagnostic aids are available to help the practitioner make a diagnosis. Among these are radiographs, electric pulp tests, thermal tests, percussion tests, test drilling, palpation, and the use of local anesthesia.

RADIOGRAPHS

Radiographs are valuable as an aid to the visualization of the presence or absence of the following:

    Deep-seated caries
        With possible pulp involvement
        With definite pulp involvement
    Deep restorations
        With liners
        Without liners
    Root fractures
    Resorptions
        Internal
        External
    Width of canal and pulp chamber
    Mineralizations and reparative dentin within
        pulp and/or root canal

Caries and Restorations

Radiographs are valuable as an aid in visualizing the depth of a carious lesion. Carious pulp exposures are detected frequently in the radiograph,

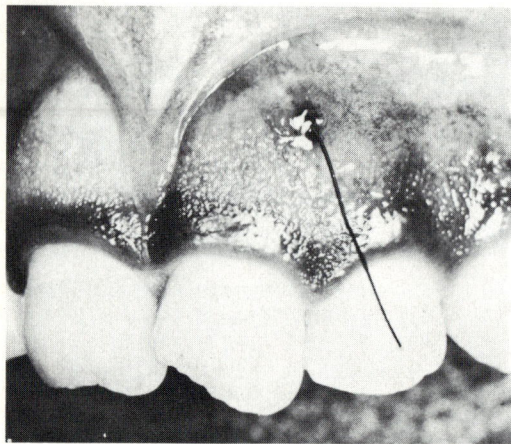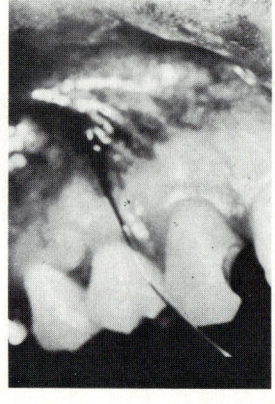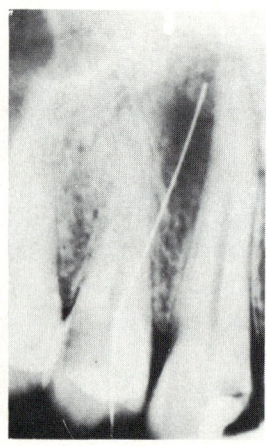

FIG. 18-3 (*Left* and *Center*) Stainless-steel wire, inserted into sinus tract. (*Right*) Radiograph shows that the wire goes to the seat of the disorder. (Bender IB, Seltzer S: The oral fistula: Its diagnosis and treatment. Oral Surg 14:1367, 1961)

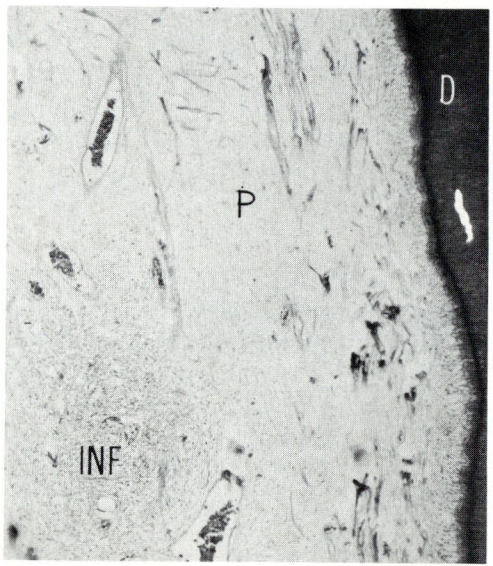

FIG. 18-4 Pulp inflammation in periodontally involved tooth. The pulp (P) of a lower cuspid has a region of chronic inflammation (INF) within it. D, dentin. ×54.

although it is sometimes difficult to ascertain the presence of an exposure from the radiographic appearance alone. When in doubt, the operator should be guided by his other findings as well as by an exploratory excavation of the lesion. When deep restorations are present, the radiograph is often a help in determining the presence or absence of liners or sub-bases under the restorations. In teeth in which liners are absent, there is reasonable suspicion of pulp involvement. If pain is present, the pulps of these teeth are probably in one of the conditions listed under Category B; hence, endodontic treatment or extraction is indicated.

Root Fractures

The presence of root fractures, particularly intra-alveolar root fractures (IARFs), which are caused by traumatic injuries, can be detected only by radiographs taken from different angulations (Bender, 1982). Orthopedists invariably take radiographs from different positions or angulations to enhance fracture detection. The type of therapy depends on pulp vitality, location of fracture, extent of fragment dislocation, degree of apical maturation, and presence or absence of symptoms. Pulpal pain is usually absent in teeth with IARFs (Bender and Freedland, 1983). Of pulps in teeth with IARFs and no pain, 75% to 80% require no therapy (Zachrisson and Jacobson, 1975; Andreasen, 1981), pointing to the probability that the pulps belong in Category A. Observation is then the course of choice. When pulp vitality is absent or if painful symptoms develop, endodontic therapy is indicated. When IARFs are more coronal and there is marked mobility of the clinical crown, or when the fracture communicates with the gingival sulcus, the pulp is in Category B (Fig. 18-5).

Resorptions

The presence of extensive resorptions, detected by radiographs, usually indicates severe pulp involvement (Fig. 18–6). Frequently, it is difficult to determine whether the resorption is internal or external in origin. In either case, the pulp is in Category B, being either chronically inflamed or necrotic. Attempts at the preservation of the pulp in such circumstances are contraindicated.

Idiopathic (Internal) Resorption. Occasionally, a "pink spot" develops in a tooth. In this condition, granulomatous tissue is formed within the pulp (Fig. 18–7). The exact etiology is unknown, but it may be related to trauma or to an unresolved pre-existing chronic pulpitis. Some of the cells of the chronically inflamed pulp begin to resorb the dentinal wall of the pulp chamber or the root canal (Fig. 18–8). The cells responsible for the resorption are mono- or multinucleated cells (dentinoclasts), which may be converted from pulpal undifferentiated connective tissue cells (Toto and Restarski, 1963) or from macrophages in granulation tissue (Gorlin and Goldman, 1970). These cells are seen occasionally in Howship's lacunae that are present at the resorbing dentinal wall. The presence of acid phosphatase and β-glucuronidase in the multinucleated cells has been demonstrated by Hasselgren and Strömberg (1976). Burstone (1953) reported an increased periodic acid-Schiff (PAS) staining reaction of the zone of dentin adjacent to the resorbed area. Possibly, the resorption occurs from outside the tooth and eventually invades the pulp chamber. A sharply outlined defect is seen in the radiograph (Fig. 18–6, top right).

Clinically, the crown of the tooth looks pinkish, because of the presence of granulomatous tissue with its numerous capillaries, together with the loss of dentin. Radicular resorptions, both internal and external, also may occur. The etiology is sometimes obscure, but both chronic total pulpitis and periodontal disease frequently are implicated.

Treatment of resorptions is difficult. Endodontic treatment must be performed (Fig. 18–6, top, center), but the outcome is always questionable. Sometimes the resorption ceases; at other times it continues in spite of removal of the pulp, pointing to the possibility that the resorption was external in origin. Upon rare occasions, a reversal of internal resorption with re-

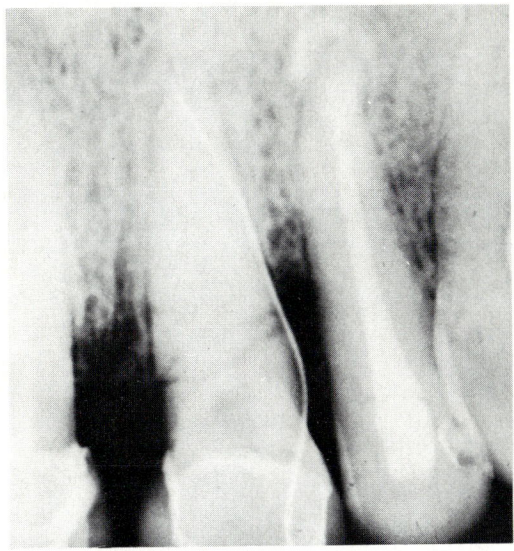

FIG. 18-5 Radiograph of upper right central incisor with root fracture. The pulp has become necrotic and a sinus tract has developed. A diagnostic wire has been inserted, prior to the taking of the radiograph. The prognosis is unfavorable.

FIG. 18-6 *(Top, left)* Resorption of the crown of an upper left central incisor; *(center)* Same tooth, after completion of endodontic therapy; *(right)* Resorption in the middle portion of the root of an upper lateral incisor. *(Bottom)* Resorption in the crown of a lower left first molar.

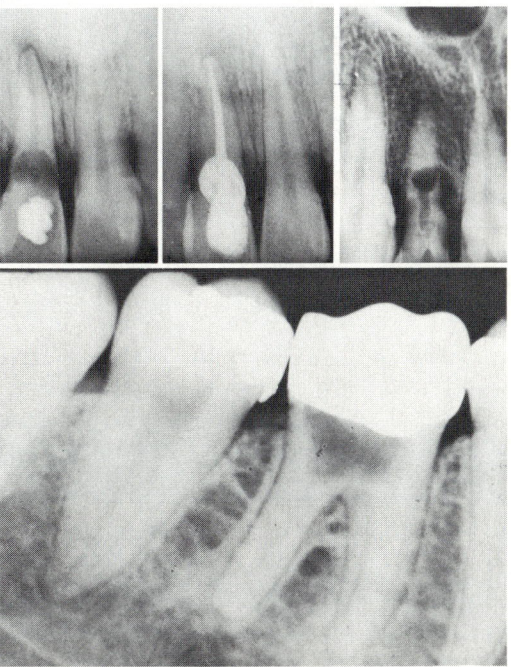

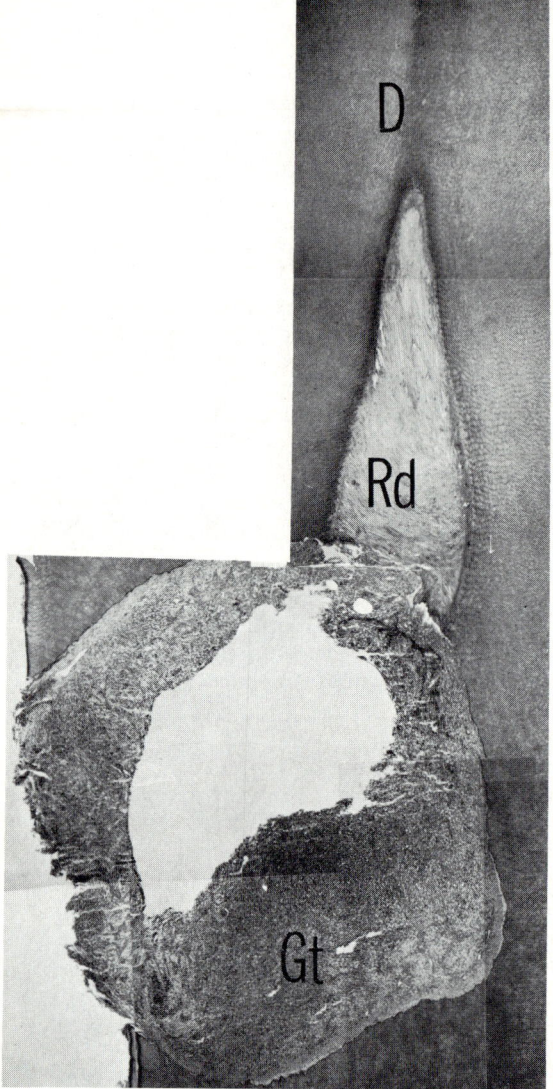

FIG. 18-7 Composite photomicrograph of a tooth with internal resorption. The dentin (D) is resorbed by granulomatous tissue (Gt). Reparative dentin (Rd) has obliterated the pulp horn. ×54.

tiate into osteodentinoblasts or odontoblasts in the presence of necrotic tissue on application of calcium hydroxide.

Width of Canal and Pulp Chamber

The width of the pulp chamber or the root canal, as seen in a radiograph, affords significant information of the status of the pulp. Excessively narrowed or widened pulp spaces, when compared with those of adjacent teeth, are definite indications of pulp pathosis. Narrowed root canals are the result of periodontal disease, previous trauma to the tooth or prior pulp capping or pulpotomy procedures, especially when calcium hydroxide has been used. Atrophied pulps are usually the end result. Unusually wide pulp spaces are indicative of previously severe pulp damage, resulting in necrosis of the pulp. This condition is sometimes found after severe trauma, such as a blow to a tooth or excessive orthodontic tooth movement (Fig. 18–10).

Mineralizations

Mineralizations within the pulp chamber or the root canals have no special significance, except that they increase in the presence of periodontal disease, after extensive operative procedures, and after traumatic injuries to teeth, with or without crown or root fractures. Perhaps of greater significance is an excessive amount of reparative dentin formation in the coronal pulp chamber. Usually, this is a sequel to severe pulp damage from previous operative procedures or trauma. Pain in such teeth is an indication that the pulp is in one of the states listed under Category B.

THERMAL TESTS

Normal responses to heat and cold tests are those in which pain is felt when the irritant is applied to the tooth but disappears as soon as the stimulus is removed. Such responses are usually indicative of uninvolved pulps. Abnormal responses are those in which pain persists after the stimulus is removed. Such abnormal responses usually are indicative of pulps in Category B. However, the usual thermal tests are not completely reliable for discerning the status of the pulp (Mumford, 1967; Teitler et al, 1972; Bhaskar and Rappaport, 1973; Fulling and Andreasen, 1976). The use of carbon dioxide snow or dichlor-difluormethane has been reported to be reliable for eliciting normal pulp vitality responses in crowned teeth and in immature

mineralization can occur with a reconstituted root canal (Fig. 18–9). Probably the undifferentiated mesenchymal cells undergo a morphologic transition, differentiating to odontoblasts, or the odontoblasts dedifferentiate to undifferentiated mesenchymal cells, which redifferentiate to odontoblasts. According to Yamamura et al (1980), different hard structures induce undifferentiated mesenchymal cells to differen-

FIG. 18-8 *(Top)* Resorption (arrows) of the dentin (D) by granulomatous tissue (Gt). E, proliferated epithelium. ×96. *(Upper middle)* Higher magnification of resorption of dentin (D). Some repair by cementum (C) is taking place. Gt, granulomatous tissue. ×240. *(Lower middle)* Higher magnification of region outlined by rectangle in picture above. Cementum (C), which is being elaborated, has trapped cells (indicated by arrows) within it. f, Fibroblasts; F, fibers. ×960. *(Bottom)* The cells of the granulomatous tissue, predominantly plasma cells (pc). ×960.

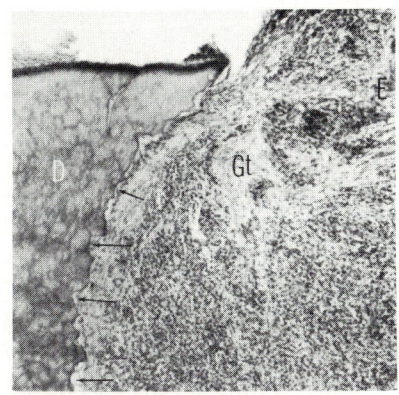
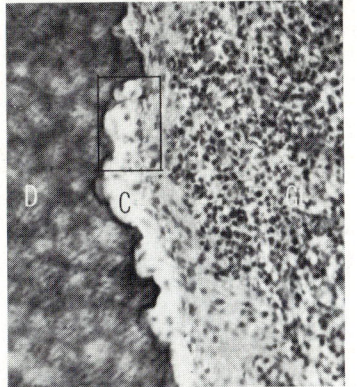
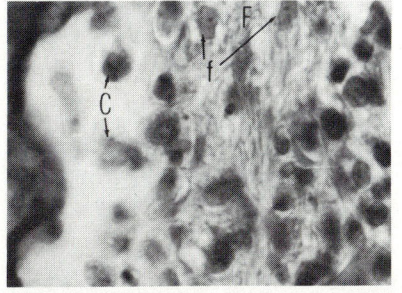
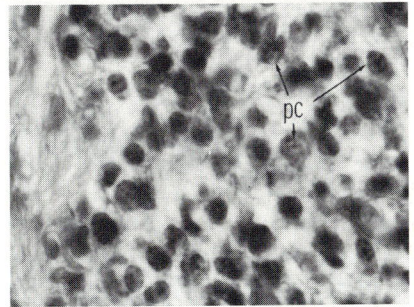

erupting permanent teeth (Andreasen, 1981). Usually, lack of response to the thermal tests occurs when the pulps are necrotic. However, the diagnosis of necrosis of the pulp is more secure when there are also no reactions to both electrical and thermal tests.

ELECTRIC PULP TESTS

Prolonged application of the electric pulp tester to the teeth of experimental animals has been shown to be harmless to the pulp (McDaniel et al, 1973). However, the electric pulp tester is a crude device, and not too much reliance should be placed upon it. Therefore, its results must be evaluated in the light of all the accumulated diagnostic data. The reader is referred to Chapter 19, Clinical Diagnosis, in which the electric pulp test and its limitations are fully discussed.

Caution should be exercised in the use of electric pulp testers, or other electrical dental equipment, such as electrocautery and electronic root canal measuring devices on patients wearing artificial pacemakers. The use of these instruments may be hazardous for such patients, possibly causing ventricular fibrillation and persistence of cardiac contraction (Starmer et al, 1971). In dogs wearing pacemakers, electric pulp testers can switch a demand pacemaker to a fixed rate (Woodworth, 1973; Wooley et al, 1974). Although it has not been proved, the battery-powered electric pulp tester may be less hazardous, since it completely isolates the circuit from the power line system. However, this type is just as unreliable for pulp testing.

PERCUSSION TEST

A positive percussion test is a fairly reliable indication of the presence of periapical tissue involvement (Category B). However, the converse

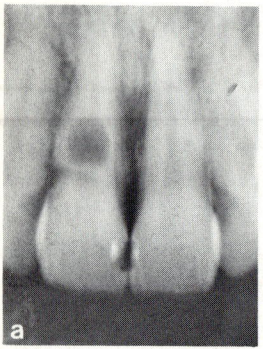 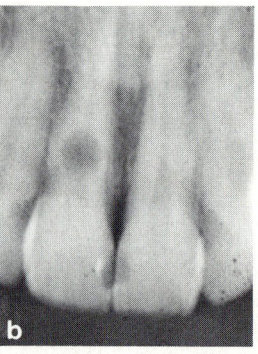 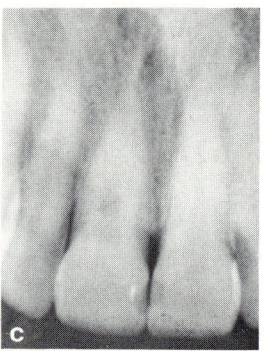 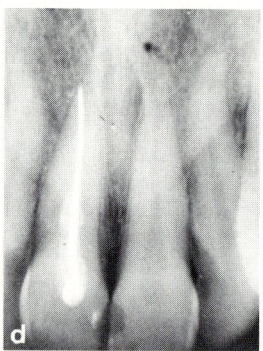

FIG. 18-9 Repair with reformation of hard structure in the root canal following initial internal resorption. (a) Radiograph at initial examination. (b) Two years later; note distinct reduction in size. (c) Eight years later, evidence of reformation continues. (d) Nine years later, patient developed an acute pulpalgia, followed by endodontic therapy. (Weisman MI, Rackley RH: Recalcification of internal resorption. J Georgia Dent Assoc 41:15, 1968)

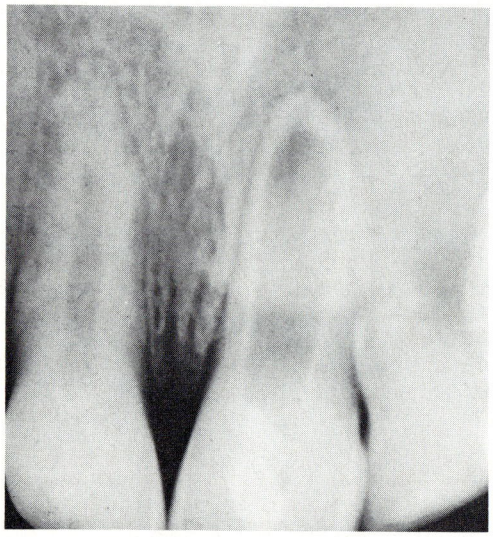

FIG. 18-10 Excessive width of pulp chamber and root canal of upper right central incisor. Due to death of the pulp cells, dentin is no longer being elaborated.

is not completely true. Lack of a positive percussion test does not give assurance that inflammation has not extended into the periapical tissues.

PALPATION TEST

Soreness of the mucosa over the root of a tooth is a reliable indication of inflammation of the periodontal ligament. The inflammation may be of pulpal origin, but it may also be the result of traumatic occlusion. If pulpal in origin, endodontic treatment or extraction is indicated.

TEST DRILLING

When teeth are covered with full crowns, or if hard tissue has formed in the pulpal space, test drilling is frequently helpful in determining pulp vitality. A sensation of pain when the dentin is pierced is an indication of the presence of a vital pulp. However, this does not imply that inflammation is absent.

ANESTHETIC TEST AND REFERRED PAIN

Local anesthesia is a significant aid in diagnosis, especially when the pain is not localized or the teeth are crowned. In the latter instance, not all of the ordinary tests can be made. Referred pain is a common characteristic of a partial pulpitis (Category B). Once the inflammation involves the apical periodontal ligament, the pain begins to localize. After necrosis of the pulp occurs, the referred pain usually stops and the correct diagnosis becomes more apparent. Occasionally, however, even teeth with necrotic pulps cause referred pain.

A direct correlation of referred pain sites with specific teeth does not exist. Pain originating from a posterior tooth may be referred to teeth of the opposite jaw on the same side, i.e., from uppers to lowers or vice versa. Upon occasion, pain from the lower molars may be referred to the ear. In such cases, local anesthesia must be employed as an aid in diagnosis. The patient should be given a mandibular block injection. If pain persists after the signs of anesthesia appear, the offending tooth is most likely in the upper jaw. If the pain disappears with the onset of symptoms of anesthesia, the offending tooth is located in the mandible.

Sites of Referred Pain

The sites of referred pain, together with the other diagnostic data, aid in locating the offending tooth. Usually, attention is directed to one or two teeth. The offending tooth is often the one with the deepest restoration. If doubt still exists, and if the pain is endurable, it is preferable to wait until the pain begins to localize.

Pulpal pain is seldom referred to the 12 anterior teeth; it is referred most often to the posterior teeth. Patients can frequently localize pain more precisely to a specific tooth in the anterior than in the posterior region. Seldom does an anterior tooth cause referred pain to the posterior region, and a posterior tooth seldom refers pain to the anterior teeth.

Anterior teeth, either upper or lower, practically never refer pain to the opposite jaw. However, posterior teeth can refer pain to the opposite arch on the same side. These observations have been corroborated by the experimental findings of Van Hassel and Harrington (1969). With the use of an electric pulp tester, they noted a 100% stimulus discrimination between corresponding teeth in the opposite jaws of the anteriors. In the posteriors, the premolars and first molars, they obtained a 95% accurate discrimination response; in the second molars, there was an 85% discrimination response. In the third molars, they found a 100% correct stimulus discrimination in 15 trials.

Pulpalgia rarely occurs simultaneously in two or more teeth, even though several teeth may become involved consecutively. Also, pain apparently does not cross the midline. Thus, if a patient has pain, for example, on the left side, the pulpal lesion is present on the same side. However, under experimental conditions, Friend and Glenwright (1968) noted that in 20 subjects (1.5% of all teeth that were electrically stimulated), on 28 occasions, the stimulated tooth was incorrectly identified across the midline of the jaws. Their findings differed from those of Van Hassel and Harrington (1969) and Sandborg (1963), who found no decussation of pain across the midline. Clinically, pain from pulpally involved teeth is practically never referred across the midline.

Accurate localization of the source of referred pain is difficult, especially if the pain is in the posterior region. Van Hassel and Harrington made an interesting clinical observation. They noted that patients often reported that when pain first started, they were fairly certain which tooth was involved. With increase in discomfort, the patient lost the ability to discriminate which tooth in the quadrant was involved. Thus, a previous history of pain in a tooth is an important clinical consideration for pain localization when the pain is referred.

Pain of Systemic Origin

Pain referred to the teeth may be of systemic origin. As a general rule, pain of dental origin is unilateral, whereas pain of systemic origin is bilateral. Pain of the latter type is observed, on rare occasions, in diabetics who may suffer from diabetic pulpalgia. Bilateral pain is also manifested in atypical facial neuralgias with specific localization in the teeth, especially in the upper molars. The complaint is most common in females past 40 years of age and may occur unilaterally.

Unilateral pain referred to the teeth may be of systemic origin. In trigeminal neuralgia, spasmodic pain occurs only unilaterally. Although trigeminal neuralgia can occur on either side, both sides of the head are not affected at the same time. This disease has a slightly greater incidence in females and is rarely observed in patients under 40 years of age (Merritt, 1973). The pain symptoms are classic: spontaneity of onset; electricitylike character; and brevity of duration. Trigger zones are present, related to the three divisions of the trigeminal nerve, the maxillary division being more commonly involved. Pain can be triggered by touching any of the zones. The patient tends to avoid the trigger zone area of each of the three divisions of the fifth nerve. This disorder creates no problem in diagnosis.

Unilateral pain referred to the teeth may be due to coronary insufficiency (angina pectoris and myocardial infarction) or sinus inflammation. Usually, in the former, pain is referred to the lower left jaw (Hurst and Logue, 1970), but it may be more intense in carious or restored teeth.

In sinusitis, pain may be localized around the apices of the upper premolars and molars. The teeth may be tender to percussion, but, usually,

TABLE 18-1
Subjective Symptoms and Objective Findings as Related to Probable Category of Treatment

TREATMENT CATEGORY	PRESENCE OR CHARACTER	SYMPTOMS AND FINDINGS	PRESENCE OR CHARACTER	TREATMENT CATEGORY
	←	**PAIN**	→	
	No	Previous history	Yes	
	No	Episodes	Frequent	
	Yes (infrequent)			
	No	Intensity	Moderate to severe	
	Yes (mild to moderate)			
	Brief	Duration	Long	
	No	On percussion	Yes	
A	No	On palpation	Yes	B
	No	Referred	Yes	
		TEST RESULTS		
Conservative procedures, designed to preserve vitality of pulp	Normal	Response to heat or cold	Abnormal	Endodontic or exodontic procedures
	Similar to that of control	Response to electric pulp tester	Different from that of control	
		PATHOLOGY		
	Shallow to moderate	Dental caries	Deep (with pain)	
	Deep (without pain)			
	No	Pulp exposure	Yes	
	No	Extensive restorations	Yes (with pain)	
	Yes (without pain)			
	Normal	Tooth color	Abnormal	
	No	Periodontal disease	Yes (with pain)	
	Yes (without pain)			
	No	Swelling	Yes	
	No	Sinus tract	Yes	
	No	Fracture	Yes (with pain and mobility)	
	Yes (with no pain or mobility)			
	No	Resorption (extensive)	Yes	
	No	Rarefaction (in radiograph)	Yes	
	←		→	

Arrows indicate progressive degree of probability in choice, or successful outcome of therapy.

they are not oversensitive to thermal changes. Pain usually increases on jumping or when the head is lowered.

Barodontalgia (Aerodontalgia)

Aerodontalgia (dental pain experienced while flying or during decompression tests) was thought to be caused by irritation of the maxillary sinuses (Shiller, 1965). However, the pulps of the teeth that react to hyperbaric conditions may be inflamed or necrotic; the pain may result from gas "bubble" formation in the blood vessels of the involved pulps under severe pressure changes. Periodontal abscesses may also be exacerbated as a result of changes in barometric pressure (Hodges, 1978). Emphysema of the facial tissues has also been reported to occur in a submariner after submergence of the submarine. The increased pressure forced the air through an exposed root canal into the soft tissues of the face and neck (Verunac, 1973).

Pain From Cracked Teeth

Pain may be caused by cracked teeth, i.e., coronal fractures involving the enamel, the dentin, and frequently the pulp. Cracks may develop in enamel from thermal tensile stresses, because transient heat is conducted much more readily in enamel than in dentin (Brown et al, 1970). Thus, when teeth are subjected to sudden temperature change, the enamel reaches the new temperature much more rapidly than the dentin. With lower temperatures, the enamel is restrained from contracting by the dentin, resulting in enamel cracks. In addition, cycling of temperatures, as occurs in daily eating and drinking, can reverse stress distribution and stress direction, eventually creating a sufficiently high stress level to cause cracking of enamel (Brown et al, 1972; Despain et al, 1974; Lloyd et al, 1978). Bachman and Lutz (1976) have reported that enamel cracks may occur following the clinical application of the carbon dioxide snow test or dichlor-difluormethane, which are used in thermal vitality tests of teeth. However, profile analysis and scanning electron studies of replicas of the enamel surface before and after the application of CO_2 snow revealed that no new cracks were created (Peters et al, 1983). Existing cracks may enlarge under masticatory forces. Posterior teeth with proximal restorations are most frequently affected. The fractures usually occur mesiodistally and are often difficult to discover. The existence of fractures may be suspected if the teeth are sensitive to thermal changes and the pressure of chewing causes discomfort.

According to Silvestri (1976), an incomplete tooth fracture may also cause a wide range of bizarre symptoms, from vague discomfort for years to a severe, constant pain or even a quick, unbearable spasm lasting for a few seconds. Cameron (1964) called this the cracked-tooth syndrome. Diagnosis is facilitated by staining with iodine or methylene blue, and by wedging of the teeth. However, teeth with IARFs seldom exhibit pulpal pain (Bender and Freedland, 1983).

Pulpitis may, on the other hand, cause symptoms resembling those of the myofascial pain dysfunction syndrome (MPD; Caulfield, 1981). Thus, careful and thorough diagnostic pulp tests should be performed to rule out pulpitis before establishing a diagnosis of MPD (Duquette and Goebel, 1973).

All clinical tests are diagnostic aids, but no single one of them can be used conclusively or exclusively for a definite diagnosis. All of the symptoms, the clinical findings and the test results must be evaluated, and the evaluation must be tempered by the experience of the operator before a clinical diagnosis can be made. In spite of all efforts, the final diagnosis may still be clouded in doubt. Under such circumstances, watchful waiting is preferable to misdiagnosis and may be necessary before clarification of the diagnosis can be made.

In Table 18–1, the relationship of subjective symptoms and objective findings to probable categories of treatment is depicted.

BIBLIOGRAPHY

Andreasen JO: Traumatic injuries of the teeth, pp 58, 140, 2nd ed. Munksgaard, Copenhagen, 1981

Bachman A, Lutz F: Schmelzsprünge durch die Sensibilitätsprüfung mit CO_2-Schnee und Dichlor-difluormethaneine Vergleichende M-vivo Untersuchung. Schweiz Mschr Zahnheilk 86:1042, 1976

Barber FE, Lees S, Lobene RR: Ultrasonic pulse-echo measurements in teeth. Arch Oral Biol 14:745, 1969

Baume LJ: Diagnosis of diseases of the pulp. Oral Surg 29:102, 1970

Bender IB: Factors influencing radiographic appearance of bony lesions. J Endodont 8:161, 1982

Bender IB, Freedland JB: Clinical considerations in the diagnosis and treatment of intra-alveolar root fractures. JADA 107:595, 1983

Bender IB, Seltzer S: Roentgenographic and direct observation of experimental lesions in bone. I. JADA 62:152, 1961

Bender IB, Seltzer S: The oral fistula: its diagnosis and treatment. Oral Surg 14:1367, 1961

Bender IB, Seltzer S: The effect of periodontal disease on the pulp. Oral Surg 33:458, 1972

Bhaskar SN, Rappaport HM: Dental vitality tests and pulp status. JADA 86:409, 1973

Brown AC, Goldberg MP: Surface temperature and temperature gradients of human teeth in situ. Arch Oral Biol 11:973, 1966

Brown WS, Dewey WA, Jacobs HR: Thermal properties of teeth. J Dent Res 49:752, 1970

Brown WS, Jacobs HR, Thompson RE: Thermal fatigue in teeth. J Dent Res 51:461, 1972

Burstone MS: The ground substance of abnormal dentin, secondary dentin and pulp decalcifications. J Dent Res 32:269, 1953

Cameron CE: Cracked-tooth syndrome. JADA 68:405, 1964

Clark GE, Walter RG, McWalter GM, Esquire RG: Pain history as a predictor of conservative deep caries treatment. J Dent Res 62:170, Abst 7, 1983

Caulfield JB: Hairline tooth fracture: A clinical case report. JADA 102:501, 1981

Despain RR, Lloyd BA, Brown WS: Scanning electron microscope investigation of cracks in teeth through replication. JADA 88:580, 1974

Duquette P, Goebel WM: Pulpitis simulating the myofascial pain dysfunction syndrome: report of three cases. JADA 87:1237, 1973

Ferguson JL: Liquid crystals. Sci Am 211:77, 1964

Fiore-Donno F: Comparisons between clinical and histopathological diagnosis of dental pulp disease. Schweiz Mschr Zahnheilk 78:1148, 1968

Friend LA, Glenwright HD: An experimental investigation into the localization of pain from the dental pulp. Oral Surg 25:765, 1968

Fry AE, Watkins RF, Phatak NM: Topical use of corticosteroids for the relief of pain sensitivity of dentine and pulp. Oral Surg 13:594, 1960

Fulling HJ, Andreasen JO: Influence of maturation status and tooth type of permanent teeth upon electrometric and thermal pulp testing. Scand J Dent Res 84:286, 1976

Gorlin RJ, Goldman HM: Thoma's Oral Pathology. St. Louis, CV Mosby, 1970

Hasselgren G, Stromberg T: Histochemical demonstration of acid hydrolase activity in internal dentinal resorption. Oral Surg 42:381, 1976

Hasler JF, Mitchell DF: Painless pulpitis. JADA 81:671, 1970

Hattyasy D: Possibilities of the conservation of the damaged dental pulp. Internat Dent J 16:63, 1963

Hodges FR: Barodontalgia at 12,000 feet. JADA 97:66, 1978

Howell RM, Duell RC, Mullaney TP: The determination of pulp vitality by thermographic means using cholisteric liquid crystals. Oral Surg 29:763, 1970

Hurst JW, Logue RB: The Heart. New York, McGraw-Hill, 1970

Johnson RH, Dachi SF, Haley JV: Pulpal hyperemia — A correlation of clinical and histologic data from 706 teeth. JADA 81:108, 1970

Kosoff G, Sharpe CJ: Examination of the contents of the pulp cavity in teeth. Ultrasonics 4:77, 1966

Lawson BF, Mitchell DF: Pharmacologic treatment of painful pulpitis. A preliminary controlled double-blind study. Oral Surg 17:47, 1964

Lloyd BA, McGinley MB, Brown WS: Thermal stress in teeth. J Dent Res 57:571, 1978

Lundy T, Stanley HR: Correlation of pulpal histopathology and clinical symptoms in human teeth subjected to experimental irritation. Oral Surg 27:187, 1969

Massler M: Therapy conducive to healing of the human pulp. In Siskin M (ed): The Biology of the Human Dental Pulp. St. Louis, CV Mosby, 1973

McDaniel KF, Rowe NH, Charbeneau GI: Tissue response to an electric pulp tester. J Prosth Dent 29:84, 1973

Merritt HH: Textbook of Neurology. 5th ed, p 366. Philadelphia, Lea and Febiger, 1973

Miles AEW, Fearnhead RW: Post mortem color changes in teeth. J Dent Res 33:735, 1954

Mitchell DF: Differential diagnosis of odontalgia. In Healy HJ (ed): Endodontics. St. Louis, CV Mosby, 1960

Mitchell DF, Tarplee RE: Painful pulpitis. Oral Surg 13:1360, 1960

Mumford JM: Reproducibility and discrimination in electric pulp testing. J Dent Res 39:1111, 1960

Mumford JM: Pain threshold of normal human anterior teeth. Arch Oral Biol 8:493, 1963

Mumford JM: Pain perception threshold and adaptation of normal human teeth. Arch Oral Biol 10:957, 1965

Mumford JM: Pain perception threshold on stimulating human teeth and the histological condition of the pulp. Brit Dent J 123:427, 1967

Mumford JM: Thermal and electrical stimulation of teeth in the diagnosis of pulpal and periapical disease. Proc Roy Soc Med 60:197, 1967

Peters DD, Lorton L, Mader CL, Augsburger RR, Ingram TA: Evaluation of the effects of carbon dioxide used as a pulpal test. I. In vitro effect on human enamel. J Endodont 9:219, 1983

Reynolds RL: The determination of pulp vitality by means of thermal and electrical stimuli. Oral Surg 22:231, 1966

Rubin RL: On the controversy of classification of caries and pulpitis. Stomatolgiia (Moskva) 46:90, 1967

Sandborg LO: Förmagen att okalisera en dental smärtretning; en experimentell-klinisk undersökning. Svensk Tandläk T 56:499, 1963

Schroeder A: Control of pain in endodontic practice, p 121. In Grossman LI (ed): Mechanism and Control of Pain. Masson Publishing Company USA, Inc, 1979

Schroeder A, Triadan H: The pharmacotherapy of pulpitis. Oral Surg 15:345, 1962

Seltzer S, Bender IB, Ziontz M: The dynamics of pulp inflammation: Correlations between diagnostic data and actual histologic findings in the pulp. Oral Surg 16:846, 969, 1963

Seltzer S, Bender IB, Ziontz M: The interrelationship of pulp and periodontal disease. Oral Surg 16:1474, 1963

Shiller WR: Aerodontalgia under hyperbaric conditions. Oral Surg 20:694, 1965

Silvestri AR: The undiagnosed split root syndrome. JADA 92:930, 1976

Starmer CF, McIntosh HD, Whalen RE: Electrical hazards and cardiovascular function. New Eng J Med 284:181, 1971

Sutton PRN: Greenstick fracture of the tooth crown. Brit Dent J 112:362, 1962

Teitler D, Tzadik D, Eidelman E, Chosack A: A clinical evaluation of vitality tests in anterior teeth following fracture of enamel and dentin. Oral Surg 36:649, 1972

Toto PD, Restarski JS: The histogenesis of pulpal odontoclasts. Oral Surg 16:172, 1963

Tyldesley WR, Mumford JM: Dental pain and the histological condition of the pulp. Dent Pract 20:333, 1970

Van Hassel HJ, Harrington GW: Localization of pulpal sensation. Oral Surg 28:753, 1969

Verunac JJ: Recurrent severe facial emphysema in a submariner. JADA 87:1192, 1973

Viener AE: Fractured teeth: A cause of odontalgia. Oral Surg 20:594, 1965

Weisman M, Rackley RH: Recalcification of internal resorption. J Georgia Dent Assoc 41:15, 1968

Woodworth JV: Hazard in dental office to pacemaker wearers. New Eng J Med 289:1039, 1973

Woolley LH, Woodworth J, Dobbs JL: A preliminary evaluation of the effects of electrical pulp testers on dogs with artificial pacemakers. JADA 89:1099, 1974

Yamamura T, Shimono M, Koike H, Terao M, Tanaka Y, Sakai Y, Inoue T, Shusaka Y, Tackikawa T, Kawahara H, Watanabe O: Differentiation and induction of undifferentiated mesenchymal cells in tooth and periodontal tissue during wound healing and regeneration. Bull Tokyo Dent Coll 21:181, 1980

Zachrisson BU, Jacobsen I: Long-term prognosis of 66 permanent anterior teeth with root fracture. Scand J Dent Res 83:345, 1975

19
CLINICAL DIAGNOSIS

In the past, pulp diseases have been classified on a clinical basis by the use of histologic terms. Traditionally, clinical and histopathologic nomenclature has been intertwined, resulting in a mishmash of misleading terms and diagnoses (Stephan, 1937; Rebel, 1954; Gardner, 1963; Harndt, 1969). For example, an acute serous pulpitis has been taken to mean that the patient has pain (hence the adjective 'acute'), that the pulp is inflamed (pulpitis), and that the character of the inflammation is nonsuppurative (serous). However, the term has also been understood to mean that, on a clinical basis, the pulp is overly sensitive to cold and that it reacts more quickly to the electric pulp tester than the pulp of a control tooth.

Other clinical diagnoses, such as hyperemia, a pathologic entity in which blood vessels are dilated and filled with erythrocytes, have brought the concept of therapy into the classification. With such a diagnosis, thermally sensitive teeth react quickly to the electric pulp tester, but symptoms disappear when a sedative dressing is placed in the teeth; presumably the pathosis is reversed.

Investigations of Mitchell and Tarplee (1960), Matsumiya et al (1962), Seltzer et al (1963), Ogilvie and Ingle (1965), Pheulpin et al (1967), Holz et al (1968), Fiore-Donno (1968), Baume (1970), Tyldesley and Mumford (1970), Hess (1970), Ehrmann (1971), and Dummer et al (1980) have demonstrated the futility of attempting to mix clinical and histopathologic classifications. Instead, the status of the pulp has been classified on the basis of clinical symptomatology plus the results of certain test procedures (Seltzer et al, 1963; Hess, 1967; Fuchs and Szymaniak, 1968). Such classifications lead only to a suggestion of treatment procedures. A calculated guess of the histologic status of the pulp can be made, but it is only a guess. To prove whether the guess is correct, either the tooth must be extracted or the pulp must be extirpated and processed for histologic examination. Histologic studies of extirpated pulps leave a great deal to the imagination, owing to the distortion, twisting, and ripping of pulp tissue that necessarily occur during removal of the pulp with a barbed broach.

Clinical diagnosis of pulp diseases involves the taking and recording of medical and dental histories, an analysis of the results of various pulp tests and radiographic findings, and a clinical oral examination.

The medical history should include a recording of past and present illnesses, congenital defects, degenerative diseases, surgical procedures, and psychiatric problems. Also included should be a record of medications the patient is currently taking—as well as pills and elixirs not usually considered by the patient to be medications, such as vitamins, antihistamines—and his smoking and eating habits.

The dental history should include the chief complaint and the history relating to the involved tooth or teeth. Among the symptoms to be recorded are the presence or the absence of pain and the previous history of pain. The characteristics of the pain, such as sharp, dull, localized, diffused, throbbing, intermittent, continuous, or referred to other regions of the head or neck, which were deemed previously to be important, have limited diagnostic value. However, the intensity of the pain, regardless of characteristics, is significant. Another symptom to be noted is sensitivity to external stimuli: is the pain increased or decreased by cold and/or heat, pressure, mastication, lying down, or sweet or sour foods? Whether or not the tooth feels elongated also should be recorded.

Clinical signs (objective symptoms) also are to be noted. Among these are the presence or absence of extraoral or intraoral swelling, sinus tract, lymph node involvement, tooth discoloration, pain on percussion, mobility, and tenderness of the apical region on palpation.

If a pulp exposure is detected, it should be recorded as well as its cause, such as caries or traumatic injury.

The presence or the absence of bases and restorations, such as silicates, resins, amalgams, foils, inlays, or others is also to be recorded.

Electric pulp and thermal tests are to be made and radiographs of the involved teeth are to be evaluated for the presence or the absence of recurrent caries, mineralization of pulp tissue, root resorptions, widened periodontal ligament spaces, and regions of rarefaction.

However, it should be emphasized that there is no clinical sign or symptom that designates the histopathologic status of the pulp with certainty. The use of electric, thermal, percussion, and palpation tests helps to establish an empirical diagnosis, but none of the tests is completely reliable. Other clinical findings, such as referred pain, mobility, and radiographic findings, are reliable for some forms of pulp pathosis, but not for others.

When the foregoing findings are correlated with histologic examinations of sections of extracted teeth, the following relationships can be discerned.

SUBJECTIVE SYMPTOMS (PATIENT'S COMPLAINTS): RELATIONSHIP OF PAIN TO HISTOLOGIC FINDINGS

Incidence of Pain

Increase in the incidence of pain parallels the increase in the severity of the histopathologic condition encountered. Thus, in the categories representing teeth with uninflamed pulps (intact-uninflamed pulp, atrophic pulp, and transitional stage) pain is present in less than one fifth of the cases. In the categories of inflamed teeth (chronic partial pulpitis with or without partial necrosis and chronic total pulpitis with partial necrosis), the incidence of pain increases sharply to three fifths of the cases. The difference beween the two groups is highly significant statistically.

The incidence of pain increases in each category, from chronic partial pulpitis through chronic partial pulpitis with partial necrosis, to chronic total pulpitis with partial necrosis.

At a still more advanced stage (total necrosis) the incidence of pain falls to about 50%, perhaps because drainage is established, and intrapulpal pressure drops, in necrotic pulps. Even here there is an established difference with respect to incidence of pain in inflamed teeth.

Previous History of Pain

The vast majority of patients with pulpalgia have a previous history of pain. Recording of a previous history of pain correlates well with the presence of destructive pulpal pathosis. Over 90% of patients in pain, when interrogated, reported that they had experienced pain in the same tooth at some time prior to their present pain experience. In at least 80% of those patients, moderate to severe pulpitis or necrosis of the pulp was found (Seltzer et al, 1963). These findings indicate that a previous history of pulpalgia is an important diagnostic means of establishing the presence of destructive pulpitis.

Intensity (Severity) and Duration of Pain

Pain is the most common symptom of a diseased pulp. In the absence of pain, most pulp pathoses remain undetected in vivo. Pain usually indicates tissue damage and, to some degree, reflects the extent of the damage. However, the psychological component of pain frequently gives a misleading picture of the severity of the underlying disease process. Fear of dentists and dental procedures frequently causes an exaggerated perception of pain, resulting in an incompatibility of symptomatology and pulpal pathosis. Under these circumstances, the severity of pain cannot be correlated with the severity of tissue change (Weiss, 1959; Mumford, 1965; Hattyasy, 1966; Rubin, 1967).

Severity and duration of pain appear to be partially related to the status of the pulp. Mild to moderate pain is usually associated with less inflamed pulps. Thus, in the intact-uninflamed, atrophic, transitional stage, and chronic partial pulpitis categories, no severe pain occurs. Severe pain and pain of long duration appear to be reliable indicators of severe pulpitis or pulp necrosis, but such symptoms are occasionally misleading (Mitchell and Tarplee, 1960). Severe pain usually indicates the presence of liquefaction necrosis or a change in intrapulpal pressure. The tissue pressure may differ at different sites of the inflamed pulp (Van Hassel, 1973). Even severe inflammation may involve only a small pulpal region (Tønder and Kvinnsland, 1983). Small abscesses may be found in one region while the rest of the pulp is histologically normal (Seltzer et al, 1963; Cardoso and Mitchell, 1971; Mumford, 1976). Thus, the most severe pain occurs when the diagnosis is chronic partial pulpitis with partial necrosis. In chronic total pulpitis, the incidence of severe pain is reduced and moderate pain is present in the greatest number of patients. In the necrosis group the pain is mild to moderate in half of the painful teeth. When vital pulp tissue is present, the pulpal cavity is not an isobaric chamber (Närhi, 1978). However, following the development of necrosis, the intrapulpal pressure drops, causing the pulp to become an isobaric chamber, one in which all regions are in hydrostatic equilibrium (Van Hassell, 1973). Thus, in the most advanced stages of pulp disease, when drainage has been established, the severity of the pain tends to decrease.

Character of Pain

Various characteristics, such as sharp, dull, intermittent, continuous, throbbing, diffuse, and others have been used to describe pulpal pain. Our studies, and those of Tyldesley and Mumford (1970) and Mumford (1976), have failed to uncover any correlation between specific pain characteristics and histopathologic status of the pulp. However, there tends to be an increased awareness of the various types of pain (sharp, dull, throbbing, localized, diffuse, intermittent, and continuous) in the categories of chronic partial pulpitis and chronic total pulpitis with necrosis. Thus, there are no characteristic or pathognomonic signs for various histopathologic states of the pulp.

In differentiating pain characteristics, a distinction can be made between dentinalgia, or dentinal pain, and pulpalgia or pulpal pain. The etiologies are different. In dentinalgia, pain is rapid in onset, sharp and lancinating and is caused by stimulating the dentin of a vital pulp. Dentinalgias are usually not provoked by pulpitides but are primarily caused by external stimuli. The stimuli are to the terminal nerve endings, composed of fast-conducting A delta fibers (Hagerstrom, 1976; Matthews, 1977; Närhi et al, 1982) that extend into the dentinal tubules from the pulp, a distance of about 150 μm. C fibers apparently do not respond to mechanical stimulation of dentin (Jyväsjärvi et al, 1981).

In pulpalgia, the pain is deep, dull, and throbbing and is usually caused by a rise in intrapulpal pressure, which follows pulpal inflammation. In the more severe pulpalgias, not only are the fast-conducting A delta fibers activated, but the deeper pulp nerves, including the slow-conducting unmyelinated C fibers, also become stimulated. Firing of the C fibers is usually associated with pulpal inflammation and heat stimulation (Närhi et al, 1982a).

Spontaneity of Pain

The occurrence of spontaneous pain appears to be an indication of severe pathosis of the deep pulpal tissues (Guthrie et al, 1965). Pain initiated by stimuli such as cold, heat, and sweets and disappearing within seconds probably indicates that nerve endings in the odontoblastic layer have been stimulated. Persistence of such pain probably indicates a more extensive inflammatory involvement.

Pain on Percussion

Pain is elicited on percussion much more frequently in all pulp conditions in which necrosis, either partial or total, is present than in those categories in which necrosis is not evident. The difference is highly significant. This appears to indicate that percussion is an important diagnostic test for detection of partial or total necrosis of pulp tissues.

A possible explanation for pain on percussion in teeth with partial pulpitis is suggested by the observation that, in some instances in which chronic pulpitis is present in the coronal portion of the pulp, the radicular pulp appears to be uninflamed except for the presence of dilated blood vessels — yet, chronic inflammation is sometimes found extending beyond the apex of the tooth and into the periodontal ligament.

The exact cause of the periapical inflammation is undetermined. The apical pulp tissue is much more fibrous than the coronal pulp tissue. This fibrous tissue apparently acts as a barrier to the further progression of inflammation from the coronal portion rootward. However, inflammation is not completely inhibited in the periapical tissues. Small regions of chronic inflammation, delineated by coarse collagen fiber bundles, are found in the central portion of the pulp. Analogously, in a periapical granuloma, dense fiber bundles are elaborated around the periphery, tending to encapsulate it. Nevertheless, chronic inflammatory cells may be found in the tissue beyond the collagen fibers, such as the marrow spaces of the bone.

The edema which accompanies the presence of inflammatory cells may be responsible for the painful reaction of the tooth to percussion.

Pain on Thermal Stimuli

In many teeth, pain is increased by thermal stimuli. However, no correlation is discernible between this symptom and the histologic diagnosis when the pain is of short duration. Pain induced by thermal stimuli, such as heat and cold, that persists after the removal of the stimulus is indicative of pulpitis or pulp necrosis (Lundy and Stanley, 1969). There does not appear to be a correlation between the type (acute or chronic) or severity (with or without liquefaction necrosis) of the pulp pathosis and the type of thermal stimulus (Reynolds, 1966). Inflamed or necrotic pulp can react to either or both, or neither of the two stimuli.

Sensitivity of short duration to thermal stimuli, is apparently increased in pulposis induced by periodontal disease (Seltzer et al, 1963). When pain persists after removal of the stimulus from periodontally involved teeth, pulpitis should be suspected.

Pain on Other Stimuli

Pain, or postoperative discomfort that occurs following insertion of metallic fillings or crowns, is often exacerbated by thermal irritation (Silvestri et al, 1977) such as ingestion of hot and cold drinks after cementation of restorations (Takahashi, 1982). Other causes of pain can be ascribed to reversible acute pulpitis (Category A). Acute pulpitis is associated with a transient rise in intrapulpal pressure. Persistent pulpal pain following restorative procedures is strongly indicative of an irreversible pulpitis (Category B).

Increased pain when the patient is lying down, eating sweet or sour foods, or submitting to tissue palpation or pressure occurs more frequently in teeth with pathologic pulp states but is not significantly greater in any specific category.

Pain and Carious Pulp Exposure

Most teeth with carious pulp exposures are painful. When the patient complains of pain to his dentist, a prediction that pulp exposure is present frequently may be made.

Mitchell and Tarplee (1960) found that pulpitis and pulp exposure are invariably associated with one another. Histologic examination reveals that, when pulps are exposed, the severity of the inflammatory response increases. Thus, in teeth with carious pulp exposure, most of the pulps either are totally necrotic or are partially or totally inflamed with partial necrosis. It is rare to find either inflammation-free or mildly pathologic states of the pulp when pulp exposures are present. The statistical relationships between pulp exposure and severity of inflammation are highly significant. These findings would contraindicate pulp capping procedures for cariously exposed pulps.

Summary

In summation, pain, although not a completely reliable indicator of the status of the pulp, can be used as a guide, together with other signs and symptoms. Clinically, the pain may be classified as mild, moderate or severe pulpalgia. The implications of such categorization are as follows: mild to moderate pulpalgia is usually associated with transitional stages, chronic partial pulpitis or atrophic pulps. Pain that arises spontaneously or persists following thermal stimulation, together with a history of previous pain, usually indicates the presence of severe pulp damage, probably irreversible by therapeutic measures. Severe pain in cariously involved teeth usually indicates pulp exposure (Mitchell and Tarplee, 1960), and severe pulp pathosis, probably with liquefaction necrosis (Seltzer et al, 1963; Künzel, 1968). Under restorations, pain usually indicates the presence of an irreversible pulpitis or pulp necrosis.

OBJECTIVE FINDINGS: RELATIONSHIP OF CLINICAL TESTS TO HISTOPATHOLOGIC FINDINGS

The Electric Pulp Test

Correlation With Classification of Pulp Disease. The conventional electric pulp tester uses high-frequency current to stimulate the nerves of the dental pulp. Most pulp testers use a fixed frequency while the voltage is varied. Current is applied to the tooth until the threshold of stimulation is reached (Millard, 1973). Some battery-powered pulp testers include sensitive, digital read-out voltmeters. Experimental models have attached digital printers activated by pushbutton controls (Stark et al, 1977). Measurement of voltage in teeth is unsatisfactory; voltage drop may vary because of variations in the electrical resistance of enamel. In addition, cracks, pits, fissures, caries, restorations, and fractures may cause variations in electrical resistance. In order to overcome such variations in resistance, a stimulator that measures current rather than voltage, has been used. Efforts to determine the pain threshold values of normal teeth have been made by Björn (1946), using a square wave stimulus of 10 milliseconds' duration every 2 or 3 seconds. Similar experiments have been conducted by Mumford, (1960, 1963), using a Nitram stimulator that gave 50 stimuli per second each of 10 milliseconds' duration and also a current square wave stimulator that had a 10 millisecond duration and a frequency of 50 stimuli per second. Of these studies, the narrowest range of oscilloscope readings of the square waves was 0.7 $\mu\text{Å}$ to 4.5 $\mu\text{Å}$. Subsequently, Mumford (1965) modified his procedure and used a 30 millisecond stimulus at 20 counts per second, applied to a larger contact area. The pain perception threshold range was then recorded as 2.2 $\mu\text{Å}$ to 20.5 $\mu\text{Å}$ — still too great to be of practical clinical value.

Pain elicited by the electric pulp tester is a poor indicator of the status of the pulp. No correlation between pain perception or reaction thresholds and the condition of the pulp has been discovered by Mumford (1965, 1967), Reynolds (1966), Lundy and Stanley (1969), Johnson et al (1970) and Matthews et al (1974). Determination of pain reaction threshold is subject to many variables related to the psyche of the patient. However, in pathologically involved pulps the reaction occurs at levels of stimulation either above or below those required for response from the control teeth (Seltzer et al, 1963). Actually, the pulp tester helps to determine pulp vitality or nonvitality and not the condition of the pulp (Cooley and Robison, 1980). However, even necrotic pulps occasionally evince painful responses to the electric pulp tester.

Pulp response to the electric pulp tester is often lacking in traumatized teeth and in developing permanent teeth. In the latter, several years elapse before the root apex closes, so that the maturation of innervation is slow. Thus, the pulpal nerves fail to terminate among the odontoblasts and reach the predentin or dentin, as occurs in the fully developed teeth in occlusion (Bernick, 1963). The lack of pulp response to electrical stimulation in immature teeth may also be attributed to the larger quantity of pulp tissue, which produces a greater electrical impedance. The amount of electric current passing through a unit area in the pulp is greatest where the pulp tissue is thinnest, i.e., where there is a lesser impedance (Hargreaves, 1973). Moreover, clinical observations appear to indicate that cutting the dentin of young permanent teeth is less painful than similar procedures in the teeth of older persons.

Thus, the electric pulp test is of some value in suggesting the possibility of an inflammatory state, but it is far from definitive. A response similar to that of the corresponding control teeth is given by more than 50% of the teeth with intact-uninflamed or mildly inflamed pulps and by 6% to 40% of the teeth with more severely inflamed pulps.

No response to the electric pulp test is given by 72% of the teeth with totally necrotic pulps, whereas teeth in all other categories usually give a response. Thus, there is a statistically significant relationship between absence of response to the pulp test and presence of a totally necrotic pulp. If a tooth does not respond, the dentist can be fairly sure that at least some necrosis is present, since only 2.3% of the teeth in all of the following groups combined — intact-uninflamed; transitional; atrophic; and chronic partial pulpitis without necrosis — fail to react to

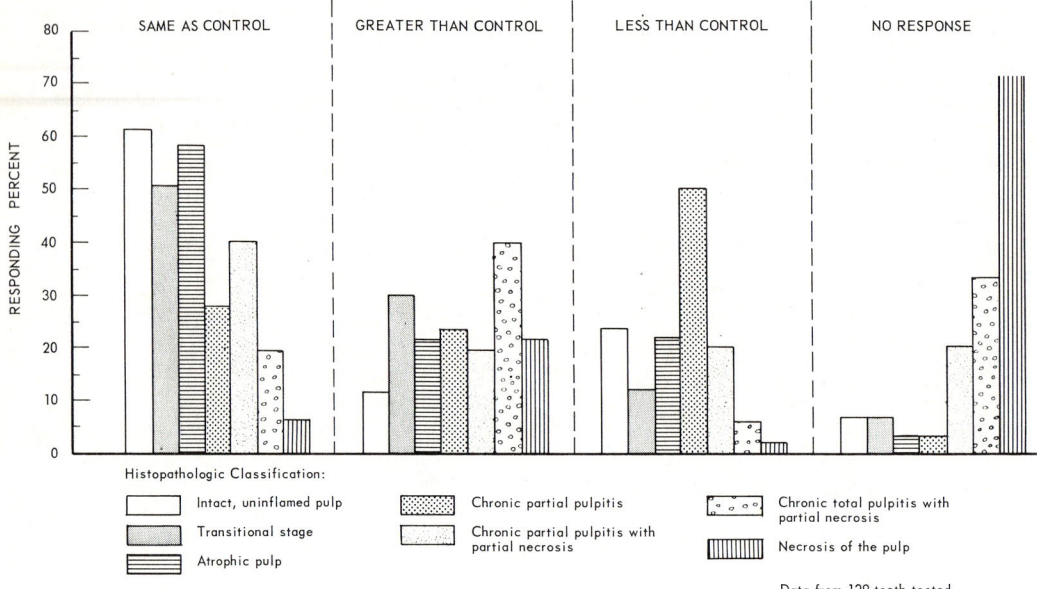

FIG. 19-1 Response to electric pulp test.

the pulp tester. The converse is not true, since 53% of the teeth in the partial and the complete necrosis groups combined do give some kind of response. The difference between these groups is statistically significant. There is no way of determining partial necrosis by means of the pulp tester.

No significant correlations with histologic diagnoses are found when the teeth respond either above or below the corresponding level of response of the control teeth (Fig. 19-1).

Control teeth often give abnormal readings. There is no way of knowing whether the control tooth has a normal pulp or whether the reactions to the pulp tester are within normal limits. For example, examination of teeth obtained by multiple extractions from the same patient often reveal some teeth with atrophic pulps and some with chronic pulpitis. Obviously, a diagnosis based on the use of an inflamed pulp as a control would be invalid; however, the operator has no way of knowing whether he has chosen a suitable control tooth without extracting it and making a histologic section. Examination of the teeth in the mouth would be inadequate, since noncarious and unfilled teeth sometimes have atrophic pulps. This may help to explain differences in the accuracy of electrodiagnosis reported by various investigators.

There appears to be no correlation between the presence or the absence of pain and the electric pulp-test reading.

Other Pulp Testing Methods

Because of the inadequacies of the electric pulp tester, other modalities have been tried in an effort to correlate some parameters of disease processes with clinical testing procedures. A historical review of many of these methods has been presented by Chambers (1982).

Ultrasonics. Attempts have been made to detect pulpitis by ultrasonic means, but with little success (Kosoff and Sharpe, 1966). The problem is that little information is available relative to the acoustic properties of dental hard tissues, mainly because of the crudity of the instrumentation. With an improved instrument, the transmission and reflection of sound from the dentinoenamel junction and from the dentin-pulp interface have been recorded (Barber et al, 1969). With continued improvement, it is conceivable that an ultrasonic diagnostic tool will be perfected.

Infrared Thermography. Alterations in the temperatures of diseased bodily structures have been detected with sophisticated infrared thermographic equipment. It has been assumed that teeth with vital pulps would have higher surface temperatures than those with necrotic pulps. However, Crandell and Hill (1966) found that, by the use of an infrared thermometer, there were no differences between the surface temperatures of teeth with normal pulps and those of pulpless teeth.

Liquid Crystals. Howell, et al (1970) have attempted to employ the color change of cholisteric liquid crystals applied to the surfaces of the teeth, as a diagnostic modality.

There are three types of liquid crystal, termed nematic, smectic, and cholisteric according to their molecular arrangement (Ferguson, 1964). The molecules of cholisteric crystals are arranged in layers. Changes in temperature or pressure alter the pitch and period of the helical structure, so that new colors are produced. Cholisteric crystals can, therefore, serve as the active elements in devices that map the distribution of temperatures. Howell and his co-workers calibrated the color changes induced in ten pulpless teeth; six of these teeth exhibited lower surface temperatures than those of control teeth. They, and Banes and Hammond (1978) concluded that thermography was a useful addition to the dentist's diagnostic armamentarium.

Thermocouples. Another method of measuring tooth surface temperature is by the use of thermocouples. Brown and Goldberg (1966) measured the surface temperatures of the 6 maxillary anterior teeth of 14 human subjects with small thermocouples. Their results showed that there was no significant difference between normal teeth and pulpless teeth. Temperature fluctuations were attributed to varying air currents. Brown and Goldberg concluded that passive conduction from the periodontal tissues was the major source of heat which determined surface temperature; tooth circulation and pulp metabolism were relatively unimportant sources of tooth temperature. On the other hand, Stoops and Scott (1976), and Banes and Hammond (1978), using a thermistor probe, showed that teeth with vital pulps have a higher surface temperature than nonvital teeth.

Thermal Tests

Extreme Cold. Pulp vitality has also been tested by the use of dry ice or carbon dioxide snow (Odontotest) and/or the refrigerant dichlor-difluormethane (Frigen). The former has been reported to give uniformly dependable vitality responses; in 1000 teeth an accuracy of 97.5% has been recorded, compared to 97.2% for electric pulp testing (Saxer, 1958).

According to Chambers (1982), the advantages of carbon dioxide snow vitality testing are its ease and speed of application and its reliability. The method has been reported to be more reliable than other methods for testing the vitality of immature developing permanent teeth and traumatically injured anterior teeth. (Fulling and Andreasen, 1976; Ehrmann, 1977). In such teeth, pulp responses are frequently absent with other testing modalities. The carbon dioxide snow test also produces a distinct vitality response in teeth covered with metal crowns, precluding the use of test drilling. The test can also be used on teeth with orthodontic appliances or large metallic fillings, conditions that may yield false responses from electrical testing. In addition, false-positive vitality reactions have not been reported in teeth with liquefaction necrosis. Ehrmann (1977) has claimed that the test is ineffective in teeth with calcified pulps or in those of elderly patients with large deposits of reparative dentin. However, Schroeder (1981) has claimed that even degenerated and atrophic pulps will react to the cold.

Although the temperature of carbon dioxide snow is $-78°C$ ($-108.4°F$), Augsburger and Peters (1981) found the intrapulpal temperature, as measured in vitro, decreased only by a mean of $15.6°C$ ($4.01°F$) for noncarious teeth. In gold-crowned teeth, the decrease was $13.2°C$ ($8.2°F$) after a 5-second exposure. Their clinical studies indicated that a 2-second exposure produced a vital response. They concluded that lack of response indicated the presence of a nonvital pulp. They also found that, despite the extremely low temperature, the test did not cause significant temperature changes in the adjacent normal or crowned teeth. Histologic studies have indicated that the pulp is not damaged by the application of the CO_2 snow test (Schiller, 1937).

Cold induced by the vapocoolant dichlor-difluormethane causes a reduction in intrapulpal temperature. As with carbon dioxide snow, this vapocoolant has also been found reliable for testing pulp vitality in immature permanent teeth.

Heat. Temperature elevation for pulp testing is usually applied through application of heated gutta-percha to the labial or buccal surface of the tooth. The temperature is not controlled by this method. Compared to the other pulp testing methods, the determination of pulp vitality is questionable.

Correlation of Thermal Tests With Histopathology

Normal Response to Heat and Cold. The majority of teeth with intact-uninflamed pulps respond normally* to heat and cold. Thus, a correlation appears to exist between a normal response to thermal tests and the presence of an uninflamed pulp. Generally speaking, a normal response to heat and cold occurs more frequently in uninflamed pulps or mildly inflamed pulps without necrosis than in pulps that are inflamed or necrotic.

Abnormal Response to Heat. There appears to be no correlation between an abnormal response to heat and the histologic diagnosis of the pulp. Even when liquefaction necrosis is present, there is no apparent increase in abnormal response to heat, compared with the response of uninflamed pulps.

Abnormal Reaction to Cold. Abnormal responses to cold are equally distributed among the pulps of teeth in all diagnostic categories. No single pathologic state of the pulp produces responses to cold more than any other state.

A small number of teeth that react to thermal stimuli respond to both heat and cold. These are distributed throughout all diagnostic categories, the greatest number being in the atrophic group.

No Response to Heat or Cold. There is a significant lack of response to thermal tests in most teeth for which the diagnosis is necrosis of the pulp. This correlates well with the lack of response to the electric pulp tests in teeth with necrotic pulps.

Radiographic Findings

Root Resorption. Although many resorptions (resulting both from periapical granulomas and from periodontal involvement) are discovered on the lateral aspects of the roots in the tissue sections, some cannot be detected radiographically. It seems that only resorptions of considerable magnitude show up in the ordinary dental radiograph. In teeth with chronic pulpitis, granulomatous tissue is often found within the root canal and resorptions of the internal surface of the wall of the root canal are found histologically, but these, too, are not often detectable by radiography.

Granulomas. There is a marked discrepancy between the results obtained from detection of granulomas by radiography and those obtained by histologic examination. Widened periodontal ligament spaces or periapical areas of rarefaction are discernible by radiograph in about half of the teeth in which granulomas are found histologically. These observations tend to confirm the fact that radiographs can reveal only those inflammatory lesions that have invaded the junction area between cortical and cancellous bone.

Caries

Shallow to moderately deep carious lesions produce no morphologically detectable pulp changes except for an increase in reparative dentin formation. As caries involves more and more primary dentin, scattered macrophages and lymphocytes occur in the coronal portion of the pulp under the involved dentinal tubules.

In deeper carious lesions that are closer to the dental pulp, increased numbers of macrophages, lymphocytes and occasional polymorphonuclear leukocytes (polys) are detected. Dilatation of blood vessels becomes apparent. Otherwise, the pulps remain structurally intact. A frank chronic inflammatory process develops in the pulp when the carious lesion is very deep. Exposure of the pulp by caries causes an acute inflammation in the region of the pulp under the exposure, together with liquefaction necrosis (abscess formation). This is overlaid on the pre-existing chronic pulpitis.

Dental caries is detected around the margins of restorations in many tissue sections in teeth in which clinical examination and radiographs do not reveal its presence. In tissue sections, occasionally, demineralized tubules are found around the margins of restorations, a condition that would permit the ingress of microorganisms or their products. Evidently, radiographic studies alone are not sensitive enough to reveal

---

* Normal reactions to thermal tests are those in which pain is elicited by the stimulus but disappears as soon as it is removed. In abnormal reactions, the pain persists after the stimulus is removed.

TABLE 19-1
Correlation of Clinical Signs and Symptoms With Histologic Diagnosis

HISTOLOGIC DIAGNOSIS	INCIDENCE OF PAIN	INTENSITY OF PAIN		PREVIOUS HISTORY OF PAIN	PAIN ON PERCUSSION	PULP EXPOSURE
		MILD TO MODERATE	SEVERE			
CATEGORY A (TREATABLE)*						
Intact-uninflamed pulp	13%	13%	—	No	4%	—
Transitional stage	11%	11%	—	No	5%	11%
Atrophic pulp	25%	25%	—	No	8%	—
Acute pulpitis	25%	25%	—	No	—	—
Chronic partial pulpitis without necrosis	42%	37%	5%	Yes	17%	21%
CATEGORY B (NONTREATABLE)*						
Chronic partial pulpitis with partial necrosis	64%	21%	43%	Yes	43%	79%
Chronic total pulpitis	78%	60%	18%	Yes	36%	78%
Total pulp necrosis	54%	29%	25%	Yes	38%	71%

Columns 1, 2, 3, and 4 are based on patient reports. Columns 5 and 6 are based on examination. Percentages are of teeth tested. Of patients in pain, 92% had a previous history of pain. Of patients with a previous history of pain, 20% had pulps in Category A and 80% had pulps in Category B.
* Categories are defined in Chap. 18, Differential Diagnosis.

the presence of caries around the margins of restorations. The presence of caries is associated with pain in many teeth. Incidence of pain increases in carious teeth in direct proportion to the increased severity of the inflammatory response.

Carious Vital Pulps With Radiographic Periapical Lesions. A general consensus exists among clinicians that teeth with radiographic periapical lesions of pulpal origin need endodontics or extraction. This long-held belief is based on the observation that periapical lesions do not heal spontaneously without root canal therapy. However, Moore (1967), Jordan et al (1978), and Cotton et al (1983) have reported that radiographic periapical lesions around a small number of carious vital teeth with symptoms classified under Category A disappear following indirect pulp capping procedures.

In the study of Jordan et al, treatment was reported to be successful in 11 of 24 teeth (45%). The success was based on the following criteria: the teeth belonged to young patients (ages 11 to 24); they gave a positive vitality response; there was no history of spontaneous or prolonged pain; thermal stimulation provoked mild pain of short duration; no pain was evoked on percussion; and care was exercised to prevent pulp exposure by the removal of carious dentin. All these factors, except the periapical radiolucency, are present in teeth in Category A, probably indicating chronic partial pulpitis.

The prognosis for conservative treatment of teeth with periapical rarefactions is distinctly less favorable. Such teeth are in the twilight zone between Category A (chronic partial pulpitis without necrosis) and Category B (chronic partial pulpitis with necrosis). The results of the above studies imply that caries-induced periapical radiolucencies are not diagnostic of pulp necrosis (Cotton et al, 1983). However, absence of an apical radiolucency does not imply that the pulp or the periapical region is free of inflammation, because the apical region may contain chronic inflammatory cells that are undetectable by ordinary radiography. An inflammatory lesion near the junctional region of the cancellous and endosteal bone can produce radiographically detectable periapical lesions (Bender, 1982). Early detection of occult periapical inflammation is facilitated by the use of a high-resolution cadmium telluride probe, which measures technetium polyphosphonate (^{99}mTC) uptake (Telfer et al, 1980).

Restorations

The incidence of pain is lower in teeth that have no restorations than in those with restorations. Thus, operative procedures might be indicated

TABLE 19-2
Correlation of Results of Clinical Tests With Histologic Diagnosis

	ELECTRIC PULP TESTS				THERMAL TESTS						HEAT AND COLD
					RESPONSE TO COLD			RESPONSE TO HEAT			
HISTOLOGIC DIAGNOSIS	GREATER THAN CONTROL	LESS THAN CONTROL	SAME AS CONTROL	NO RESPONSE	NORMAL	ABNORMAL	NO RESPONSE	NORMAL	ABNORMAL	NO RESPONSE	NO RESPONSE
CATEGORY A (TREATABLE)*											
Intact-uninflamed pulp	11%	22%	61%	6%	74%	11%	15%	75%	10%	15%	5%
Transitional stage	31%	13%	50%	6%	56%	22%	22%	50%	22%	28%	17%
Atrophic pulp	21%	21%	58%	0	53%	28%	19%	50%	39%	11%	3%
Acute pulpitis	†	†	†	†	†	†	†	†	†	†	†
Chronic partial pulpitis without necrosis	22%	50%	28%	0	50%	27%	23%	50%	36%	14%	9%
CATEGORY B (NONTREATABLE)*											
Chronic partial pulpitis with partial necrosis	20%	20%	40%	20%	33%	33%	34%	25%	25%	50%	25%
Chronic total pulpitis	40%	7%	20%	33%	21%	21%	58%	25%	20%	55%	50%
Total pulp necrosis	22%	0	6%	72%	11%	11%	78%	11%	6%	83%	78%

Percentages are of teeth tested.
* Categories are defined in Chap. 18, Differential Diagnosis.
† Not tested.

as a cause of pulp inflammations and consequent pain. The incidence of pain increases with the severity of the inflammatory response found in the pulps under the restorations.

In most teeth with restorations, histologically demonstrable chronic pulpitis apparently persists for long periods without symptoms. In many instances, the presence of inflammatory cells, together with reparative dentin, appears to indicate that the terminal stage of resolution of the lesion is being reached. Many teeth with chronic partial pulpitis are symptomless. Even teeth with a partial pulpitis with partial liquefaction necrosis are occasionally without symptoms. Similarly, symptoms are present infrequently in teeth with a chronic total pulpitis with partial necrosis. One third of the teeth with restorations and total pulp necrosis give no painful symptoms. The incidence and the severity of pain apparently are greater in teeth with restorations than in those without restorations, but the differences are not statistically significant.

Tables 19–1 and 19–2 summarize the data on which the foregoing discussion is based. These charts will enable the diagnostician to make a probable correlation of the clinical signs and symptoms with the results of various tests and with the histopathologic diagnosis of the pulp state.

CLASSIFICATION FOR CLINICAL DIAGNOSIS

A classification of pulpal conditions, based on clinical symptoms, has been developed by Morse et al (1977). In general, the categories are valid, but as in all biologic conditions, there are variations. The classifications are as follows:

Vital asymptomatic: A pulpal condition, usually called normal, in which the pulp responds to thermal and electrical tests in a manner similar to that of a corresponding control tooth. The patient usually reports no adverse symptoms.

Hypersensitive dentin: A pulpal condition, with no apparent histologic changes, in which the patient feels pain when the dentin is exposed to touch from a dental explorer, fingernail, or toothbrush and to thermal or other stimuli. However, the pain disappears within a few seconds after the stimulus is removed.

Inflamed-reversible: A pulpal condition, commonly induced by dental caries and operative procedures, in which the patient responds to thermal or osmotic stimuli such as sweet or sour foods or fluids, but the symptoms disappear when caries or other irritants are removed and a sedative dressing is placed. Symptoms do not usually occur spontaneously and do not last for more than a few seconds. In some instances, symptoms may be absent.

Inflamed/degenerating without radiolucent periapical area — irreversible: A pulpal condition, usually caused by deep dental caries or restorations, in which spontaneous pain may occur or be precipitated by thermal or other stimuli. The pain is usually moderate to severe and lasts for a long time (minutes to hours). Radiographs show no periapical changes. Endodontic therapy is indicated for this and the following three categories.

Inflamed/degenerating with radiolucent periapical area — irreversible: A pulpal condition, similar to that just mentioned, but in which periapical or lateral radiographic changes are evident.

Necrotic without radiolucent periapical area: A pulpal condition in which there may or may not be spontaneous moderate to severe pain, or pain elicited by various stimuli such as thermal, percussion, or palpation. Response to various testing modalities (thermal and electrical) is usually absent. Radiographic changes are not evident.

Necrotic with radiolucent periapical area: Periapical or lateral periodontal radiographic changes are evident in this pulpal condition. Otherwise, it is similar to the previous category.

CLASSIFICATION FOR THERAPEUTIC PURPOSES

A diagnosis of the extent of pulpal involvement in pulposis or pulpitis is difficult; it is easier to determine from clinical findings that a pulp is necrotic. Despite the difficulty in correlating clinical and histologic findings, the clinician must make a diagnosis of the status of the pulp, inasmuch as correct diagnosis dictates proper treatment. The diagnosis implies a prediction, based on clinical judgment, of the type of pulp treatment indicated and its probable outcome. Such a prediction has led to the designation of pulp diseases as reversible or irreversible; treatable or nontreatable; pulps indicated for pulp capping or conservative pharmacotherapy; or pulps indicated for extirpation or root canal therapy (Szymaniak and Pankiewicz, 1968; Pilz, 1969; Baume, 1970; Dummer et al, 1980). Such designations are empirical and cannot be proved by presently available investigative modalities (Hattyasy, 1966). The evaluation of symptoms can only permit an educated guess as to whether or not the pulp can be treated and saved. Correlations between clinical symptoms and histopathology are difficult and fraught with error. Although symptoms such as severe pain, or swelling, are usually indicative of severe pulp damage, this does not always hold true.

The basic premise of all clinical classifications is that pulps exhibiting no symptoms or mild to moderate symptoms (predominantly pain) are judged to be amenable to therapy, with a reasonable chance for recovery. When symptoms are severe, the pulp is usually judged to be beyond repair.

Our findings have led us to the conclusion that the most significant factor in determining whether or not a diseased pulp is amenable to therapy is the presence of an abscess. Such a determination may usually be made on the following criteria: there has been a history of previous pain; there is no reaction to pulp tests; the results of electric tests differ markedly from those of control teeth; pain is spontaneous, severe and long lasting, and thermal irritants or tests evoke severe pain that persists after removal of the stimulus. In addition, clinical findings such as tooth elongation, mobility, sensitivity to percussion and palpation, the presence of swelling or a sinus tract are further evidence of severe pulp pathoses that are nontreatable. Thus, the course of treatment is based on clinical judgment.

However, there is no sure way to determine afterward whether that judgment was correct. Even clinically successful pulp therapy, which apparently has vindicated the judgment of the therapist, does not actually confirm that judgment. Should symptoms be relieved and should the pulp remain relatively free of symptoms and maintain its vitality, such therapy might be considered to have been successful in resolving preexisting pulp inflammation. However, there is no sure way of knowing what the condition of the pulp was at the time of treatment. Conversely, should pain or swelling develop subsequent to treatment, either the treatment may have been unsuccessful, or the diagnosis may have been incorrect—the pulpitis being so severe that it could not be reversed.

Actually, there is no way of determining whether the diagnosis or the treatment was incorrect. The pulp might not have been inflamed initially, or the inflammation might persist without symptoms, or the pulp might have become necrotic without symptoms. Inflammation may have been induced by the manipulative procedures or medicaments applied, or the pulp may have been subsequently irritated by new or recurrent caries, leaky restorations or trauma. Thus, unsuccessful pulp therapy that terminates in endodontic treatment or extraction does not necessarily mean that the clinical judgment was incorrect.

Clinical judgment has, therefore, dictated pulp therapy. With respect to the treatment of deep-seated carious lesions, two schools of thought have emerged. One school believes that the cariously involved tooth always has a pulp inflammation. In such cases, caries should be excavated completely, even if pulp exposure results (Waechter, 1966; Langeland and Langeland, 1968; Kröncke, 1970). The other school believes that, rather than risk pulp exposure by complete excavation of caries, indirect pulp capping is desirable (Jordan and Suzuki, 1971; Jordan et al, 1978). Such a belief is based on findings that the deep layers of carious dentin are sterile and the pulp is not infected or inflamed until almost or actually exposed (Reeves and Stanley, 1966; Massler, 1967; Schroeder, 1968; Shovelton, 1968). There is no lack of evidence to support the contentions of both groups.

In our view, the clinical evidence already enumerated, which indicates the presence of severe pulpal pathosis, dictates a treatment policy of pulp extirpation and endodontic therapy. In the absence of such evidence, therapeutic management by indirect pulp capping is the preferable regimen. In such cases, efforts should be made to maintain pulp vitality, even though chronic pulp inflammation may persist. The vitality of the pulp should be maintained as long as possible, in the absence of evidence that chronic pulp inflammation is harmful to the well-being of the organism. The defensive capacity of the pulp is thereby retained.

BIBLIOGRAPHY

Augsburger RA, Peters DD: In vitro effects of ice, skin refrigerant, and CO_2 snow on intrapulpal temperature. J Endodont 7:110, 1981
Bachman A, Lutz F: Schmelzsprünge durch die Sensibilitätsprüfung mit CO_2-Schnee und Dichlor-difluormetheine vergleichende in-vivo-Untersuchung. Schweiz Mschr Zahnheilk 86:1042, 1976
Banes JD, Hammond HL: Surface temperatures of vital and non-vital teeth. J Endodont 4:106, 1978
Barber FE, Lees S, Lobene RR: Ultrasonic pulse-echo measurements in teeth. Arch Oral Biol 14:745, 1969
Baume LJ: Diagnosis of diseases of the pulp. Oral Surg 29:102, 1970
Bender IB: Factors influencing the radiographic appearance of bony lesions. J Endodont 8:161, 1982
Brown AC, Goldberg MP: Surface temperature and temperature gradients of human teeth in situ. Arch Oral Biol 11:973, 1966
Chambers IG: The role and methods of pulp testing in oral diagnosis: A review. Int Endo J 15:1, 1982
Cooley RL, Robison SF: Variables associated with electric pulp testing. Oral Surg 50:66, 1980
Cotton W, Langeland W, Burmeister JA, Farrell PE: Evaluation of carious teeth with apical radiolucencies for indirect pulp capping. J Dent Res Abst 62:216, Abst 424, 1983
Crandell CE, Hill RP: Thermography in dentistry: A pilot study. Oral Surg 21:316, 1966
Dummer PMH, Hicks R, Huws D: Clinical signs and symptoms in pulp disease. Int Endo J 13:27, 1980
Ehrmann EH: Pulp testers and pulp testing with particular reference to the use of dry ice. Aust Dent J 22:272, 1977
Ferguson JL: Liquid crystals. Sci Am 211:77, 1964
Fiore-Donno F: Comparaisons entre le diagnostic clinique et histo-pathologique des pulpopathies. (Comparisons between clinical and histopathological diagnosis of dental pulp diseases.) Schweiz Mschr Zahnheilk 78:1148, 1968
Fulling HJ, Andreasen JO: Influence of maturation status and tooth type of permanent teeth upon electrometric and thermal pulp testing. Scand J Dent Res 84:286, 1976
Hagerstam G: The origin of impulses recorded from dentinal cavities in the tooth of the cat. Acta Physiol Scand 97:121, 1976
Hargreaves JA: Responses of intradental nerve fibers to stimulation of dentine and pulp. Acta Physiol Scand 115:173, 1982
Hargreaves JA: The traumatized tooth: In Siskin M (ed): The Biology of the Human Dental Pulp, p 414. St. Louis, CV Mosby, 1973
Hattyasy D: Possibilities of the conservation of the damaged dental pulp. Internat Dent J 16:63, 1966
Hess J-C: Conceptions nouvelles de pathologie et de therapeutique pulpaires. (Current concepts of pulp pathology and therapy.) Rev Franc Odontostomat 14:61, 1967
Hess J-C: Endodontie. Paris, Libraire Maloine SA, 1970
Holz J, Fiore-Donno G, Baume LJ: Contrôles biologiques des matériaux d'obturation: Normalisation des méthodes experimentales et des critéres d'évaluation. Rev Mens Suisse Odonto-stomat 78:307, 1968
Howell RM, Duell RC, Mullaney TP: The determination of pulp vitality by thermographic means using cholisteric liquid crystals. Oral Surg 29:763, 1970
Johnson RH, Christensen GJ, Stigers RW, Laswell HR: Pulpal irritation due to the phosphoric acid component of silicate cement. Oral Surg 29:447, 1970
Johnson RH, Dachi SF, Haley JV: Pulpal hyperemia—a correlation of clinical and histologic data from 706 teeth. JADA 81:108, 1970
Jordan RE, Suzuki M: Conservative treatment of deep carious lesions. J Canad Dent A 37:337, 1971
Jordan RE, Suzuki M, Skinner DH: Indirect pulp-capping of carious teeth with periapical lesions. JADA 97:37, 1978
Jyväsjärvi E, Närhi M, Huopaniemi T: Warm receptive mechanisms in the pulp and dentin of the cat. CED and Scand division of IADR Abstracts. Abst #168, 1981
Kosoff G, Sharpe CJ: Examination of the contents of the pulp cavity in teeth. Ultrasonics 4:77, 1966
Kröncke A: Das Schmerzsymptom bei Erkrankungen der Pulpa. Oest Z Stomat 65:162, 1968
Kröncke A: Treatment of deep carious lesions. Internat Dent J 20:238, 1970
Langeland K, Langeland LK: Cutting procedures with minimized trauma. JADA 76:991, 1968
Lundy T, Stanley HR: Correlation of pulpal histopathology and clinical symptoms in human teeth subjected to experimental irritation. Oral Surg 27:187, 1969
Massler M: Pulpal reactions to dental caries. Internat Dent J 17:441, 1967
Matsumiya S, Suzuki A, Takuma S: Atlas of Clinical Oral Pathology. Tokyo, Tokyo Dental College Press, 1962
Matthews B: Responses of intradental nerves to electrical and thermal stimulation of teeth in dogs. J Physiol 264:641, 1977
Matthews B, Searle BN, Adams D, Linden R: Thresholds of vital and non-vital teeth to stimulation with electric pulp testers. Brit Dent J 137:352, 1974
Millard HD: Electric pulp testers. JADA 86:872, 1973
Mitchell D, Tarplee R: Painful pulpitis. Oral Surg 13:1360, 1960
Moore DL: Conservative treatment of teeth with vital pulps and periapical lesions: A preliminary report. J Pros Dent 18:476, 1967
Morse DR, Seltzer S, Sinai I, Biron G: Endodontic classification. JADA 94:685, 1977
Mumford JM: Reproducibility and discrimination in electric pulp testing. J Dent Res 39:1111, 1960
Mumford JM: Pain threshold of normal human anterior teeth. Arch Oral Biol 8:493, 1963
Mumford JM: Pain perception threshold and adaptation of normal human teeth. Arch Oral Biol 10:957, 1965
Mumford JM: Relationship between the pain-perception threshold of human teeth and their histological condition of the pulp. J Dent Res 44:1167, 1965 (abst)
Mumford JM: Thermal and electrical stimulation of teeth in the diagnosis of pulpal and periapical disease. Proc Roy Soc Med 60:197, 1967
Mumford JM: Toothache and Oral Facial Pain. Edinburgh, Churchill-Livingstone, 1976
Närhi MVO: Activation of dental pulp nerves of the cat

and dog with hydrostatic pressure. Proc Finn Dent Soc 74:Suppl V, 1978

Närhi MVO, Hirvonen TJ, Hakumäki MOK: Activation of intradental nerves in the dog to some stimuli applied to the dentine. Arch Oral Biol 27:1053, 1982

Närhi MVO, Hirvonen TJ, Hakumäki MOK: Responses of intradental nerve fibres to stimulation of dentine and pulp. Acta Physiol Scand 115:173, 1982

Obwegeser H, Steinhauser E: Ein neues Gerät zur Vitalitätsprüfung der Zahne mit Kohlensäureschnee. Schweiz Mischr Zahnheilk 73:1001, 1963

Ogilvie AL, Ingle JI: An Atlas of Pulpal and Periapical Biology. Philadelphia Lea & Febiger 1965

Pheulpin J-L, Fiore-Donno G, Baume L-J: Les inflammations pulpaires: Leurs diagnostics clinique et histopathologique. Rev Mens Suisse Odonto-stomatol 77:701, 1967

Pilz W: Die klinische Pulpitisdiagnostik unter pathohistologischem oder symptomatologischem Aspekt. (Clinical diagnosis of pulpitis with the pathohistological or symptomatological approach.) Deutsche Stomatol 19:120, 1969

Reeves R, Stanley HR: The relationship of bacterial penetration and pulpal pathosis in carious teeth. Oral Surg 22:59, 1966

Reynolds RL: The determination of pulp vitality by means of thermal and electrical stimuli. Oral Surg 22:231, 1966

Saxer A: Die Vitalitätsprüfung der Zähne. Med Diss, Zurich, 1958

Schiller F: Ist die Vitalitätsprüfung mit Kohlensäureschnee Unschädlich? Ost Z Stomat 35:1056, 1937

Schroeder A: Endodontics—Science and Practice, p 15. Chicago, Quintessence, 1981

Schroeder A: Indirect capping and treatment of deep carious lesions. Internat Dent J 18:381, 1968

Seltzer S, Bender IB, Ziontz M: The dynamics of pulp inflammation: Correlations between diagnostic data and actual histologic findings in the pulp. Oral Surg 16:846, 969, 1963

Seltzer S, Bender IB, Ziontz M: The interrelationship of pulp and periodontal disease. Oral Surg 16:1474, 1963

Shohar I, Mahler Y, Samueloff S: Dental pulp photoplethysmography in human beings. Oral Surg 36:915, 1973

Shovelton DS: A study of deep carious dentine. Internat Dent J 18:392, 1968

Silvestri AR, Cohen SN, Wetz JH: Character and frequency of discomfort immediately following restorative procedures. JADA 95:85, 1977

Stanley HR, Swerdlow H, Driscoll EJ: Minimizing pulpal reactions with prednisolone therapy. J Oral Therap Pharmac 2:1, 1965

Stark MM, Kempler D, Pelzner RB, Rosenfeld J, Leung RL, Mintatos S: Rationalization of electric pulp-testing methods. Oral Surg 43:598, 1977

Stoops LC; Scott D, Jr: Measurement of tooth temperature as a means of determining pulp vitality. J Endodont 2:141, 1976

Szymaniak E, Pankiewicz H: Wspoklzesne pognady na kliniczna diagnostyke za palen' miazgi. (Current views on the clinical diagnosis of pulp inflammations.) Czas Stomat 21:381, 1968

Takahashi N: Thermal conductive analysis of restored teeth by finite element method. J Oral Rehab 9:83, 1982

Telfer N, Abelson SH, Witmer RR: Role of bone imaging in the diagnosis of active root canal infection. 6:570, Endodont 1980

Tyldesley WR, Mumford JM: Dental pain and the histological condition of the pulp. Dent Pract Dent Rec 20:333, 1970

Van Hassel HJ: Physiology of the human dental pulp. In Siskin M (ed): The Biology of the Human Dental Pulp, p 16. St. Louis, CV Mosby, 1973

Waechter R: Caries profunda. Deutsche Zahnärztl Zeit 21:601, 1966

INDEX

An f *following a page number indicates a figure; a* t *represents tabular material.*

Abacus bodies, 46, 47f, 82, 84f
Abrasion, dental, 329
Abscess
  periodontal, 370
  pulpal, 184, 184f, 187, 258, 286, 287
Accessory canals, 303–305, 304f, 305f
Acetylcholine
  as neurotransmitter, 132, 134, 145–146
  in pain induction, 145
  vasodilation from, 111, 115
Acetylcholinesterase, 120, 145, 146
Acid etchants, 218–219, 219f
Acid etching, 227
Acid phosphatase
  in caries, 176
  of odontoblasts, 94
  in pulp capping and pulpotomy, 291
  in pulposis, 309
  in tooth development, 3, 4
Acidophilia, 41
Acidulated sodium fluoride, 222
Acromegaly, 33, 74
Acrylic resin crowns, 246
Acrylic resins, 225, 240, 241f, 248
Actinomyces, 177
Adenosine monophosphate, cyclic, 157–158
Adenosine triphosphatases
  of odontoblasts, 94
  in tooth development, 3, 4
Adhesive restorative resins, 241
Adrenal insufficiency, 74
Adrenaline, 115
Adrenergic fibers, 134, 146
Adrenocorticotropic hormone, 72, 74, 168–169
Adrenoreceptors, 115
Aerodontalgia, 370
Aging, of pulp, 79, 81f, 271, 271f
  cellular components in, decreased, 325
  circulation with, 126, 126f, 327–328
  clinical correlations of, 345–346
  dead tracts with, 327
  dentin matrix mineralization with, 332, 333f
  dentinal sclerosis with, 325–326, 326f, 327f
  dystrophic mineralizations with, 339–340, 339f, 340f
  fibers with, 97, 98f, 325, 345
  fibroblasts in, 325
  nerves in, 328
  odontoblasts in, 325
  reparative dentin in, 329–333, 329f
  reparative dentinogenesis with, 331–333, 332f, 333f
  secondary dentin in, 328–329, 328f
Aging theories, 324–325
Air spray, 203
Alcian blue stain, 41–42

Alcohol, 218
Alkaline phosphatase
  in caries, 176
  deficiency of, 27
  of odontoblasts, 94
  in pulp capping and pulpotomy, 291, 292f, 294f
  in pulpal repair, 263
  in pulposis, 309
  in tooth development, 3, 4, 5, 42–43
Alveolar bone, 2
Amalgam restorations, 243–246, 245f, 248
Ameloblastomas, 12
Ameloblasts, 2, 17
Amelogenesis imperfecta, 22–23, 23f
Anachoresis, 189–190
Anaphylatoxin, 155
Anesthetic test in differential diagnosis, 368–371
Anesthetics
  general, 125
  local, 124–125
Anodontia, 20–22, 21f
Antibiotics
  for pulp capping and pulpotomy, 296
  tooth development affected by, 28–31, 31f, 32f, 33f
Antibodies, 162–165, 165f, 166f
  pulpal production of, against caries, 179–181, 182f, 183f
  in pulpal repair, 264
Antigens, 162, 163, 165f, 166
  caries, 179–181
  in pulpal repair, 264
Anti-inflammatory agents, 154
Apexification procedures, 297–298, 297f
Arachidonic acid, 153, 154
Argyrophilic fibers, 52
Arterial supply to teeth, 105, 106f
Arterioles, pulpal, 106, 107f, 108
  in control of blood flow, 112, 115f, 116f, 118f
  innervation of, 140
Arthus reactions, 187, 264
Artifacts, 346, 346f
Ascorbic acid. See Vitamin C
Aspirin
  action of, 154
  topical application of, to dentin, 145
Atrophy, pulpal, 338, 338f
  from caries and operative procedures, 338–339
  histology of, 350f, 351, 351f
  from periodontal disease, 308f, 309–311, 310f, 311f, 339
Attrition, dental, 326, 327f, 329, 329f
Autonomic nervous system, 133
Axon, 131

Bacteremia, 191
Bacteria
  in anachoresis, 189–190
  dentinal invasion of, 174, 174f, 176f, 177
  marginal leakage and percolation for entry of, 248
  in pulpal exposure, 179, 180f, 190f
  pulpal invasion of, 190f
    via anachoresis, 189–190
    via cariously exposed pulp, 189
    via drugs, 270
    via periodontal involvement, 191
    via pressure, 190–191
    via systemic infection, 192
Barodontalgia, 370
Basophilia, 41
Bell stage of tooth development, 2, 3f, 4f, 6f
Bifid crown, 21
Blood supply
  arterial, to teeth, 105, 106f
  in dentinogenesis, 42
  to developing tooth, 10–11, 12f
  in pulpal repair, 167
  pulpal. See Circulation of pulp
  veinous drainage from, 105, 106f
B lymphocytes, 162–163, 163f
Bradykinin, 115, 118, 155
Bud stage of tooth development, 1, 2f
Burkitt's lymphoma, 101
Burs
  nature of, effects based on, 201
  size of, effects of, 202–203

Calcium
  in aging theories, 324
  in dentinogenesis, 43, 45, 46, 51
  in nerve impulse, 132
  parathyroid hormone and, 33, 75
  placental transport of, 19
  tetracycline chelation with, 28
  in vitamin D deficiency, 18
Calcium acid phosphate, 224, 224f
Calcium chloride, 145
Calcium fluoride, 220
Calcium hydroxide
  with acid etchants, 219
  as cavity liner, 226–227, 227f
  as cement, 231
  with composite resin restorations, 241
  for crown and bridge cementations, 246, 247
  dentinal sclerosis from, 326
  for desensitization of teeth, 224
  microbial death with, 177

with pin insertion, 206
  in pulp capping, 188–189, 289–291
  in pulpotomy, 289–291
Calcium monofluorophosphate, 226
Calcospherites, 56, 56f, 332, 333f
Cap stage of tooth development, 1–2, 2f, 5f
Capillaries, pulpal, 106, 108, 108f, 113, 117f–119f
  in lymphatic system, 121, 122
  with mechanical exposure, 282, 283f
  in pulpitis, 255–257, 257f
  scaling and root planing affecting, 314–315
  in transcapillary exchange, 110–111, 111f
  types of, 109–110
  ultrastructure of, 109, 109f, 110f, 114, 119f
Carbon dioxide snow test, 379
Carboxylate cement, 206
Caries
  brown pigmentation of dentin with, 176, 178
  in clinical diagnoses, 380–381
  defense against, 177–178, 178f, 179f
  in dentin, 173–177
    microorganisms in, 176–177, 176f
    morphology of, 173–176, 174f–176f
  dentinal remineralization with, 60
  in differential diagnoses, 361, 363–364
  dystrophic mineralizations with, 340–343, 341f–343f
  in enamel, 173
  etiology of, 173
  immunologic reaction to, 179–181, 182f, 183f
  incidence of, with aging, 59
  pulp capping with, indirect, 188–189, 189f, 190f
  pulpal reaction to, 178–187, 180f, 181f, 188f
  pulpitis from, 181–187, 184f–186f
  radiation, 275–276, 277
  reparative dentin under, 329
  sodium fluoride and stannous fluoride for, 222, 223f
Catecholamines, 115
Cathepsins, 155, 168
Cavit, 232
Cavity liners, 225–227
  for amalgam restorations, 243–244
  for composite resins, 241
Cavity preparations
  cleansing and drying medicaments for, 218–219, 218f, 219f
  dentinal tubule exposure via, 196
  depth of, 197–199, 197f, 198f
  dry, 201
  extensiveness of, 205–206, 205f, 206f
  pulpal damage from, 268
Cell-mediated immunity, 159

Cell rests of Malassez, 10
Cementoblasts, 64
Cementoenamel junction, 10
Cements and bases, 227–232, 246–247
Cementum, 2, 314
Cervical glands, 121
Chemotaxis, 155–157, 258–260
Chickenpox, 14
Chlorhexidine, 218
Cholinergic fibers, 134, 145–146
Chondroblasts, 64
Chondroitin sulfatase, 98, 168
Chondroitin sulfate, 168
  in connective tissue, 68, 78, 79, 98
  in pulp capping and pulpotomy, 291, 293f, 294f
Chymotrypsin, 157
Circulation of pulp
  aging effects on, 126, 126f
  anesthetics affecting, 124–125
  blood flow rate in, 120, 121f
  blood flow regulation in, 111–121
  capillaries in. See Capillaries, pulpal
  chemical regulation of, 115–116
  endodontic therapy affecting, 125, 126f
  function of, 105–106
  inflammation affecting, 127–128
  lymphatic, 121–124, 122f, 123f
  with mechanical exposure, 282, 283f
  microvascular network for, 106–108, 108f
  osteotomy affecting, anterior, 126–127
  periodontal disease effects on, 126, 127f
  in pulpitis, 255–257, 257f
  in pulposis, 309
  scaling and root planning affecting, 314–315
  sensory nerve activity and, 140
  structural and functional heterogeneity in, 120
  studies of, 111–114, 114f–118f, 120–121
  systemic circulation and, 105, 106f
  temperature changes affecting, 125, 201
  vasoconstriction in, 116–117, 120f
  vasodilation in, 117–120
Citric acid, 218, 219
Cleansing medicaments, 218–219, 218f, 219f
Clotting, 155
Cobalt radiation, 278
Colchicine, 31
Collagen
  in aging theories, 324
  in caries, 176
  composition of, 66–67
  dentin, 53–54
  growth hormone effects on, 74
  in inflammation, 75
  nutritional disorders affecting, 18

Collagen (continued)
  in odontoblast polarization, 42
  precursors of, 42
  preparations of, for pulp capping and pulpotomy, 291–292
  as primary component of connective tissue, 64
  pulpal, 97
  resorption of, 78
  tooth, 67
  in wound healing, 169–170
Collagen fibers, 64
  connective tissue, 64–66, 65f, 66f
  pulpal, 96–97, 98f
    with aging, 345
    around capillaries, 109
    distribution of, 344
    with inflammation, 184, 187
    in repair process, 167, 264
Collagenases, 155, 157
  in caries, 175
  in inflammation, 168
Colloidal iron stain, 42
Complement system
  activation of, 155
  effects of, 164
  in immune and allergic reactions, 163–164
Composite resins, 225, 240–241, 248
Concrescence of roots, 21–22
Congenital defects, 20–28
Connective tissue
  cells of, 69–71, 69f–71f
  collagen fibers of, 64–67, 65f, 66f
  elastic fibers of, 68
  formocresol effects on, 294, 295
  ground substance of, 68–69
  hormonal effects on, 72–75, 73f
  infection affecting, 75
  irritants of, reaction to, 266, 266f
  nutrition affecting, 71–72
  reticular fibers of, 67–68, 67f, 68f
  systemic factors affecting, 71–75
Coolants, 203–204
Copalite, 225
Copper amalgam, 245–246
Corticosteroids. See Steroids
Cortisol, 72, 168–169
Cortisone, 73–74, 99, 169
Cracked teeth, 370–371
Cretinism, 32
Crown and bridge procedures, 246–247, 269–270
Crown fractures, 207
Crystals in pulp tests, liquid, 379
Curettage effects, 314–316
Cutting instruments, 201

Cyanoacrylates, 230–231, 296
Cyclooxygenase, 153
Cytoplasm of cells, 69
  neurons, 131, 141
  odontoblasts, 80–83, 84f–86f

Dead tracts, 327
Defense cells, 95–96
Dendrites, 131
Dens in dente, 25, 27f
Dens invaginatus, 25, 27f
Dental caries. See Caries
Dental epithelium, inner and outer, 1, 2, 3f, 9–10
Dental history, 374
Dental lamina, 1, 2, 2f
Dental papilla, 1, 2, 2f, 3f, 9–11
Dental pulp. See Pulp
Dental sac, 2
Denticles, 343–344, 344f
Dentin
  aging effects on, 58–59
  amino acid content of, 53–54
  bacterial invasion of, 174, 174f, 176f, 177
  burns of, from rotary instruments, 199, 200f, 204
  carious, 173–177
    demineralization of, 176, 177
    dentinal tubule response to, 177–178, 178f
    microorganisms in, 176–177, 176f
    morphology of, 173–176, 174f–176f
    stannous fluoride effect on, 222, 223f
  chemical structure of, 53–54, 59t, 60t
  collagen of, 67
  composition of, 51
  dead tracts in, 327
  drying of, 203
  dysplasia of, 25, 26f, 27f
  dystrophic mineralization of, 339–343, 339f–343f
  fibers of, 52, 53f
  formation of. See Dentinogenesis
  hypersensitive, 220–225, 383
  innervation of, 138, 141–143, 141f–144f
  interglobular, 56, 56f
  intertubular, 48, 49, 50–51, 174, 178
  iontophoresis of therapeutic solutions through, 221–222
  irregular or amorphous, 178
  mantle, 5, 42
  matrix formation of, 331–332
  metabolic interchanges involving, 59–60, 59t, 60t
  peritubular, 47

in caries, 174, 178
    crystal structure of, 50–51
    mineralization of, 47–48, 48f, 49, 49f
  pressure effects on, 268, 268f
  properties of, 52
  pulpal fluid flow through, 196
  in pulposis, 309, 338
  remineralization of, 189
  reparative, 178, 181, 196, 196f
    under caries, 329–330
    in chronic inflammation of pulp, 263, 264f
    depth of cavity preparation vs formation of, 198, 198f, 199
    local factors affecting formation of, 334–336
    with pulpal aging, 329–331, 329f
    with pulpal exposure, 287, 288, 288f
    under restorations, 330–331, 331f
    in root canals, 331
    with silicate restorations, 238
    systemic factors affecting formation of, 336–338
  sclerosis of, 60, 94, 181, 226–227
    drugs causing, 326
    with pulpal aging, 325–326, 326f, 327f
  secondary, 54, 54f
  sensitivity of, 140–141, 219
  shavings of
    in dentin bridge formation, 334
    in pulp capping and pulpotomy, 291
  sodium fluoride effect on, 221
  sterilizing agents for, 215–218, 216f, 217f
  transparent, 94
Dentinal tubules, 80, 81f
  calcium fluoride effect on, 220
  calcium hydroxide effect on, 189, 226, 227
  in caries, 174, 175, 176f, 177–178, 178f
  cavity preparation exposure of, 196
    nerve endings in, 141, 146f
    odontoblastic process in, 80, 141, 146f
    phenol effects on, 215
    silicate restorations affecting, 238
    silver nitrate effect on, 216, 217f
    width of, 57f, 58–59, 58f
Dentinoenamel junction, 9, 10f, 198, 198f
Dentinogenesis, 4–10, 6f–11f
  autoradiography of, 55–57, 55f–57f
  diabetes affecting, 101
  experimental, 332–333
  hydroxyapatite crystals in, 49–51, 52f, 56, 56f
  initiation of, 41–42
  mechanism of, 42–52, 43f–53f
  mineralization in, 42–46
    fluorosis in, 337
    hormonal influences on, 338
    of intertubular dentin, 48, 49
    lag phases in, 51
    neonatal factors affecting, 336–337, 336f
    nutritional influences on, 337–338
    operative manipulations affecting, 334–336
    of peritubular dentin, 47–48, 48f, 49, 49f
    pulpal inflammation affecting, 334, 335f
    radiation affecting, 336
  peritubular matrix in, 47–48, 48f, 49f
  with pulpal aging, 331–333
  rate of, 54
  rhythmic deposition in, 51–52
  steroidal therapy affecting, 99
Dentinogenesis imperfecta, 23–25, 23f, 24f
Dentinoid, 5
Deoxyribonucleases, 167–168
Deoxyribonucleic acid (DNA), 69
Dermatan sulfate, 78, 79, 98
Desmosomes, 83
Diabetes
  inflammation and, 169
  pulpal effects of, 99–101
  pulpalgia with, 369
Diagnoses
  accuracy of, 384
  anesthetic tests for, 368–371
  canal width and pulp chamber in consideration of, 366, 368f
  caries consideration in, 361, 363–364, 380–381
  clinical, 373–384
  differential, 361–371, 370t
  electric pulp tests for, 367, 377–378, 378f
  mineralizations in consideration of, 366
  objective findings for, 362–363, 377
  palpation tests for, 368
  percussion tests for, 367–368
  pulpalgia in, 361–362, 374–376
  radiographs for, 363–366, 380
  restoration considerations in, 363–364, 381–383
  root fractures in consideration of, 364
  root resorption in consideration of, 365–366, 365f, 366f, 367f
  subjective findings for, 361–362, 374–376
  test drilling for, 368
  for therapeutic purposes, 383–384
  thermal tests for, 366–367, 379–380
Dichlor-difluormethane, 379
Differentiation of cells, 79
Diffusion in transcapillary exchange, 111
Diphenylhydantoin, 31
Diphosphopyridine nucleotide diaphorase, 3
Dodecyldiaminoethyl glycine, 218
Down's syndrome, 20
Drills, 199–200

Dropsin, 227
Drugs
　affecting pulp capping and pulpotomy, 284
　dentinal pain affected by, 145
　facilitating bacterial invasion of pulp, 270
　for microorganisms in dentinal tubules, 177
　in pulp capping and pulpotomy, 289–297
　temperature changes and, 125
　tooth development affected by, 28–31, 31f, 32f, 33f
Dysplasia, pulpal, 26
Drying medicaments, 218–219, 218f, 219f

Ectodermal dysplasia, 25
Edema
　in inflammation, 155
　in pulpitis, 256
Elastic fibers, 68
Electric pulp tests, 367, 377–378, 378f
Electrosurgery, 202
Emboli, pulpal, 218
Enamel
　carious, 173, 178
　dry cavity preparation effects on, 201
　pulpal fluid flow through, 196
Enamel formation, 2, 11–12, 13f, 13t
　ameloblasts in, 2
　hypoplasia in, 15, 16f, 17f
　infections affecting, 14
Enamel hypoplasia
　brain injury and, 336–337
　hereditary, 22–23
　from traumatic injury during tooth development, 15, 16f, 17f
Enamel organ, 1, 2f
Enamel pearls, 22, 22f, 309, 311f
Enamel pulp, 1
Endodontic therapy
　apexification, 297–298, 297f
　hemorrhage from, 125, 126f
　for periapical lesions, 381
　periodontal disease affected by, 317
　pulp capping. See Pulp capping
　pulpal disease classification for, 383–384
　pulpotomy. See Pulpotomy
　radiation and, 276
Endoperoxides, 153
Enzymes
　as inflammatory response mediators, 155–157, 167–168
　lysosomal, 167
　in pulp capping and pulpotomy, 291, 292f, 294f

　in pulpal inflammation, 266
　in tooth development, 3–4
Eosinophils, 71
Epinephrine
　in local anesthetics, 124
　as neurotransmitter, 134
　vasoconstriction from, 111, 115
Epithelium
　inner and outer dental, 1, 2, 3f, 9–10
　oral, 1, 2f
Erosion, dental, 326
Estrogen, 33, 75, 168
Ethylenediaminetetraacetic acid, 218, 218f
Eugenol
　pulpal effect of, 216–218
　zinc oxide and. See Zinc oxide and eugenol
Exposure, pulpal, 179
　carious, 179, 180, 181, 184, 184f, 187, 190f, 285, 285f, 353f
　in differential diagnosis, 362
　histopathology of, 286–289, 287f, 288f
　mechanical, 268–269, 269f, 282–283, 283f, 286–289, 286f
　pain and, 376
　pulp capping and pulpotomy for, 281, 282, 283–284

Fabry's disease, 101
Facial neuralgias, 369
Fat cells, 70f, 71
Fibers, pulpal, 78, 79, 96–97, 96f–98f
Fibrin, 155, 168
Fibrinogen, 155
Fibrinolysin, 168
Fibrinolysis, 155
Fibroblasts
　calcium hydroxide effect on, 226
　collagen synthesis in, 64, 78
　elastic fibers from, 68
　formocresol effects on, 294
　glycoprotein synthesis in, 78
　histology of, 69–70, 69f, 70f
　in inflammation, 75
　pulpal, 78–79, 79f, 80f, 82f, 99
　　with aging, 325
　　with inflammation, 187
　　in repair process, 167, 264
　stress affecting, 73
　beneath zone of Weil, 95
Fibromas, odontogenic, 12
Fibronectin, 5, 70, 78, 82, 90
Fibrosis, 344–345, 345f
Fistulas, 317

Fluorescence antibody techniques, 164–165
Fluoride cavity liners, 226
Fluorosis, 337
Formaldehyde preparations, 294–295
Formocresol, 294–295
Fractures
 amalgam restoration, 244
 crown, 207
 root, 207–208, 208f, 364, 365f
Frigen, 379
Frohlich syndrome, 33
Fusion of teeth, 21

Gemination, 21, 21f
Genetic factors
 in aging theories, 324
 in anodontia, 21
 in dentinal dysplasia, 24
 in dentinogenesis imperfecta, 23
 in enamel hypoplasia, 22
 in pulpal dysplasia, 26
 in regional odontodysplasia, 26
 in taurodontism, 25
 in tooth development, 20
 in tricho-dento-osseous syndrome, 26
Gerontology, 324
Gigantism, 74
Glass ionomer cements, 231–232, 292–294
Glucocorticoids, 72, 99, 169
 effects on pulp, 222
Glucose-6-phosphate dehydrogenase, 3
Glutaraldehyde, 295–296
Gold foil, 242–243, 243f, 244f
Gold inlays, 241–242
Gonadal hormones, 33–34
Granulation tissue, 159, 160f, 167, 169
 with carious pulpal exposure, 184, 185f
 in pulpal repair, 263
 in pulpitis, 260, 261f
Granuloma, 163, 167
 from periodontal disease, 312
 from pulpal exposure, 287, 287f
 from pulpal inflammation, 317, 319f, 354
 radiographs of, 380
Ground substance, pulpal, 97–99
Growth hormone, 33, 74
Guanosine monophosphate, cyclic, 158
Gutta percha
 pulpal reaction to, 232
 in thermal tests, 380

Hageman factor, 154–155
Halide ions in inflammation, 155–157

Hand instruments, 202
Hand-Schüller-Christian disease, 101
Heat and pressure effects, 200–201, 282
Hemidesmosomes, 83
Hemorrhage, pulpal, 205, 206f, 282
Heparin, 68, 78
Hereditary diseases, pulpal, 101
Hereditary enamel hypoplasia, 22–23, 23f
Hereditary opalescent dentin, 23–25, 23f, 24f
Hertwig's epithelial root sheath, 10, 10f
Histamine, 115
 in dentin sensitivity, 148
 in inflammatory response, 153
 in pain induction, 145
 in pulpal inflammation, 256
Histiocytes, 70–71, 95
Histologic classification of pulpal diseases, 349–360
 acute pulpitis, 352f, 353–354
 atrophic pulp, 350f, 351, 351f
 chronic pulpitis, 354–357, 355f–358f
 correlated to clinical tests, 377–383, 381t–382t
 difficulties in, 359–360
 necrotic pulp, 357–359, 359f
 transitional stage to pulpitis, 351–353, 352f
Hormones
 affecting pulp, 99–101
 connective tissue affected by, 72–75
 controlling blood flow, 111
 dentin mineralization affected by, 338
 in inflammation, 168–169
 pulp capping and pulpotomy affected by, 284
 tooth development affected by, 31–34
Humoral immunity, 162
Hutchinsonian teeth, 14
Hyaluronic acid, 68, 98, 168
Hyaluronidase, 75, 98, 168
Hydrocortisone, 72
Hydrogen peroxide, 155, 218
Hydrolytic enzymes, 3
Hyperpituitarism, 33
Hypersensitivity reactions, 187
Hyperthyroidism, 32
Hypoparathyroidism, 33
Hypophosphatasia, 27, 28f, 29f
Hypophosphatemia, 28, 30f
Hypothyroidism, 32

Immune response, 162–165, 154f, 165f
 in aging theories, 324–325
 to formocresol, 295
 in pulpal repair, 264
 in pulpitis, 187

Immunity
  cell-mediated, 159
  humoral, 162
Immunoglobulins, 162–165
  pulpal production of, against caries, 179–181, 182f, 183f
  in pulpal repair, 264
Impressions, 209–210, 209f, 246
Incisors
  dilaceration of, 15, 17f
  in syphilis, 14
Infections
  connective tissue affected by, 75
  cortisone affecting resistance to, 73
  inflammation and, 170–171
  from pulpal exposure, 189, 190f
  in tooth development, 14
Inflammation
  acute, 152–159
  cell mediators in, 153–154, 154f
  chronic, 159–161
  connective tissues in, 75
  cyclic AMP in, 157–158
  cyclic GMP in, 158–159
  defense cells in, 159–161, 160f, 161f
  diabetes and, 169
  endothelial lining changes with, 152
  enzymes in, 167–168
  hormones in, 168–169
  infection and, 170
  as mechanism for repair, 165–167
  plasma mediators in, 154–157, 156f–159f
  pulpal. See Pulpitis
  resolution of, factors in, 271f, 272
  stasis in, 152, 153f
  suppurative or purulent, 157
Inflammatory cells
  in histologic classification of pulp diseases, 349–350, 351–353
  in pulpal exposure, 287
  in pulpitis, 267
Inner dental epithelium, 1, 2, 3f, 9–10
Iontophoresis, 221–222
Irritants, pulpal, 215
  chemical, 215–232
  cumulative effects of, 267–272, 270f
  mechanical and thermal, 195–212
  microbial, 173–192
  radiant, 274–278

Kallikreins
  in inflammation, 155
  in pain perception, 147

Kinins, plasma, 147, 155
Krabbe's leukodystrophy, 101

Lactate dehydrogenase, 3–4
Lactobacilli, 177
Laser beam, 277
Lateral canals, 303–305, 304f, 305f
Leakage, marginal, 247
Leukemia, 101
Leukocytes, polymorphonuclear, 71, 73
  in inflammatory response, 154, 155–157, 156f, 157f
  in pulpal abscess, 184
  in pulpal exposure, 287
  in pulpitis, 179, 258, 259f
Leukotrienes, 153, 154
Ligamental injection, 124–125
Lincomycin, 31
Lymph and lymph nodes, 121
Lymphatic system
  capillaries of, 121
  clotting effects on, 155
  in dental pulp, 121–122, 122f, 123f
  in drainage of oral structures, 121, 122f
  function of, 121
  in intrapulpal pressure, 122–124
Lymphocytes, 71
  function of, 162
  in immune system, 162
  in inflammation, chronic, 159
  in pulpal inflammation, 181, 185f, 186f, 187, 260, 262, 262f
Lymphokines, 153, 162, 163
Lymphotoxin, 163

Macrophage inhibitory factor, 163
Macrophages
  of connective tissue, 70–71, 71f
  in inflammation, chronic, 159, 160f, 161f
  pulpal, 95, 96
    in pulpitis, 181, 184, 185f, 186f, 187, 260, 262, 262f
  in repair process, 264
Macula adherens, 86
Magnesium, 19
Malassez, cell rests of, 10
Mandibular vein, 105
Mantle dentin, 5, 42
Mast cells, 71, 71f, 73, 74, 96
  in inflammation, 153, 154f
  in pulpitis, 260

Maxillary artery, internal, 105
Maxillary vein, internal, 105
Measles, 14
Membrana preformativa, 2
Metabolic interchanges, pulpal, 59
Metachromasia, 41
Metarterioles, 108, 108f
Methylcellulose liners, 226
Microcirculation of pulp. *See* Circulation of pulp
Microorganisms
  in anachoresis, 190
  in bacteremia, 191
  in carious dentin, 176–177
  with indirect pulp capping, 188–189
  in periodontal disease, 313–314
  in pulpal exposure, 179, 180f
  zinc oxide and eugenol effect on, 217
Micropinocytosis, 111
Microradiography, 48–49
Microtubules
  of odontoblastic processes, 83
  in tooth development, 9, 31
Molars, mulberry, 14
Monocyte chemotactic factor, 163
Monocytes, 159
Mucopolysaccharidase, 99
Mucopolysaccharides, 68, 98
Mulberry molars, 14
Myeloperoxidase, 155
Myxedema, 74–75
Myxomas, odontogenic, 12

Necrosis, pulpal, 187
  electric pulp test of, 377
  from formocresol, 295
  histologic classification of, 357–359, 359f
  pain with, 377
  with periodontal disease, 312
  from periodontal treatment, 315, 316
  with pulpitis, 258, 354, 356f
  radiolucent periapical area and, 383
  from root fracture, 208
  from silicate restorations, 238
  sinus tracts and, 363
  from traumatic injury, 207
Neonatal line, 19–20, 20f, 336, 336f
Neoplasms, 12–14
Nerve fibers
  in dentin, 141–143, 142f, 143f, 145–146
  electrical activity from, 144–145, 145f
  myelinated vs unmyelinated, 131, 133, 133f
  pulpal, 136–138, 138f, 139f
  stimulation of, 131

Nerve impulses, 131
  eugenol effect on, 216–217
  strontium chloride effect on, 224
Nerve supply
  aging effects on, 328
  to developing tooth, 11
  affecting intrapulpal pressure, 124
  in pulpal circulation regulation, 108, 109f, 115, 116–120
    identification of, by labeling, 138–140
    vascular relationships of, 140
  to teeth, 134–140, 135f–139f
Neural conduction, 131–134
Neuralgias, 369
Neuron, 131
Niemann-Pick disease, 101
Nociceptors, 133
Nodes of Ranvier, 131
Noradrenaline, 115
Norepinephrine
  as neurotransmitter, 134
  in vasoconstriction, 115
Nutrition
  connective tissue affected by, 71–72
  dentin mineralization affected by, 337–338
  pulp capping and pulpotomy affected by, 284
  pulpal effects of, 99
  tooth development affected by, 17–19, 19f
  in wound healing, 169–170

Occlusion, traumatic, 208
Odontoblasts
  aging effects on, 325
  alcohol effects on, 218
  associated cells of, 141–142, 141f
  in caries, 174, 178
  cavity preparations affecting, 196–197, 198, 252–253, 254f
  collagen synthesis in, 64, 94
  dentinal injury to, affecting pulp, 90, 94
  in dentinal receptor mechanism for pain perception, 143–144
  in dentinogenesis, 2, 4–9, 18, 41, 44f, 45f, 80
  dry cavity preparation affecting, 201
  fluorosis effect on, 337
  function of, 94
  in hydrodynamic theory of pain perception, 146–147
  as mesenchymal syncytium, 90, 95f
  morphologic variations of, 80
  nerve endings associated with, 141–143, 143f, 144f, 145, 146, 146f
  nucleolus of, 80

Odontoblasts (continued)
  nucleus of, 80, 82f, 84f, 90, 94f
  operative procedures affecting, 90, 94, 95f
  origin of, 41
  palisading, 252, 253f
  polarization of, 42
  postextraction changes in, 253–254
  along predentin border, 82, 86f
  pulpal, 80–95, 83f
    communications between, 90–95, 94f, 95f
    cytoplasm of, 80–83, 85f, 86f
    intercellular junctions of, 83–86.
    junctional complexes of, 86, 91f–93f
    nucleus of, 80, 82f, 84f, 90, 94f
    processes of, 83, 87f–90f
  rotary instrument speed affecting, 199–200
  silicate restorations affecting, 238
  steroidal therapy affecting, 99
  in transducer mechanism of pain perception, 145
Odontodysplasia, regional, 26–27, 28f
Odontotest, 379
Opalescent dentin, 23–25, 24f, 25f
Operative procedures
  for amalgam restorations, 243–246
  bacteremia associated with, 191
  cavity preparations. See Cavity preparations
  coolants in, 203–204
  cutting instruments in, effects based on type of, 201
  dentin mineralization affected by, 334–335, 335f
  gold foils, 242–243, 243f
  gold inlays, 241–242
  with hand instruments, 202
  heat and pressure of, 200–201
  iatrogenic pulpitis from, 195–197
  inflammatory agents released due to, 256
  marginal leakage and, 247–248, 247f
  marginal percolation and, 248
  odontoblastic damage and displacement from, 252–253, 254f
  physical trauma from, 207–210
  with pins, 206
  pulpal reactions to, sequence of, 254, 256f
  pulpal rebound response to, 206–207
  pulpitis from, 252–272
  reparative dentin formation with, 260, 261f
  rotary instrument speed in, 199–200
  size of wheels and burs in, 202
  smear layer from, 202–203, 218
Oral epithelium, 1, 2f
Orangewood sticks, 225
Orthodontics, 210–212, 210f, 211f
Osteoblasts, 64
Osteoclasts, 95
Osteodentin, 336, 336f
Osteotomy, anterior, 126–127
Oxidative enzymes, 3–4

Pain, pulpal
  autonomic nervous system transmission of, 133
  barodontalgia, 370
  from cracked teeth, 370–371
  in diagnoses, 361–362, 374–376
  nerve fibers for, 133
  from periodontal disease, 317–319
  from pulpal vs periodontal lesions, 320
  of pulpitis, 254, 354, 371
  referred, 368–369
  sensory receptors for, 133–134
  substances inducing, 145
  of systemic origin, 369–370
  theories on perception of, 140–148
    dental nerve stimulation, 141–143, 141f–144f
    dentinal receptors in, 143–146, 145f
    hydrodynamic, 146–147
    polypeptides and neurotransmitters in, 147–148
Palpation test, 368
Parachlorophenol, camphorated, 216
Parathyroid hormone, 33, 75
Penicillin, 216
Percolation, 248
Percussion test, 367–368
Periapical lesions, 381, 383
Pericytes, 96, 109, 109f
Periodic Acid Schiff stain, 41
Periodontal abscess, 370
Periodontal disease
  age correlated to, 319
  bacterial invasion of pulp via, 191
  from developmental radicular groove, 309–311
  in differential diagnosis, 363
  dystrophic mineralizations with, 340–343
  pain with, 317–319
  pulpal effects of, 306–308, 307t
    atrophic changes, 308f, 309–311, 310f, 311f, 339
    in circulation, 126, 127f
    inflammation, 270
    inflammatory changes, 311–312, 312f, 313f, 314f
    resorption, 312, 315f
    from toxic products, 312–314

pulpal lesions affecting, 317, 318f, 319f
thermal responses and, 319
Periodontal ligament, 2
blood supply to, 11
cortisone effects on, 74
pulpal lesions affecting, 317
radiation effects on, 275
Periodontal treatment, 314–317
Periodontium
dental sac in development of, 2
protein deficiency affecting, 101
pulpal inflammation affecting, 317
radiation effects on, 275
Phenol, 215, 216f
Phosphate, 75
Phospholipase, 153
Phosphoric acid, 218, 229, 230, 240
Pins, 206, 246
Pit and fissure sealants, 227
Pituitary hormones, 33, 72, 73f
Pituitary senility, 33, 338
Plaque, dental, 173
Plasma cells, 71
function of, 161, 165f, 166f
in inflammation, chronic, 159
from lymphocyte differentiation, 162–163, 164f
in pulpitis, 181, 185f, 187, 260, 262f, 263
Plasmin, 155, 164
Plasminogen, 155
Platelet-activating factor, 153–154
Platelets in inflammation, 153–154
Polishing restorations, 208–209
Polyacrylic cements, 230, 230f
Polycarboxylate cements, 296
Polymorphism of teeth, 20
Polystyrene liners, 226
Porphyria, congenital, 28
Potassium chloride, 145
Potassium fluorozirconate, 226
Potassium nitrate, 224–225
Precapillaries, 108
Predentin, 5, 42, 83, 101
in caries-induced pulpitis, 179
nerve endings in, 142, 144f
in pulpal repair, 263–264, 264f
Primordial cyst, 14
Procollagen, 66
Progeria, 33, 338
Progesterone, 168
Pronase, 157
Prostacyclin, 153
Prostaglandins
in inflammatory response, 153, 159
in pain perception, 148

Proteins
in complement system activation, 155
cortisone affecting metabolism of, 73–74
enzymes. See Enzymes
nutritional importance of, 17, 71–72
pulpal effects of deficiency of, 101
in pulpal repair, 170
as serous exudate, 155
synthesis of, cellular, 69
Pterygoid plexus, 105
Pulp capping
age and status of pulp affecting outcome of, 284–286, 285f
antimetabolites affecting, 284
in differential diagnosis, 362, 363f
drugs in, 289–297
exposure affecting, size and location of, 283–284
hormonal disturbances affecting, 284
indications for, 281
indirect, 188–189, 189f
marginal leakage affecting, 284
nutritional deficiencies affecting, 284
potassium nitrate for, 225
Pulp tests
anesthetic, 368
drilling in, 368
electric, 367, 377–378, 378f
liquid crystals in, 379
palpation, 368
percussion, 367–368
of pulpal vs. periodontal lesions, 321
thermal, 366–367, 379–380
thermocouples in, 379
thermography, 378–379
ultrasonic, 378
Pulpal pain. See Pain, pulpal
Pulpal–periodontal syndrome, 319–322
Pulpalgia. See Pain, pulpal
Pulpitis
acute, 184
histologic classification of, 352f, 353–354
from operative procedures, 254–260, 255f–261f, 266
blood cells in, 258–260, 259f, 260f
from caries, 179, 180, 181–187
under caries, 178–179, 180f, 181–187, 181f, 186f
chemotaxis in, 258–260, 259f, 260f
chronic, 187
from caries, 181, 184, 184f, 185f, 187
histologic classification of, 354–357, 355f–358f
from operative procedures, 260–263, 261f, 263f, 267, 267f

Pulpitis *(continued)*
    circulation affected by, 127–128
    dentin mineralization affected by, 334, 335f
    depth of cavity preparation vs degree of, 199
    from gold inlays, 242
    ground substance alterations with, 98
    hyperplastic, 354, 362
    iatrogenic, 195–197
    inflammatory cells in, 181, 184, 185f, 186f, 187
    odontoblasts in, 254, 256, 257f
    from operative procedures, 252–272
    pathophysiology of, 256–258, 258f
    from periodontal disease, 312
    pressure with, 98
    prevention of, reasons for, 195–196
    from pulpal exposure, 268–269, 269f
    root resorption from, 265f, 266, 266f
    from silicate restorations, 238
    swelling with, 362
    transition to, 351–353, 352f
    ulcerative, 17
    vascular changes with, 255–256, 257f
Pulposis, 309–311, 338–339
Pulpotomy
    age and status of pulp affecting outcome of, 284–286, 285f
    antimetabolites affecting, 284
    for crown fracture, 207
    drugs in, 289–297
    exposure affecting, size and location of, 283–284
    histopathology of, 286–289, 287f, 288f
    hormonal disturbances affecting, 284
    indications for, 281–282
    marginal leakage affecting, 284
    nutritional deficiencies affecting, 284
    root resorption with, 287
Pus, 157

Radiation
    cellular effects of, 274
    cobalt, 278
    dental effects of, 274–276, 275f, 276f
    dentin mineralization affected by, 336
    laser beam, 277
    radium, 277, 278f
    strontium, 278
    tooth development affected by, 34–35, 34f, 35f, 274
Radioautography, 55–57, 55f–57f
Radiographs
    for clinical diagnoses, 380
    in differential diagnosis, 363
    of periapical lesions, 381, 383
    in pulpal–periodontal syndrome diagnosis and treatment, 321–322
Radium, 277, 278f
Ranvier, nodes of, 131
Raschkow, plexus of, 11, 137, 138f
Rebound response, 206–207
Repair, pulpal, 165–167
    after exposure, 287
    enzymes in, 266
    predentin changes in, 263–264, 264f
    proteins in, 170
    root resorption in, 265f, 266
    vitamins in, 169–170
Restorations, marginal leakage around, 247
Reticular fibers, 67–68, 67f, 68f
    around capillaries pulpal, 109
    pulpal, 96, 96f
Reticulin, 67, 97
    fibers of, pulpal, 78
Reticulinase, 168
Ribonucleases, 167–168
Ribonucleic acid (RNA), 69, 80, 131, 161
Rickets, 19, 19f, 28
Root
    in apexification procedures, 297–298, 297f
    development of, 10, 11f
    developmental groove of, 309–311
    fracture of, 207–208, 208f, 364, 365f
    radiation effects on, 274, 275
    resorption of, 265f, 266, 266f
        in differential diagnosis, 365–366, 365f–367f
        from granulomas, 317
        from periodontal disease, 312, 315f
        from pulpotomy, 287
        radiographs of, 380
Root canals
    in differential diagnosis, 366
    lateral and accessory canals of, 303–305, 304f, 305f
    reparative dentin in, 331
Rotary instruments, effect on pulp, 199–202, 202f
Rubella, 14

Salivary glands, 275
Scaling, 314–316
Scarlet fever, 14
Scurvy, 72, 170
Serotonin, 117
    in dentin sensitivity, 148
    in inflammatory response, 153, 514

Serous exudate, 155
Sickle cell anemia, 23, 101
Silicate restorations
   cavity liners for, 225, 226, 240
   marginal leakage with, 240
   pulpal effects of, 238–240, 293f
Silver nitrate, 145, 215–216, 217f, 220
Simmond's syndrome, 33
Sinus tracts, 320f, 321, 363
Sinusitis, 369
Slow-reacting substance of anaphylaxis, 154
Snow-capped teeth, 22
Sodum fluoride, 220–221, 220f, 221f, 222, 223f
Sodium monofluorophosphate, 222
Sodium silicofluoride, 222
Somatotropin, 74
Stannous fluoride, 222, 223f, 245–246
Stellate reticulum, 1, 2, 3f, 4f
Steroids, 72, 99
   anti-inflammatory activity of, 154, 168–169
   dentinal sclerosis from, 326
   in pulp capping and pulpotomy, 292–294
Stratum intermedium, 2, 4f
Streptodornase, 168
Streptokinase, 168
Stress hormones, 72–74
Strontium chloride, 145, 224
Strontium exposure, 278
Stuart-Prower factor, 155
Sturge-Weber disease, 101
Substance P, 118–120
   in pain perception, 147–148
   in pulpal inflammation, 256
Succinic dehydrogenase, 3
Supernumerary teeth, 21, 21f
Suppuration, pulpal, 258, 259f
Swelling, 363, 364f
Synapse, 132, 132f
Synaptic cleft, 132
Syphilis, 14

Taurodontism, 25, 27f
Tawa ascites tumor, 101
Temperature, tooth
   affecting pulpal circulation, 125
   with bleaching, 202
   with coolants, 204
   with dry cavity preparations, 201
   with electrosurgery, 202
   in impression taking, 209–210
   with polishing restorations, 208–209
   pulpal nerves affected by, 145
   thermocouple measurement of, 379

Temporal vein, superficial, 105
Tetracycline staining, 19, 28–31, 31f–33f, 59–60
Thermal insulation, bases for, 228
Thermal tests
   in clinical diagnoses, 379–380
   in differential diagnosis, 366–367
   histopathology correlated to, 380
   periodontal disease affecting, 319
Thermocouples in pulp tests, 379
Thermography, infrared, 378–379
Thromboplastin, tissue, 155
Thromboxane, 153
Thyroid hormones, 31–32
   connective tissue affected by, 74–75
   pulp affected by deficiency of, 101
Thyroid-stimulating hormone, 74
Thyrotropin, 74
Thyroxine, 74–75
Tissue stains, 41–42
T lymphocytes
   macrophages and, 159
   morphology of, 162, 162f
   origin, course and function of, 162, 163f
Tocopherol, 19
Tomes' fibers, 83, 88f, 94
Tomes' granular layer, 56, 57f
Tooth
   arterial blood supply to, 105, 106f
   bleaching of, 202
   cracked, 370–371
   desensitization of, agents for, 220–225
   innervation of, 134–140, 135f–139f
      identification of, by labeling, 138–140
      vascular relationships to, 140
   movement of, 210–212, 210f, 211f
   radiation effects on, 274–276, 275f, 276f
   traumatic injury to, 207, 207f
   veinous drainage from, 105, 106f
Tooth development
   bell stage of, 2, 3f, 4f, 6f
   blood supply in, 10–11, 12f
   bud stage of, 1, 2f
   cap stage of, 1–2, 2f, 5f
   changes in, due to birth, 19–20, 20f
   congenital defects affecting, 20–28, 21f–30f
   drugs affecting, 28–31, 31f, 32f, 33f
   enamel formation in, 11–12, 12f, 13f, 13t
   enzymes in, 3–4
   hormones affecting, 31–34
   infections affecting, 14, 14f, 15f
   neoplasms relating to, 12–14
   nutritional disorders affecting, 17–19, 19f
   odontoblasts and dentin formation in, 4–11, 6f–11f
   radiation affecting, 34–35, 34f, 35f

Tooth development *(continued)*
  tooth sizes in, 12
  trauma affecting, 15–17, 15f–18f
Tooth size
  with congenital defects, 20
  genetic factors in, 12
Trauma
  pulpal damage from 207–210, 207f–209f
  tooth development affected by, 15–17, 15f–18f
Tricalcium phosphate, 291
Tricho-dento-osseous syndrome, 25–26
Trigeminal nerve, 134, 135f
Trigeminal neuralgia, 369
Trigeminal spinal tract nucleus, 134, 135f
Triphosphopyridine nucleotide diaphorase, 3
Trypsin, 157, 164
Tumor metastasis to pulp, 101–102
Turner tooth, 14, 15f

Ultrasonic pulp tests, 378

Varnishes, 225–226, 245
Vasoactive intestinal peptide, 148
Vasoconstruction, 116–117
  with local anesthetics, 124
  norepinephrine in, 115, 116
Vasodilation, 117–120
  with dry cavity preparation, 201
  in pulpal inflammation, 256–257, 258
Veinous drainage from teeth, 105, 106f
Venules, 110, 223
  pulpal, 106, 108
Vinblastine, 31
Vincristine, 31
Viral infection
  pulpal effects of, 101
  tooth development affected by, 14
Vitamin A, 17–18, 337
Vitamin C
  connective tissue affected by, 72
  dentin mineralization affected by, 337
  pulpal fibroblasts affected by, 99, 100f
  in pulpal repair, 169–170
  in tooth development, 18

Vitamin D, 18–19, 337–338
Vitamin E, 19
Vitamin deficiencies
  affecting connective tissue, 72
  affecting pulp, 99, 100f
  affecting tooth development, 17–19
  dentin mineralization affected by, 337–338
  pulp capping and pulpotomy affected by, 284
  in wound healing, 169–170
Von Korff fibers, 9, 42, 46f, 47f, 67f, 68, 96f, 97

Water spray, 203–204
Weil, layer of, 95, 122
Wheel size, 202–203, 202f
Wound healing, 167, 169

Zinc chloride, 145
Zinc oxide and eugenol
  with amalgam restorations, 245
  with calcium hydroxide, 227
  cavity depth as criteria for use of, 199
  as cavity liner, 226, 228
  with composite resin restorations, 241
  dentinal demineralization from, 229
  in indirect pulp capping, 188–189
  marginal seal with, 228, 229f
  microbial death from, 177
  modified cements of, 229
  for pin cementation, 206
  for pulp capping and pulpotomy, 296–297, 296f
  pulpal reaction to, 228, 228f
  as temporary filling material, 228
Zinc phosphate cement
  calcium hydroxide with, 226, 229
  cavity depth in consideration of use of, 199
  with composite resin restorations, 241
  for crown and bridge cementations, 246
  for pin cementation, 206
  pulpal effects of, 229–230, 230f
  with zinc oxide and eugenol cavity liner, 226, 229
Zone of Weil, 95, 122
Zonula adherens, 86
Zonula occludens, 86